The Durability of Vascular and Endovascular Surgery

The Durability of Vascular and Endovascular Surgery

Edited by

RM GREENHALGH MA MD MChir FRCS

Professor of Surgery
Head of Department of Vascular Surgery
Imperial College School of Medicine
Charing Cross Hospital
London

Editorial Commentaries by
JANET T POWELL MD PhD
and
C VAUGHAN RUCKLEY ChM FRCSE

W B SAUNDERS COMPANY LTD
London · Philadelphia · Toronto · Sydney · Tokyo

W B Saunders Company Ltd 24–28 Oval Road
London NW1 7DX

The Curtis Center
Independence Square West
Philadelphia, PA 19106-3399, USA

Harcourt Brace & Company
55 Horner Avenue
Toronto, Ontario M8Z 4X6, Canada

Harcourt Brace & Company, Australia
30–52 Smidmore Street
Marrickville, NSW 2204, Australia

Harcourt Brace & Company, Japan
Ichibancho Central Building, 22-1 Ichibancho
Chiyoda-ku, Tokyo, 102, Japan

This book is printed on acid-free paper

A catalogue record for this book is available from the British Library.

ISBN 0-7020-2540-2

Editorial and Production Services by Jane Duncan
10 Barley Mow Passage, London W4 4PH

Typeset by Phoenix Photosetting, Chatham, Kent
Printed in Great Britain at the University Press, Cambridge

Contents

DO POPULATION STUDIES AND NATIONAL REGISTRIES PROVIDE EVIDENCE OF DURABILITY IN OUR PATIENTS?

WHAT IS THE INFLUENCE OF PHARMACOLOGICAL AGENTS?

THE DURABILITY OF VENOUS PROCEDURES

PERIPHERAL VASCULAR DURABILITY CONTROVERSIES

THE DURABILITY OF ENDOVASCULAR AORTIC ANEURYSM REPAIR

WILL FUTURE DURABILITY OF XENOGRAFTS BE DIFFERENT?

SOME HISTORICAL OBSERVATIONS ON DURABILITY

Contributors

Dr M Akhil Abdul-Hamid, MRCS
Department of Surgery
Derbyshire Royal Infirmary
London Road
Derby DE1 2QY, UK

Dr Omran Abdul-Khoudoud, MD
Division of Vascular Surgery
Union Memorial Hospital/Helix Health
330 North Calvert Street
Suite 570
Baltimore MD 2128
USA

Dr Eric Allaire, MD
Service de Chirurgie Vasculaire
Hopital Henri Mondor
51 Ave du Marechal de Lattre de Tassigny
94010 Creteil
France

Dr Alexandre d'Audiffret, MD
Service de Chirurgie Vasculaire
Hopital Henri Mondor
51 Ave du Marechal de Lattre de Tassigny
94010 Creteil
France

Dr Klaus Balzer, MD
Chefarz der Gefasschirurgischen Klinik
Evangelisches Krankenhaus
Wertgasse 30
45468 Muhlheim
Germany

Mr Jonathan D Beard, MB BS BSc ChM FRCS
Sheffield Vascular Institute
Northern General Hospital
Herries Road
Sheffield S5 7AU, UK

Professor Jean-Pierre Becquemin, MD
Service de Chirurgie Vasculaire
Hopital Henri Mondor
51 Ave du Marechal de Lattre de Tassigny
94010 Creteil
France

Dr Hugh G Beebe, MD
Jobst Vascular Center
2109 Hughes Drive
Toledo
Ohio 43606
USA

Dr Gianni Belcaro, MD PhD
Director of Angiology
Vascular Surgery & Clinical Trials Unit
Pierangeli Clinic
Pescara
Italy

Professor Peter RF Bell, MD FRCS
Department of Surgery
University of Leicester
Robert Kilpatrick Building
Leicester LE2 7LX, UK

Professor D Bergqvist, MD PhD
Department of Surgery
Academic Hospital
S-751 85 Uppsala
Sweden

Professor Giorgio M Biasi, MD FACS
Department of Vascular Surgery
Bassini Teaching Hospital
University of Milan
Via Massimo Gorki 50
20092 Cinisello Balsamo
Milan, Italy

Mr Stephen D Blair, MS FRCS
Department of Vascular Surgery
Arrowe Park Hospital
Arrowe Park Road
Upton, Wirral
Merseyside L49 5PE, UK

Dr Jan D Blankensteijn, MD
Division of Vascular Surgery G 04 232
University Hospital Utrecht
Heidelberglaan 100
3508 CX Utrecht
The Netherlands

Dr Amman Bolia, MB ChB DMRD FRCR
Department of Radiology
Leicester Royal Infirmary NHS Trust
Leicester LE1 5WW, UK

Mr Andrew W Bradbury, BSc MD FRCSEd
Vascular Surgery Unit
Department of Clinical & Surgical Sciences
The Royal Infirmary
Edinburgh EH3 9YW, UK

Ms Julie Brittenden, MD FRCSG
Vascular Surgery Unit
Dept of Clinical & Surgical Sciences
The Royal Infirmary
Edinburgh EH3 9YW, UK

Dr Ivo AMJ Broeders, MD
Division of Vascular Surgery G 04 232
University Hospital Utrecht
Heidelberglaan 100
3508 CX Utrecht
The Netherlands

Professor Kevin G Burnand, MS FRCS
Department of Surgery
St Thomas' Hospital
Lambeth Palace Road
London SE1 7EH, UK

Mr Kenneth Callum, MS FRCS
Department of Surgery
Derbyshire Royal Infirmary
London Road
Derby DE1 2QY, UK

Mr Bruce Campbell, MS FRCP FRCS
Department of Surgery
Royal Devon & Exeter Hospital
Barrack Road
Exeter EX2 5DW, UK

Dr T Coddington, BSc (Eng) MRCP BSc MB BS MRCS MARCP LMSSA AMIEE AIED
Oak Tree Lane Centre
Oak Tree Lane
Selly Oak
Birmingham B29 6JA, UK

Dr Frank J Criado, MD
Chief, Division of Vascular Surgery
Union Memorial Hospital/Helix Health
330 North Calvert Street
Suite 570
Baltimore MD 2128
USA

Mr Alun H Davies, MA DM FRCS
Department of Vascular Surgery
Charing Cross Hospital
Fulham Palace Road
London W6 8RF, UK

Dr Mario DeNunzio, MRCP FRCR
Department of Radiology
Derbyshire Royal Infirmary
London Road
Derby DE1 2QY, UK

Dr Pascal Desgranges, MD
Service de Chirurgie Vasculaire
Hopital Henri Mondor
51 Ave du Marechal de Lattre de Tassigny
94010 Creteil
France

Dr Anthony Dorling, MB BS PhD
Department of Immunology
Imperial College School of Medicine
Hammersmith Hospital
Du Cane Road
London W12 0HS, UK

Professor Bert C Eikelboom, MD
Division of Vascular Surgery G 04 232
University Hospital Utrecht
Heidelberglaan 100
3508 CX Utrecht
The Netherlands

Dr J Elfström, MD
Department of Surgery
University Hospital
S-751 85
Uppsala
Sweden

Dr Mary Ellis, BSc
Principal Vascular Technologist
Department of Surgery
Charing Cross Hospital
Fulham Palace Road
London W6 8RF, UK

Ms Karen Ferguson, BN
Department of Surgery
Charing Cross Hospital
Fulham Palace Road
London W6 8RF, UK

Dr SA Ferrari, MD
Department of Vascular Surgery
Bassini Teaching Hospital
University of Milan
Via Massimo Gorki 50
20092 Cinisello Balsamo
Milan, Italy

Dr Guy Fishwick, FRCS, FRCR
Department of Radiology
Clinical Sciences Building
Leicester Royal Infirmary
Leicester LE2 7LX, UK

Professor Francis Gerald R Fowkes, PhD FRCPE
Wolfson Unit for Peripheral Vascular Diseases
University of Edinburgh Medical School
Teviot Place
Edinburgh EH8 9AG, UK

Dr Peter A Gaines, MRCP FRCR
Department of Radiology
Northern General Hospital
Herries Road
Sheffield S5 7AU, UK

Mr George Geroulakos, MD FRCS DIC PhD
Department of Vascular Surgery
Charing Cross Hospital
Fulham Palace Road
London W6 8RF, UK

Mr Jonathan Golledge, MChir FRCS
Department of Surgery
Charing Cross Hospital
Fulham Palace Road
London W6 8RF, UK

Mr Marcel A Goodman, FRACS
Endovascular Unit
Royal Perth Hospital
Perth
Western Australia

Professor Roger M Greenhalgh, MD FRCS
Department of Surgery
Charing Cross Hospital
Fulham Palace Road
London W6 8RF, UK

Dr Maura B Griffin, MSc DMU DCR
Department of Vascular Surgery
St Mary's Hospital
Praed Street
Paddington
London W2 1NY, UK

Mrs Alison W Halliday, MS FRCS
Consultant Vascular Surgeon
Epsom General Hospital
Dorking Road
Epsom
Surrey KT18 7EG, UK

Mr Ahmed Hamsho, FRCS
Department of Vascular Surgery
Arrowe Park Hospital
Arrowe Park Road
Upton, Wirral
Merseyside L49 5PE, UK

Mr Peter L Harris, MD FRCS
Consultant Vascular Surgeon
Royal Liverpool Hospital
Prescott Street
Liverpool L7 8XP, UK

Mr David E Hartley, FIR
Endovascular Unit
Royal Perth Hospital
Perth
Western Australia

Dr B Hedberg
Department of Surgery
University Hospital
S-751 85
Uppsala
Sweden

Dr David Hinwood, MRCP FRCR
Department of Radiology
Derbyshire Royal Infirmary
London Road
Derby DE1 2QY, UK

Professor Brian R Hopkinson, ChM FRCS
Department of Vascular Surgery
University Hospital
Queens Medical Centre
Nottingham NG7 2UH, UK

Dr S Horsch, MD
Chefarz der Gefasschirurgischen Klinik
Evangelisches Krankenhaus
Wertgasse 30
45468 Muhlheim
Germany

Dr Leif Panduro Jensen, MD
Department of Vascular Surgery RK
Rigshospitalet 3111
9 Blegdamsvej
DK2100
Copenhagen
Denmark

Dr K Wayne Johnston, MD FRCS(C)
Department of Vascular Surgery
The Toronto Hospital
Eaton Building, 5-309
200 Elizabeth Street
Ontario M5G 2C4
Canada

Dr Paula L Kirby, BSc PhD
Department of Vascular Surgery
Charing Cross Hospital
Fulham Palace Road
London W6 8RF, UK

Professor Andries J Kroese, PhD
Department of Vascular Surgery
Aker Hospital
University of Oslo
Oslo
Norway

Mr Michael MD Lawrence-Brown, FRACS
Suite 33
Mount Medical Center
146 Mounts Bay Road
Perth 6000
Western Australia

Professor Robert I Lechler, MB ChB MRCP PhD FRCP FRCPath
Department of Immunology
Imperial College School of Medicine
Hammersmith Hospital
Du Cane Road
London W12 0HS, UK

Dr Gillian C Leng, BSc MB ChB MD
Dept Primary Care & Population Sciences
Royal Free Hospital
Rowland Hill Street
London NW3 2PF, UK

Mr Andrew F Lennox, MSc FRACS
Vascular Surgical Unit
St Mary's Hospital
Praed Street
Paddington
London W2 1NY, UK

Mr P Lintott, MB ChB FRCS
Academic Surgical Unit
QEQM Wing
St Mary's Hospital
Paddington
London W2 1NY, UK

Dr K-G Ljungström, MD
Department of Surgery
University Hospital
S-751 85
Uppsala
Sweden

Professor Nicholas London, MB ChB MRCP MD FRCS
Department of Surgery
University of Leicester Medical School
Leicester, UK

Professor Charles McCollum, FRCS MD
Department of Surgery
South Manchester University Hospital
Nell Lane
West Didsbury
Manchester M20 8LR, UK

Mr James May, MD
Endovascular Research Unit
Department of Surgery
Blackburn Building D06
University of Sydney
New South Wales 2006
Australia

Ms Felicity J Meyer, MA FRCS
Department of Surgery
St Thomas' Hospital
Lambeth Palace Road
London SE1 7EH, UK

Mr Timothy Mims
Division of Vascular Surgery
Union Memorial Hospital/Helix Health
330 North Calvert Street
Suite 570
Baltimore MD 2128
USA

Dr P Mingazzini, MD
Department of Vascular Surgery
Bassini Teaching Hospital
University of Milan
Via Massimo Gorki 50
20092 Cinisello Balsamo
Milan, Italy

Dr Frans L Moll, MD PhD
Department of Surgery
St Antonius Hospital
Koekoekslaan 1
CM Nieuwegein
The Netherlands

Dr Robert P Mun, PhD
Department of Chemical Engineering
Curtin University of Technology
Perth
Western Australia

Mr Roddy Nash, MD FRCS
Department of Surgery
Derbyshire Royal Infirmary
London Road
Derby DE1 2QY, UK

Professor Andrew N Nicolaides, MS FRCS
Department of Vascular Surgery
St Mary's Hospital
Praed Street
Paddington
London W2 1NY, UK

Dr Rudolf P Tutein Nolthenius, MD
Department of Surgery
St Antonius Hospital
Koekoekslaan 1
CM Nieuwegein
The Netherlands

Professor Lars Norgren, MD PhD
Department of Surgery
University Hospital
S-221 85 Lund
Sweden

Dr P Örtenwall, MD
Department of Surgery
University Hospital
S-751 85 Uppsala
Sweden

Dr Tomas Pfeiffer, MD
Clinic for Vascular Surgery & Kidney Transplant
Chirurgische Klinik und Poliklinik der Heinrich-Heine-Universitat
40225 Dusseldorf
Moorenstrasse 5
Germany

Professor Janet T Powell, MD PhD
Professor of Vascular Biology
Charing Cross Hospital
Fulham Palace Road
London W6 8RF, UK

Mr Frank J Prendergast, FRACS
Endovascular Unit
Royal Perth Hospital
Perth
Western Australia

Dr D Raithel, MD
Chefarz der Gefasschirurgischen Klinik
Eunngelisches Krankenhaus
Wertgasse 30
45468 Muhlheim
Germany

Mr Ganesh Ramaswami, PhD FRCS
Department of Vascular Surgery
St Mary's Hospital
Praed Street
Paddington
London W2 1NY, UK

Dr Punit S Ramrakha, BA BM ChB MRCP
Department of Clinical Pharmacology
Imperial College School of Medicine
Hammersmith Hospital
Du Cane Road
London W12 0HS, UK

Dr Lutz Reiher, MD
Clinic for Vascular Surgery & Kidney
Transplant
Chirurgische Klinik und Poliklinik der
Heinrich-Heine-Universitat
40225 Dusseldorf
Moorenstrasse 5
Germany

Mr Antonio Rosales, PhD
Department of Vascular Surgery
Aker Hospital
University of Oslo
Oslo
Norway

Professor C Vaughan Ruckley, MB ChM FRCSE
Vascular Surgery Office
Department of Surgery
The Royal Infirmary of Edinburgh
Edinburgh EH3 9YW, UK

Dr Tarun Sabharwal, MB BS
Specialist Registrar in Radiology
Charing Cross Hospital
Fulham Palace Road
London W6 8RF

Dr A Sampaolo, MD
Department of Vascular Surgery
Bassini Teaching Hospital
University of Milan
Via Massimo Gorki 50
20092 Cinisello Balsamo
Milan, Italy

Mr Marcos Sanchez, MD
Division of Vascular Surgery
Union Memorial Hospital/Helix Health
330 North Calvert Street
Suite 570
Baltimore MD 2128
USA

Professor Wilhelm Sandmann
Klinik fur Gefasschirurgie und
Nierentransplant
Chirurgische Klinik und Poliklinik der
Heinrich-Heine-Universitat
40225 Dusseldorf
Moorenstrasse 5
Germany

Dr H Scholz, MD
Chefarz der Gefasschirurgischen Klinik
Evangelisches Krankenhaus
Wertgasse 30
45468 Muhlheim
Germany

Professor Torben Veith Schroeder, MD DMSc
Department of Vascular Surgery RK
Rigshospitalet 3111
9 Blegdamsvej
DK2100
Copenhagen
Denmark

Dr Guillem Seban, MD
Service de Chirurgie Vasculaire
Hopital Henri Mondor
51 Ave du Marechal de Lattre de Tassigny
94010 Creteil
France

Dr James B Semmens, PhD
Centre for Health Services Research
Department of Public Health
University of Western Australia
Nedlands
Western Australia 6907

Mr Kishore Sieunarine, FRACS
Endovascular Unit
Royal Perth Hospital
Perth
Western Australia

Mr Dominic Slade, FRCS
Department of Surgery
South Manchester University Hospital
Nell Lane
West Didsbury
Manchester M20 8LR, UK

Professor Carl Erik Slagsvold, PhD
Department of Vascular Diagnostics
Aker Hospital
University of Oslo
Oslo
Norway

Dr Felicity B Smith, PhD
Wolfson Unit for Peripheral Vascular Diseases
University of Edinburgh Medical School
Teviot Place
Edinburgh EH8 9AG, UK

Mr Jason J Smith, FRCS
Department of Surgery
Barnet General Hospital
Wellhouse Lane
Barnet
Herts EN5 3DJ, UK

Mr Nigel J Standfield
Room BN1/10, 1st Floor B Block North
Division of Surgery, Anaesthesia & Intensive Care
Imperial College School of Medicine
Hammersmith Campus
DuCane Road
London, UK

Mr Gerard Stansby, MChir FRCS
Academic Surgical Unit
QEQM Wing
St Mary's Hospital
Paddington
London W2 1NY, UK

Dr S Sternjakob, MD
Department of Vascular Surgery
Bassini Teaching Hospital
University of Milan
Via Massimo Gorki 50
20092 Cinisello Balsamo
Milan, Italy

Dr Thomas J Tegos, MD
Department of Vascular Surgery
St Mary's Hospital
Praed Street
Paddington
London W2 1NY, UK

Dr Stephen M Thomas, MRCP FRCR
Sheffield Vascular Institute
Northern General Hospital
Herries Road
Sheffield S5 7AU, UK

Mr Matthew M Thompson, MD FRCS
Department of Surgery
Clinical Sciences Building
Leicester Royal Infirmary
Leicester LE2 7LX, UK

Professor Jonathan B Towne, MD
Medical College of Wisconsin
9200 West Winconsin Avenue
Milwaukee WI 53226
USA

Dr T Troëng, MD
Department of Surgery
University Hospital
S-751 85
Uppsala
Sweden

Dr Jos C van den Berg, MD
Department of Radiology
St Antonius Hospital
Koekoekslaan 1
CM Nieuwegein
The Netherlands

Dr Greg van Schie, FRACR
Endovascular Unit
Royal Perth Hospital
Perth
Western Australia

Mr Stuart R Walker, MB BS FRCS
Specialist Registrar
Department of Vascular and Endovascular Surgery
University Hospital
Queens Medical Centre
Nottingham NG7 2UH, UK

Dr Eric Wellons, MD
Department of Vascular Surgery
Union Memorial Hospital/Helix Health
330 North Calvert Street
Suite 570
Baltimore MD 2128
USA

Dr Jan J Wever, MD
Division of Vascular Surgery G 04 232
University Hospital Utrecht
Heidelberglaan 100
3508 CX Utrecht
The Netherlands

Professor Geoffrey H White, MD
Endovascular Research Unit
Department of Surgery
Blackburn Building D06
University of Sydney
New South Wales 2006
Australia

Mr John HN Wolfe, MS FRCS
Vascular Surgical Unit
St Mary's Hospital
Praed Street
Paddington
London W2 1NY, UK

Preface

Indications in Vascular and Endovascular Surgery, the companion to this title, was published a year ago and had a very good reception. It has proved to be an extremely popular title. From that book and the symposium about that topic at Charing Cross, London in 1998, it emerged that the durability of technical procedures is the uppermost issue in the minds of many vascular surgeons and radiologists. Consequently we have chosen this topic which both reflects the progression of disease in the vessels themselves and the durability of the devices and procedures used for improvement.

Therefore there are several portions of this book covering the subject of durability of vascular and endovascular surgery. First, we feel that it is necessary to examine the life expectancy of various patients who have vascular disease and we learn much from population studies and national registries. Later, there is a need to predict the place of xenotransplantation as it will affect our surgical options for the future. Pharmacological manipulation is aimed at improving the natural history of vascular disease both in the primary and in the secondary prevention aspects. We must also ask ourselves to what extent drug therapy enhances vascular and endovascular technology outcomes.

The rest of the book is concerned with vascular problems, both arterial and venous where procedures are performed on 'shifting sands'. In other words, we could perhaps expect a more durable result if we were sure in the first place that the architecture and state of the blood vessels would stay the same as at the time of vascular and endovascular intervention. Unfortunately, we are not at liberty to make this assumption. Vascular and endovascular procedures are chosen therefore with the knowledge that the blood vessels themselves are unlikely to stay the same and frequently the strength and weakness of the procedures are affected by changes in the blood vessels around and close to where the intervention has taken place.

The authors have been chosen from the point of view of their own knowledge of their subject, but they are also asked to review the subject, and reference important contributions from other centres and to focus their chapters on the issues raised here which form the reasons for this book.

I am very fortunate to be able to include the expert commentaries on individual chapters by Professor Janet Powell and Professor Vaughan Ruckley; these have brought a new dimension to the book.

I am extremely grateful to WB Saunders for arranging that Seán Duggan is able to continue working on their behalf for this series of books.

RM Greenhalgh

ARE ENDOVASCULAR METHODS AS DURABLE AS OPEN PROCEDURES?

The durability of subintimal angioplasty

Amman Bolia, Peter RF Bell and Nicholas London

INTRODUCTION

Although this chapter primarily addresses the durability of subintimal percutaneous transluminal angioplasty (S-PTA), because the technique is not widely practised, we will begin by describing its history, its indications and the details of the technique itself. Our first S-PTA was performed in 1987 in a 58-year-old claudicant with a 10-cm left popliteal artery occlusion.[1] Following a successful subintimal angioplasty, the patient was symptom free for 9½ years until he died of other causes. Since this first case, S-PTA has been used in over 700 femoropopliteal occlusions. The long-term outcome on the first 200 occlusions have been reported.[2] In addition S-PTA has been used extensively for tibial occlusions[3–6] and also there has been some experience in iliac,[7] profunda, brachial,[8] axillary and subclavian artery occlusions. S-PTA has made a major impact on the treatment of claudicants[2] and is our first line treatment for up to 60% of patients with critical ischaemia.[6,9–11]

INDICATIONS

Femoropopliteal occlusion

Very short (less than 3cm) or recent occlusions (less than 3 months old) and narrow vessels with extensive diffuse disease (less than 4mm in diameter) are excluded from the subintimal approach. Short occlusions can be treated transluminally and diffuse disease in small vessles responds relatively adversely. However, if dissection occurs while attempting the transluminal approach, subintimal recanalization is pursued. Subintimal recanalization is generally applicable in the following situations:

1. *Occlusions of long standing*. An occlusion that has been present for a long period of time becomes hard, rendering itself impossible to deal with intraluminally. A dissection occurs readily in such situations.
2. *Hard occlusions*. An occlusion is hard when the feel imparted to the guidewire is such that an intraluminal approach is impossible.
3. *Long occlusions*. The longer the occlusion, the more difficult it is to maintain intraluminal position with the guidewire.
4. *Diffuse and tandem disease*. An occlusion in an underlying diffusely diseased artery does not allow the guidewire to be negotiated intraluminally throughout the length of the occlusion.

5. *Previously failed intraluminal approach.* A dissection is likely to ensue where a previous intraluminal approach has failed.
6. *The presence of a large proximal collateral.* When a large collateral is present at the origin of an occlusion,[1] the resultant anatomy may lack the necessary 'stump' to allow engagement of a guidewire. S-PTA allows such an unfavourable anatomy to be dealt with, by initiating a dissection above the collateral. The dissection follows the main vessel, thus avoiding entry into the collateral.
7. *Flush superficial femoral artery occlusions.* Flush occlusions with a very small stump or no stump at all can be treated by S-PTA.
8. *Successful recanalization following a perforation.* If a perforation of the superficial femoral artery occurs during an attempted intraluminal approach, subsequent attempts at crossing the lesion may result in the guidewire following the same path leading into the perforation. However, using the extraluminal approach, one can avoid the site of the perforation, by choosing a different route within a dissection, in order to achieve a successful recanalization.[12]
9. *Calcified vessels.* The presence of moderate to heavy calcification is generally regarded as unfavourable for angioplasty due to the hardness of the occlusion. Attempts at intraluminal recanalization of such a hard occlusion result in the wire taking the path of least resistance, which is in a dissection. Using S-PTA, many such lesions can have a favourable outcome.
10. *Long stenoses.* Long stenoses generally have a poor outcome with intraluminal angioplasty. In view of the favourable long-term results of S-PTA, many of the long superficial femoral artery stenoses are now recanalized using S-PTA. An ideal lesion for S-PTA is when there is a reasonably disease-free segment in the proximal superficial femoral artery and the distal superficial femoral artery, but a long segment of diffuse stenosis in between. S-PTA allows exclusion of this diseased segment from the neolumen, thus allowing possibly improved long-term outcome.
11. *Failed bypass graft.* In patients in whom femoropopliteal graft has become occluded, it may be possible to recanalize the original femoropopliteal occlusion using S-PTA.[13]

Popliteal occlusions extending into tibial arteries

S-PTA allows the recanalization of a popliteal occlusion that extends into one or more of the runoff vessels. If all three runoff vessels are suitable distally, then it is possible to recanalize the entire trifurcation.[5]

Tibial occlusions

The majority of patients with critical limb ischaemia have tibial arterial disease. Most occlusions of tibial arteries can be treated with S-PTA, provided there is a reasonable artery distally to which the dissection has to be extended. Favourable factors are that the distal artery is 'smooth' on angiography and disease free. Factors that are less favourable are small, diffusely diseased distal artery and heavy calcification. One or more tibial occlusions can be recanalized at the same time,[5] depending on whether there are suitable favourable factors for each one.

TECHNIQUE

The principle behind the technique is to dissect intentionally into the subintimal space and the whole length of the dissection is dilated with a balloon.

Femoropopliteal occlusions

An ipsilateral antegrade puncture of the common femoral artery is made for occlusions that begin near the origin of the superficial femoral artery. With subintimal approach, a very small stump (5mm or even less) is all that is required. When there is a reasonable length of the superficial femoral artery available proximally, the puncture is usually made selectively into the superficial femoral artery itself. A 5F (Van Andel type, Cook Ltd, Letchworth, UK) predilating catheter is introduced antegradely up to the origin of the occlusion. Heparin (5000 units) and tolazoline (12.5mg) are injected before crossing the lesion. Tolazoline, a vasadilator, helps to dilate the distal vessels and reduces the possibility of spasm during the procedure. A straight floppy guidewire (3cm floppy, 180cm long and 0.035 inch diameter ; Boston Scientific, UK) is used to enter the occlusion. The tip of the wire is directed towards the arterial wall, taking care to avoid any large collaterals. Sometimes this requires either curving the tip of the of the guidewire or using a preshaped catheter (Cobra). The wire/catheter combination is then advanced into the occlusion and in the majority of cases, the wire/catheter combination advances into the path of least resistance which is in a dissection. Entry in the subintimal space is confirmed by injection of a small volume of dilute contrast medium. Omnipaque 200 (Nycomed, Oslo) is diluted to half strength for this purpose. Once in the subintimal space, the guidewire moves freely, encountering little resistance. The straight guidewire is now replaced by a tapered tip J wire (1.5mm J, 180cm long, 0.035 inch diameter; Boston Scientific, UK). The length of the occlusion is traversed either by forward pressure on the J wire or by advancing the catheter with a J wire protruding from it. The entire crossing of the occlusion is performed using the road map facility on the digital subtraction angiography (DSA) equipment if available. This allows the monitoring of the path of the guidewire and displays the exact length of the occlusion. When the catheter tip is 2–3cm from the distal end of the occlusion, the catheter is retracted 2–3cm and the J wire manipulated to form a large loop.

It is this large loop in the guidewire that enables the re-entry into the true arterial lumen distally by use of forward pressure on the loop. The resistance to forward pressure will suddenly decrease once the true lumen has been entered. Sometimes, the procedure results in a dissection having to be extended further than the end of the occlusion in order to achieve re-entry. This is usually of no consequence to the patient unless some major collateral has been compromised without achieving re-entry. In order to avoid this possibility, the most important and major collaterals that are feeding the artery beyond the occlusion should be avoided. A good example of such a collateral is the one often present at the level of the mid-popliteal artery having arisen from a branch of the profunda artery. It is important that if this is the only feeding vessel to the distal vasculature, that its origin is not compromised by the dissection, especially during the early phase of the learning curve. Damage to this important collateral, and subsequent failure to re-enter the artery distally may result in flow compromise and a possible emergency situation, whereby arterial reconstructive surgery may be required to restore distal circulation to the limb.

Once the lesion has been crossed, a 5 French balloon catheter (usually 5 or 6mm in diameter) is inflated throughout the entire length of the subintimal channel using approximately 10–12 atmospheres of pressure and 15-second inflations at a time. Any residual stenosis of more than 30% is balloon dilated repeatedly until satisfactory result in achieved. Any impairment of flow as seen by contrast injection is rectified by multiple inflations using higher pressures in the balloon. At the conclusion of the procedure, a further dose of tolazoline (12.5mg) is given. This facilitates peripheral vasodilation and reduces peripheral resistance. It helps to enhance the flow through the recanalized segment.

Asprin, if not contraindicated, is prescribed for patients who have had a successful recanalization, the usual dose being 150mg daily for 3 months. Oral anticoagulants are not prescribed.

Tibial arteries

Short occlusions are usually crossed easily intraluminally, but subintimal recanalization is applicable in longer occlusions of 3cm or more. The technique for crossing the lesions is basically similar to the approach used in femoropopliteal occlusions, except that we prefer to use a hydrophilic guidewire (180cm long, 0.035 inch diameter and angled; Terumo Ltd, Tokyo, Japan). Once again, the aim is to form a loop in the guidewire towards the end of the occlusion. From experience, a loop is very helpful in achieving luminal re-entry. Because the intima becomes thinner in the distal arterial tree, it is usually not difficult to re-enter the true lumen in the distal tibial vessels. Balloon dilatation is performed in a similar manner to the femoropopliteal segment. A 5 French 2cm long, 3mm diameter balloon is used to achieve dilatation using 10 to 12 atmospheres of pressure at 15-second inflations at a time. Repeated inflations may be necessary if a satisfactory result has not been achieved. Should spasm occur despite the injection of tolazoline, 100-μg boluses of intra-arterial nitroglycerin are administered (up to a maximum of 500 μg).

RESULTS

Femoropopliteal occlusions

The first 200 procedures in 176 patients over a period of 64 months were carried out between 1987 and 1992 and have been reported elsewhere.[2] The results are presented here briefly. Of the 176 patients, the mean age was 68 (22–92) years, 130 (74%) were males, 33 (19%) were diabetics, 62 (35%) were hypertensive and 61 (35%) were smokers.

Technical success was defined as recanalization with 30% or less residual stenosis and antegrade flow at the conclusion of the procedure. Technical failures resulted from inability to either enter, traverse or exit the subintimal space. The common reasons for abandoning the procedure were usually failure to progress with the catheter in a heavily calcified vessel, or an occurrence of a perforation, or failing to re-enter the lumen distally. Major complications were defined as those that altered the patient's clinical state, whereas minor complication did not. Patient follow-up consisted of clinical examination and ankle brachial pressure index (ABPI) only. These were performed at 24 hours, 1, 3, 6, 9 and 12 months and thereafter at 6-monthly intervals. Patency was analysed by looking at primary patency only and the factors influencing reocclusion were examined by investigating the effect on the haemodynamic patency of technically successful procedures. Haemodynamic patency required that the ABPI rose by more than 0.10 within 24 hours and did not fall more than 0.15 from the post-procedure level. Symptomatic patency required that claudication distance improved by at least 50%, the resolution of rest pain or healing of ulcers and minor amputations.

Technical success rate and complications

The technical success rate was 80% (159/200) and there were no significant differences between the technical success and failure groups with the respect to the incidence of diabetes, critical ischaemia/claudication, occlusion site or occlusion length. The technical success rate for occlusions less than 10cm was 81%, for occlusions 11–20cm was 83%, and for occlusions more than 20cm was 68%, with no significant statistical difference in terms of ability to recanalize a short or a long occlusion. There were two major (1%) and 13 minor complications (6.5%). The major complications were one retroperitoneal and one scrotal haematoma and although both required surgical evacuation there were no long-term sequelae. The minor complications were two groin haematomas, seven distal emboli and four vessel perforations. The groin haematoma resolved spontaneously. Two of the perforations required no treatment and two were treated by embolization using embolization coils. Of the seven distal emboli, six were aspirated using an 8 French non-tapered aspiration catheter and in addition one required regional fibrinolysis with streptokinase (5000 units per hour) for 24 hours. There were no deaths or limb loss directly related to the subintimal angioplasty procedure. The 30-day mortality was 3/200 (1.5%), all three deaths resulting from myocardical infarction.

Figure 1 shows an excellent long-term outcome in a patient with 50-yard claudication.

After this study period, the subsequent 275 procedures were analysed (unpublished results). There were 31 failures (11%), thus a success rate of 89%. The mean length of occlusion in this group was 15cm.

The failures in these 31 procedures were due to failure to re-enter distally in 15 (5%), heavy calcification in six (2%), perforation in four (1.5%), fresh occlusion in two

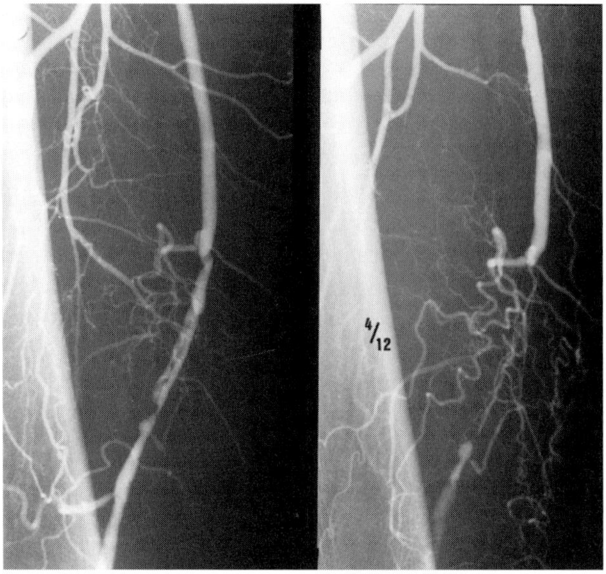

(a) (b)

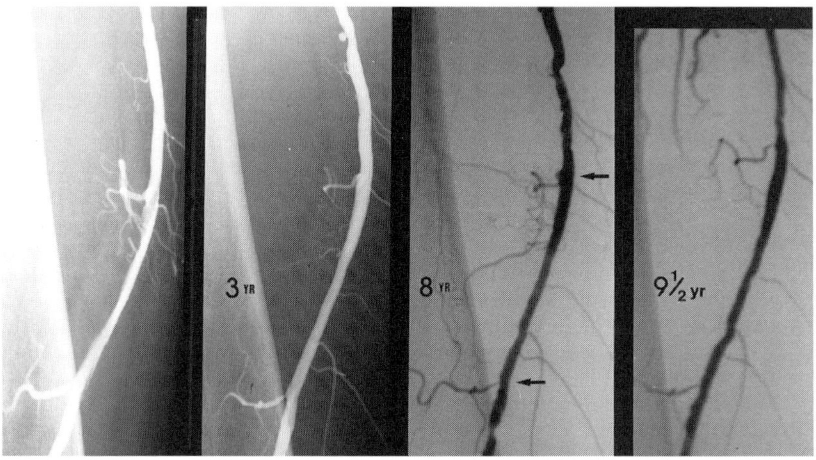

(c) (d) (e) (f)

Fig. 1. This patient has 50-yard claudication in the right leg. (a) Atheromatous disease and possible fresh thrombus is present at the level of the adductor canal. Angioplasty was not attempted in view of the possible fresh clot. (b) The occlusion had 'matured', at 4 months. (c) S-PTA was carried out. Notice the eccentric lumen and the smooth dissection channel. (d) 3 years later there is no evidence of recurrence of disease in the angioplastied segment but some disease is present in the proximal part of the vessel. Interestingly, some branch vessels have developed in the angioplastied segment. (e) 8 years later minor irregularities are present in the recanalized segment but extensive disease has developed in the rest of the artery. (f) 9½ years later again the recanalized segment shows minor disease but the rest of the artery shows more diffuse and extensive atheromatous disease.

(1%) and damage to important collaterals without reconstitution of flow in four (1.5%). In these four cases, emergency bypass surgery was required. There were ten embolic complications, of which eight were aspirated percutaneously, and the other two were haemodynamically not significant. Surgical embolectomy was not required in any case.

Patency

The long-term symptomatic and haemodynamic patencies of all 200 procedures (i.e. analysed on an 'intention to treat' basis) and of the 159 technical successful procedures are shown in Figs 2 and 3. The haemodynamic patencies at 12 and 36 months for all procedures were 56% and 46% respectively; the symptomatic patencies were 58% and 48%. The haemodynamic patencies at 12 and 36 months for technically successful procedures were 71% and 58% respectively. The symptomatic patencies were 73 and 61%; 3% of the technically successful procedures failed within 24 hours.

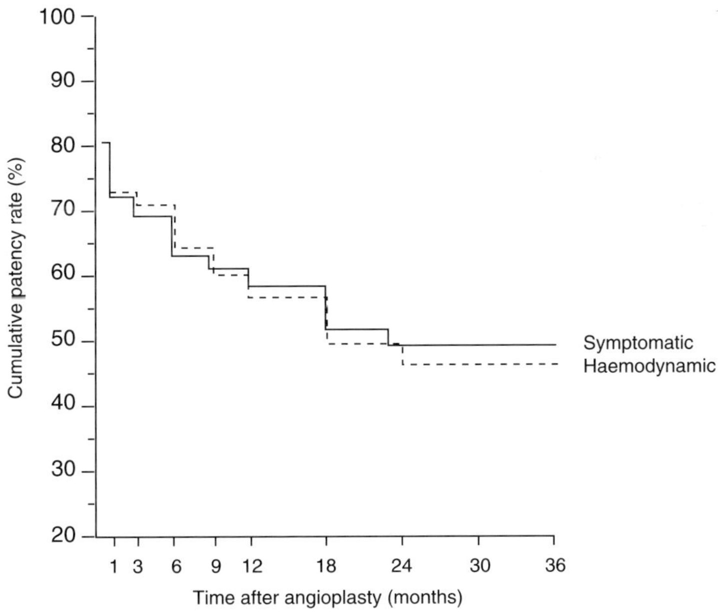

Number at risk

200	109	82	60	43	36	25	Haemodynamic
200	112	87	64	46	39	27	Symptomatic

Fig. 2. Cumulative haemodynamic and symptomatic patencies for all 200 attempted subintimal angioplasties.

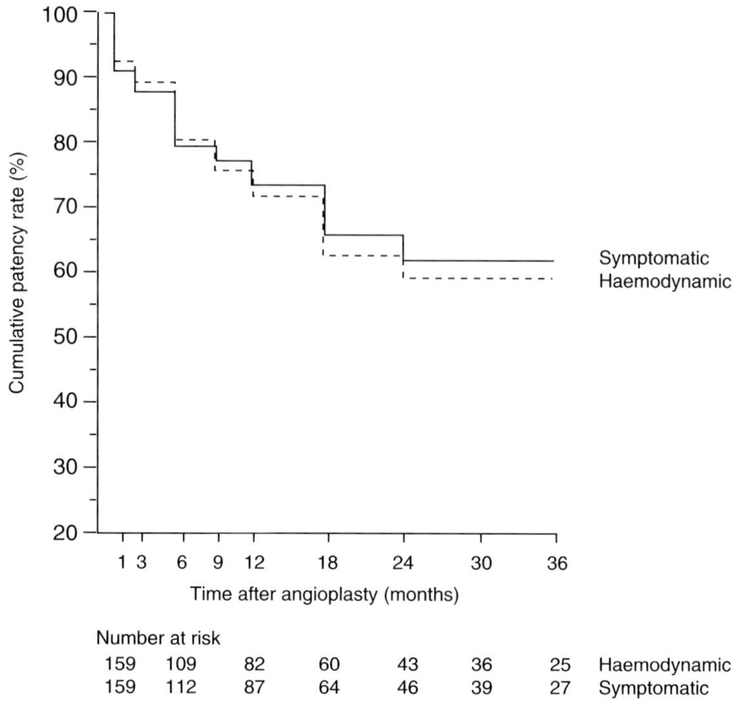

Fig. 3. Cumulative haemodynamic and symptomatic patencies of the 159 technically successfully procedures.

Tibial occlusions

The published literature on angioplasty of tibial lesions is limited, and a few available series have combined the treatment of stenoses and occlusion.[14–18] A small study carried out at the Leicester Royal Infirmary of tibial occlusions treated by S-PTA has been published elsewhere.[6] A total of 32 infrapopliteal artery occlusions in 28 critically ischaemic limbs in 27 patients have been recanalized by S-PTA; 25 (89%) of the treated occlusions were of a single vessel, whereas in three limbs (11%) multiple occlusions were recanalized. The median (range) length of occlusion was 7 (2–30) centimetres. Of the 28 limbs, four (14%) had rest pain, 17 (61%) had ulceration and seven (25%) had gangrene. The immediate technical success rate was 26 of 32 (81%) occlusions.

There were no failures at 24 hours and 30-day mortality was 0. Three complications included one puncture-related retroperitoneal haematoma that required surgical intervention, a vessel perforation that was of no consequence to the patient, and was regarded as a failed procedure and one distal embolization after a successful recanalization that was aspirated percutaneously.

Although long-term results are not available yet, the 1-year haemodynamic and symptomatic patencies were 50% and 54% respectively.

In patients with critical limb ischaemia, tibial vessel patency is only desirable to relieve rest pain, heal ulceration or demarcate gangrene to allow localized surgery.

In the majority of cases S-PTA allows this to happen (Fig. 4).

The impact of S-PTA on critical ischaemia

S-PTA has made a significant impact on the treatment of chronic critical limb ischaemia at the Leicester Royal Infirmary. A recent prospective survey of all critical limb ischaemia patients who presented at the Leicester Royal Infirmary was carried out during the 12-month period in 1994.[10] There were 222 referrals in 188 patients.

This survey showed that the majority of the patients were treated with angioplasty (42%); 6% of the patients had a combined treatment of angioplasty and surgery (minor amputations) and 24% of the patients had reconstructive surgery; 17% of the patients were treated conservatively and 10% had primary amputation.

The mean (range) hospital stay for patients treated by surgery was 16 (3–97) days, for angioplasty 4.5 (1–73) days, and amputation, 18 (7–91) days.

The in-hospital mortality rate was 10% with a limb salvage rate of 79%. The complication rate of PTA requiring surgery was 5.5%.

A further prospective 12-month study was carried out as a continuation of this previous study.[11] The aim of the study was to assess and compare the efficacy of PTA and surgery in the treatment of severe lower limb ischaemia. Of the 188 patients (222 critically ischaemic limbs) complete 12-month follow-up data could be obtained in 180 patients (187 limbs).

The overall 12-month patient survival was 75%. The 12-month survival rates for surgery and angioplasty were significantly higher (91% and 78% respectively) compared with those of primary amputation and conservative management (57% and 52% respectively).

The overall 12-month limb salvage rate was 71%. The limb salvage for patients treated with either PTA or surgery was 76% (Fig. 5).

The policy to attempt PTA whenever possible enables 46% of the patients in the study to be revascularized by this modality compared with a national average of 22%.[19] Furthermore, the limb salvage rates for PTA compare very favourably with surgery.[11]

The data from this study strongly supports the use of PTA as first-line treatment for severe limb ischaemia with no major evidence that PTA is detrimental to later surgery if required. In the context of a 12-month survival of 75% and a 3-year survival of only 50–60%, a long-term solution is not what many of these elderly frail patients require. This study highlights that as a minimally invasive procedure, PTA serves the majority of patients very well, with a short hospital stay, and 12-month limb salvage rates that equate with those achieved by surgery.

CONCLUSION

S-PTA offers a high success and low complication rates and good long-term patencies in patients with femoropopliteal occlusions, presenting with intermittent

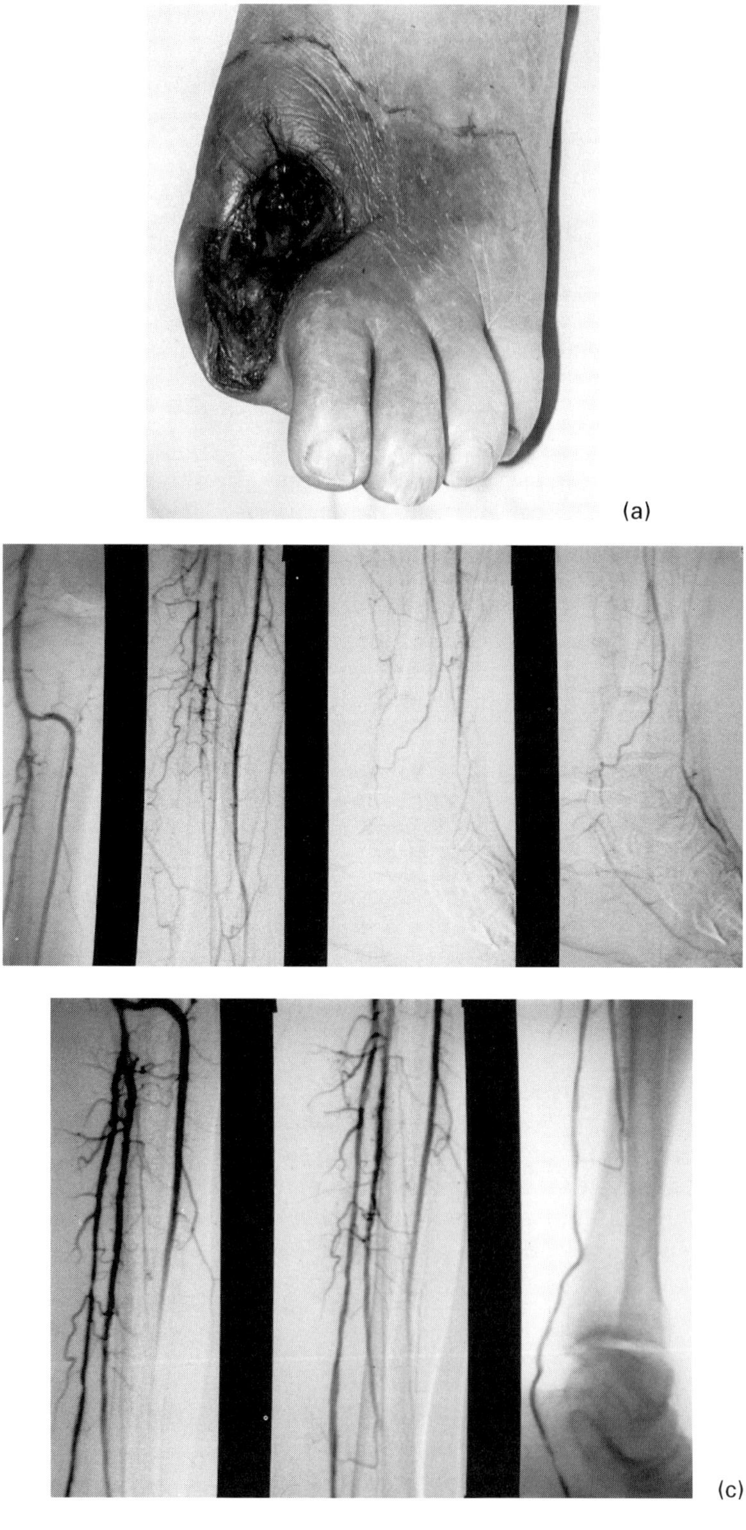

(a)

(b)

(c)

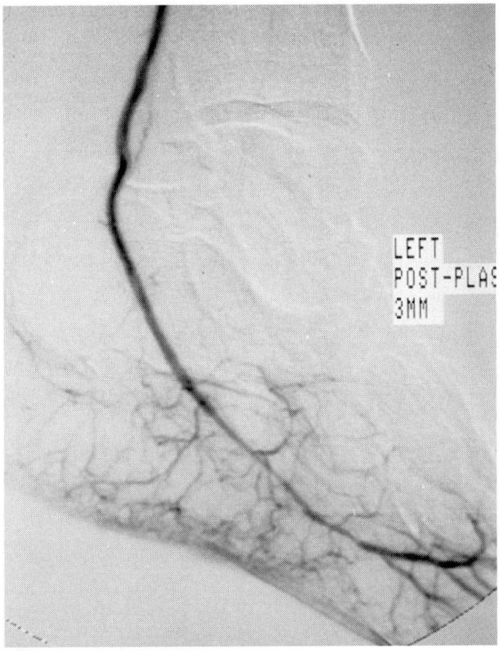

(d)

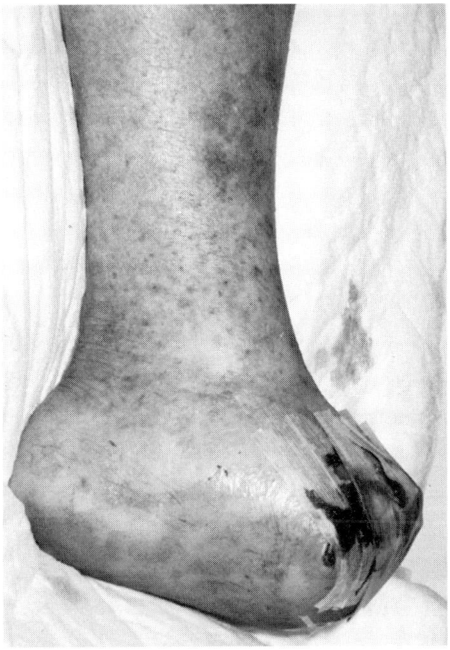

(e)

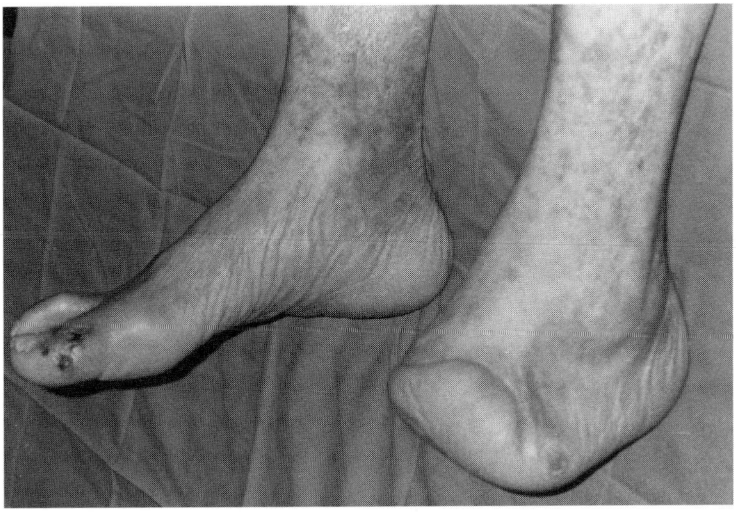

(f)

Fig. 4. This patient had an amputation of the big toe for gangrene, in the presence of a dorsalis pedis pulse. (a) The gangrene was extending further into the foot. (b) A diagnostic arteriogram showed a good anterior tibial artery but this was occluded at the level of the dorsalis pedis artery. All the other runoff vessels were partly or totally occluded but there was filling of the lateral plantar arch. (c) Attempt was made to recanalize the peroneal and the posterior tibial arteries. (d) Excellent flow was established in the foot following a successful recanalization of the posterior tibial artery. (e) The amputation was limited to the forefoot thus avoiding a below knee amputation. (f) At 3½ years, despite reocclusion of the previously recanalized tibial arteries, the patient is asymptomatic and there are no signs of ischaemia in the left leg but the right toe is showing ischaemic ulceration on the big toe.

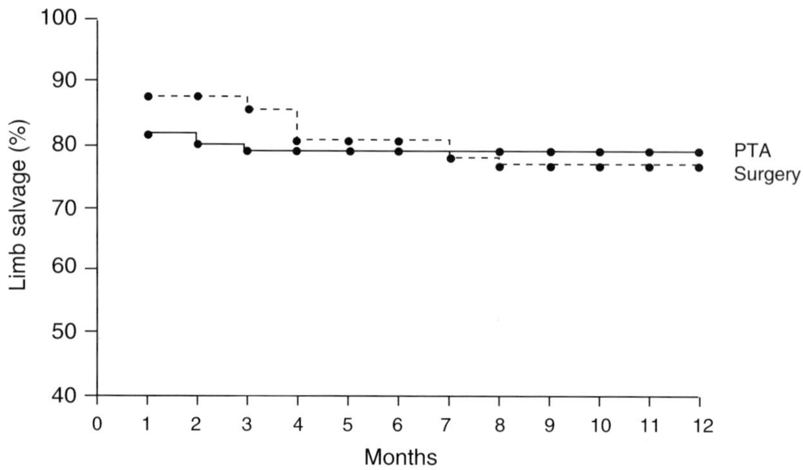

Number at risk

84	65	64	62	60	56	53	50	49	49	49	49	47	PTA
57	48	48	47	43	43	43	42	40	40	40	40	40	Surgery

Fig. 5. Limb salvage for surgery and PTA standard error less than 10% at all time points.

claudication or critical ischaemia. No specialized equipment or materials are necessary. It does not require extensive experience by the operator. The technique is inexpensive and therefore could potentially have widespread application, as an alternative to bypass surgery.

In elderly patients presenting with critical limb ischaemia and tibial occlusions, S-PTA is safe, effective and inexpensive. It therefore offers an excellent alternative to distal reconstructive surgery for the treatment of tibial artery occlusion in patients with critical limb ischaemia. The data from a study carried out at Leicester Royal Infirmary[10,11] strongly support the use of PTA as first-line treatment for severe lower limb ischaemia, with no major evidence that PTA is detrimental to later surgery if required. PTA offers a short hospital stay[10] and 12-month limb salvage rates that equate with those achieved by surgery.[11]

REFERENCES

1. Bolia A, Miles KA, Brennan J, Bell PRF: Percutaneous transluminal angioplasty of occlusions of the femoral and popliteal arteries by subintimal dissection. *Cardiovasc Intervent Radiol* **13**: 357–363, 1990
2. London NJM, Srinivasan R, Sayers RD *et al.*: Subintimal angioplasty of femoropopliteal artery occlusion: The long-term results. *Eur J Vasc Surg* **8**: 148–155, 1994
3. Bolia A, Sayers RD, Thompson MM, Bell PRF: Subintimal and intraluminal recanalization of occluded crural arteries by percutaneous balloon angioplasty. *Eur J Vasc Surg* **8**: 214–219, 1994

4. Varty K, Bolia A, Naylor AR *et al.*: Infrapopliteal percutaneous transluminal angioplasty: A safe and successful procedure. *Eur J Vasc Endovasc Surg.* **9**: 341–345, 1995
5. Nydahl S, London NJM, Bolia A: Technical report: Recanalization of all three infrapopliteal arteries by subintimal angioplasty. *Clin Radiol* **51**: 366–367, 1996
6. Nydahl S, Hartshorne T, Bell PRF *et al.*: Subintimal angioplasty of infrapopliteal occlusions in critically ischaemic limbs. *Eur J Vasc Endovasc Surg* **14**: 212–216, 1997
7. Bolia A, Fishwick G: Recanalization of iliac artery occlusion by subintimal dissection using the ipsilateral and the contralateral approach. *Clin Radiol* **52:** 684–687, 1997
8. Bolia A, Nasim A, Bell PRF: Percutaneous extraluminal (subintimal) recanalization of a brachial artery occlusion following cardiac catheterization. *Cardiovasc Intervent Radiol* **19**: 184–186, 1996
9. London NJM, Varty K, Sayers RD *et al.*: Percutaneous transluminal angioplasty for lower limb critical ischaemia. *Br J Surg* **82:** 1232–1235, 1995
10. Varty K, Nydahl S, Butterworth P *et al.*: Changes in the management of critical limb ischaemia. *Br J Surg* **83**: 953–956, 1996
11. Varty K, Nydahl S, Nasim A *et al.*: Results of surgery and angioplasty for the treatment of chronic severe lower limb ischamia. *Eur J Vasc Endovasc Surg* **16:** 159–163, 1998
12. Nasim A, Sayers RD, Dunlop P *et al.*: Intentional Extraluminal recanalization of the femoropopliteal segment following perforation during percutaneous transluminal angioplasty. *Eur J Vasc Endovasc Surg* **12**: 246–249, 1996
13. Nasim A, Sayers RD, Bell PRF, Bolia A: Recanalization of the native artery following failure of a bypass graft. *Eur J Vasc Surg* **10:** 125–127, 1995
14. Bakal CW, Sprayege N, Scheinbaum K *et al.*: Percutaneous transluminal angioplasty of the infrapopliteal arteries: Results in 53 patients. *Am J Roent* **154:** 171–174, 1990
15. Schwarten DE: Clinical and anatomical considerations for nonoperative therapy in tibial disease and the results of angioplasty. *Circulation* **83** (Suppl I): 86–90, 1991
16. Schwarten DE, Cutliff WB: Arterial occlusive disease below the knee:treatment with percutaneous transluminal angioplasty performed with low-profile catheters and steerable guide wires. *Radiology* **169:** 71–74, 1988
17. Flueckiger F, Lammer J, Klein GE *et al.*: Percutaneous angioplasty of crural arteries. *Acta Radiologica* **33:** 152–155, 1992
18. Buckenham TM, Loh A, Dormandy JA *et al.*: Infrapopliteal angioplasty for limb salvage. *Eur J Vasc Surg* **7:** 21–25, 1993
19. Harris PL for The Vascular Surgical Society of Great Britain and Ireland: Critical limb ischaemia: management and outcome. Report of a national survey. *Eur J Vasc Endovasc Surg* **10:** 108–113, 1995

Commentary

The authors described their first subintimal percutaneous transluminal angioplasty (S-PTA) in 1987 and since then, they have performed it in a number of areas, but the durability of their femoropoliteal reconstructions are very notable. Of the 200 procedures attempted, 159 were described as technically successful and in the figures the authors use the term 'symptomatic' as well as 'haemodynamic' patency. By symptomatic I assume they mean that the patient remains free of original symptoms, but of course, without checking by imaging, it is possible for a patient to be symptom-free and not necessarily to have a patent procedure. However, the figures show that the haemodynamic and symptomatic patencies run side by side. In comparison with surgery, PTA seems to be doing quite well over a very short follow-up period and this is clearly a technique which must be noted and we must all look out for the long-term durability of this novel technique as the results come in. *RMG*

The durability of iliac and femoral angioplasty

Julie Brittenden and Andrew W Bradbury

INTRODUCTION

Angioplasty, with or without deployment of a stent, is now an accepted part of the armamentarium of vascular surgeons and interventional radiologists managing lower limb ischaemia of all severities. This is perhaps remarkable given the almost complete absence of controlled data indicating its superiority over alternative treatment modalities, either in clinical or cost-effectiveness terms. As previously discussed,[1] it may be that one has to look beyond science to understand the primary reasons for the emergence of angioplasty in this field. Be that as it may, constraints on health care spending world-wide and increased patient 'consumerism' mean that the various health care systems in which we work have to adapt rapidly to new pressures and expectations. Treatments that cannot be shown to be clinically and economically worthwhile will no longer be funded, and patients will not accept risk without evidence of benefit. How then will angioplasty and stenting fare in this new environment ?

Despite the widespread acceptance of angioplasty, there is no doubt that many (if not all) vascular surgeons used to visualizing the inside of atherosclerotic vessels find it difficult to believe that such a vessel simply forced open, or intentionally dissected,[2] with a balloon will remain patent for any meaningful period of time. There are, therefore, important questions to be addressed regarding not only the safety but also the durability of percutaneous transluminal angioplasty (PTA) in the iliac and femoral segments; and whether this can be significantly improved by the use of stents.

The authors are aware of a large literature reporting uncontrolled anatomic and haemodynamic patency rates after angioplasty and stenting for various grades of lower limb ischaemia.[3] However, having reviewed this literature and examined in detail the results of our own large prospectively studied cohort of patients undergoing iliac and femoral PTA ± stents, we have taken the view that such data provide a disappointingly small amount of useful information regarding the durability of the procedures because:

1. Without a control group for comparison the reported outcomes are virtually meaningless; how does one know if the procedure has significantly positively or negatively impacted the natural history of the underlying condition in question?[4]
2. The only end-point that really matters is the symptomatic outcome. Haemodynamic patency, assessed by measurement of ankle brachial pressure index (ABPI), or anatomic patency assessed by follow-up angiography or duplex ultrasound, while of some academic interest, are much less clinically relevant.

When discussing the management of lower limb ischaemia, it is important to divide patients into three broad groups; namely, intermittent claudication (IC), subcritical limb ischaemia (SCLI)[5] and critical limb ischaemia (CLI).[6] Patients in these groups have quite different prognoses with so-called 'conservative' therapy and to group such patients together, as has been done in the past, is now scientifically unacceptable .[7,8]

It is a widely held view amongst vascular surgeons and interventional radiologists that PTA ± stenting in the aortoiliac segment is inherently more successful in terms of clinical outcome than PTA of the femoropopliteal segment. Perusal of the available literature provides surprisingly little support for this contention. Thus, although the haemodynamic and anatomic patency of interventions in the aortoiliac segment may be greater than those performed at an infrainguinal site, it remains to be seen whether this truly leads to a superior symptomatic outcome in the long term. Nevertheless, for the purposes of this chapter, the two territories are considered separately.

The aim of this chapter is to address three fundamental questions; namely, is there any evidence that:

1. PTA ± stenting provides a more durable relief of symptoms than best medical therapy in patients with intermittent claudication and SCLI; or more a durable prevention of amputation than femorodistal bypass in patients with CLI.
2. Interventions at the aortoiliac segment are more durable than those at the femoral level.
3. Does the deployment of a stent in the iliac segment provide a more durable outcome than PTA alone? The authors have taken the view that femoral artery stenting with present technologies is associated with unacceptably poor results and will not, therefore, be discussed.[9,10]

INTERMITTENT CLAUDICATION

Natural history

There are certain well established facts regarding the epidemiology[11] and natural history[12] of IC against which the success or failure of PTA ± stenting in the treatment of the condition must be gauged.

1. IC affects up to one in 20 middle aged people and its prevalence increases with advancing age.
2. The prognosis, as far as the leg is concerned, is largely benign with less than 10% of claudicants ever requiring intervention to prevent limb loss and less than 1% per year progressing to amputation.
3. The prognosis as far as risk of premature cardiovascular death is concerned is high. Claudicants have an annual mortality in the region of 5–10% which is 2–3 times greater than that of an age- and sex-matched non-claudicant population. Most of these deaths result from myocardial infarction and stroke.
4. Best medical therapy, comprising exercise and cardiovascular risk factor reduction, results on average in a 180% increase in walking distance[13–15] and a reduction in risk of death by up to one-third.[16,17]

As a result, any treatment for IC must be widely applicable and applied, must focus on the life not the limb, be of proven clinical benefit and durability, relatively inexpensive, and above all safe. How well does PTA meet these criteria ?

Randomized controlled trials

Astonishingly, there are only two published randomized controlled trials, comprising only 118 patients, comparing angioplasty and medical therapy with medical therapy alone in the management of IC.

The Edinburgh study

Of 600 consecutive new patients referred with unilateral claudication undergoing duplex ultrasound and/or angiography, only 10% were considered suitable for PTA by consultant interventional radiologists. Thus, 62 patients with iliac stenosis or short segment femoral stenosis or occlusions were randomized to best medical therapy (advice regarding exercise and smoking and aspirin) or best medical therapy and angioplasty. At 6 months follow-up, walking distances, ABPI, and duplex patency rates were significantly greater in the angioplasty group; and pain scores assessed by the Nottingham Health Profile quality of life questionnaire were significantly lower. However, at 2 years, there were no differences between the groups with regard to patient reported or treadmill maximum walking or onset to claudication distances; or in quality of life parameters and ABPI. The authors reasonably concluded that 'in a selected group of claudicants with relatively discrete iliofemoral disease, the addition of angioplasty did not confer benefit in terms of perceived or measured walking distance, ABPI or quality of life.[18]

The Oxford study

This trial, which was reported in two phases, compared angioplasty with a supervised exercise programme in 56 patients with iliofemoral disease. In the angioplasty group, there were significant increases in the mean ABPI at 3, 6, and 9 months but no corresponding significant increase in mean walking distance. Conversely in the exercise group, there were significant and progressive increases in the mean walking distances at 6, 9 and 12 months but no increase in mean ABPI.[19] At 6-year follow-up in 37 patients, there were no differences between the two groups.[20]

Comment

Perhaps not surprisingly these studies have been criticized for their small size and methodology. Nevertheless, they are all that is currently available and provide the only credible data with regard to the durability of PTA in this patient group. The validity of these two independent studies is further strengthened by the fact that the results are almost identical; both trials indicate that, although there may be a short-term advantage to PTA in some patients, this is not durable in the medium term. Three further points are worthy of comment:

1. Although there was no clinical benefit of PTA at 2 years in the Edinburgh study, duplex ultrasound examination performed at that time did demonstrate

significantly fewer occluded arteries and a lesser degree of stenosis in the PTA group. This serves to demonstrate the irrelevance of anatomic and haemodynamic measures of patency on which so may previous uncontrolled studies base their conclusions.
2. Both studies included patients with iliac and femoral disease. Unfortunately, the numbers are too small to allow statistically meaningful subgroup analysis. However, in patients with disease confined to the superficial femoral artery, the Oxford group noted that exercise training resulted in a greater improvement in claudication than angioplasty. This may because collateral formation is more effective at the infrainguinal site.
3. Unless investigators follow up their patients in the medium and long term (3–5 years) they may get a falsely optimistic view of the success of their intervention.

ILIAC ANGIOPLASTY AND STENT DEPLOYMENT

Uncontrolled data

Although a number of large uncontrolled studies have shown no additional benefit from stent deployment (Table 1),[22–30] a recent meta-analysis performed by Bosch and colleagues[21] has suggested that the durability of iliac angioplasty can be improved by the routine or selective use of stents. They analysed six angioplasty and eight stent studies, comprising a total of 2216 patients, published since 1990. The immediate technical success rate was 91% in the angioplasty group and 96% in the stent group; post-procedure mean ABPI was significantly higher in the stented patients and morbidity and mortality were similar in both groups. In patients with claudication the 4-year patency rates for angioplasty were 53% for stenoses and 54% for occlusive lesions. Corresponding figures for stented patients were 77% and 61% respectively. They therefore concluded that deployment of a stent reduces the early

Table 1. A comparison of iliac angioplasty with or without stent placement

	Patients	*Occlusion (%)*	*Critical ischaemia (%)*	*Follow-up (years)*	*Primary patency (%)*
Angioplasty only					
Jeans[22]	180	6.1	27	4	58
Jorgensen[23]	150	0	29	5	68
Stokes[24]	53	0	67	5	76[a]
Tegtmeyer[25]	200	1.8	42	4	87
Stent placment					
Henry[26]	184	9.2	7.1	4	86
Long[27]	61	44	6.3	4	41
Martin[28]	140	8.8	23	2	71
Strecker[29]	114	25	13	3	95
Vorwerk[30]	109	0	1.7	4	82

[a]Results in patients with claudication only

re-occlusion rate by about 40%. However, no data with regard to medium-term clinical outcome were provided and the lack of association between 'patency' and symptomatic outcome has already been discussed. Furthermore, these studies included a mixture of patients with IC, SCLI and CLI such that it is difficult to draw any firm conclusions about the appropriateness or durability of iliac stent placement from this analysis.

Randomized controlled trials

To date, only two randomized control trials, have compared angioplasty and stent placement in the management of iliac occlusive disease. Unfortunately, neither has included a 'best medical treatment only' arm.

The Richter study

This study has only appeared in abstract form in German[31] and the present authors have been unable to obtain details of randomization and study design. However, the cumulative 'clinical success' rate at 5 years in the angioplasty and stent group was reported as 70% and 93% respectively.

The Dutch trial

This trial[32] compared routine with iliac selective stenting (based on the presence of a residual pressure gradient > 10mmHg) in 279 patients with IC and an iliac stenosis greater than 50% on angiography. In the selective group, stents were deployed in 59/136 (43%) patients. The initial haemodynamic success rate was similar in both groups at 81–82%, as was the complication rate. The mean follow-up was 9.3 months; 2-year follow-up was only available in 37/143 (26%) patients in the iliac stent group and 34/136 (25%) patients in the selective stent group. In these patients the clinical success rate was 77–78%, and the patency rates were 70–71%. However, 43% of the patients in the primary stent group and 35% of the patients in the selective stent group still had symptoms of claudication at 2 years. Quality of life improved significantly in both groups following intervention, but there were no differences between the two groups. The study therefore appears to show no difference in the immediate and 2-year technical and clinical outcome between the two treatment strategies. Although this trial provides by far the most credible data currently available with regard to the utility and durability of iliac stenting in IC, the study does have a number of limitations; namely, the short duration of follow-up, the large number of stents deployed in the selective group, the small number of occlusive lesions (8%), and the absence of a 'best medical treatment only' arm for comparison.

The main take-home message from this trial appears to be that further trials are required, possibly comparing the clinical and cost-effectiveness of four different treatment strategies: conservative management, angioplasty alone, angioplasty with selective stenting on the basis of well established and pre-determined indications, and routine stenting. Until such a trial is conducted, one cannot be certain whether intervention of any kind confers additional benefit over 'best medical therapy' in terms of durable symptoms relief in IC, and if so whether this durability can be further augmented in certain cases by placement of a stent. The logistical difficulties and expense of conducting such a trial of sufficient power to provide a statistically meaningful result at a minimum of 2-year follow-up would, of course, be enormous. However, given the increasing pressure on health services spending one can easily imagine a situation where, without hard data to support the efficacy of PTA ± stent placement in IC, funding for these expensive interventions will simply not be forthcoming – especially as we know limb loss from claudication is rare and local arterial intervention does not appear to impact positively on the excess cardiovascular mortality suffered by this group of patients.

The Edinburgh experience with iliac intervention

General trends

In Edinburgh, since 1982, a designated clinic has been used to follow-up patients who have undergone surgical and endovascular interventions for lower limb ischaemia. A prospectively gathered computerized data base has been generated by this clinic and a preliminary analysis of this data base forms the basis of the local data to be presented. Between 1982 and 1989 and also 1990 and 1997 there has been a fourfold increase in the number of angioplasties performed annually for claudication; a significant increase in the number of procedures performed in the femoral segment (19% vs 42%), as well as a significant increase in the number of procedures performed for occlusive as opposed to stenotic disease (3% vs 14%, both $p < 0.001$ χ^2 with Yates correction). Despite the increased number of more distal and morphologically unfavourable lesions being treated there has been no significant increase in the initial clinical (7% vs 11%) or technical (both periods 6%) failure rate. Furthermore, major morbidity, defined as that sufficiently severe to delay hospital discharge, has fallen significantly (11% vs 6%, $p<0.05$, χ^2 with Yates correction). The proportion of patients requiring unplanned surgical revascularization for either complications of angioplasty or poor immediate clinical or technical remains is 1-2% in both time periods.

Angioplasty only vs unilateral stent deployment

The number of iliac angioplasties performed for IC shows a gradual increase through the 1980s with a peak in activity around 1992-3. However, once the results of the Edinburgh study became available locally in 1994, the numbers of procedures undertaken declines dramatically (Fig. 1). Since 1991, there has been an 11-fold increase in the number of unilateral iliac stents being deployed. These data exclude bilateral iliac, so-called 'kissing', stents (which will be considered separately below), as well as those patients who underwent iliac angioplasty ± stenting prior to a planned infrainguinal bypass procedure.

Patients undergoing angioplasty alone or angioplasty and stenting are compared in Table 2. It is important to emphasize that these two groups were not randomized and that the indications for use of stents were not strictly defined. In many cases the decision to stent or not simply reflects the personal preferences of the individual radiologist. Nevertheless, these data do provide useful comparisons regarding the

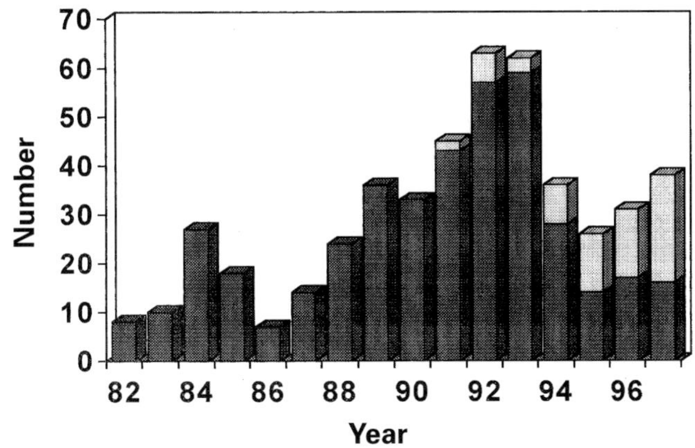

Fig. 1. Number of iliac PTA: dark areas (n=234) and stents: lighter area (n=67) performed each year in patients with claudication. No stents prior to 1991.

durability of PTA ± stenting in our centre. Patients with occlusions were significantly more likely to undergo stenting. There were no differences in the male to female ratios, median ages, or sites of procedure. The technical failure rates (as defined by the interventional radiologist undertaking the procedure) were the same in each group, but the clinical failure rate (no improvement in symptoms at time of discharge from hospital or first clinic review) was significantly higher in the angioplasty only group. The unplanned surgical revascularization rate (operative procedures

Table 2. Patient characteristics and initial outcome of iliac angioplasty versus stents in claudicants

1991–1997	*PTA* *n=234*	*Stent* *n=63*	*p value*[b]
Male:female ratio	3.3:1	3.4:1	NS
Median age (range)	57 [44–63]	51 [33–]	NS
Immediate clinical failure rate	33 (14%)	3 (5%)	p<0.05
Technical failure rate	14 (5%)	5 (8%)	NS
Unplanned surgical revascularization	6 (3%)	2 (3%)	NS
	3 FFXO	1 ABG	
	1 ABG, 2 IFB	1 IFB	
Morbidity[a]	8 (3%)	5 (8%)	p<0.01
Occlusion/stenosis	20 (8%)	19 (27%)	p < 0.03
Common iliac/external iliac/both	74% / 26% / 3%	78% / 22% / 7%	NS
Symptomatic outcome at 6 weeks			
Improved / no change / worse	71% / 16% /13%	86% / 7% / 7%	p < 0.001
Symptomatic outcome at last follow-up			
Improved / no change / worse	63% / 18% / 19%	69% / 17% / 14%	NS

[a] Results in patients with claudication
[b] χ^2 with Yates correction; FFXO: femoral to femoral cross-over; ABG: aortobifemoral graft; IFB: iliofemoral bypass; PTA: percutaneous transluminal angioplasty
NS: not significant.

performed as a consequence of technical failure, clinical failure or complications) was the same in each group. Major morbidity (defined as that severe enough to delay hospital discharge) was significantly higher in the stented patients, although the number of adverse events was small. At 6 weeks follow-up, patients who had undergone stenting reported a significantly better clinical outcome. However, in the medium term, this early clinical advantage to stenting had disappeared; despite the stented group having been followed for a shorter period of time (stent group: median 15, range 2–62 months; angioplasty only group: median 27, range 2–102, months). Patients undergoing intervention for occlusive lesions had a poorer clinical outcome. Thus, in the angioplasty only group, 36% of patients with a treated occlusion reported a deterioration in their walking distance at last follow-up compared with only 18% in those with a treated stenosis. In the stent group, the difference was even more marked, the figures being 31% and 8% respectively reporting a deterioration. There was no significant difference in outcome between common and external iliac procedures although the numbers in each subgroup are small and the possibility of a type II error cannot be excluded.

Bilateral 'kissing' stents

Bilateral iliac stents which oppose in the distal aorta, so-called 'kissing' stents, have been deployed in 15 claudicants. The procedure was initially clinically successful in 14 patients, and failed in one patient who underwent an aortobifemoral graft during the same admission. Technical problems occurred in an additional four patients with one patient requiring surgical repair of a false aneurysm and a further patient undergoing successful endovascular treatment for popliteal and anterior tibial embolus. Twelve patients reported an initial improvement in their claudication distance. Fourteen patients have been followed up for a median of 15 (range 3–58) months, and to date five patients have occluded stents, three bilaterally. Stents occluded at 3,5,13,29 and 30 months post-insertion. Two patients have undergone, and a further patient is due to undergo, aortobifemoral grafting.

Comment

Although flawed by lack of randomization and the absence of predetermined indications for stent placement, these prospectively gathered data comparing the clinical durability of iliac angioplasty and stenting for claudication do reflect the situation in the real world and may be similar to those experienced by workers in other vascular units. What they show is a dramatic increase in the use of iliac stents since their introduction in 1991 such that, in 1997, more claudicants underwent stent placement than PTA alone in the aortoiliac segment. It is important to emphasize that this introduction of stents was haphazard, uncontrolled and not based on any scientific data suggesting that this was the correct thing to do. Why then did it happen? Presumably, it was partly due to the novelty of the devices coming on the market as well as the intense marketing pressure exerted on vascular surgeons and interventional radiologists by the manufacturers. However, it may also represent our response to the disappointing clinical results obtained with regard to iliac angioplasty alone in the Edinburgh controlled trial. Unfortunately, despite the increased expense entailed, these data suggest that iliac stenting has little if any thing to offer over and above angioplasty in terms of durable relief of the symptoms of claudication. Indeed, what is remarkable about the data is how closely the clinical outcomes of our claudicants undergoing angioplasty and stent placement mirror those of claudicants which we have elected to treat conservatively, despite the fact that on balance those put forward for intervention have less extensive, more discrete lesions. Thus, it is hard to convince oneself that, with the exception of those patients who suffered major morbidity as a direct or indirect consequence of their procedure, either iliac PTA or stenting has impacted the natural history of claudicating patient in the medium term

FEMORAL ANGIOPLASTY

The Edinburgh experience with femoral angioplasty

The numbers of femoral PTAs performed, mirrors closely the numbers of iliac interventions (Fig. 2) Since 1989, 238 primary femoral angioplasties for claudication have been performed, of which the majority (193, 81%) were performed for stenotic lesions. When compared with iliac interventions, patients undergoing femoral angioplasty for IC were more likely to be male and to be older (Table 3). There was no significant difference with respect to immediate technical and clinical failure rates or major morbidity. At 6-week follow-up improvement in claudication distance was reported by 76% of patients but at a median follow-up of 26 (range 2–110) months, only 60% said their symptoms were better than they were prior to intervention.

It is difficult to compare these data with those published in the literature as many previous studies have either combined femoral, iliac and popliteal lesions; or have included patients with IC, SCLI and CLI. However, Stanley and colleagues[33] have

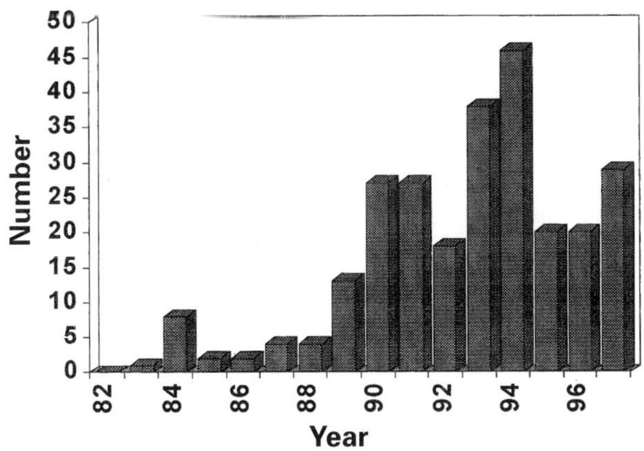

Fig. 2. Number of femoral PTA (n=259) performed each year in patients with claudication

Table 3. Characteristics and clinical outcome of patients undergoing femoral angioplasty

1989–1997	*Claudication n=238*	*Subcritical Ischaemia n=124*	*Critical ischaemia n=90*
Male:female ratio	3:1	1.1:1	1:1
Median age (range)	64 [39–83]	71 [37–94]	71 [40–92]
Clinical failure rate	27 (11%)	13 (10%)	18 (20%)
Technical failure rate	16 (7%)	9 (7%)	8 (9%)
Major morbidity	14 (6%)	6 (5%)	2 (2%)
Mortality (30 day)	0	0	2 (2%)
Symptomatic outcome at 6 weeks			
Improved / no change / worse	76% / 12% / 12%	67% / 23% / 10%[a]	NA
Symptomatic outcome at last follow-up			
Improved / no change / worse	60% / 20% / 20%	44% / 11% / 44%[a]	NA

NA: not available at present. [a]Excludes those who have required surgical revascularization or amputation.

reported a roughly comparable but retrospective study of 176 patients who underwent angioplasty of the superficial femoral or popliteal artery for claudication (74%) or critical ischaemia (26%). The overall cumulative patency rate at 12 months was 46% and the limb salvage rate was 95%. Due to the high initial failure rate and poor patency, the authors recommended that angioplasty should not be used to treat claudication.

Comment

Many, if not all, of the conclusions drawn above with respect to the durability of iliac interventions are equally applicable to femoral angioplasty. Thus, the morbidity and immediate failure rate are similar and the clinical outcome in terms of durable symptom-relief almost identical. There appears to be no evidence, therefore, that iliac interventions are inherently more successful than femoral angioplasties, despite the fact that iliac patency rates in anatomic and haemodynamic terms are generally accepted to be superior. The observation in Edinburgh that apparently successful iliac stenting is associated with about the same outcome, as far as the patient is concerned, as angioplasty of the superficial femoral artery again suggests that these interventions may have little or no effect on the natural history of IC in the medium and long term in the majority of patients.

SEVERE LIMB ISCHAEMIA

Definitions

There are two possible reasons why certain groups of surgeons and interventional radiologists believe angioplasty to be the first-line treatment of all patients with severe limb ischaemia, while others report disappointing results and advocate femorodistal bypass if technically possible.[34–44] First, the former have superior endovascular technique and expertise. Second, and perhaps more likely, the two groups are comparing 'apples and pears'. This, while subintimal angioplasty may represent a significant advance in the management of lower limb ischaemia, to date only a minority of interventional radiologists appear to have mastered the technique. What is certain, however, is that a better means of stratifying patients with severe limb ischaemia (SLI) is required so that like can be compared with like for the purposes of future controlled trials. Wolfe and Wyatt[5] have done a great service to this area by highlighting the important differences in outcome between subcritical and critical limb ischaemia.

Critical limb ischaemia

As defined by the Second European Consensus document[6] CLI comprises either 1) persistent recurring rest ischaemic rest pain requiring strong (opiate) analgesia for more than 2 weeks and an ankle systolic blood pressure of <50mmHg; or 2) ulceration or gangrene of the foot or toes and an ankle systolic blood pressure of <50mmHg. In such patients, the implication is that, without urgent revascularization either by surgery or endovascular therapy, the limb will be lost and/or the patient die.

Subcritical limb ischaemia

Can be defined as the presence of rest pain without tissue loss and an ankle systolic blood pressure which is frequently greater than 50mmHg. Such patients are on the borderline between severe claudication and full-blown CLI and are frequently encountered in vascular clinics. It is a common observation that such patients may respond to best medical therapy comprising risk factor modification and/or heparinization, and can be tipped back towards claudication. Indeed, limb salvage rates as high as 64% at 12 months following conservative management have frequently been reported.[5]

Effect of strategy on outcome of percutaneous transluminal angioplasty for severe limb ischaemia

If a vascular unit's management strategy for severe limb ischaemia includes a low threshold for performing PTA in patients with SCLI then, as the natural history of the condition is relatively benign and more akin to the claudicant population, they are likely to be able to report excellent limb salvage rates following their interventions. By contrast, if unit strategy is to treat SCLI medically and to only intervene surgically or by endovascular means when conservative treatment has clearly failed, then the results of PTA in that situation are likely to be less impressive. Similarly if that unit's strategy for CLI is femorodistal bypass where possible, reserving endovascular therapy for those who are 'non-reconstructable', then the results of angioplasty are likely to be disappointing. Unfortunately, at the present time, there are no controlled data to help the clinician decide whether angioplasty or femoro-bypass surgery is the most clinical and cost-effective means of treating patients with SCLI and CLI.

As surgery and angioplasty should be viewed as complementary not competing modalities the question then becomes one of strategy – which modality does one attempt first ? Although a well constructed vein bypass with good run-in, run-off and conduit is likely to have a better anatomic patency than angioplasty, given the limited life expectancy of these patients and the imperfect relationship between anatomic patency and limb loss, by performing femorodistal bypass one might be 'buying' additional years of the patency the patient simply does not require; and at the cost of increased morbidity and mortality when compared with PTA. By contrast, angioplasty while being associated with poorer anatomic patency may buy time for the patient until death from other causes, repeat angioplasty or until collaterals develop; and all this at potentially a fraction of the cost, morbidity and mortality of surgery. It is against this background that any consideration of the durability of angioplasty in the management of severe limb ischaemia must be considered.

Randomized controlled trials

To date, there have been no randomized control trials which have specifically compared angioplasty with surgery in patients with severe limb ischaemia. The Veterans Administration (VA) trial randomized 255 male patients to either surgery or angioplasty.[7] Unfortunately aortoiliac and infrainguinal disease were not analysed separately and 75% of the procedures were performed for claudication. Holm and colleagues,[8] randomized 102 patients with predominantly IC or SCLI to either angioplasty or surgery. There were no differences in outcome at 1-year follow-up, but again patients with iliac and infrainguinal disease were not analysed separately.

The Health Technology Assessment arm of the UK National Health Service has recently funded a multicentre randomized controlled trial to compare the clinical cost-effectiveness of a 'surgery first' with an 'angioplasty first' strategy in the management of severe limb ischaemia. The trial will be conducted in centres throughout Scotland and the north of England and the administration will be based at the Vascular Surgery Unit, Edinburgh University. Patients who could be treated by either angioplasty or surgery will be randomized to either angioplasty first or surgery first (Fig. 3). Patients with significant aortoiliac disease will be excluded unless inflow can be corrected, and randomization will be stratified to separate SCLI from CLI. As well as the primary clinical end-points (death, limb loss) there will be a quality of life and health economic assessment of the two modalities. The trial will run for 5 years and will hopefully answer some of the difficult questions outlined above with regard to the durability of each strategy. Readers wishing further information should contact the senior author

The Edinburgh experience with interventions for severe limb ischaemia

General trends

The difficulties in obtaining credible data on the durability of iliac and femoral PTA ± stenting in the management of severe limb ischaemia without the confines of a well

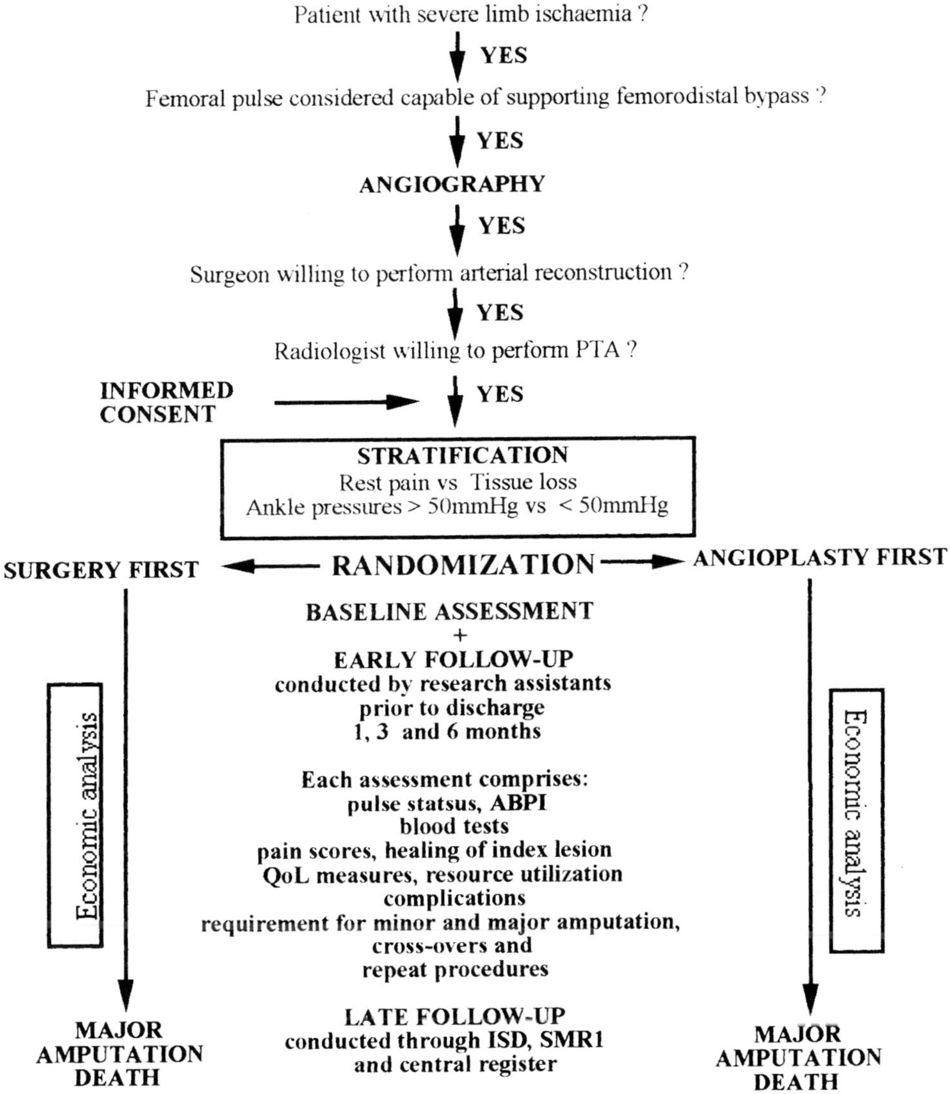

Fig. 3. Outline of multicentre randomized controlled trial to compare a 'surgery first' versus 'angioplasty first' strategy in the management of severe limb ischaemia.

constructed and funded randomized controlled trial are amply demonstrated by our own attempts to analyse the data from this unit. Disappointingly, despite the existence of a dedicated follow-up clinic and a member of medical staff to run it, as well as the prospective gathering of information into a computerized data base, the heterogeneous nature of the severe limb ischaemia patient group together with their high levels of co-morbidity leading to non-attendance at clinic, but high rates of admission to other services, means few firm conclusions can be drawn about the

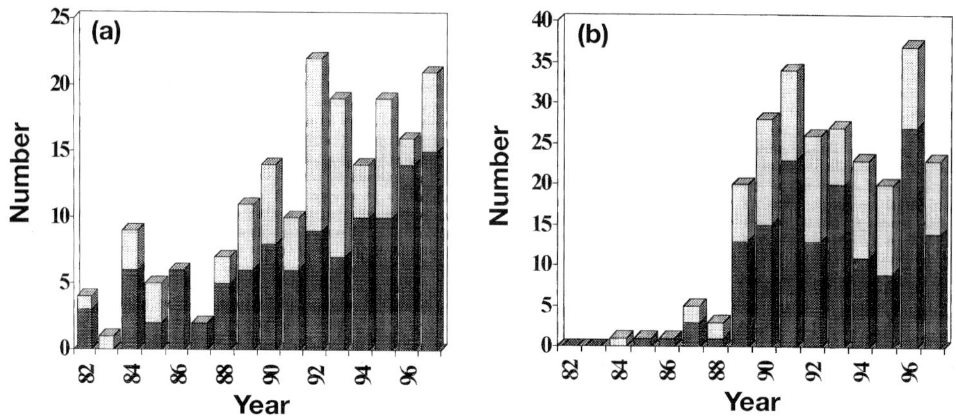

Fig. 4. Number of iliac (a) and femoral (b) PTA performed each year for critical (light areas) and subcritical (dark areas) ischaemia.

indication for endovascular therapy and its durability. However, as with the claudicant group, there have been some interesting changes in activity and practice over the last 15 years; reliable data on immediate outcomes and morbidity are also available. Thus, prior to 1989, although the overall number of interventions for SCLI and CLI was small, most were performed in the aortoiliac segment. Since then there has been a dramatic increase in the numbers performed, particularly at the femoropopliteal level. Overall, angioplasties for SCLI exceed those for CLI (Fig. 4).

Femoral angioplasty

Between 1989 and 1997, femoral angioplasties were performed for SCLI and CLI in 124 and 90 patients respectively (Table 3).

Subcritical limb ischaemia

In the SCLI group, there was a technical and immediate clinical failure rate of 7% and 10% respectively, and a major morbidity of 5%. Failure of the procedure to improve rest pain lead to early surgical revascularization in only three (2%) patients. Furthermore, major amputation was performed in only three (2%) patients during the same admission. At first clinic follow-up, 67% were improved, 23% reported no change and 10% said they were worse. The median follow-up in the patients who did not undergo post-procedure revascularization or amputation was a median of 9 (range 1–83) months, with 58% of patients being followed up for 6 months and 41% for more than a year. In those patients followed up for more than 6 months, 44% of patients reported an improvement in their symptoms, 11% no change and 44% a deterioration. However, within a year of angioplasty 15% of the patients underwent amputation, of which 59% were located below and 18% above knee. Further revascularization surgery was performed in 4% of patients.

Table 4. Iliac angioplasty for critical and subcritical ischaemia: Patient characteristics and immediate outcome

1989–1997	*Subcritical ischaemia n=79*	*Critical ischaemia n=60*
Male:female ratio	1.6:1	1.28:1
Median age (range)	67 (38–85)	68 (47–89)
Immediate clinical failure rate	8 (10%)	9 (15%)
Technical failure rate	4 (5%)	4 (7%)
Salvage revascularization	3 (4%)	3 (5%)
Major morbidity	7 (9%)	3 (5%)
Mortality (30 day)	1 (1.3%)	1 (2%)
Symptomatic outcome at 6 weeks[a]		
Improved/no change/worse	69% / 22% / 9%[a]	NA
Symptomatic outcome at last follow-up[a]		
Improved/no change/worse	45% / 21% / 34%[a]	NA

NA: not available at present. [a]Excludes those who have required surgical revascularization or amputation.

These data confirm the relatively benign nature of SCLI and suggest that, at least in the short term, angioplasty can relieve rest pain in a significant proportion of patients. However, as in claudication, the medium-term results are less impressive. As only a minority of patients with recurrent of rest pain refractory to conservative management had a pattern of disease that was amenable to repeat angioplasty and required either amputation or surgical revascularization, one must address the question of whether at least a proportion of these patients would have been better served by surgery in the first instance.

Critical limb ischaemia

The technical and immediate clinical failure rates were high at 9% and 20% respectively. However, the major morbidity and 30-day mortality rate were both low at 2%. Although surgical revascularization was performed in only two (2%), minor and major amputations were performed during the same admission in 28% and 10% of patients respectively. This probably reflects the fact that most of these patients had been considered for PTA because they were considered surgically 'unreconstructable'. During follow-up, amputations were performed in a further 17% of patients – of which 79% were major. Further information on the outcome of this patient cohort is being sought.

Iliac angioplasty

Since 1989, 79 patients have undergone iliac angioplasty for SCLI and 60 for CLI.

Subcritical limb ischaemia

Overall, 23% of iliac angioplasties in patients with SCLI were performed to provide inflow for planned distal bypass (n = 12) or femorofemoral cross-over grafts (n = 6).

All bar one were performed for stenotic lesions. Initial outcome, morbidity and salvage revascularization rates are shown in Table 4. At 4-week follow-up, 69% patients said their rest pain had improved and only 9% felt it was worse. Excluding those patients who underwent either planned or unplanned surgery subsequent to their angioplasty, the medium follow-up is 8 months, with 69% of patients being followed up for more than 6 months and 38% for more than 12 months. In those patients followed up for 6 months or longer, 45% reported an improvement in their symptoms but 34% said they had suffered a deterioration. No amputations were performed within 30 days of the procedure. During follow-up, major leg amputation was required in only three patients (5%), two patients underwent aortobifemoral grafting, one patient a femoral-popliteal bypass and there were four deaths.

Critical limb ischaemia

The patient characteristics were similar to those with SCLI (Table 4). The technical and clinical failure rates were slightly higher, and occlusive lesions accounted for 10% of the total. Planned revascularizations were performed in 17 (29%) patients. Distal amputations were performed in 11 (19%) patients within 30 days of the procedure.

Comment

It is difficult to ascertain the indications for angioplasty in this group of patients as such a high proportion of the procedures were combined with surgery, or performed to allow healing of a distal amputation site. Follow-up in remaining patients is incomplete, and only 5% underwent later revascularization in our unit, suggesting that these patients had significant morbidity or no surgically correctable disease. The end-points in these patients are amputation and death, and it is unclear what role angioplasty may have in delaying either.

SUMMARY

Intermittent claudication

Current data suggest that:

1. Angioplasty does not provide a more durable relief of symptoms than best medical therapy, although it is possible that a proportion of patients will derive a short-term (6/12) improvement in walking distance.
2. Angioplasty does not reduce the excess cardiovascular mortality. Suggestions that successful angioplasty will allow the patient to walk further and that this, in turn, may improve the cardiac prognosis are purely speculative.
3. Angioplasty may not be inherently more successful at the iliac segment. Although it is likely that haemodynamic and anatomic patency rates are better than in the femoral segments, this may not be associated with a more durable relief of symptoms.
4. Femoral stenting is not durable.

5. Selective iliac stenting may improve haemodynamic patency and clinical outcome when compared with angioplasty alone. However, at present, data are conflicting and the precise indications for stent placement have not been adequately defined.
6. With present technology and techniques, 'kissing' stents appear to have a high occlusion rate and should be used with caution in claudicants, especially as acute occlusion of such stents seems to lead frequently to the requirement for aortoiliac reconstruction.
7. Angioplasty and stenting are associated with a significant incidence of major morbidity (5–10%) although mortality appears to be rare.

Subcritical limb ischaemia

Current data suggest that:

1. Iliac angioplasty ± stenting can be achieved with a morbidity, clinical and technical failure rate similar to that obtained in patients with claudication.
2. Iliac angioplasty ± stenting has a useful role in providing inflow for bypass procedures.
3. Iliac and femoral interventions appear to relieve rest pain and reduce the requirement for major limb amputation and bypass surgery in the medium term in a significant proportion of patients. However, as in claudication, medium-term durability is questionable. Furthermore, as discussed above, it is possible that many patients with SCLI would have had an equally satisfactory outcome with 'best medical therapy' only in the first instance.

Critical limb ischaemia

In our own patients with CLI the clinical failure rate and amputation following angioplasty was high. Similarly disappointing results have been reported by other workers who have employed endovascular therapy in patients with true CLI, especially where there is tissue loss as well as rest pain. Although, in many of these patients angioplasty may have been the only treatment option, the question that must be addressed is whether at least a proportion of such patients would have been better served by primary amputation.

CONCLUSIONS

As is the case with most reviews of interventional techniques whether they be vascular or endovascular, the 'take-home' message is that the procedure will almost certainly work well in some patients and almost certainly fail in others. Although, to an extent, common sense and clinical experience will allow the clinician to decide which category their particular patient is in, it is undoubtedly the case that without further controlled trials many fundamental questions pertinent to everyday practice regarding the durability of iliac and femoral angioplasty remain unanswered and currently unanswerable.

REFERENCES

1. Bradbury AW, Ruckley CVR: Angioplasty for lower limb ischaemia: time for randomised controlled trials. *Lancet* **347**: 277–228,1996
2. Bolia A, Sayers RD, Thompson MM, Bell PRF: Subintimal and intraluminal recanalisation of occluded crural arteries by percutaneous balloon angioplasty. *Eur J Vasc Surg* **8**: 214–219, 1994
3. Hunink MGM, Meyerovitz MF: Infra-inguinal percutaneous transluminal angioplasty. *Advances in Vascular Surgery* Vol 2 pp.135–159. St Louis: Mosby-Year Book Inc, 1994
4. Robers C, Torgerson D. Randomisation methods in controlled trials. *Br Med J* **317**:1301, 1998
5. Wolfe JHN, Wyatt MG: Critical and sub-critical limb ischaemia. *Eur J Vasc Endovasc Surg* **13**: 578–582,1997
6. Second European Consensus Document on Critical Limb Ischaemia: *Eur J Vasc Surg* **6** (Suppl A): 1–32, 1992
7. Wolf GL, Wilson SE, Cross AP: Percutaneous transluminal angioplasty versus operation for peripheral arteriosclerosis. *J Vasc Surg* **9**: 1–9, 1989
8. Holm J, Arfridsson B: Chronic lower limb ischaemia. A prospective randomised controlled trial comparing the 1-year results of vascular surgery and percutanous transluminal angioplasty (PTA). *Eur J Vasc Surg* **5**: 517–522, 1991
9. Vroegindeweji D, Vos LD, Tielbeek AV *et al.*: Balloon angioplasty combined with primary stenting versus balloon angioplasty alone in femoropopliteal obstructions: A comparative randomized study. *Cardiovasc Intervent Radiol* **20**: 420–425, 1997
10. Gray BH, Olin JW: Limitations of percutaneous transluminal angioplasty with stenting for femoropopliteal arterial occlusive disease. *Semin Vasc Surg* **10**: 8–16, 1997
11. Fowkes FGR, Housely E, Cawood EH *et al.*: Edinburgh artery study: prevalence of asymptomatic and symptomatic peripheral arterial disease in the general population. *Int J Epidemiol* **20**: 384–392, 1991
12. McDermott MM, McCarthy W: Intermittent claudication. The natural history: *Surg Clin N Am* **75**: 581–591, 1995
13. Regensteiner JG: Exercise in the treatment of claudication: assessment and treatment of functional impairment. *Vasc Med* **2**: 238–242, 1997
14. Brandsma JW, Robeer BG, van den Heuvel S *et al.*: The effect of exercises on walking distance of patients with intermittent claudication:a study of randomised clinical trials. *Phys Ther* **78**: 278–286, 1998.
15. Robeer GG, Brandsma JW, van den Heuvel SP *et al.*: Exercise therapy for intermittent claudication: a review of the quality of randomised clinical trials and evaluation of predictive factors. *Eur J Vasc Endovasc Surg* **15**: 36–43, 1998
16. Antiplatelet Trialist Collaboration: Secondary prevention of vascular disease by prolonged antiplatelet treatment. *Br Med J* **296**: 320–331, 1998
17. Pederson TR, Kjekshus J, PyoralaK *et al.*: Effect of simvastatin on ischemic signs and symptoms in the Scandinavian Simvastatin Survival Study (4S). *Am J Cardiol* **81**: 333–335, 1998
18. Whyman MR, Fowkes FGR, Kerracher EMG *et al.*: Is intermittent claudication improved by percutaneous transluminal angioplasty ? A randomised controlled trial. *J Vasc Surg* **26**: 551–557, 1997
19. Creasy TS, McMillan PJ, Fletcher EW *et al.*: Is percutaneous transluminal angioplasty better than exercise for claudication? Preliminary results from a prospective randomised trial. *Eur J Vasc Surg* **4**: 135–140, 1990
20. Perkins JM, Collin J, Creasy TS *et al.*: Exercise training versus angioplasty for stable claudication. Long and medium term results of a prospective, randomised trial: *Eur J Vasc Endovasc Surg* **11**: 409–413, 1996
21. Bosch JL, Hunink MG: Meta-analysis of the results of percutaneous transluminal angioplasty and stent placement for aortoiliac occlusive disease. *Radiology* **204**: 87–96, 1997
22. Jeans WD, Cole SE, Horrocks M *et al.*: Angioplasty gives good results in critical limb

ischaemia. A 5-year follow-up in patients with known ankle pressure and diabetic status having femoropoplteal dilatations. *Br J Radiol* **67**: 123–128, 1994
23. Jorgensen B, Skovgaard N, Norgard J *et al.*: Percutaneous transluminal angioplasty in 226 iliac artery stenoses: role of the superficial femoral artery for clinical success. *VASA* **21**: 382–386, 1992
24. Stokes KR, Strunk HM, Campbell DR *et al.*: Five-year results of iliac and femoropopliteal angioplasty in diabetic patients. *Radiology* **174**: 977–982, 1990
25. Tegtmeyer CJ, Hartwell GD, Selby JB *et al.*: Results and complications of angioplasty in aortoiliac disease. *Circulation* **83**: 153–160, 1991
26. Henry M, Amor M, Ethevenot G *et al.*: Palmaz stent replacement in iliac and femoropopliteal arteries: primary and secondary patency in 310 patients with 2–4-year follow-up. *Radiology* **197**: 167–174, 1995
27. Long AL, Sapoval MR, Beyssen BM *et al.*: Strecker stent implantation in iliac arteries: patency and predictive factors for long-term success. *Radiology* **194**: 739–744, 1995
28. Martin EC, Katzen BT, Benenati JF *et al.*: Multicentre trial of the wallstent in the iliac and femoral arteries. *J Vasc Intervent Radiol* **6**: 841–842, 1995
29. Strecker EP, Hagen B, Liermann D *et al.*: Iliac and femoropopliteal vascular occlusive disease treated with flexible tantalum stents: *Cardiovasc Intervent Radiol* **16**: 158–164, 1993
30. Vorwerk D, Gunther RW, Schurman K *et al.*: Aortic and iliac stenoses: follow-up results of stent replacement after insufficient balloon angioplasty in 118 cases. *Radiology* **198**: 45–48, 1996
31. Richter GM, Roeren T, Noeldge G *et al.*: Initial long-term results of a randomized 5-year study: iliac stent implantation versus PTA. *VASA* (Suppl) **35**: 192–193, 1992
32. Tetteroo E, van der Graaf Y, Bosch JL *et al.*: Randomised comparison of primary stent placement versus primary angioplasty followed by selective stent placement in patients with iliac-artery occlusive disease. Dutch Iliac Stent Trial Study Group. *Lancet* **351**: 1153–1159, 1998
33. Stanley B, Teague B, Raptis S *et al.*: Efficacy of balloon angioplasty of the superficial femoral artery and popliteal artery in the relief of leg ischaemia. *J Vasc Surg* **23**: 679–685, 1996
34. Nydahl S, Hartshorne T, Bell P *et al.*: Subintimal angioplasty of infrapopliteal occlusions in critically ischaemic limbs. *Eur J Vasc Endovasc Surg* **14**: 212–216, 1997
35. Ray SA, Minty I, Buckenham TM *et al.*: Clinical outcome and restenosis following percutaneous transluminal angioplasty for ischaemic rest pain or ulceration. *Br J Surg* **82**: 1217–1221, 1995
36. London NJM, Srinivasan R, Naylor AR *et al.*: Sub-intimal angioplasty of femoropopliteal artery occlusions: the long-term results. *Eur J Vasc Surg* **8**: 148–155, 1994
37. Buckenham TM, Loh A, Dormandy JA *et al.*: Infrapopliteal angioplasty for limb salvage. *Eur J Vasc Surg* **7**: 21–25, 1993
38. Currie IC, Wakely CJ, Cole SEA, *et al.*: Femorpopliteal angioplasty for severe limb ischaemia. *Br J Surg* **81**: 191–193, 1994
39. Cooper JC , Welsh CL: The role of percutaneous transluminal angioplasty in the treatment of critical limb ischaemia. *Eur J Vasc Surg* **5**: 261–264, 1991
40. Blair JM, Gewertz BL, Moosa H *et al.*: Percutaneous transluminal angioplasty versus surgery for limb-threatening ischaemia. *J Vasc Surg* **9**: 698–703, 1989
41. Varty K, Nydahl S, Butterworth P *et al.*: Changes in the management of critical limb ischaemia. *Br J Surg* **83**: 953–956, 1996
42. Varty K, Nydahl S, Bolia A *et al.*: Surgery or angioplasty for critical limb ischaemia. *Br J Surg* **84** (Suppl 1):1 (abstract 0) 1997
43. Sivanathan UM, Browne TF, Thorley PJ *et al.*: Percutaneous transluminal angioplasty of tibial arteries. *Br J Surg* **81**: 1282–1285, 1994
44. London NJM, Varty K, Sayers RD *et al.*: Percutaneous transluminal angioplasty for lower-limb critical limb ischaemia. *Br J Surg* **82**: 1232–1235, 1995

Commentary

In this chapter the randomized trials are described and the Edinburgh experience with iliac and femoral angioplasty is described. The authors have summarized the current data for intermittent claudication and subcritical and critical ischaemia very carefully. For intermittent claudication, even the iliac segment has a question mark for angioplasty and femoral stenting is described as 'not durable'. The 'kissing' stent technique is given short shrift and the authors state that angioplasty and stenting are associated with significant incidence of major morbidity.

The authors are positive of the value of iliac angioplasty to provide a better inflow for downstream bypass procedures for subcritical ischaemia and they state that iliac and femoral interventions relieve rest pain and reduce the need for amputation and bypass surgery. However, they seem disappointed with the results of angioplasty for critical ischaemia. *RMG*

The value of the ankle brachial pressure index in predicting the durability of femoropopliteal angioplasty

Jonathan Golledge, Karen Ferguson, Mary Ellis, Tarun Sabharwal, Alun H Davies, Roger M Greenhalgh and Janet T Powell

INTRODUCTION

The indications for femoropopliteal angioplasty are controversial.[1,2] Angioplasty is commonly used to treat intermittent claudication, although randomized comparisons with supervised exercise have shown equivalent results.[1,2] Endovascular therapies may be attractive in patients with critical ischaemia since they often have many other medical problems; however, these patients usually have poor infrageniculate vessels and therefore can expect a less durable result.[3]

Irrespective of the indications for angioplasty a durable outcome is desirable. Outcome is better for patients with claudication rather than critical ischaemia,[3] short rather than long stenoses or occlusions,[4] and good runoff.[5] Assessment of the technical adequacy of angioplasty has only recently come to attention. A number of methods are used, including palpation of pulses, measurement of ankle pressure, completion angiogram, colour duplex and intravascular ultrasound.[6–8] The relative value of these is the subject of this chapter. However, prior to concentrating on this area the causes of angioplasty failure and methods of outcome assessment are discussed, since it is only by an appreciation of these that the results of femoropopliteal angioplasty can be understood.

CAUSES OF FAILURE OF ANGIOPLASTY

Failure to cross the stenosis or occlusion, complications requiring abandonment of the procedure, immediate occlusion or failure to achieve adequate dilatation of the stenosis or occlusion lead to technical failure in 5–25% of patients depending on lesions treated.[4,9] Early thrombosis of the angioplasty site in the first few days has been demonstrated in up to 8% of patients.[10] Failure between 1 and 12 months following angioplasty is usually attributed to restenosis of the angioplasty site. All patients develop some reduction of lumen diameter compared with the post-angioplasty dimension. However, it is only when such narrowing becomes flow limiting that restenosis is significant. A 50% or greater reduction in lumen diameter occurs in 30–50% of patients.[11,12] Failure during this intermediate time may also result from the presence of flow limiting lesions which were wrongly felt to be not significant or inappropriate to treat, e.g. as they required distal bypass in patients with claudication only. Later failure is a result of progression of the underlying atherosclerotic disease. The latter two causes of failure have to date received relatively little attention and appear to have been underrated.

OUTCOME MEASURES IN FEMOROPOPLITEAL ANGIOPLASTY

The outcome of angioplasty has been assessed by patients' symptoms, palpation of pulses, measurement of ankle pressure, and imaging of the angioplasty site using angiography or duplex.[13] Outcome results differ depending which measurement is used.[14] Recently attempts have been made to give a more comprehensive assessment of symptomatic outcome using quality of life methods, but as yet no specific questionnaire exists for peripheral vascular disease.[15] Measurement of the ankle pressure has been used to assess the haemodynamic outcome. An improvement of 0.1–0.15 in the ankle brachial pressure index (ABPI) compared with pre-angioplasty value has been usually required for haemodynamic success to be recorded.[13,16] The Society for Vascular Surgery has suggested guidelines for reporting outcome of angioplasty based on symptomatic and haemodynamic outcome.[13] Changes in the lower limb are graded on a scale of 7, from +3 to -3. A grade of +3 indicates marked improvement in symptoms and an ABPI>0.9. Grade +2 indicates a moderate improvement in symptoms and an improvement in ABPI of >0.1. Grade +1 implies a small improvement in symptoms without significant improvement in ABPI. Grade 0 indicates no change, while -1 to -3 indicate graded deterioration in symptoms. However, since symptomatic and haemodynamic outcome may differ this is difficult to implement in all cases. Information on the angioplasty site itself and thus the restenosis rate can only be provided from duplex or angiography, although the development of magnetic resonance and computerized tomographic angiography may provide alternative techniques.

INITIAL ASSESSMENT OF ANGIOPLASTY

Immediate assessment of the technical adequacy of angioplasty has the potential role of identifying patients requiring further balloon dilatation, alternative endoluminal or operative procedures to achieve optimum outcome. Although, to date no quality control technique has been shown to improve outcome. Traditionally the technical adequacy of angioplasty has been measured by the completion angiogram, a technically successful procedure being defined as a residual stenosis of less than 30%.[13] Palpation of pulses provides a very simple assessment of technical success, but this is a rather subjective measure. Measurement of the ABPI provides an equally simple assessment of outcome which is more objective. The cuff pressure required to occlude flow in the pedal arteries is compared with the brachial pressure. This has been shown to be a reproducible test with 95% confidence intervals of around 0.15.[17] This test has long been used in the assessment of patients presenting with lower limb ischaemia but the value of ABPI in outcome assessment has been questioned in some areas. For example ABPI has a sensitivity and specificity of only around 70% in detecting vein graft stenoses, much lower than that of colour duplex.[18] However, ankle pressure does have the advantage over duplex in assessing the overall perfusion of the limb in contrast to techniques which image the angioplasty site only, and as such might be expected to give a better guide to symptomatic success.

CHARING CROSS SERIES

Patients and angioplasty

In order to illustrate the use of some of these initial outcome assessment methods a consecutive series of 74 patients undergoing femoropopliteal angioplasty at Charing Cross is discussed. Only patients with symptoms of persistent and incapacitating intermittent claudication (43), rest pain (4) and tissue loss (ulcer 24, gangrene 3), associated with single, short (<10 cm) stenoses or occlusions of the superficial femoral or popliteal artery were selected for the study. Following angioplasty a completion angiogram was performed and any residual narrowing measured. Colour duplex imaging of the angioplasty site and measurement of the ABPI were performed 24 hours after angioplasty. Follow-up, including assessment of symptoms, palpation of pulses, measurement of ABPI and duplex surveillance of the angioplasty site, was performed 3, 6, 9 and 12 months after angioplasty.

Outcome assessment

Outcome was assessed at 1 year separately in terms of symptoms, improvement in ankle pressure, and development of restenosis. Symptomatic success was defined as resolution of the presenting symptom at 1 year. Thus patients presenting with claudication had to be asymptomatic, while those with rest pain, ulceration or gangrene needed resolution of these conditions without major limb loss, repeat angioplasty or surgery to be considered successful. If patients died within 1 year of angioplasty without requiring intervention for symptoms they were excluded from the univariate analyses (n=5). Haemodynamic success was defined as maintenance of an improvement of ≥0.15 in ABPI after 1 year. If pre-angioplasty ABPI was 0.85-0.9 maintenance of an index of ≥1 was accepted as success. While, if a significant improvement in ABPI was achieved and the patient died during follow-up (n=1) or underwent further vascular intervention to the limb (n=1) the patient was excluded from univariate analyses. Restenosis was recorded when the velocity ratio through the angioplasty site V2/V1≥2.5.

Initial outcome of angioplasty (Fig. 1)

In 67 patients (91%) angioplasty was technically successful. In two patients (one presenting with claudication and one an ulcer) it was not possible to cross the occlusion with a guidewire (one later required an endarterectomy). Acute thrombosis at the angioplasty site occurred in two patients (both of these had presented with ulceration). Both patients were treated with intra-arterial thrombolysis unsuccessfully (see below). In three patients (one treated for rest pain

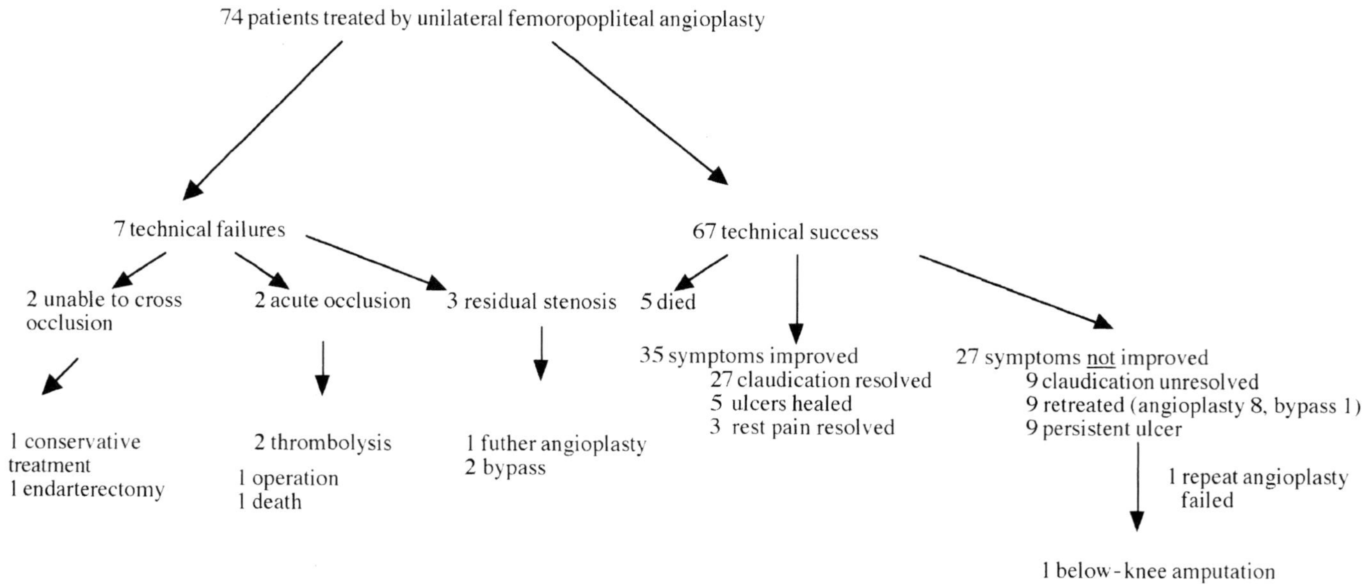

Fig. 1. Outcome of femoropopliteal angioplasty.

and two for claudication) completion angiograms demonstrated a residual stenosis of ≥50%. Two of these patients underwent bypass surgery and the third was treated by repeat angioplasty.

One of the patients receiving thrombolysis after angioplasty, developed haemorrhage from the femoral puncture site which required operative repair of the artery. Thrombolysis succeeded in clearing the angioplasty site thrombosis in the second patient. However, the treatment was complicated by small bowel infarction. This patient died 3 weeks after angioplasty. Five other patients developed a small groin haematoma, all of which resolved without intervention and did not require blood transfusion.

Outcome at 1 year

Five patients died during follow-up, two at 1 and three at 3 months (ankle pressure had not been improved by angioplasty in three of these patients). For 35 (51%) patients symptoms improved, while for 34 (49%) angioplasty failed to improve symptoms (Table 1, Fig. 1). Nine of the 43 patients presenting with intermittent claudication still had symptoms at 1 year, seven further patients presenting with claudication had required intervention (bypass two, endarterectomy one, repeat

Table 1. Characteristics of patients in relation to symptomatic outcome at 12 months following femoropopliteal angioplasty

	Improvement	*No improvement*	*p value*
Number	35	34	
Age	70 (50–86)	74.5 (58–87)	0.07
Male	21	20	0.92
Presenting complaint:			
intermittent claudication	27	16	0.04 (0.01)[a]
rest pain	3	1	
tissue loss (ulcer or gangrene)	5	17	
Haemodynamics and assessment of angioplasty:			
ABPI pre	0.65 (0.3–0.9)	0.57 (0.2–0.9)	0.18
ABPI post	1.0 (0.64–1.0)	0.83 (0.33–1.0)	0.008
Δ ABPI	0.26 (0–0.7)	0.2 (–0.3–0.6)	0.09
residual stenosis (angiography, %)	14 (0–30)	15.5 (0–100)	0.19
velocity ratio (day 1)	1.3 (0.6–7.1)	1.5 (0–3.5)	0.90
ABP1<0.8 at 1 day	5	14	0.01
ABPI<0.9 at 1 day	12	21	0.02
Δ ABPI<0.14	5 (33)	13 (32)	0.02
Δ ABPI<0.25	8 (28)	17 (27)	0.01

Improvement was defined as resolution of the presenting symptom at 1 year (see Methods). Technical failures (n=7) are included but five patients who died without adequate follow-up are excluded. Numbers in parentheses for change (Δ) in ABPI represent total in each group who could be classified: i.e. their pre-angioplasty ABPI did not preclude a positive result. Numbers for continuous variables are medians and range (in brackets). Values are compared with chi-squared (nominal variables) and Mann-Whitney U test (continous variables). [a]Chi-squared analysis for intermittent claudication or not as presenting symptom.

angioplasty four) for symptomatic restenosis (four) or technical failure (three), while for 27 patients claudication had resolved. Of the 24 patients presenting with ulceration, technical failure was reported for three (see above), three patients had died at 1 month and three at 2 months, four patients underwent repeat angioplasty for restenosis, in five patients the ulcer healed whilst nine patients had persistent ulceration. Of the four patients presenting with rest pain, bypass was performed in one (following technical failure), and the three remaining patients were asymptomatic at 1 year. Of the three patients presenting with gangrene, two died at 3 months and one developed restenosis, repeat angioplasty failed and this patient required a below-knee amputation.

Favourable haemodynamic outcome was achieved in 41 (58%) patients, while in 30 (42%) patients no improvement (n=26) or deterioration (n=4) in ankle pressure occurred (Table 2). Twenty of the 67 patients undergoing technically successful angioplasty later developed restenosis: eight within 3 months, nine further patients within 6 months, two at 9 months and two at 12 months. By life-table analysis the

Table 2. Characteristics of patients who had a good and poor haemodynamic outcome within 12 months of femoropopliteal angioplasty

	≥0.15	*No improvement*	*p value*
Number	41	30	
Age	68 (51–87)	75 (50–86)	0.01
Male	27	18	0.61
Presenting complaint:			
intermittent claudication	22	19	0.57 (0.42)[a]
rest pain	3	1	
tissue loss (ulcer or gangrene)	16	10	
Diabetes	7	12	0.03
Lesion:			
severity (%)	83 (50–100)	67 (50–100)	0.002
length (cm)	0.9 (0.1–10)	1.0 (0.1–10)	0.85
occlusion	15	4	0.03
Haemodynamics and assessment of angioplasty:			
ABPI pre	0.59 (0.3–0.9)	0.68 (0.27–0.9)	0.13
ABPI post	1.0 (0.64–1.0)	0.8 (0.33–1.0)	0.0002
Δ ABPI	0.29 (0.1–0.7)	0.12 (-0.3–0.37)	<0.0001
residual stenosis (angiography, %)	10 (0–40)	22.5 (0–100)	0.01
velocity ratio (day 1)	1.3 (0.6–7.1)	1.5 (0–3.5)	0.89
ABP1<0.8 at 1 day	4	17	<0.0001
ABPI<0.9 at 1 day	14	21	0.003
Δ ABPI<0.14	5 (41)	16 (27)	<0.0001
Δ ABPI<0.25	7 (35)	19 (22)	<0.0001

Technical failures (n=7) are included. Excluded were one patients who died at 3 months at which stage there was an improvement in ABPI, one patient who was operated on for a residual stenosis despite an improvement in ABPI and one patient who had a pre-angioplasty ABPI of 0.92 (see Methods). Numbers in parentheses for change (Δ) in ABPI represent total in each group who could be classified: i.e. their pre-angioplasty ABPI did not preclude a positive result. Numbers for continuous variables are medians and range (in brackets). Values are compared with chi-squared (nominal variables) and Mann-Whitney U test (continous variables). [a]Chi-squared analysis for intermittent claudication or not as presenting symptom.

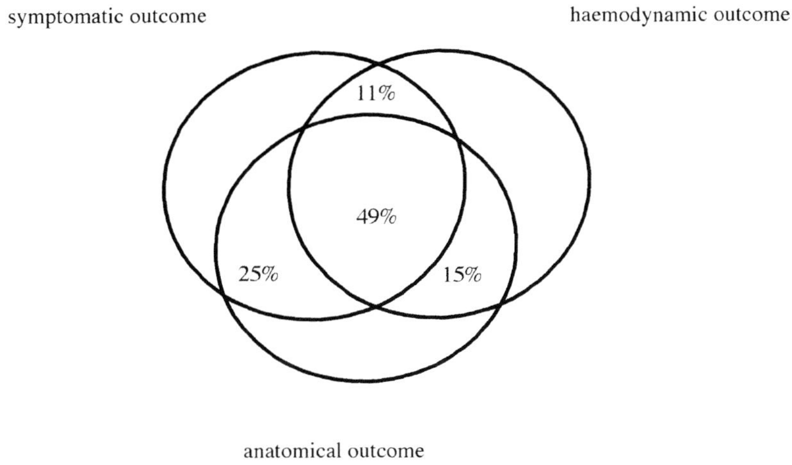

Fig. 2. Comparison of outcomes of femoropopliteal angioplasty assessed by symptomatic, haemodynamic and anatomical result.

restenosis rate at 6 months was 29% and 39% at 1 year. Seven of the patients developing restenosis underwent repeat angioplasty with technical success. However, one patient later required a below-knee amputation (see above) and one further patient underwent femoropopliteal bypass with relief of symptoms

While symptomatic, haemodynamic and anatomical results were clearly related, success by one criteria did not always predict success for the other two definitions. For the 61 patients in which outcome could be classified by all three definitions comparison of results is illustrated in Fig. 2. There was agreement in outcome by all three definitions for only 30 (49%).

Value of immediate post-angioplasty assessment in predicting outcome at 1 year

The residual stenosis measured on the completion angiogram was not predictive of symptomatic outcome or restenosis, but did suggest patients more likely to have haemodynamic failure at 1 year (Tables 1 and 2). Duplex of the angioplasty site at 24 hours was not helpful in predicting outcome by any criteria. The most powerful predictor of outcome at 1 year was the ABPI 24 hours after angioplasty (Tables 1 and 2). On stepwise multiple regression analysis the 24-hour ABPI was the only variable predicting symptomatic outcome, p=0.0004, haemodynamic outcome, p=0.002, and restenosis, p=0.003, at 1 year. A 24-hour ABPI of ≥0.9 had a sensitivity of 66%, a specificity of 62%, a positive predictive value of 64% and a negative predictive value of 64% in predicting symptomatic outcome at 1 year. The change in ABPI following angioplasty was also an important factor, an improvement in ABPI≥0.25 had a sensitivity of 80%, a specificity of 86%, a positive predictive value of 90% and a negative predictive value of 73% in predicting haemodynamic outcome at 12 months. The 24-hour ABPI was also predictive of restenosis. Life-table analysis demonstrated

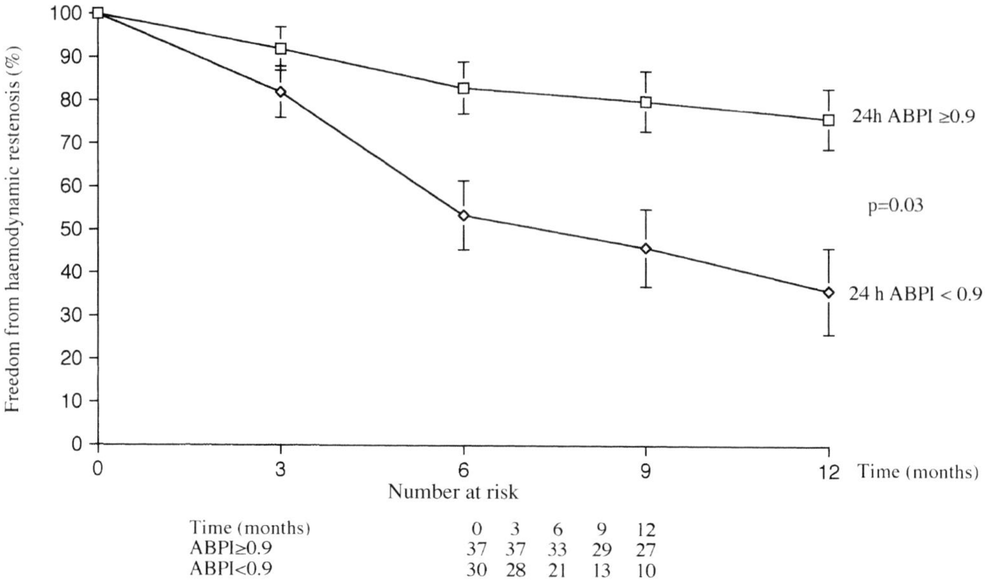

Fig. 3. Ankle brachial pressure index assessed at 24 hours following femoropopliteal angioplasty predicts development of restenosis. Freedom from haemodynamic restenosis is shown for patients with an ABPI≥0.9 (□) and an ABPI<0.9 (◇) at 24 hours. Vertical lines are error bars and numbers at risk are also shown.

that 24% of patients with a 24-hour ABPI≥0.9 compared with 64% of patients with a 24-hour ABPI<0.9 developed restenosis by 12 months, $p=0.03$ (Fig. 3).

Other factors determining outcome

Patients presenting with intermittent claudication rather than tissue loss or rest pain had more favourable symptomatic outcomes (Table 1). Haemodynamic outcome at 1 year was significantly worse in older patients, and patients with diabetes (Table 2). Patients with occlusions successfully treated by angioplasty did well even though the median lesion length was greater for occlusion, 2.0 (0.2–10) cm, than stenosis, 0.7 (0.1–10) cm, $p=0.0002$.

QUALITY CONTROL IN FEMOROPOPLITEAL ANGIOPLASTY

Having appropriately selected a patient for femoropopliteal angioplasty the next goal is to carry out optimal balloon dilatation. Most commonly the completion angiogram has been used as quality control. However, data from our study and others would suggest that the post-angioplasty angiogram is a poor guide to the late success of the procedure.[7,19] Duplex ultrasound has been used with mixed success, with some studies identifying patients likely to fail in the first year,[7,19] while other investigators have found no role for duplex as quality control.[20] Of the three tests of technical adequacy of angioplasty we assessed, only the ABPI at 24 hours proved a reliable predictor of outcome at 1 year (Tables 1 and 2, Fig. 3). Since angiography and duplex are recognized as being accurate means of assessing arterial disease this finding is surprising. Ankle pressure gives a guide to the overall peripheral perfusion, which is not available from visualizing the angioplasty site alone. Thus in addition to identifying patients in which a lesion has been inadequately dilated, the ankle pressure may also identify those in which another lesion is flow limiting. Recognition of such deficits at an early stage could alter patient management in order to improve outcome. The reduction of restenosis rate in patients with favourable post-angioplasty ankle pressure most likely relates to the known association between poor runoff and restenosis.[21]

Other techniques which have been used to assess the initial outcome of angioplasty include intravascular ultrasound (IVUS) and magnetic resonance angiography. Van der Lugt and colleagues assessed the value of IVUS in predicting outcome of 147 patients treated by femoropopliteal angioplasty.[8] Intravascular ultrasound findings were not useful in predicting symptomatic or haemodynamic outcome at 6 months; however, IVUS-measured area stenosis after angioplasty was predictive of restenosis at 6 months.

ACHIEVING OPTIMAL RESULTS IN FEMOROPOPLITEAL ANGIOPLASTY

At present, symptomatic and haemodynamic success at 1 year following femoropopliteal angioplasty would appear to be only around 50%, depending on

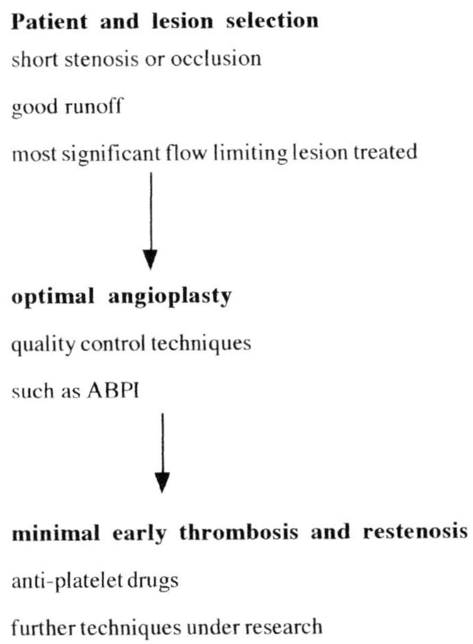

Fig. 4. Approaches to improve outcome of femoropopliteal angioplasty.

case mix.[12,16] Figure 4 suggests an algorithm for achieving optimal results. Our data suggests that the 24-hour ABPI, in contrast to more elaborate techniques such as duplex surveillance, predicts the outcome of femoropopliteal angioplasty at 12 months. Clearly, technical excellence in the performance of angioplasty does contribute to a higher ABPI and there is therefore a need to achieve an 'on table' measure at the time of angioplasty completion which correlates with 24-hour ABPI, and can thus be used to guide the balloon dilatation. However, the condition of the upstream and downstream arteries are also important determinants of the 24-hour ABPI, which is predictive of success at 12 months.

REFERENCES

1. Perkins JST, Collin J, Creasy TS *et al.*: Exercise training versus angioplasty for stable claudication . Long and medium term results of a prospective randomised trial. *Eur J Vasc Endovasc Surg* **11:** 409–413, 1996
2. Wyman MR, Fowkes FGR, Kerracher EMG *et al.*: Intermittent claudication is not improved by percutaneous transluminal angioplasty – A randomised controlled trial. *Br J Surg* **84:** 571, 1997
3. Capek P, Mclean GK, Berkowitz HD: Femoropopliteal angioplasty. Factors influencing long term results. *Circulation* **83:** 170–180, 1991
4. Matsi PJ, Manninen HI, Soder HK *et al.*: Percutaneous transluminal angioplasty in femoral artery occlusions: primary and long-term results in 107 claudicant patients using femoral and popliteal catheterisation techniques. *Clin Radiol* **50:** 237–244, 1995
5. Hunink MGM, Donaldson MC, Meyerovitz MF *et al.*: Risks and benefits of femoropopliteal percutaneous balloon angioplasty. *J Vasc Surg* **17:** 183–194, 1993
6. El-Bayer H, Roberts A, Hye R *et al.*: Determinants of failure in superficial femoral artery angioplasty. *Angiology* **43:** 877–885, 1992
7. Mewissen MW, Kinney EV, Bandyk DF *et al.*: The role of duplex scanning versus angiography in predicting outcome after balloon angioplasty in the femoropopliteal artery. *J Vasc Surg* **15:** 860–866, 1992
8. Van der Lugt A, Gussenhoven EJ, Pasterkamp G *et al.*: Intravascular ultrasound predictors of restenosis after balloon angioplasty of the femoropopliteal artery. *Eur J Vasc Endovasc Surg* **16:** 110–119, 1998
9. Johnston KW: Femoropopliteal arteries: reanalysis of results of balloon angioplasty. *Radiology* **183:** 767–771, 1992
10. Nyamekye I, Sommerville K, Raphael M *et al.*: Non-invasive assessment of arterial stenoses in angioplasty: A comparison with angiography. *Eur J Vasc Endovasc Surg* **12:** 471–481
11. Becquemin J-P, Cavillon A, Haiduc F: Surgical transluminal femoropopliteal angioplasty: Multivariate analysis outcome. *J Vasc Surg* **19:** 495–502, 1994
12. Tielbeek AV, Rietjens E, Buth J *et al.*: The value of duplex surveillance after endovascular intervention for femoropopliteal obstructive disease. *Eur J Vasc Endovasc Surg* **12:** 145–150, 1996
13. Rutherford RB, Becker GJ: Standards for evaluating and reporting the result of surgical and percutaneous therapy for peripheral vascular disease. *Radiology* **181:** 277–281, 1991
14. Matsi PJ, Manninen HI: Impact of different patency criteria on long term results of femoropopliteal angioplasty: Analysis of 106 consecutive patients with claudication. *JVIR* **6:** 159–163, 1995
15. Chetter IC, Spark JI, Dolan P *et al.*: Quality of life analysis in patients with lower limb ischaemia: Suggestions for European Standardisation. *Eur J Vasc Endovasc Surg* **13:** 597–604, 1997

16. Alback A, Biancari F, Schmidt S *et al.*: Haemodynamic results of femoropopliteal percutaneous transluminal angioplasty. *Eur J Vasc Endovasc Surg* **16:** 7–12, 1998
17. Fisher CM, Burnett A, Makeham V *et al.*: Variation in measurement of ankle-brachial pressure index in routine clinical practice. *J Vasc Surg* **24:** 871–875, 1996
18. Davies AH, Magee TR, Tennant SG *et al.*: Criteria for identification of the 'at-risk' infrainguinal bypass graft. *Eur J Vasc Endovasc Surg* **8:** 315–319, 1994
19. Spijkerboer AM, Nass PC, de Valois JC *et al.*: Evaluation of femoropopliteal arteries with duplex ultrasound after angioplasty. Can we predict results at one year? *Eur J Vasc Endovasc Surg* **12:** 418–423, 1996
20. Sacks D, Robinson ML, Marinelli DL, Perlmutter GS: Evaluation of the peripheral arteries with duplex US after angioplasty. *Radiology* **176:** 39–44, 1990
21. Maca T, Ahmadi R, Derfler K *et al.*: Elevated lipoprotein (a) and increased incidence of restenosis after femoropopliteal PTA. Rationale for the higher risk of recurrence in females? *Atherosclerosis* **127:** 27–34, 1996

Commentary

The importance of these data is that outcome of angioplasty at 12 months is predicted by 24-hour ankle brachial pressure index. The ABPI is an overall assessment of the arterial status of the ankle level. One of the factors which will lead to a high ABPI is a successful technical angioplasty. This is not the only factor. What really is required is a measure of the success of angioplasty at the time of the procedure which also predicts durability. To assess ABPI at the same time as angioplasty is of dubious value because sometimes it takes a period before the ABPI stabilizes. All in all, these data suggest that if an angioplasty is performed technically well, it is more likely to be durable. *RMG*

Is popliteal and tibial angioplasty effective for critical ischaemia?

Ken Callum, M Akhil Abdul-Hamid, Roddy Nash, David Hinwood and Mario DeNunzio

INTRODUCTION

The indications for below-knee angioplasty and the wisdom of such procedures were considered in *Indications in Vascular and Endovascular Surgery*.[1,2] Conclusions were that tibial angioplasty has lagged behind that in other vessels because of an erroneous perception that there is a high complication rate, that it is difficult to do a bypass after failed angioplasty and that the long-term results are poor. These reports are not necessarily correct. Case selection is paramount, but percutaneous transluminal angioplasty (PTA) can be used for short lesions in possibly around 10% of patients with critical ischaemia.[2] Alternatives are amputation, medical treatment or bypass surgery, which with a good vein and good runoff remains the gold standard, and yet may have troublesome complications.

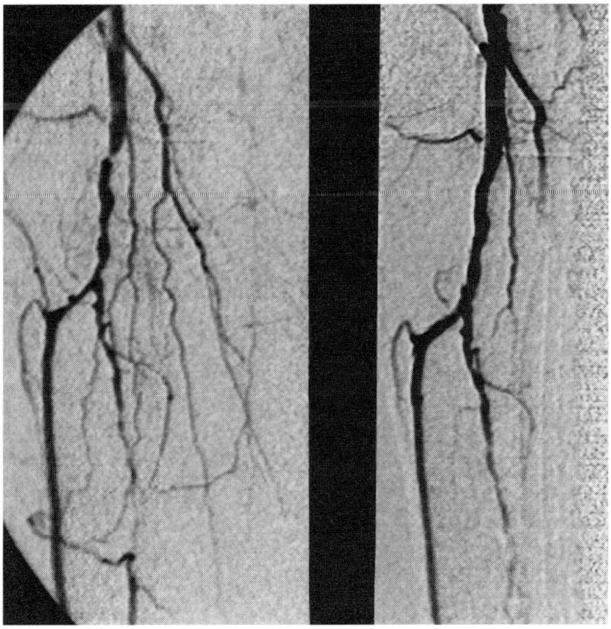

Fig. 1. A typical popliteal and tibial angioplasty.

There are no randomized trials of these treatment options and indeed there would be considerable logistical problems to such a trial. There is a pressing need for better stratification of the risks and problems in this area if we are going to be able to compare like with like.[3]

If we try to answer the question as to whether popliteal and tibial angioplasty are effective for critical ischaemia, this immediately prompts two further questions. First: What do we mean by 'critical ischaemia'? and second: What do we mean by 'effective'? Do we mean relieving symptoms, preventing amputation, maintaining vessel patency, or are we talking about cost-effectiveness? In addition we need to consider complications, durability and the ability to repeat the procedure or if it fails to perform a bypass. These factors will be discussed in turn and illustrated by our experiences in Derby. Figure 1 shows a typical popliteal and tibial angioplasty.

CRITICAL ISCHAEMIA

In the past, attempts were made to define critical ischaemia in terms of ankle systolic blood pressure associated with rest pain and tissue loss.[4] However, definitions based on blood pressure measurements have little clinical relevance[5] and no definition of critical ischaemia can predict which diabetics, with their added problems of susceptibility to infection, will need an amputation.[6] Critical limb ischaemia has been defined clinically as chronic or acute-on-chronic ischaemia that endangers the whole or part of the leg.[7] Thus it means the degree of ischaemia that would necessitate amputation in the absence of revascularization. This is a vague definition because no one could leave a patient who was thought to need an amputation with a treatable lesion. However, up to 18% of patients with 'critical ischaemia' who are unsuitable for revascularization do not require amputation.[7] Presumably some patients did not truly have critical ischaemia while others may have developed sufficiently good collaterals.

In comparing different treatments accurately it is essential to have some more precise definition of critical ischaemia. This prompted Wolfe and Wyatt[8] to stratify leg ischaemia into high and low risk with respect to subsequent outcome. They used the terms critical and subcritical ischaemia depending on whether there was tissue loss and an ankle pressure of less than 40mm Hg. Few of the studies on the effect of tibial angioplasty have used quite such strict criteria, and many relied on the clinical definition of persisting rest pain, ulceration or gangrene.[10–13] Thus complete agreement on the precise definition of critical ischaemia continues to elude us, but a single definition that has stood the test of time is that given by Wolfe[9] that patients with critical ischaemia should meet one of the two following criteria:

1. Rest pain and an ankle systolic pressure of less than 40mm Hg.
2. Rest pain with ulceration and/or gangrene.

WHAT IS MEANT BY 'EFFECTIVE'?

Relief of symptoms

On the face of it this would appear to be a good indicator of effectiveness. However, some patients with a patent reconstruction still persist in having rest pain and gangrene, presumably due to more distal disease. This is particularly likely in diabetics where microvascular disease and infection play a part. Conversely some patients with critical ischaemia do experience a spontaneous improvement as collaterals develop. Nevertheless relief of symptoms is a good indicator and is what matters most to the patient. However, this is subjective and therefore it is difficult to obtain really reliable information.

Limb salvage

All patients with critical ischaemia, by definition, face amputation. Avoidance of major amputation (below knee or higher) is the ultimate goal, providing the patient has a reasonably functioning pain-free limb. The same comments regarding symptoms apply in that most vascular surgeons have experienced patients with patent femoropopliteal bypass grafts who have still required amputation. Likewise there are occasions when a graft occludes after functioning for several months. The patient who may have been in agony prior to the reconstruction remains symptom free even though the graft has failed. This again is presumably due to the development of collaterals as a stenosis develops gradually. Although there is a failure of reconstruction, to the patient it is still a success.

Amputation (and also death) are the most clear-cut end-points with which no one can argue. The whole object of limb salvage surgery is to keep the patient alive and avoid amputation where possible. Thus these are by far the most important criteria with which to measure effectiveness, even if they are not always the most accurate way of assessing patency of a reconstruction.

Vessel patency

To the purist this is what matters in assessing efficacy, even if not to the patient or practising clinician who are interested in keeping life and a functioning pain free limb. There may, however, be difficulties in assessing patency, particularly in tibial vessels. Doppler ankle systolic pressures are helpful, but may be unreliable particularly in diabetics. Duplex scan is excellent for the femoral and popliteal arteries, but is more difficult in tibial vessels and is operator dependent.

Digital subtraction angiography via the arterial route is reliable for tibial vessels, but it is invasive, and is not justifiable for routine surveillance. The intravenous route rarely gives clear enough imaging of the distal vessels, and the volume required may cause problems in elderly patients with a tendency to heart failure. A combination of clinical, Doppler ankle pressures and duplex examination give the best all round assessment of vessel patency, with arteriography reserved for intended intervention.

Cost-effective

Angioplasty has been estimated to cost approximately £500 compared with £3000 for a reconstruction.[14] However, in our hospital the cost of tibial angioplasty is nearer £700 and this can be more if small-diameter coronary-derived balloons are used. Following angioplasty patients can normally go home the next day thus reducing the cost.[15] Angioplasty would therefore appear to be very cost-effective. However, patients requiring tibial angioplasty are often frail with rest pain or ulceration and, therefore, admission may be longer increasing the overall cost. A study of the cost of managing lower limb-threatening ischaemia[16] showed no difference between angioplasty and bypass surgery when the total cost of the patient care over the following year was considered. The implication was that they needed further vascular interventions though this was not actually stated. The biggest single cost was length of stay in hospital which was frequently prolonged because of slow progress with rehabilitation or delay in discharge because of inappropriate housing or inadequate support. Of the different groups they looked at, those having angioplasty were on average the oldest and almost a third were diabetics compared with almost a quarter of those having surgery. They estimated for amputation, outpatient visits, transport, District Nurse and home care. They did not include the cost of permanent residential care, and previous studies have shown this is much more likely to be required after amputation than successful limb salvage.[17]

Certainly there seems little doubt that with angioplasty the procedure itself is cheaper than reconstruction and the length of the stay shorter. It may be that the poorer risk patients are selected for angioplasty. The question of whether it is cost-effective depends therefore on the longer term results and is discussed later.

Complications

As previously mentioned, there has been a view that the tibial vessels are 'tiger country'.[18] There is a perception that there is a high complication rate.[1] However, the success of infrapopliteal angioplasty has been improved since the advent of new technologies, including low-profile balloons and steerable hydrophilic guidewires,[12,19,20] the treatment of spasm with vasodilators such as nitroglycerin or calcium channel blockers[21] and the use of digital subtraction and road mapping.[21] There have now been numerous reports of tibial angioplasty with very low complication rates.[1,2,12,13,22–25] When complications such as local occlusion or distal embolization do occur they may be corrected by thrombolysis or aspiration.[19,26–28] Thus it seems that the much anticipated and feared serious potential complications of distal small vessel PTA has been grossly exaggerated.[1]

Durability

Durability of the procedure

This of course is the theme of this book and therefore the most important issue to answer here. Most studies have presented their results as primary patency, secondary patency following a repeat PTA and limb salvage which in some patients

Table 1. Primary and secondary patency and limb salvage in previous studies.

Ref.	*No of patients*	*Length of follow-up*	*Primary patency*	*Secondary patency*	*Limb salvage*
Löfberg[28]	82	3 years	36	44	72
Sivananthan[12]	38	3 years	54	–	–
Varty[29]	38	2 years	68	79	77
Bergqvist[2]	82	3 years	36	44	72
Criado *et al.*[1]	26	23 months	46	–	80

was obtained with a bypass procedure. Most give results at 2 or 3 years, with primary patency varying from 36 to 68%, secondary patency from 44 to 79% and limb salvage from 72 to 80% (Table 1).[1,2,12,28,29]

There was no evidence that early or late failure of PTA prejudiced either a repeat PTA or subsequent bypass surgery.[1,2,13,30,31]

While the 3-year limb salvage rate following repeat PTA and/or by-pass surgery of 72–80% are acceptable, the primary patency rates are not so good. The counter argument is that there are few properly conducted studies showing the long-term efficacy of PTA or its superiority over other methods of treatment.[32] There are strong arguments for conducting a carefully planned randomized controlled trial comparing angioplasty with other treatments.[33] One of the problems with comparing tibial angioplasty with distal bypass graft, would be finding a sufficient number of patients who would be suitable to be randomized for either treatment.

Durability of the patient

Numerous studies over the years have alluded to the poor long-term outlook of patients with critical ischaemia.[34] Some cynics would say that if a study on patients with critical ischaemia reports more than 50% still alive 5 years later then the patients did not truly have critical ischaemia. Death may follow surgery, particularly amputation, but is more commonly due to associated cardiac or cerebrovascular disease. With this rather poor long-term outlook it becomes relatively less important to have a procedure with really good long-term results. A relatively non-invasive treatment such as angioplasty can give acceptable limb salvage, albeit with a further angioplasty in some or a subsequent bypass operation in a small proportion of others.

POPLITEAL AND TIBIAL ANGIOPLASTY AT THE DERBYSHIRE ROYAL INFIRMARY: A 4-YEAR REVIEW

A retrospective audit of primary popliteal and tibial angioplasty performed for critical ischaemia during the period 1994–1997 was carried out. Patients had rest pain and reduced ankle systolic pressure or ischaemic ulcers and gangrene fulfilling the criteria described earlier.[9]

Method

Under local anaesthesia (5–10ml of 1% lignocaine) an antegrade puncture of the ipsilateral common femoral artery (CFA) or occasionally the proximal superficial femoral artery (SFA) is performed. If patients have a femorodistal graft then this can be punctured just proximal to the knee where it may be palpable or by using ultrasound guidance.

Adequate opiate analgesia is required for patients with rest pain to ensure that they are comfortable and can keep still during the procedure.

A 5F introducer sheath is inserted at the puncture site. Angiography can be performed via the side port of the sheath or via a straight catheter positioned in the popliteal artery. Digital subtraction angiography with a 'road mapping' facility is required especially for crossing complex lesions. Prior to crossing the diseased segment the patient is anticoagulated with heparin 3000–5000 units and nitroglycerin 100–200 μg is given to prevent vasospasm.

To cross crural vessel lesions we usually use a hydrophilic guidewire (Terumo Corporation, Tokyo, Japan) in conjunction with a straight catheter. Once the lesion has been crossed the straight catheter is exchanged for a 3mm balloon on a 5F shaft. Occasionally in very small vessels or for very distal lesions a 2mm or 2.5mm balloon on a 3F shaft is required over a 0.018 inch guidewire. Check angiography is performed via the side port of the sheath with the wire left across the lesion in case repeat angioplasty is required.

Systemic anticoagulation is not routinely given post-procedure, but all patients should receive 75 mg of aspirin daily.

Success of PTA was judged radiologically and clinically using the criteria recommended by the SVS/ISCVS.[35–37] Follow-up was clinical, with Doppler pressures and duplex scan where possible. Death, major amputation (below knee or higher) and further PTA or reconstruction were clinical outcomes.

RESULTS

During the 4-year period a total of 39 patients had distal angioplasties for critical ischaemia. There were 20 males and 19 females. The average age was 72 and 20 of the patients were diabetics. Also, 21 patients had more proximal PTAs, usually the superficial femoral, in addition to the popliteal or tibial angioplasties. A total of 13 patients had multiple distal angioplasties so that in all 54 PTAs were performed, 29 in the popliteal and 25 in the tibial vessels. Of the latter, six were in the tibioperoneal trunk, six in the posterior tibial, 11 in the anterior tibial and two in the peroneal.

The technical success rate was remarkable with only one failure, which was successful 2 weeks later when the procedure was repeated. There were no immediate serious local complications though one patient had troublesome bleeding which settled with prolonged pressure, and one further patient had a popliteal artery thrombosis which cleared with local thrombolysis. There were however 10 early failures within 30 days and this carried a bad prognosis for life and limb. Of these 10 patients, three had an amputation (one of the three patients died), on the same admission. Three more died on the same admission and a further three died some months later.

The mean length of follow-up was just under 18 months with a range from less than a month to 4 years. In addition to the four early deaths there were eight later ones. There were seven major amputations and a further six patients had successful repeat angioplasties. Thus with a mean follow-up period of 18 months the primary patency rate was 38%, secondary patency rate was 54% and limb salvage rate 82%. These results are comparable with those of Criado *et al.*[1] and Bergqvist.[2]

There are also two case reports to present:

Patient VR a diabetic male born 30.5.46.

In 1992 this patient had a left below-knee amputation for a gangrenous foot. In August 1994 he presented with gangrene of all the toes of the right foot. A right superficial femoral PTA was performed with good revascularization (Fig. 2) and the toes were amputated (Fig. 3). This subsequently healed satisfactorily and has remained healthy.

Since then he has been followed up with 4-monthly visits to the vascular laboratory for Doppler ankle pressures and duplex scans. He has had a total of seven further PTAs of the superficial femoral or popliteal artery and tibioperoneal trunk with good result 4 years later (Fig. 4).

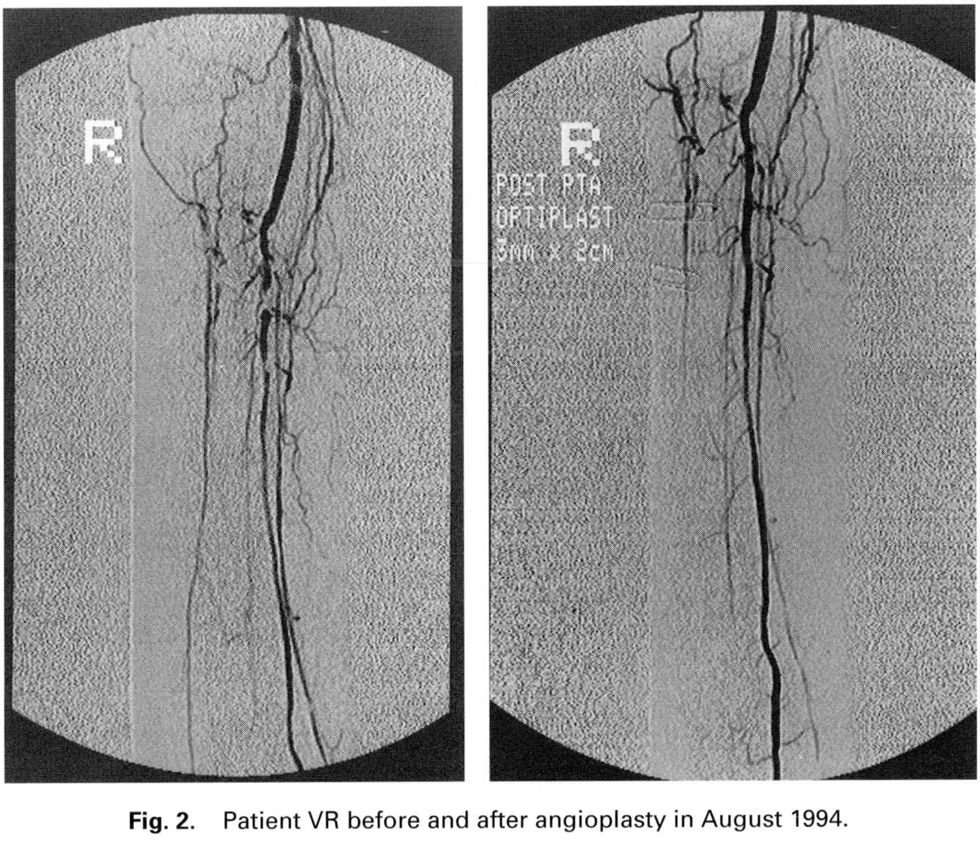

Fig. 2. Patient VR before and after angioplasty in August 1994.

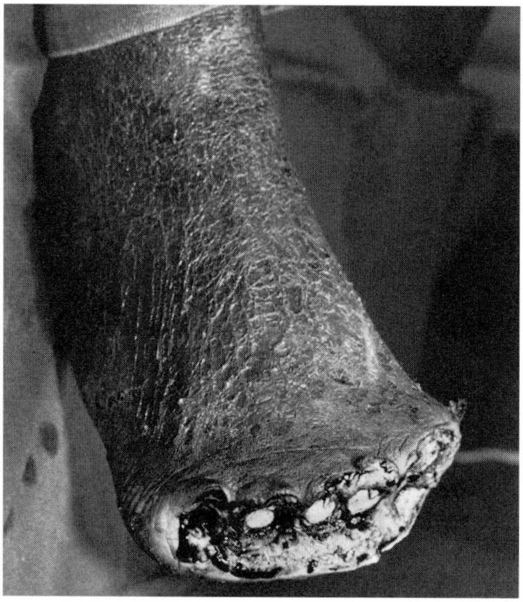

Fig. 3. Patient VR during amputation of his toes which was performed under local anaesthetic block at the ankle. The bones were trimmed back slightly more prior to completion and the wound subsequently healed satisfactorily.

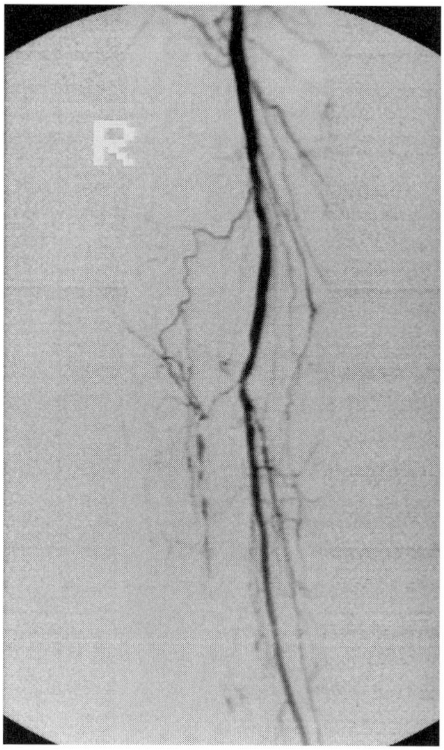

Fig. 4. The same vessels as Fig. 2, 4 years later.

Patient HV a diabetic male born 17.11.35.

In November 1992 this patient had a right below-knee amputation which became infected and was converted to an above-knee amputation in December 1992.

In January 1993 he developed critical ischaemia in the left foot and a left popliteal and proximal anterior tibial angioplasty was performed with good result. He too has had 4-monthly Doppler pressures and duplex scans. He has had further femoral or popliteal PTA since then and he too is independent and walking with his right limb prosthesis. Figure 5 shows the films taken before and after the original PTA in 1993 and a repeat angiogram 3 years later.

If one estimates an angioplasty at £500, a 24-hour hospital stay at £200 and each visit to the vascular laboratory at £5 then just under £5000 has been spent on the first patient to keep his leg for the last 4 years. Just under £3000 has been spent on the second patient to keep his leg for the last 5 years. Both these two patients are still doing well at the time of writing and would consider the procedures to have been both effective and cost-effective.

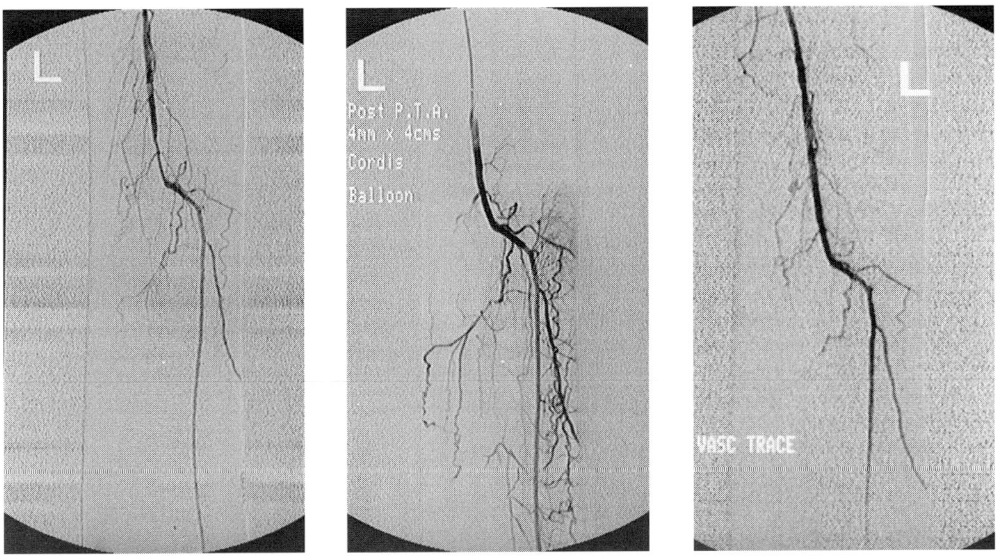

Fig. 5. Left and middle: films taken before and after distal popliteal and anterior tibial angioplasty. Right: the same vessel 3 years later.

SUMMARY AND CONCLUSION

Is popliteal and tibial angioplasty effective for critical ischaemia? The answer is a qualified 'yes'. Most of the studies have not had a particularly good primary patency rate except for those of Bolia *et al.*, with subintimal angioplasty,[10] described in the first chapter. The secondary patency rates after further PTA are a little better, but still not wonderful, but the limb salvage is really quite worthwhile. In some, the extra patency has been with bypass surgery and in others presumably it has been due to the development of collaterals.

Angioplasty can be repeated, almost as often as one likes, as illustrated by our two case histories. There is no increased problem with a subsequent femorotibial bypass if the angioplasty should fail. The complication rates are low.

The procedure itself is undoubtedly cheaper than a bypass or amputation and there will usually be a much shorter length of stay. However, doubt has been cast about the longer term value for money, although this may simply be a reflection that the most severely diseased patients tend to be selected for PTA for critical ischaemia. Some more work on this aspect of the cost of tibial angioplasty would be of interest.

Because the results with subintimal tibial angioplasty seem to be so much better than with the intraluminal it seems important that other centres should try this method and report their results as has already been alluded to.[3] The problem is that many radiologists feel the subintimal technique is more difficult.

There is still sufficient doubt about the place of angioplasty or bypass, that a properly conducted randomized controlled trial is long overdue.[33] This would be particularly difficult in the tibial section because of the problem of finding a sufficient number of patients who were felt suitable to be randomized to either treatment. However, it should be possible with a large multicentre trial, although there is an argument for trying to establish more widely whether we should be doing subintimal or transluminal angioplasty before comparing with surgery.

REFERENCES

1. Criado FJ, Twena M, Abdul Khadoud O, Al-Soufi B: What are the indications for endovascular procedures below the knee? In: Greenhalgh RM (Ed) *Indications in Vascular and Endovascular Surgery* pp. 367–383. London: WB Saunders, 1998
2. Berqvist D, Karacagil S, Lofberg AM: In: Greenhalgh RM (Ed) Is angioplasty below the knee joint wise? *Indications in Vascular and Endovascular Surgery* pp. 353–366. London: WB Saunders, 1998
3. Hopkinson BR: Editorial comment. In: Greenhalgh RM (Ed) *Indications in Vascular and Endovascular Surgery* p. 382. London: WB Saunders, 1998
4. Second European Consensus document on chronic critical limb ischaemia: *Eur J Vasc Endovasc Surg* **6** (Suppl A): 1–32, 1992
5. Thomson MM, Sayers RD, Varty K *et al.*: Chronic critical leg ischaemia must be redefined. *Eur J Vasc Endovasc Surg* **7**: 420–426, 1993
6. Tyrell MR, Wolfe JHN: Critical leg ischaemia: An appraisal of clinical definitions. *Br J Surg* **80**: 177–180, 1993
7. Audit Committee of the Vascular Surgical Society of Great Britain and Ireland: Recommendations for the management of chronic critical lower limb ischaemia. *Eur J Vasc Endovasc Surg* **12**: 131–135, 1996
8. Wolfe JHN, Wyatt MG: Critical and subcritical ischaemia. *Eur J Vasc Endovasc Surg* **13**, 578–582, 1997
9. Wolfe JHN: The definition of critical ischaemia – is this a concept of value? In: Greenhalgh RM, Jamieson CW, Nicolaides AN (Eds) *Limb Salvage and Amputation for Vascular Disease* pp. 1–10. London: WB Saunders, 1988
10. Bolia A, Sayers RD, Thompson MM, Bell PRF: Subintimal and intraluminal recanalisation of occluded crural arteries by percutaneous balloon angioplasty. *Eur J Vasc Endovasc Surg* **8**: 214–219, 1994

11. Nydahl S, Hartshorne T, Bell PRF *et al.*: Subintimal angioplasty of Infrapopliteal occlusions in critically ischaemic limbs. *Eur J Vasc Endovasc Surg* **14**: 212–216, 1997
12. Sivananthan UM, Browne TF, Thorley PJ, Rees MR: Percutaneous transluminal angioplasty of the tibial arteries. *Br J Surg* **81**: 1282–1285, 1994
13. Varty K, Nydahl S, Bolia A *et al.*: Results of surgery and angioplasty for the treatment of chronic severe lower limb ischaemia. *Eur J Vasc Endovasc Surg* **16**: 159–163, 1998
14. Cheshire NJ, Noone MA, Davies L *et al.*: Economic options and decision making in the ischaemia limb. *Br J Surg* Abstr VSS **78**: 371, 1991.
15. Holm J, Arfvidsson B, Jivegard L *et al.*: Chronic lower limb ischaemia: A prospective randomised controlled study comparing the by-pass results of vascular surgery and percutaneous angioplasty. *Eur J Vasc Surg* **5**: 517–522, 1991
16. Singh S, Evans L, Datta D *et al.*: The costs of managing lower limb-threatening ischaemia. *Eur J Vasc Endovasc Surg* **12**: 359–362, 1996
17. Hosie KB, Kockelberg R, Newbury-Ecob RA *et al.*: A retrospective review of the outcome of patients over 70 years of age considered for vascular reconstruction in a district general hospital. *Eur J Vasc Surg* **4**: 313, 1990
18. Ferguson JM, Stonebridge PA: Endovascular Surgery. *J Roy Coll Surg Edin* **41**: 223–231, 1996
19. Schwarten DE, Cutcliff WB: Arterial occlusive disease below the knee: treatment with percutaneous transluminal angioplasty performed with low-profile catheters and steerable guide-wires. *Radiology* **169**: 71–74, 1988
20. Casarella WJ: Percutaneous transluminal angioplasty below the knee: new techniques, excellent results. *Radiology* **169**: 271–272, 1988
21. Gordon RL, Ring EJ: Below knee angioplasty. *Persp Vasc Surg* **2**: 67–74, 1989
22. Ray SA, Minty I, Buckenham M *et al.*: Clinical outcome and restenosis following percutaneous transluminal angioplasty for ischaemic rest pain or ulceration. *Br J Surg* **82**: 1217–1221, 1995
23. Peregrin JH, Kovác J, Krajicková D *et al.*: Percutaneous transluminal angioplasty of the infrapopliteal arteries: the technical success and 1-year clincial results. *J Int Radiol* **13**: 77–81, 1998
24. Buckenham TM, Loh A, Dormandy JA, Taylor RS: Infrapopliteal angioplasty for limb salvage. *Eur J Vasc Surg* **7**: 21–25, 1993
25. Wack C, Wölfle KD, Loeprecht H *et al.*: Perkutane Ballon dilatation bei isolierten Läsionen der Unter schenkelarteriess mit Kritischer Beinischämic. *VASA* **23**: 30–34, 1994
26. Schwarten DE: Clinical and anatomical considerations for non-operative therapy in tibial disease and the results of angioplasty. *Circulation* **83** (Suppl 1): 86–90, 1991
27. Bakal CW, Spraynegan S, Scheinbaum K *et al.*: Percutaneous transluminal angioplasty of the infra-popliteal arteries: results in 53 patients. *Am J Roent* **154**: 717–724, 1990
28. Löfberg A-M, Lörelius L-E, Karacagıl S *et al.*: The use of below-knee percutaneous transluminal angioplasty in arterial occlusive disease causing chronic limb ischaemia. *Cardiovasc Intervent Radiol* **19**: 317–322, 1996
29. Varty K, Bolia A, Naylor AR *et al.*: Infrapopliteal percutaneous transluminal angioplasty: A safe and successful procedure. *Eur J Vasc Endovasc Surg* **9**: 341–345, 1995
30. Holm J, Arfviddson B, Jivegard L *et al.*: Chronic lower limb ischaemia. A prospective randomised control study comparing the 1 year result of vascular surgery and PTA. *Eur J Vasc Endovasc Surg* **5**: 517–522, 1991
31. Wilson SE, Wolf GL, Cross AP: Percutaneous transluminal angioplasty versus operation for peripheral arteriosclerosis. *J Vasc Surg* **9**: 698–703, 1989
32. Porter JM: Endovascular Arterial intervention:expression of concern. *J Vasc Surg* **21**: 955–957, 1995
33. BradburyAW, Ruckley CV: Angioplasty for lower limb ischaemia:time for randomised control trials. *Lancet* **347**: 277, 1996
34. Dormandy JA, Thomas PRS: What is the natural history of a critically ischaemic patient with or without his leg? In Greenhalgh RM, Jamieson CW, Nicolaides AN (Eds) *Limb Salvage and Amputation for Vascular Disease*, pp 11–26. London: WB Saunders, 1998
35. Standards of Practice Committee of the Society of Cardiovascular and Interventional

Radiology: Guidelines for percutaneous transluminal angioplasty. *Radiology* **177**: 619–626, 1990
36. Ahn SG, Rutherford RB, Becker GJ *et al.*: Reporting standards for lower extremity arterial and endovascular procedures. *J Vasc Surg* **17**: 1103–1107, 1993
37. Rutherford RB: Standards for evaluating results of interventional therapy for peripheral vascular disease. *Circulation* **83** (Suppl 1): 6–11, 1991

Commentary

This is a further report from a busy practical centre in which the authors praise the subintimal angioplasty technique and imply that it is superior. Nevertheless, they are using a conventional technique and feel that it has some place in the management of critical ischaemia, both in terms of popliteal and tibial angioplasty. They call for a random controlled trial against surgery, the current goal standard, but recognize that such a controlled trial could be very difficult because of the great variation in the cases. *RMG*

The use of high resolution ultrasound in the prediction of restenosis following lower limb angioplasty and the implications for stenting

Andrew F Lennox, Maura B Griffin, Ganesh Ramaswami, Thomas J Tegos and Andrew N Nicolaides

INTRODUCTION

Ever since its original description in 1964 by Dotter and Judkins percutaneous transluminal angioplasty (PTA) has become increasingly popular as a result of its low morbidity, mortality and reduced hospital stay in comparison with surgery.[1] However, the long-term efficacy of PTA is limited by restenosis at the site of angioplasty in 20–30% of patients. Several animal species have been used to investigate the pathogenesis of atherosclerotic disease and also for the study of restenosis, in order to identify pharmacological agents that could potentially reduce the incidence of these conditions.[2]

To date, although many groups have demonstrated reduction in incidence of restenosis in animal models, such a reduction has not been successfully reproduced in humans. One of the main reasons for the failure of animal experiments to predict outcome in man is that modelling a truly advanced atherosclerotic lesion in animals is difficult; also the beneficial effects of drugs that work in the animal model cannot be easily extrapolated to the human situation. Reducing the incidence of restenosis would have significant benefits not only to the individual patients who could have longer symptomatic improvement in addition to avoiding further interventions, but would also have important implications for the cost of treating lower limb peripheral vascular disease. It has been proposed by Calliff in 1990 that by modestly reducing the incidence of restenosis following coronary angioplasty in the USA from approximately 33% to 25%, an annual saving of $450 million could result.[3]

The ability to predict stenotic lesions that are at a higher risk of developing restenosis following PTA would provide a valuable tool in improving the outcome of this minimally invasive procedure. Patients who could be identified prior to the PTA with a potentially high incidence of subsequent restenosis could either be offered alternative interventions such as stenting or atherectomy, although it is yet to be proven that these methods have a better long-term benefit in the lower limb than conventional balloon angioplasty.

High resolution duplex ultrasound provides a useful non-invasive investigation to assess atherosclerotic lesions both prior to and following PTA, and can be used to study the natural history and fate of plaques over the course of time. High resolution duplex ultrasound has been proposed as a potential method of determining plaque characteristics that can be associated with better patency rates.[4]

KNOWN FACTORS ASSOCIATED WITH RESTENOSIS FOLLOWING PERCUTANEOUS TRANSLUMINAL ANGIOPLASTY

Several studies have investigated the factors that are predictive of long-term successful outcomes following lower limb angioplasty. Johnston in 1987 presented the results of almost 1000 PTA procedures with an initial success of 88.6%, which fell to 48.2% at 5 years, and by using multiple regression analysis was able to identify the following indicators of a good long-term outcome:[5]

- symptoms (intermittent claudication compared with resting ischaemia);
- site of the angioplasty that is being performed (common iliac compared with the femoropopliteal segments);
- severity of the lesion (stenosis compared with occlusion);
- run-off vessels below the knee (two or three vessels compared with no patent tibial arteries).

Subsequent studies have corroborated the findings that PTA below the inguinal ligament has poor results. In addition, age was found to be predictive of better outcome. Varty examined the outcome in 40 infrapopliteal PTA procedures, with 20 patients being treated for claudication and the other 20 for critical limb ischaemia.[6] Although he found a 90% early 3-month improvement of symptoms there was a 59% primary and 79% secondary patency at 2 years with a 77% limb salvage rate in the critically ischaemic limbs at 1 year.

Albäck more recently demonstrated in a series of 95 patients that there was a significantly better success rate following PTA in claudicants than patients with critically ischaemic legs (83% vs 70% initial success and 61% vs 38% success at 2 years, $p=0.03$). This difference was particularly obvious in patients with poor run-off scores (as determined by the SVS/ISCVS Reporting Standards criteria).[7]

One of the main limitations in interpreting these results is the outcome criteria used to determine a 'successful' procedure. Initial angiographic improvement, reduction of symptoms, improvement of clinical grade, increase of ankle brachial pressure index (ABPI), improvement of distal pulses, change in Doppler velocity waveform from monophasic to biphasic or triphasic and increasing of the treadmill exercise distance are all useful parameters indicating the effect of the PTA. However, they give little information regarding the fate of the plaque that has been treated. In order to determine the long-term changes and the growth of plaques following the controlled injury initiated by balloon dilatation, it is necessary to follow the individual plaques over time rather than the symptoms or the haemodynamic effects that they produce. The following section will discuss the ability of high resolution duplex ultrasound to study lesions treated by PTA to determine when plaques restenose and the rate of growth during that process.

THE CONTRIBUTION OF INTRAVASCULAR ULTRASOUND

In recent years attempts have been made to assess outcome following PTA of the lower limbs[8,9] and coronary vessels (PTCA)[10,11] using intravascular ultrasound

(IVUS). This methodology enables 360° cross-sectional imaging of the vessel and plaque being treated, and provides information which is much more accurate than angiography regarding the immediate post-angioplasty residual plaque morphology and luminal area. IVUS also gives a better insight into the mechanisms of plaque disruption, medial rupture and dissection that result in the compression and redistribution of plaque during PTA. Although much work with the IVUS has been applied in coronary disease it has not been able to predict restenosis.[12]

Although IVUS has been used in lower limb disease the number of studies available is rather small. Gussenhoven has demonstrated in 31 patients that IVUS images taken *prior* to PTA had no quantitative or qualitative relationship to later problems with patency.[13] The EPISODE trial, which included 137 patients was able to conclude that those plaques which eventually developed restenosis were associated with a lesser increase in immediate luminal area, a greater proportion of 'hard' plaque, an increased amount of dissection and also a reduced incidence of medial rupture.[8] Arko has also used IVUS in addition to arteriography to assess the adequacy of stent deployment in aortoiliac occlusive disease.[9] He found that despite an acceptable angiogram IVUS was able to identify 40% of stents post-deployment to be underexpanded requiring further intervention. This group had no incidence of restenosis at a mean follow-up of 28 months compared with 25% in the group that had angiography without an IVUS examination.

In addition to the lack of strong data supporting its use in the femoropopliteal segments, the main controversy with IVUS is the added costs, which may or may not be offset by any improvements in patency. Furthermore, the inability to repeat the studies at regular intervals following PTA due to its invasive nature limits its use as a research tool.

THE PREDICTION OF RESTENOSIS

Various haemostatic, rheological and lipid factors have also been investigated in the past to determine their relationship with the development of coronary artery restenosis following PTA. Elevated levels of fibrinogen at 6 months[14] and low levels of high density lipoproteins (HDL),[15] were associated with an increased post PTCA restenosis. Lipoprotein(a) levels, total cholesterol, thrombin–antithrombin complexes and antiplasmin–plasmin complex have not been shown to predict subsequent restenosis.[16] Relatively little work has been done along these lines in lower limb angioplasty, but recently Price in 1997 reported the results of 102 patients undergoing aortoiliac and femoropoliteal PTA, and found that in the 26% of lesions that had restenosed at 2-3 years there was no evidence that pre-procedural levels of factors such as whole blood viscosity, plasma viscosity, haematocrit, von Willebrand factor, fibrin D-Dimer or plasminogen activator inhibitor-1 were predictive of this complication compared with the group whose lesions remained patent.[17] Only the mean plasma fibrinogen level was able to reach statistical significance between the two groups, with the levels being marginally lower in the patients with restenosis (3.31 g/l vs 3.75 g/l).

Despite the data published, there is no reliable method prior to PTA of predicting those patients who will have a higher incidence of subsequent restenosis. The ability to predict a subgroup or subgroups with high or low incidence of restenosis would have important implications in management.

HIGH RESOLUTION ULTRASOUND IN THE ASSESSMENT OF LOWER LIMB ARTERIAL DISEASE

Peripheral vascular disease (PVD) has traditionally been investigated by angiography which provides information about the vessel lumen. Some inferences can be made about the arterial wall depending on the outline of a stenosis but angiography does not provide direct information about the thickness of the arterial wall or plaque consistency or asymmetry.

In the last 10 years duplex scanning has become a useful diagnostic modality in lower limb vascular disease. It provides non-invasive anatomical and physiological information to such an extent that angiography has become unnecessary in the majority of patients.[18,19] Changes in cross-sectional area of the vascular lumen can be determined by means of peak systolic velocity (PSV) at the site of stenosis and its immediate normal vicinity, that is peak systolic velocity ratio (PSVR).[20] A recent meta-analysis by Koelemay in 1996 looked at the 95% confidence intervals of sensitivity and specificity in the aorto-iliac, femoropopliteal and infrapopliteal tracts.[21] For a stenosis greater than or equal to 50% or occlusion the results were 86 (80–91)% and 97 (95–99)% for the aortoiliac segment, 80 (74–85)% and 96 (94–98)% for the femoropopliteal segment, 83 (59–96)% and 84 (69–93)% respectively for the infrapopliteal arteries. For planning operative treatment most surgeons feel that diagnostic angiography is mandatory especially when the patient needs a femorodistal reconstruction but not for making a decision to operate or not operate. The meta-analysis results based on 71 studies confirmed that duplex scanning is an accurate, non-invasive test for the assessment of arterial occlusive disease in the aortoiliac and femoropopliteal segments in patients with claudicating or critical ischaemia. There was no difference in the accuracy between duplex scanning and angiography to detect a significant stenosis or occlusion. This is the reason duplex scanning is replacing angiography for the determination of treatment stategy especially in patients with localized lesions as these can be treated by PTA. More recently, Sensier in 1998 suggested that because of its inherent limitations angiography may no longer be considered to be the 'gold standard' even for the infrapopliteal segment and although further research is needed in this area their study showed that assessment of this vasculature by ultrasonography appears to be an effective replacement of arteriography for the majority of patients.[22]

Many radiologists now accept patients for angioplasty based on duplex findings without prior diagnostic angiography. It is performed at the same time as the angioplasty thereby avoiding unnecessary duplication. This practice decreases the complication rate and is more convenient for the patients. In addition duplex scanning has a high negative predictive value, so that significant lesions in the aortoiliac and femoropopliteal segments can be reliably excluded. As a result, in many centres the number of diagnostic angiograms and the waiting lists are reducing.

Ultrasound has been introduced in the angiography suite and velocity measurements at the site of stenosis before and immediately after angioplasty are used to indicate the effectiveness of the procedure. In the presence of high velocities, indicating a sub-optimal dilatation, the operator may perform further dilatations until a satisfactory result is obtained.[23] Furthermore, some authors have used ultrasound not only to detect lesions suitable for PTA, but also have performed the PTA under ultrasound control.[24]

THE ROLE OF DUPLEX SCANNING IN THE NATURAL HISTORY OF RESTENOSIS FOLLOWING PERCUTANEOUS TRANSLUMINAL ANGIOPLASTY

It has now become necessary to study the natural history of plaques after PTA in patients rather than animal models in order to understand the mechanisms and factors that produce restenosis and the timing of the latter. The key to natural history studies is the performance of frequent measurements to collect information about rate, time and geometry of plaque growth thereby allowing one to observe the local changes in the arterial wall that lead to the remodelling of the plaque.

Angiographic imaging provides valuable morphologic data but does not yield precise information regarding residual flow abnormality or pressure gradient at the PTA site.[25] IVUS complements angiography by providing information on plaque consistency as indicated earlier. However, the expense and associated risks of angiography and IVUS restrict its use for serial follow-up examinations.

In contrast, ultrasound is non-invasive and can be used frequently, even daily, if necessary to provide information both on lumen and plaques. In addition to the size of the plaque it provides information on plaque echodensity and texture.

As indicated above, duplex scanning has become accepted as a new method of diagnosing the presence, severity and extent of PVD. In many centres clinical decisions are made solely on the results of duplex scanning. This has become possible because technology has provided ultrasonic images with high resolution and velocity measurements which are highly reproducible.[4] In our department, radiologists accept patients for PTA on the basis of duplex.

In Mewissen's study duplex scanning played a significant role in the immediate haemodynamic evaluation of the PTA site because of its ability to identify severe residual stenoses undetected by angiography. It demonstrated that angiography could not predict normalization of flow haemodynamics after balloon angioplasty. The presence of a functional stenosis identified by duplex scanning despite a normal angiogram was predictive of clinical deterioration and PTA failure. Finally, normalization of flow haemodynamics in the treated arterial segment correlated with PTA durability.[23]

A recent addition to the grading of restenosis and plaque thickness on duplex scanning is the ability to study the morphology of the plaque. A recent concensus on the morphology of atherosclerotic carotid bifurcation plaques has indicated that high resolution ultrasound can be used to characterize plaques and that echodensity and texture may have prognostic implications.[26] Regular borders, echogenicity and a homogenous texture are characteristics of stable plaques. Irregular borders, echolucency and heterogenous texture characterize those that are potentially unstable.[27]

More recently it has been suggested that computer assisted methods of plaque characterization using digital image processing can provide measurements that may be as important as the degree of stenosis in predicting clinical outcome.[28] The technique of image standardization recently developed by our department has made the measurement of plaque echodensity reproducible. Echodensity is an index of the amount of fibrous tissue and by inference plaque stability/instability. This methodology has been applied to plaques in the lower limb arteries and in addition the feasibility of monitoring restenosis following PTA using high resolution ultrasound has been demonstrated. Local factors, such as plaque morphology, and their association with success or failure of angioplasty, has been investigated and a number of features have been shown to predict restenosis.[4]

METHOD OF NORMALIZATION AND DIGITAL IMAGE PROCESSING

Tissue echodensity and texture are very important features of ultrasonic images. However, two significant impediments for accurate qualitative and quantitative assessments of echodensity and texture are recognized. First, density perception by the human eye is very unreliable in evaluating echodensity. Ultrasound is very subjective. The operator adjusts the gain and settings to what he or she perceives as optimum in relation to surrounding tissues and ambient light in the examination room. Secondly comparison of images obtained using different gain settings is difficult. Therefore a method that would allow normalization of such images is essential if comparisons and reproducible measurements are to be made. A method has now been developed that can achieve this.[28]

Plaque images can be transferred to a personal computer and normalized using linear scaling and two reference points: blood, which is black, and adventitia, which is white. Blood is assigned a grey value in the range of 0–5 and adventitia 185–195. All other grey shades are adjusted accordingly on a linear scale (0 = absolutely black; 255 = absolutely white) the slope of which is then defined by the above two reference points, blood and adventitia. Normalization of the image will ensure that plaque echodensity and texture measurements will be independent of brightness and contrast of the images. This is a novel application of digital image processing in the field of atherosclerotic plaque imaging.

Plaque echodensity can be measured by the grey scale median (GSM) of the pixels of the plaque and texture can be expressed by measurements such as Kurtosis (K) of the histogram distribution of the pixels, contrast, and entropy using standard algorithms. A low K value indicates a heterogenous plaque; a high K value indicates a homogenous plaque. (See Appendix for more details of image recording, capture and normalization).

In addition to echodensity and texture measurements the velocity and plaque thickness measurements can be obtained using ultrasound. An increase in the PSVR (> 2.0) at the site of angioplasty is the criterion used to determine restenosis.

Thus weekly or monthly repetition of these measurements can provide information on the rate of plaque growth and structure.

RESTENOSIS AFTER PERCUTANEOUS TRANSLUMINAL ANGIOPLASTY: A HUMAN MODEL

In a recent study 23 patients with 40 stenoses (>70% and <5cm in length) in the iliac and femoropopliteal segments were studied by duplex scanning before PTA, on day 1, weekly for 8 weeks, 3 months, 6 months and at 1 year. Changes in the following parameters over time in the post-angioplasty period and their inter-relationship were compared for analysis of results (a) total plaque thickness (mm) (sum of anterior + posterior components of the plaque), (b) minimal luminal diameter (MLD) (mm), (c) peak systolic velocity ratio (PSVR), (d) rate of plaque 'growth': changes in plaque thickness plotted over time and (e) absolute plaque 'growth' (mm) (plaque thickness at final visit or at time of restenosis subtracted from plaque thickness on day 1 after angioplasty) and the PSVR as illustrated in Fig.1. A PSVR > 2.0 was used to indicate restenosis. Measurements on transverse images were also performed to identify the full extent of the plaque in case of extension onto the lateral or medial walls. Colour was also used in order to outline extremely echolucent plaque, which may be difficult to visualize using B-mode alone.

After the exclusion of 10 stenoses as a result of calcification which made imaging impossible, and failed procedures, 30 stenoses in 17 patients were included for analysis. Interobserver variability for the above 30 stenoses was performed with the following results: the correlation coefficient and mean absolute difference limits of agreement were r = 0.99, 0.06 ± 0.26 mm, (95% CI 0.46–0.58) mm for plaque thickness;

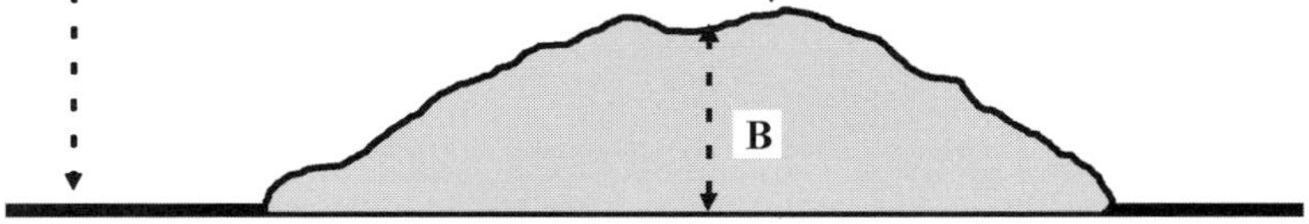

A = Anterior component of plaque.
B = Posterior component of plaque.
C = Minimal lumen diameter.
D = Proximal lumen diameter.
V1 = Pre-stenotic velocity.
V2 = Velocity at site of stenosis.

Fig. 1. Diagrammatic representation of ultrasound parameters calculated at the site of stenosis.

r = 0.97, -0.03 ± 0.46 mm, (95% CI -0.49–0.43 mm) for MLD and r = 0.98, 0.04 ± 0.31, (95% CI -0.27–0.35) for PSVR. Of these 30 stenoses, six were in the common iliac, two in the external iliac, one in the profunda, 20 in the superficial femoral and one in the popliteal arteries. The follow-up of these plaques demonstrated the feasibility of using ultrasound to study the development of restenosis.

During this follow-up, two distinct groups were observed. Plaques that had grown more than 2 mm had sustained 'growth' until week 24; this remained unchanged at 1 year. However, where 'growth' was less than 2 mm the maximum thickness was reached at week 6.The incidence of restenosis was far greater in the first group (62%) than the second group at 24% (p = 0.03). This study also demonstrated that there are situations where plaque 'growth' was not synonymous with restenosis as illustrated in Fig. 2. Due to plaque geometry, the lumen of the vessel was maintained because the anterior and posterior components of the plaque grew asymmetrically.

The relationship between absolute plaque 'growth' (plaque thickness on final visit or at time of restenosis subtracted from plaque thickness on day 1 after angioplasty) and PSVR is shown in Fig. 3. However, analysis of data showed that in stenosis (a) angioplasty was inadequate and only showed a 32% increase in MLD. In five stenoses (b) plaque growth was more than 2 mm in an asymmetric configuration. Figure 4 summarizes the relationship between absolute plaque 'growth' and restenosis after exclusion of these six stenoses (r = 0.63).

The overall prevalence of restenosis (PSVR >2) was 40% at 24 weeks remaining unchanged at 1 year. This is in keeping with the findings of the critical period of restenosis being 3–5 months for lesions in the coronary arteries.[29,30] In the iliac

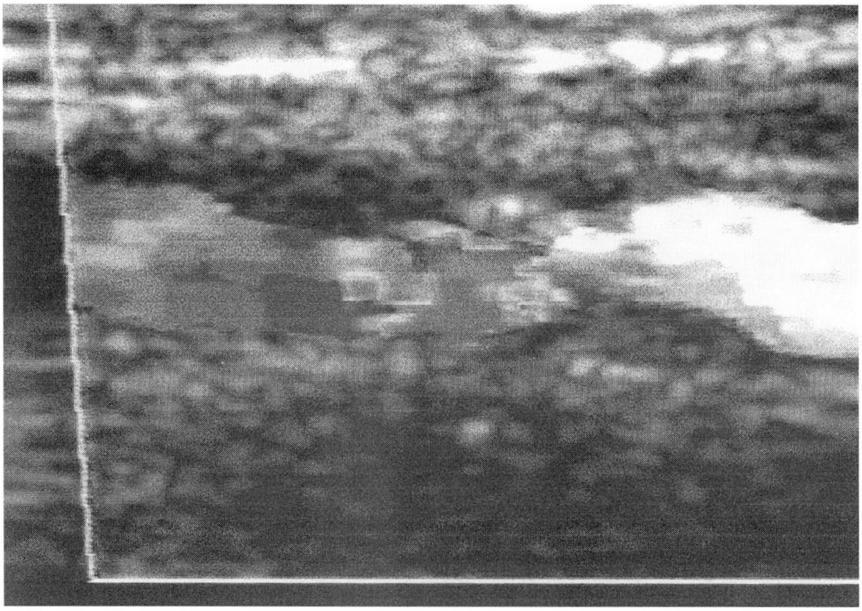

Fig. 2. Asymmetric plaque growth following PTA demonstrating maintenance of luminal diameter without restenosis.

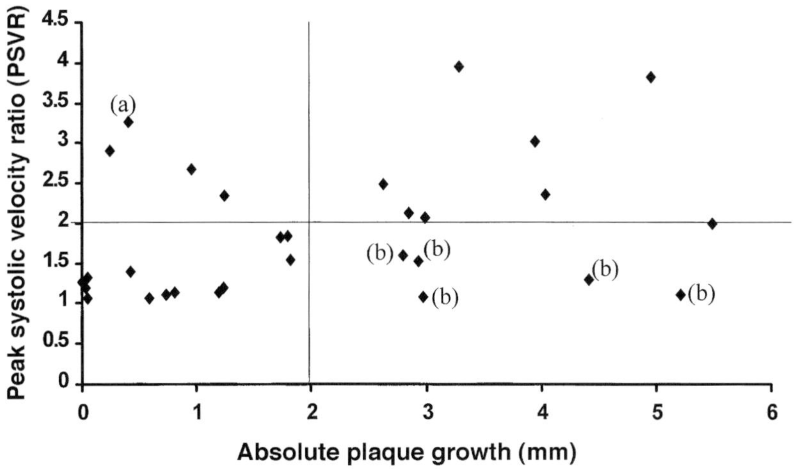

Fig. 3. The relationship between absolute plaque 'growth' and PSVR in the follow-up period. An increase in PSVR > 2.0 signified restenosis.

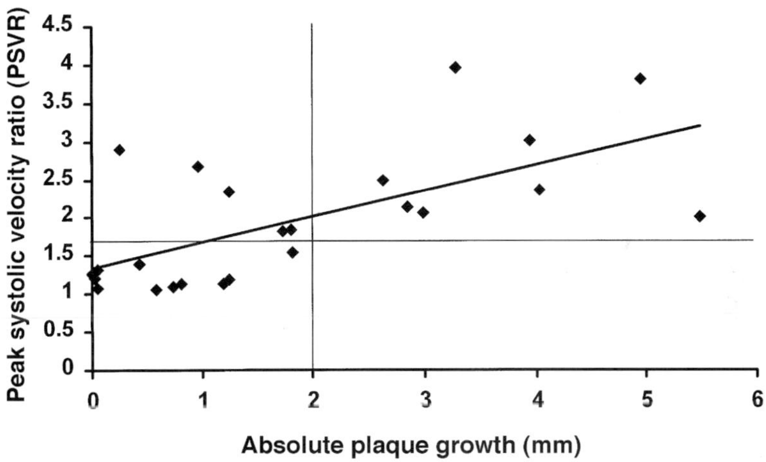

Fig. 4. The relationship between absolute plaque 'growth' and restenosis (PSVR > 2.0) in the follow-up period after the exclusion of six stenoses (one due to poor dilatation, five due to asymmetric plaque 'growth') r = 0.63.

segment, the restenosis rate was 50% (4/8) and in the femoropopliteal segment 36% (8/22). Of the lesions that restenosed, 33% recurred before week 8 and the remaining 67% between weeks 8 and 24. This may be due to different mechanisms involved in the restenosis process; thrombus formation in the early lesions and smooth muscle hyperplasia in the late ones. The lack of histological verification limits the drawing of further conclusions. There were no cases of restenosis between weeks 24 and 52 (1year).

It was then decided to determine the value of ultrasonic plaque characterization in identifying a 'high risk' group of patients at risk of restenosis, prior to PTA. Using the methodology outlined in the Appendix, all baseline B-mode images were standardized and a grey scale median value was assigned to each plaque. When a stenosis had both an anterior and posterior component, an average of two medians was taken. The reproducibility of grey scale median measurements was assessed and inter-observer variability showed a coefficient of correlation (r) of 0.93 and the 95%CI was 4.1–5.9.

RELATIONSHIP BETWEEN PLAQUE GREY-SCALE MEDIAN AND IMMEDIATE OUTCOME AFTER ANGIOPLASTY

The plaque GSM of the stenoses subjected to angioplasty ranged from 6 to 71 (mean 31.3 ± 17.9) i.e. from echolucent to very echogenic (fibrous) plaques. Figure 5a shows an example of an echolucent plaque with a GSM of 17 in the superficial femoral artery. Figure 5b shows the same plaque day 1 after angioplasty; the anterior and posterior plaque having reduced in thickness with a resultant increase in the MLD and subsequent decrease in PSVR. Figure 6a is an example of a fibrous plaque with a GSM of 41 and Fig. 6b represents the same plaque on day 1 after PTA. The anterior plaque has not reduced in thickness as much as the previous example; however the MLD has increased quite considerably, resulting in a fall of the PSVR.

It was found that when the GSM was less than 25, the absolute reduction in plaque thickness (mm) on day 1 was significant ($p < 0.03$) as shown in Table 1 compared with a GSM greater than 25. It would appear that the lower the GSM, the more effective was the process of plaque compression by the angioplasty balloon. This could be explained simply by the fact that plaques with a GSM of less than 25 being more echolucent due to their higher content of cholesterol and therefore more compressible than plaques with a GSM greater than 25 as a result of fibrous tissue. There was no relationship between GSM and increase in MLD and percentage decrease in PSVR at the site of angioplasty. This is possibly due to the fact that irrespective of the nature of the plaque, angioplasty achieves its effect; by compression in echolucent plaques and by vessel wall dilatation in the very fibrous plaques.

Table 2 shows the relationship between plaque GSM and restenosis based on the increase in PSVR > 2.0. Statistical significance ($p < 0.001$; with Yates correction) was demonstrated between the two groups. When the plaque GSM was less than 25 (echolucent), the incidence of restenosis was 12% in comparison with 78% seen in those plaques with a GSM greater than 25 (echogenic). Figure 7 shows the relationship between plaque GSM and PSVR ($r = 0.66$). Indeed, when the GSM was greater than 30 the restenosis rate was 100%. However there was no correlation between plaque GSM and absolute plaque 'growth'. This could be explained by the combination of 'growth' and vessel wall recoil in plaques with a GSM greater than 25 resulting in lumen loss and restenosis.

One important message from this study was the higher prevalence of restenosis in plaques with a higher GSM. On the basis of these measurements therefore it may be possible to determine who will be at greater risk of restenosis prior to PTA thus allowing better selection of lesions for angioplasty with better therapeutic results.

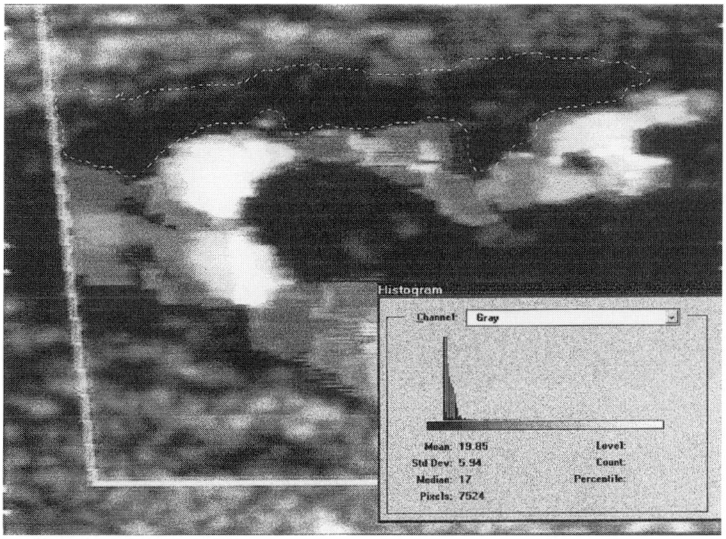

(a)

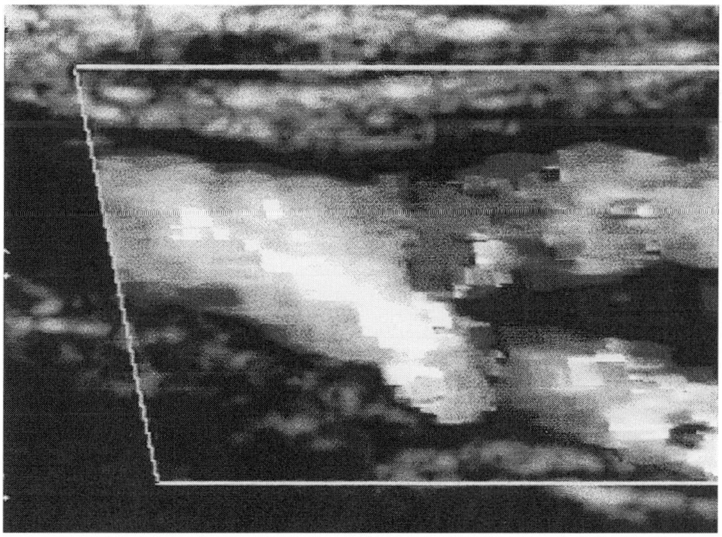

(b)

Fig. 5. a) Flow image of superficial femoral artery stenosis pre-angioplasty with the echolucent plaque outlined and GSM calculated by computer analysis. b) Day 1 following successful PTA showing increase in luminal diameter due to compression of the plaque components.

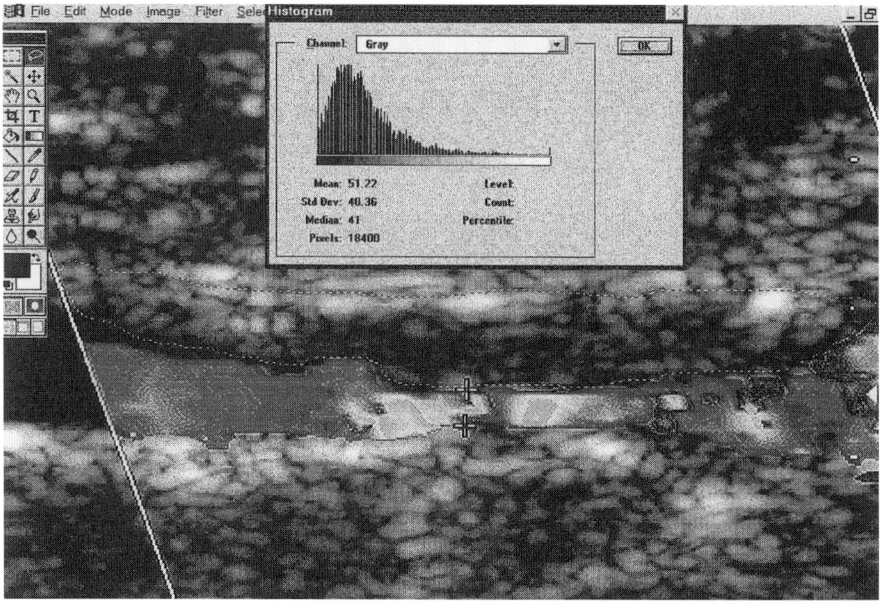

(a)

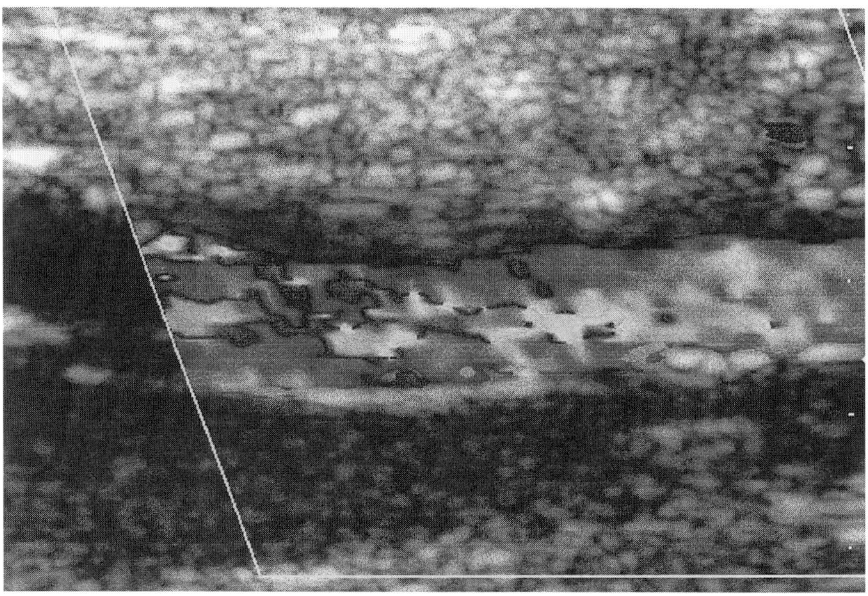

(b)

Fig. 6. a) Flow image of superficial femoral artery stenosis pre-angioplasty with the echogenic (fibrous) anterior plaque outlined and GSM calculated by computer analysis. b) Day 1 following successful PTA showing increase in luminal diameter due to vessel wall dilatation and minimal compression of the plaque.

Table 1. The relationship between plaque grey-scale median (GSM) and reduction in plaque thickness on day 1 following angioplasty

	Plaque GSM		
	< 25	*>25*	*p (t-test)*
Plaque thickness (mm) (pre-angioplasty) (A)	5.6 ± 2.2	5.2 ± 2.2	NS
Plaque thickness (mm) (day 1 after angioplasty) (B)	2.2 ± 1.7	3.3 ± 0.9	NS
Absolute decrease in plaque thickness (mm) (A - B)	3.3 ± 1.8	1.8 ± 1.6	< 0.03

NS = Not significant

Table 2. The relationship between grey-scale median (GSM) and restenosis (PSVR > 2.0) for the 31 lesions undergoing PTA

	No stenosis (PSVR < 2.0)	*Stenosis (PSVR > 2.0)*	*Total*
Plaque GSM <25	15	2 (11.8%)	17
Plaque GSM >25	3	11 (78.8%)	14
Total	18	13	31

p < 0.001 (with Yate's correction)

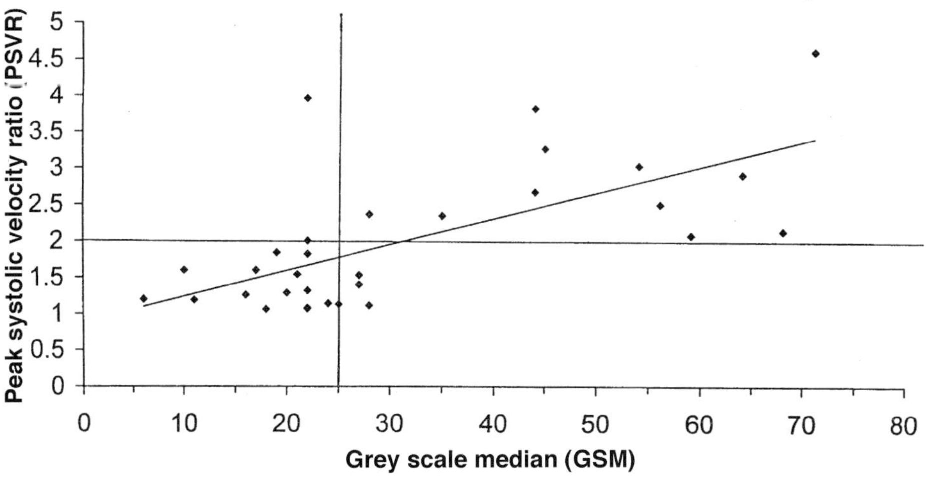

Fig. 7. Relationship between plaque GSM and PSVR in the post-angioplasty period indicating a higher incidence of restenosis in patients with echogenic plaques (GSM > 25)

CLINICAL IMPLICATIONS FOR LOWER LIMB ARTERIAL STENTING

Intravascular metallic stents have received most attention in recent years as a way to prevent early recurrence after endovascular procedures. They were initially advocated to reduce early occlusion or restenosis after PTA of the coronary or peripheral arteries and also gained acceptance for the 'salvage' of vessels following an acute dissection, intimal flaps or thrombosis. Stents can be either self-expanding or balloon expandable depending on the properties of the metal framework of the mesh, and they function by avoiding the elastic recoil of the vascular stenoses and also provide internal support for the artery.[31] The role of stent placement in the lower limb arteries remains controversial, particularly in regard to the use of primary stenting as treatment for stenosis. Stents have been used in the aortoiliac segments with excellent immediate and mid-term patency results (see Table 3).[32–37] A randomized study comparing stents with PTA in the iliac vessels showed cumulative 4-year patency rates of 94% and 69% respectively;[38] however, other series would favour higher patency rates greater than 80% for PTA alone.[39]

Neointimal hyperplasia and restenosis can be demonstrated in the patients following stent insertion with duplex scanning as seen in patients within our study group; however they often do not achieve haemodynamic significance due the larger calibre and flow rate through these vessels compared with the femoropopliteal segments. In these more distal vessels there have only been a small number of studies assessing the results of stenting (Table 3), demonstrating excellent early success of more than 95% but patency of only 50–80% at 1–2 years.[35,38,40,41] Only one randomized study has compared primary stenting with PTA and not demonstrated any benefit with the stenting procedure.[38] To date, indications for femoral stenting have been the same as for iliac stenting, with the potential advantage of the ability of treating in-stent restenosis or occlusion with either PTA or atherectomy. Although there was

Table 3. Results of iliac and femoral stenting procedures

Author	*No*	*Primary patency (%)*	*Late patency (%)*	*Follow-up (months)*
Iliac				
Palmaz *et al.* 1992[32]	587	100	84	24
Rabbia *et al.* 1993[33]	156	98	96	9
Henry *et al.* 1993[34]	148	100	91	20
Strecker *et al.* 1993[35]	114	100	95	36
Vorwerk *et al.* 1992[36]	125	98	89	24
Strunk *et al.* 1993[37]	118	98	67	36
Femoral				
Sapoval *et al.* 1992[40]	22	95	49	12
Do-dai-do *et al.* 1992[38]	52	81	69	12
Strecker *et al.* 1993[35]	84	100	80	12
Henry *et al.* 1993[41]	108	98	72	20

initial concern that external compression at the knee or hip joint may cause kinking or fracturing of the device, this does not appear to be a major practical limitation.[42]

At present, the long-term benefits compared with PTA remain unproved and selective use of stents would appear appropriate, especially when the extra costs are considered. Insight into the identification of patients who are more susceptible to the development of restenosis has been demonstrated using high resolution ultrasound in the studies presented within this chapter. This work is valuable not only in the prediction of which patients may have poor prognosis with PTA, but may also provide a subgroup that can be identified *prior* to the angioplasty who could benefit from a primary stenting procedure. If failure of long-term patency is due to excessive elastic recoil and minimal compression of the stenotic plaque, the extra support obtained with stent placement may limit these forces. Neointimal hyperplasia may continue to be a problem in these patient groups, and new therapies including pharmacological agents, gene therapy and intraluminal radiation may hold the key to ultimately reducing the incidence of this complication thereby improving patency of endovascular procedures. The methodology using duplex that has been described would also have the benefit of identifying 'higher risk' patients for the development of restenosis who could be used in randomized studies to assess the effects of these new treatment modalities. In this situation the results against a control group would be more apparent and thus could be performed in studies with a smaller number of patients.

REFERENCES

1. Dotter CT, Judkins MP: Transluminal treatment of arteriosclerotic obstructions: descriptions of a new technique and a preliminary report of its application. *Circulation* **30**: 654–670, 1964
2. Lafont A, Faxon D: Why do animal models of post angioplasty restenosis sometimes poorly predict the outcome of clinical trials? *Cardiovasc Res* **39**: 50–59, 1998
3. Calliff RM, Ohman E, Fid DJ *et al.*: Restenosis: the clinical issues. In: Topol EJ (Ed) *Textbook of Interventional Cardiology*. Philadelphia: WB Saunders Co, 1990
4. Ramaswami G, Dhanjil S, Nicolaides AN *et al.*: Restenosis after percutaneous transluminal angioplasty: a human model. *Am J Surg* **176**: 102–108, 1998
5. Johnston KW, Rae M, Hogg-Johnston SA *et al.*: 5-Year results of a prospective study of percutaneous transluminal angioplasty. *Ann Surg* **206**: 403–413, 1987
6. Varty K, Bolia A, Naylor AR *et al.*: Infrapopliteal percutaneous transluminal angioplasty: a safe and successful procedure. *Eur J Vasc Endovasc Surg* **9**: 341–345, 1995
7. Albäck A, Biancari F, Schmidt S *et al.*: Haemodynamic results of femoropopliteal percutaneous transluminal angioplasty. *Eur J Vasc Endovasc Surg* **16:** 7–12, 1998
8. Van Sambeek MRH, Gussenhoven EJ, Van der Lugt A *et al.*: Is the use of intravascular ultrasound essential for femoropopliteal balloon angioplasty and stenting. In: Greenhalgh RM (Ed) *Indications in Vascular and Endovascular Surgery*. London: WB Saunders Co, 1997
9. Arko F, Mettauer M, Mc Collough R *et al.*: Use of intrasvascular ultrasound improves long-term clinical outcome in the endovascular management of atherosclerotic aortoiliac occlusive disease. *J Vasc Surg* **27**: 614–23, 1998
10. Jain SP, Jain A, Collins TJ *et al.*: Predictors of restenosis: A morphometric and quantitative evaluation by intravascular ultraound. *Am Heart J* **128**: 664–673, 1994
11. Iwabuchi M, Haruta S, Taguchi A *et al.*: Intravascular ultrasound findings after successful primary angioplasty for acute myocardial infarction: Predictors of abrupt occlusion. *J Am Coll Cardiol* **30**: 1437–1434, 1997

12. Peters RJG, Kok WE, DiMario C *et al.*: Prediction of restenosis after coronary balloon angioplasty *Circulation* **95**: 2254–2261, 1997
13. Gussenhoven EJ, Van der Lugt A, Pasterkamp G *et al.*: Intravascular ultrasound predictors of outcome after peripheral balloon angioplasty. *Eur J Vasc Endovasc Surg* **10**: 279–288, 1995
14. Montalescot G, Ankri A, Vicaut E *et al.*: Fibrinogen after coronary angioplasty as a risk factor for restenosis. *Circulation* **92**: 31–38, 1995
15. Shah PK, Armin J: Low density lipoprotein level is associated with increased restenosis rate after coronary angioplasty. *Circulation* **85**: 1279–1285, 1992
16. Alaigh P, Hoffman CJ, Korlipara G *et al.*: Lipoprotein(a) level does not predict restenosis after percutaneous transluminal coronary angioplasty. *Thromb Vasc Biol* **18**: 1281–1286, 1998
17. Price JF, Mamode N, Smith FB *et al.*: Haemostatic and rheological factors as predictors of restenosis following percutaneous transluminal angioplasty. *Eur J Vasc Endovasc Surg* **14**: 392–398,1997
18. Pemberton M, Nydahl S, Hartshorne T *et al.*: Colour-coded duplex imaging can safely replace diagnostic arteriography in patients with lower-limb arterial disease. *Br J Surg* **83**: 1725–1728, 1996
19. Legemate DA, Teeuwen C, Hoeneveld H, Eikelboom BC: Value of duplex scanning compared with angiography and pressure measurement in the assessment of aortoiliac arterial lesions. *Br J Surg* **78**: 1003–1008, 1991
20. Moneta GL, Yeager RA, Antonovic R, Hall LD *et al.*: Accuracy of lower extremity arterial duplex mapping. *J Vasc Surg* **15**: 275–284, 1992
21. Koelemay MJW, DEN Hartog D, Prins MH *et al.*: Diagnosis of arterial disease of the lower extremities with duplex ultrasonography. *Br J Surg* **83**: 404–409, 1996
22. Sensier Y, Fishwick G, Pemberton M *et al.*: A comparison between colour duplex ultrasonography and arteriography for imaging infrapopliteal arterial lesions. *Eur J Vasc Endovasc Surg* **15**: 44–50, 1998
23. Mewissen MW, Kinney EV, Bandyk D *et al.*: The role of duplex scanning versus angiography in predicting outcome after balloon angioplasty in the femoropopliteal artery. *J Vasc Surg* **15**: 860–866, 1992
24. Ramaswami G, Al-Kutoubi A, Nicolaides AN *et al.*: Peripheral transluminal angioplasty under ultrasound guidance: Initial clinical experience and prevalence of lower limb lesions amenable to ultrasound-guided angioplasty. *J Endovasc Surg* **2**: 27–35, 1995
25. Barnes WR: Non-invasive diagnostic assessment of peripheral vascular disease. *Circulation* **3**: 20–27, 1991
26. Widder B, Pault K: Mophological characteristics of carotid artery stenosis by ultrasound duplex scanning. *Ultrasound Med Biol* **16**: 349–354, 1990
27. El-Barghouty N, Geroulakos G, Nicolaides AN *et al.*: Computer assisted carotid plaque characterisation. *Eur J Vasc Endovasc Surg* **9**:389–393, 1995
28. Elatrozy T, Nicolaides AN, Tegos T *et al.*: The effect of B-mode ultrasonic image standardisation on the echodensity of symptomatic and asymptomatic carotid bifurcation plaques. *Int Angiol* **17**: 179–186, 1998
29. Nobuyoshi M, Kimura T, Nosaka H *et al.*: Restenosis after successful percutaneous transluminal angioplasty: Serial angiographic follow up of 229 patients. *J Am Coll Cardiol* **12**: 616–623, 1988
30. Serruys PW, Luijten HE, Beatt KJ *et al.*: Incidence of restenosis after successful coronary angioplasty: a time-related phenomenon. A quantitative angiographic study in 342 consecutive patients at 1,2,3 and 4 months. *Circulation* **77**: 361–371, 1988
31. Becker GJ: Intravascular stents: General principles and status of lower extremity arterial applications. *Circulation* **83**: 122–136, 1991
32. Palmaz JC, Laborde JC, Rivera FJ *et al.*: Stenting of the iliac arteries with the Palmaz stent:experience from a multicentre trial. *Cardiovasc Intervent Radiol* **15**: 291–296, 1992
33. Rabbia C, Rossato D, Savio D, Margarita G: Lo dtenting percutaneo nel trattamento delle lesion steno-ostruttive iliache. Esperienza con stent Palmaz in 156 pocedure. *Radiol Med (Torino)* **86**: 308–315, 1993
34. Henry M, Amor M, Ethevenot G, Henry I: Percutaneous peripheral rotational ablation

using the Rotablator: Immediate and mid-term results. Single centre experience with 148 lesions treated. *Int Angiol* **12**: 231–237, 1993
35. Strecker EP, Hagen B, Liermann D *et al.*: Iliac and femoropopliteal vascular occlusive disease treated with flexible tantalum stents. *Cardiovasc Intervent Radiol* **16**: 158–165, 1993
36. Vorwerk D, Gunther RW: Stent placement in iliac artery lesions: three years of clinical experience with the Wallstent. *Cardiovasc Intervent Radiol* **15**: 285–291, 1992
37. Strunk HM, Schild HH, Duber C *et al.*: Ergebnisse angiographischer verlaufskontrollen nach percutaner stentimplantaion in beckenarterien mit vergleich zwischen Wall-und Palmaz stent. *Rofo Fortschr Geb Rontgenstr* **159**: 251–257, 1993
38. Do-dai-do, Triller J, Wolpoth BH *et al.*: A comparison study of self-expandable stents vs ballon angioplasty alone in femoropopliteal artery occlusions. *Cardiovasc Intervent Radiol* **15**: 306–312, 1992
39. Van Andel GJ, Van Erp WFM, Krepel VM, Breslau PJ: Percutaneous transluminal dilatation of the iliac artery: Long-term results. *Radiology* **156**: 321–323, 1985
40. Sapoval MR, Long AL, Raynaud AC *et al.*: Femoropopliteal stent replacement: long-term results. *Radiology* **184**: 833–838, 1992
41. Henry M, Amor M, Ethevenot G *et al.*: Long-term follow-up of femoral stenting with Palmaz stent: a single centre experience. Presented at the VIth International Congress for Endovascular Intervention, Phoenix, 1993
42. Sigwart U: Stents: a mechanical solution for a biological problem? *The 1996 Grüntzig Lecture. Eur Heart J* **18**: 1068–1072, 1997

APPENDIX

Method of image normalization

The steps of the image normalization protocol are as follows:

1. *Discard colour information.* The colour information in the digitized image is omitted so that all the processing and analysis is performed on images in grey mode rather than in RGB (red, green, blue) mode.
2. *Measurement of the GSM of blood.* An area of noiseless blood is selected. Using the histogram facility in the programme, the median grey level value of the selected pixels is obtained.
3. *Measurement of the GSM of adventitia.* An echodense piece of adventitia is selected. The measurements of the GSM are made at the brightest part of the adventitia and on the same arterial wall as the plaque. Only the innermost 2/4 of the adventitia are selected along a horizontal band. Areas of low echoes within the band are included.
4. *Measurement of the GSM of plaque.* A temporary logarithmic scaling of the whole image is performed in order to reveal detail in the dark areas and allow a better visualization of the plaque surface. Subsequently the plaque is outlined on the original image and the GSM of the selected area is measured.
5. *Image normalization.* Algebraic (linear) scaling of the whole image is performed using the 'curves' facility of the software. The grey scale is adjusted so that the GSM of blood is in the range of 0–5 (as close to 0 as possible) and that of adventitia in the range of 185–195 (as close to 190 as possible). Thus the grey values of all pixels in the normalized image will change according to the new linear scale defined by the reference values for blood and adventitia.

6. *Measurement of the GSM of blood and adventitia in the normalized image*. Steps 2 and 3 are repeated on the normalized image to ensure that the GSM of blood and adventitia is in the range of 0–5 and 185–195 respectively. If this is not the case the original image is used and steps 2–6 are repeated.
7. *Measurement of the GSM of the plaque in the normalized image*. The plaque is outlined and the GSM of the selected pixels measured. Because the distribution of the grey values of the pixels in the selected area is usually skewed, the median rather than the mean is used for all measurements.

A number of prerequisites should be observed and applied during duplex image acquisition: full dynamic range, linear post-processing curve, TCG curve vertical through the lumen of blood, ultrasonic beam at right angles to the arterial wall, ability to outline the whole plaque proximally and distally, minimization of noise in the blood and availability of an echodense section of adventitia at the vicinity of the plaque. The images are recorded on video and the still images are digitized off-line on a personal computer (PC) using a commercially available video grabber card. Also, it is possible to directly digitize still images on a magneto-optical disk and transfer them to a PC.

By using the full dynamic range the maximum number of grey levels are available. Because the normalization of the image is achieved by linear scaling the original image obtained by the duplex should not be subjected to post-processing curves available to many duplex instruments which are not as close to linear as possible. Although the TGC curve should be sloping so that the grey tones of tissues are the same irrespective of depth, it should be vertical through blood. Because there is relatively little attenuation of ultrasound by blood, this will ensure that the adventitia of the anterior and posterior vessel wall will be of equal brightness.

Ultrasonic images are the result of reflections from tissue interfaces. Adventitia being a key reference point in the normalization process, would provide the optimum image only if the ultrasonic beam is at right angles to it. The operator should ensure optimum image magnification so that the whole plaque is included in the image with a clearly visualized section of adventitia in the vicinity of the plaque. The gain should be adjusted so that areas of blood (vessel lumen) are free of noise. Lack of such an area would make image normalization impossible.

The ability to record images for plaque characterization using the above methodology requires training. For a person experienced in vascular ultrasound this can be achieved in a couple of days. Learning digital image processing of plaques makes the ultrasonographer aware of the essential prerequisites for image acquisition and results not only in a higher quality of images but also in a higher number of images suitable for plaque analysis being obtained.

Commentary

If only we could know in which patients arterial lesions are likely to recur after angioplasty, results would be so much better and more durable. Those which tend to recur might or might not benefit from stent. Any new information in this direction is most valuable. This group have used grey scale median (GSM) of plaque type to attempt to predict where it is easy to squash arterial lesions and to achieve a good result. The authors state that with a low GSM, the process of plaque compression by angioplasty balloon is more effective. These are the more echolucent plaques with higher cholesterol content and seem to be more compressible. This is certainly a start and raises the distinct possibility that plaque type as measured by duplex scan, could steer the clinical procedure in the future. *RMG*

Single centre comparison of iliac artery surgical reconstruction compared with angioplasty with and without stenting

Lutz Reiher, Tomas Pfeiffer and Wilhelm Sandmann

INTRODUCTION

Percutaneous transluminal angioplasty (PTA) with or without application of stents is nowadays generally regarded as standard treatment of short length arterial occlusive disease (AOD) of iliac arteries. In our practice, however, we see an increasing number of patients with restenosis in iliac vessels after this treatment. In order to estimate the efficacy of surgical and endovascular approaches in this region we analysed our patients treated by thrombendartectomy or PTA and followed the results for durability.

PATIENTS

From January 1988 until April 1994, 256 patients were treated for stenosis or occlusion of iliac arteries either by thrombendartectomy (TEA) of the aortic bifurcation or of iliac arteries (184 patients) or PTA of iliac arteries (72 patients). Preoperative or preinterventional data are summarized in Table 1. The decision whether to perform PTA or TEA was taken in a conference of vascular surgeons and interventional radiologists: PTA was applied in patients with short segmental

Table 1. Patients' characteristics and stage of arterial occlusive disease before TEA or PTA

	TEA		*PTA*	
No of patients	184		72	
No of lower extremities	234		76	
Sex	m 131	w 53	64	10
Mean age	60.7 (28–85) years		57.0 (29–78) years	
	n	%	*n*	%
Claudication	119	64.7	34	97.1
Rest pain	28	15.2	2	5.7
Necrosis or gangrene	39	21.2	0	

TEA: Thrombendartectomy.
PTA: Percutaneous transluminal angioplasty.

stenosis of common or external iliac arteries; within the area of arterial bifurcations, it was avoided. Also, PTA was not performed, if the iliac arteries were occluded. A stent was placed in six cases to keep the dilated segment open.

The mean age ot the patients in the TEA group, which contained relatively more patients with severe limb ischaemia, was slightly higher, than in the PTA group but risk factors were numerous in the two groups (Table 2). In 50 patients of the surgical group, including 48 patients with disease of the aortic bifurcation, the iliac arteries were reconstructed on both sides. This never happened in the angioplasty group, because the disease was more limited. In 104 surgical patients there was an additional arterial reconstruction in the groin or below (Table 3). Again, the arterial

Table 2. Risk factors and history

	TEA		*PTA*	
	n	%	*n*	%
Smoking	137	74.5	30	85.7
Cerebrovascular disease	103	56.0	9	25.7
Hypertension	98	53.3	21	60.0
Hyperlipidemia	86	46.7	15	42.9
Coronary heart disease	69	37.5	20	57.1
Diabetes	43	23.4	8	22.9
History of myocardial infarction	41	22.3	8	22.9
Patients with 1 or 2 risk factors	68	37	8	22.9
Patients with 3 or more risk factors	116	63	27	77.1
Patients with previous operation of concerned vessels	13	7	1	2.9
Patients with previous balloon angioplasty of concerned vessels	10	5	1	2.9

TEA: Thrombendartectomy.
PTA: Percutaneous transluminal angioplasty.

Table 3. Site of TEA/PTA and additional operations

	TEA		*PTA*	
	n	%	*n*	%
Site of TEA/PTA				
aortic bifurcation	48		0	
Common iliac artery	162		8	
External iliac artery	160		18	
Internal iliac artery	20		0	
Location of PTA not specified in protocol[a]			56	
No of patients with additional operations	104	56.5	0	
TEA or patch plasty of arteries in the groin	79			
Bypass to femoral or below-knee arteries	56			
Renal artery TEA	8			

TEA: Thrombendartectomy.
PTA: Percutaneous transluminal angioplasty.
[a] No differentiation was made between common or external iliac artery.

disease in the PTA group was less extensive and distal reconstructions were not necessary.

METHODS

Patients' clinical records were reviewed for the stage of disease, risk factors, therapeutic procedures, and early outcome. Patients were invited for an outpatient examination, for interview about their further postoperative/postinterventional course, a duplex examination of their iliac and groin arteries, and measurement of ancle pressure indices.

EARLY RESULTS

As many patients of the PTA group were sent to our radiologists from other hospitals or teams we had preinterventional information in only 36 cases. There were two deaths in the surgical group within 30 days of operation but no deaths in the PTA group. The attempt to dilate an iliac artery stenosis was not successful in one case. We observed an early occlusion of the operated or dilated arteries in eight and five cases respectively (Table 4).

Table 4. Early complications after TEA and PTA

Early postoperative complications in 50 patients	*TEA*		*PTA*	
	n	%	*n*	%
Death (< 30 days)	2	1.1	0	
Occlusion of lower arteries	12	6.5	0	
Wound infection (delayed healing)	10	5.4	0	
Occlusion at site of TEA	8	4.3	5	6.6
Bleeding, requiring reoperation	7	3.8	0	
Others	9	4.9	0	

TEA: Thrombendartectomy.
PTA: Percutaneous transluminal angioplasty.

LATE RESULTS

During the follow-up there were further interventions below the groin, and more major amputations in the TEA group, but fewer late deaths (Fig.1), and fewer secondary operations at the site of the primary endarterectomy (Table 5). The re-examination revealed more patent iliac arteries in the surgical group but we found only a trend and no statistical difference if compared with PTA (Table 6).

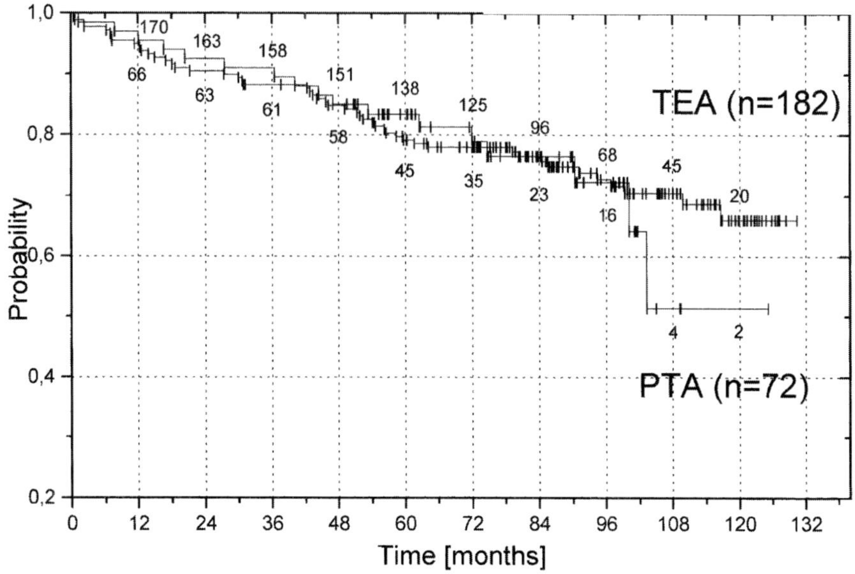

Fig. 1. Kaplan-Meyer survival analysis of 182 patients undergoing thrombendartectomy (TEA) and percutaneous transluminal angioplasty (PTA) of the iliac arteries.

Table 5. Events during follow-up

	TEA		*PTA*	
	n	*%*	*n*	*%*
Death during follow-up	67	36.4	14	19.4
Follow-up examination	67	36.4	31	43.1
Examination refused	43	23.4	19	26.4
Lost to follow-up	5	2.7	8	11.1
Secondary intervention at site of TEA/PTA	19	8.1	8	10.5
Major amputation during follow-up	6	2.6	1	1.3
Further intervention below the groin	19	8.1	4	5.3

TEA: Thrombendartectomy.
PTA: Percutaneous transluminal angioplasty.

Table 6. Late results after TEA/PTA

Follow-up examination	*TEA*		*PTA*	
	n	*%*	*n*	*%*
No of patients	67	36.4	31	43.1
No of concerned legs	93	39.7	34	44.7
Patent iliac arteries	55	59.1	14	41.2
Moderate stenosis	19	20.4	13	38.2
Severe stenosis	5	5.4	4	11.8
Occlusion	4	4.3	1	2.9
Second intervention during follow-up	10	10.8	2	5.9

DISCUSSION

The anatomic distribution and extent of arteriosclerosis was greater in the surgery group; nevertheless there was a higher iliac patency rate in this group. This was also found in other studies.[1,2] The anatomic distribution of arteriosclerosis has a high impact on results of therapy, of both types.[3–5] As mentioned above, the indication for PTA was only made in cases of a favourable anatomic situation. Patients with more widespread disease were assumed to be candidates for surgery.

CONCLUSION

Only a prospective randomized study could clearly compare these groups but we can draw some conclusions from our findings.

At present we see no reason to change our policy as to the indication for angioplasty or surgery: PTA has poorer long-term results despite being performed for milder diseases. There is no logic in performing angioplasty in more elderly patients with worse risks as restenosis is more likely in our view.

REFERENCES

1. Becquemin JP, Cavillon A, Allaire E *et al.*: Iliac and femoropopliteal lesions: Evaluation of balloon angioplasty and classical surgery. *J Endovasc Surg* **2:** 42–50, 1995
2. Wilson SE, Wolf GL, Cross AP: Percutaneous transluminal angioplasty versus operation for peripheral arteriosclerosis. *J Vasc Surg* **9:** 1–9, 1989
3. Labode JC, Palmaz JC, Rivera FJ *et al.*: Influence of anatomic distribution of atherosclerosis on the outcome of revascularization with iliac stent placement. *J Vasc Intervent Radiol* **4:** 513–521, 1995
4. Johnston KW: Iliac arteries: reanalysis of results of balloon angioplasty. *Radiology* **186:** 207–212, 1993
5. Oertli D, Wigger P, Landmann J *et al.*: Long-term results after open and semiclosed thrombendarterectomy for aortoiliac occlusive disease. *Eur J Vasc Endovasc Surg* **11:** 432–436, 1996

Commentary

The value of this experience is that it is a single centre experience but as the authors have said, angioplasty or surgical endarterectomy are performed for totally different indications. In addition, patients with angioplasty have many data gaps because they are referred to radiologists and this is typical of the experience of many vascular surgeons. The authors correctly conclude that the only way to know the answer in terms of durability comparisons would be to perform a random controlled trial, but they imply that such a trial would be inappropriate because they would prefer to use balloon angioplasty for unilateral lesions and for mild lesions. On the other hand, they are inclined to surgery for more severe lesions. It is much the same story here as it is for renal artery stenosis. Sometims it is just extremely difficult to achieve an equipoise view in the minds of surgeons and patients so that a random controlled trial can be performed. Perhaps one important finding is mentioned by the authors which is that despite surgical patients having more severe arterial disease, the patency of surgical patients is better than that of angioplasty patients. They therefore imply that if a patient is quite sick, it may not necessarily always be the right move to call for the lesser procedure of angioplasty because in their opinion, restenosis occurs more frequently in that group. They imply that their view is towards surgery and removal of the disease once and for all rather than relying upon angioplasty which they imply is fraught with restenosis. This is the prejudiced view which emerges from this chapter from a single centre experience, but the authors are quite fair in making plain that their experience of surgery and angiography are of completely different groups of patients. *RMG*

The durability of percutaneous transluminal angioplasty of the renal artery

George Geroulakos and Gianni Belcaro

INTRODUCTION

Renal artery stenosis may be the cause of hypertension, impairment of renal function and decreased survival. Only 4% of patients with hypertension have non-essential hypertension and in the majority of them the hypertension is related to renovascular disease.[1] By definition, ischaemic nephropathy represents extraparenchymal renal artery obliterative disease in association with decreased renal excretory function. The precise prevalence of ischaemic nephropathy is not known. Similarly it is unknown how often it progresses to end-stage renal failure. However, in a series of 182 patients with irreversible renal failure on dialysis, a renovascular cause for their renal failure was found in 16.5%.[2]

The goals of renal artery angioplasty are to cure the renovascular hypertension and to improve or stabilize renal function. The first percutaneous transluminal renal artery angioplasty (PTRA) was reported in 1978 by Gruentzig.[3] Since then refinements in balloon catheter technology, the introduction of digital subtraction angiography which decreased the length of the procedure and the contrast load and the wide experience gained with this technique in various centres, have contributed to the establishment of PTRA as an important option for the management of selected patients with renal artery stenosis. The aim of this chapter is to review the literature on the long-term results of PTRA. Rutherford has suggested that long-term results should not only be presented in the best possible light with initial failures excluded and we would agree with this perspective.[4]

INITIAL TECHNICAL SUCCESS

There is no uniform agreement on what constitutes technical success which is determined from the immediate post-PTRA angiogram. Martin *et al.*[5] in a large series of 110 patients who underwent PTRA defined as technical success the safe crossing and dilatation of the stenosis with no major morbidity, a residual stenosis of less than 50% and a residual pressure gradient of less than 10%. By contrast, Weibull defined as technical success the total elimination of the stenosis, while the treatment was deemed a technical failure if this result was not achieved.[6] In another study on the clinical outcome of PTRA in 320 patients, success was defined as residual stenosis of 30% or less and failure was defined as residual stenosis that exceeded 30% or the inability to reach or cross the lesion.[7] This unfortunate absence of universally accepted reporting standards makes comparisons at times difficult. However, if we assume that the underlying disorder is atherosclerosis it is important to recognize that the technical failure rate of first angioplasty in medical centres with the most experience averages 12% (range 0–25%).[8]

Ostial atherosclerotic lesions are associated with a high incidence of technical failure. A stenosis is considered ostial if the proximal 4mm of the renal artery lumen is involved.[5] These lesions may be the result of a well localized atherosclerotic plaque at the origin of the renal artery. This type of stenosis responds well to PTRA. Extensive atherosclerotic changes of the lumen of the aorta can also produce a stenosis at the ostium of the renal artery. Angioplasty of these stenoses is associated with a high incidence of elastic recoil. An increased percentage of successful outcome of ostial PTRA depends on the ability to differentiate between these two types of lesions which is often imposible.

In patients with postostial lesions the technical success rate has been excellent. These lesions, however, comprise only 15–20% of all atherosclerotic renal artery lesions.[9]

In a large series of 250 attempted PTRA the technical success for unilateral ostial atherosclerosis was 29% (4/14) while the success for postostial atherosclerosis was 94.5% (103/109) which was statistically highly significant ($p<0.001$).[10]

Also, PTRA is highly effective for treating patients with fibrous dysplasia of the renal arteries. In a meta-analysis of 370 patients with fibrous dysplasia of the renal arteries who presented with secondary hypertension, PTRA was considered technically successful in 94% (324/345) of the 345 patients in whom the data were available.[11] Patients with fibrous dysplasia of the renal arteries tend to be younger and healthier than patients with atherosclerotic renal artery disease.

COMPLICATIONS

Renal angioplasty may be considered a safe procedure only when immediate access to surgical expertise is available and safe routines for dealing with complications are established.[12] Trauma to the renal artery requiring emergency surgery may occur. These complications may make surgery more difficult and occasionally a nephrectomy may be indicated. Martin *et al.*[5] in a series of 110 patients with PTRA reported four patients who developed occlusion of the renal artery during the PTRA. Three were treated with a bypass graft and one with a thrombectomy.

The experience of others has been similar. In a smaller series of 50 patients who underwent PTRA for renovascular hypertension three patients required surgical intervention for technical failures. One had an aortorenal bypass and two underwent nephrectomies.[13]

Mortality rates associated with PTRA are approximatelly 2% (range 0–29).[5,7,10,14,15] Reported causes of death include diffuse cholesterol embolization,[7,14,16] retropertitoneal haematoma,[14] cerebrovascular accident[7] and complications related to aortic surgery.[7] A detailed analysis of complications of PTRA in four large series is given in Table 1. The most common complication in these series was contrast-induced acute renal failure. The acute renal impairement is temporary but permanent chronic renal failure requiring dialysis is a very small but real risk.[7,14]

Table 1. Complications secondary to renal artery angioplasty

	Bonelli[7]	*Martin*[5]	*Beart*[10]	*Canzanello*[14]
Number of patients	320	120	202	100
Deaths within 30 days	7			3
Subintimal dissections	18		1	1
Renal artery perforations /ruptures	4		2	
Main renal artery thrombosis	2	3	3	2
Renal embolization	2		5	7
Other embolization	1			1
Haematoma treated with surgery	2	2		
Cerebrovascular accident	1	1		
Myocardial infarction	1			
Acute renal failure	18	4	6	30

LONG-TERM RESULTS AFTER PTRA FOR RENAL ARTERY STENOSIS

Anatomic results

In most studies the durability of PTRA is reported on the basis of functional outcome rather than anatomic results. Thus the long-term results are based on the effect of this procedure on the blood pressure and serum creatinine. The lack of documentation on the anatomic outcome in most studies is due to the reluctance of most clinicians to perform repeat arteriography mainly because of the invasive nature of this modality and the risk of contrast-induced nephrotoxocity. On the other hand, duplex ultrasonography, which is a non-invasive technique of proven validity in documenting the natural history of renal artery stenosis, has not so far gained wide acceptance because it is a technically difficult examination and the good results reported in selected centres have not been universally reproduced.

There is a poor correlation following PTRA, between functional clinical outcome and anatomic results. Angiographic stenosis may recur without relapse of the hypertension. In one study, follow-up angiography (2–18 months) in 18 patients showed restenosis of the renal artery in seven. Relapse of the hypertension was observed in only three patients.[17] Tullis *et al.*[18] recently reported a series of 18 patients with renovascular hypertension who underwent PTRA and were followed up for a mean of 28 months with duplex. Two patients were cured, five of six who improved had a final duplex stenosis greater than 60% and six of ten failures had a final duplex diagnosis of normal renal arteries. Therefore, studies based on clinical outcome alone without a follow-up imaging examination cannot determine the anatomical durability of PTRA.

Restenoses are more frequently seen in renal arteries presenting with mild residual stenosis compared with those without a residual stenosis as determined by duplex on day 2 following PTRA.[19] Table 2 summarizes the anatomical intermediate and long-term outcome of PTRA. It demonstrates that in five series the cumulative incidence of restenosis after a first successful PTRA is 25% for a mean follow-up of 20 months.

Table 2. Restenosis after a first PTRA

Author/year	*No. of renal arteries*	*Length of follow-up (months)*	*Method of follow-up*	*Restenosis rate (%)*
Weibull 1991[23]	71	56	Angiography	55
Plouin 1993[20]	92	8.8	Angiography	16
Tullis 1997[18]	40	12	Duplex	18
Jensen 1995[12]	180	12	Angiography	13
Baumgartner 1997[19]	63	12	Duplex	27
TOTAL	446	20		25

Effect on hypertension

The functional outcome of PTRA on blood pressure is evident primarily in more effective control with fewer medications rather than cure. Bonelli reported the clinical outcome of PTRA in 320 patients and observed that the maximum benefit on the blood pressure occurred in the 48-hour period after angioplasty.[7] He concluded that if the post-PTRA result is not optimal, further long-term improvement is unlikely.

In all studies definition of cure of hypertension after PTRA required that patients were able to stop taking antihypertensive medication. In addition, in most studies, cure was considered a diastolic blood pressure of 90 mm Hg or less, thus ignoring the contribution of the systolic blood pressure component. Only a few reports considered as clinically cured, patients with resultant systolic blood pressure of 140 mm Hg and diastolic pressure of 90 mm Hg or less.[7,19] The definitions of improvement are complex and more variable. These are based on a percentage fall in the blood pressure and a reduction in medication. Improvement is usually defined as either a 15% reduction in the diastolic pressure or a diastolic pressure less than 90 mm Hg with the patient taking less antihypertensive medication than before the procedure. Ramsay in a review of published series on the blood pressure response to angioplasty observed that no study used exactly the same definition for improvement.[21] Standardization of reporting definitions including consideration of antihypertensive medication is essential in future studies.

A summary of data from six series on the long-term results of PTRA on hypertension in patients with atherosclerotic renal artery stenosis is shown in Table 3. Baseline patient characteristics which have been reported as predictors of reduced benefit from PTRA on hypertension include insulin-dependent diabetes, symptoms or history of atherosclerosis in other organs, age older than 70 years,[5] unilateral renal artery stenosis in patients who have a decreased renal artery end-diastolic ratio in the contralateral kidney[22] and a long duration of treatment with antihypertensive medication.[7]

Table 4 shows the effect of PTRA on hypertension in patients with fibromuscular dysplasia of the renal artery. The cumulative percentage of patients who were cured or improved from this procedure is 87% over a mean follow-up of 28 months. These excellent results can be well compared with those of reconstructive vascular surgery. Therefore PTRA is currently considered as the initial treatment of choice for patients with fibromuscular dysplasia of the main renal artery.[24]

Table 3. Blood pressure response to PTRA in patients with atherosclerotic renal artery stenosis

Author/year	*No. of patients*	*Cure (%)*	*Improved (%)*	*Follow-up (months)*
Canzanello 1989[14]	100	4	39	29
Beart 1990[10]	141	28	32	25.1
Weibull 1991[23]	61	15	75	56
Bonelli 1995[7]	188	8.4	61.6	33.3
Von Knorring 1996[13]	27	11	74	48
Baumgartner 1997[19]	35	8.6	45.7	12
TOTAL	552	11	54	32

Table 4. Blood pressure response to PTRA in patients with fibromuscular renal artery stenosis

Author/year	*No. of patients*	*Cure (%)*	*Improved (%)*	*Follow-up (months)*
Sos 1983[25]	31	59	33	16
Beart 1990[10]	19	58	21	25
Tegtmeyer 1991[24]	66	39	59	39
Jensen 1995[12]	30	36	43	12
Bonelli 1995[7]	120	22	63	42.5
Von Knorring 1996[13]	11	45	55	48
TOTAL	277	42	45	28

Effect on renal function

Renal artery stenosis may be associated with impairment of renal function. Natural history studies have shown that progression of renal artery stenosis occurs at a rate of approximately 20% per year. Progression to occlusion is associated with a marked decrease in kidney length.[26] There is no evidence at present that this natural history can be improved by PTRA. However, in a number of patients, PTRA may produce a durable improvement or stabilization of the renal function. A 15% reduction in serum creatinine in the most recent follow-up is assumed to represent significant improvement in renal function. An increase of greater than 15% in serum creatinine indicates deterioration in renal function and stabilization is considered when postoperative creatinine in the last follow-up visit is within 15% of the preoperative level. Using the above criteria, Weibull *et al.*[23] in a series of 23 patients with renal impairement who were treated with PTRA, showed improvement of the serum creatinine in 16 (49%) patients. In 13 (39%) patients renal function was stabilized while in four (12%) it deteriorated at the end of 12 months follow-up. Similar findings were reported by Baumgartner[19] in a series of 22 patients with impaired renal function who underwent PTRA: 12(54%) improved and in six (28%) the renal function was stabilized at the end of 12 months follow-up.

CONCLUSION

Since the first PTRA in 1978, a number of well documented reports have given us a better understanding of the merit of PTRA and its role in the management of renovascular disease. There is now general agreement that PTRA should be the initial treatment of choice for patients with non-ostial stenosis and renal artery fibromuscular dysplasia. Both technical and functional results are very good and are comparable with surgery for this group of patients.[27–29] By contrast, the evidence is less clear for patients with ostial stenosis. This group comprises the majority of patients with atherosclerotic renovascular disease. In these patients PTRA is associated with a high incidence of elastic recoil and restenosis due to intima hyperplasia or recurrent atherosclerotic disease. Some have advocated stenting for ostial stenosis.[30] However, a number of recent series have reported modest results at follow-up following a high immediate technical success.[18,31]

Finally it should appreciated that PTRA is not a benign procedure. Complications can occur and be serious occasionally leading to death, emergency surgical revascularization of the kidney or nephrectomy.

REFERENCES

1. Working Group on Renovascular Hypertension: First report on the Working Group on Renovascular Hypertension. *Arch Intern Med* **147**: 820–829, 1987
2. Mailloux LU, Bellucci AG, Mossey RT *et al.*: Predictors of survival in patients undergoing dialysis. *Am J Med* **84**: 855–862, 1988
3. Gruentzig A, Kuhlmann U, Vetter W *et al.*: Treatment of renovascular hypertension with percutaneous transluminal dilatation of a renal artery stenosis. *Lancet* **i**: 801–802, 1978
4. Rutherford RB: Reporting standards for long-term results of vascular surgery. In Yao J, Pearce W (Eds) *Long-term Results in Vascular Surgery* pp. 1–8. Stamford CT: Appleton and Lange, 1993
5. Martin L, Cork RD, Kaufman SL: Long-term results of angioplasty in 110 patients with renal artery stenosis. *JVIR* **3**: 627–632, 1992
6. ibull H, Bergqvist D, Bergentz SE *et al.*: Percutaneous transluminal renal angioplasty versus surgical reconstruction of atherosclerotic renal artery stenosis: A prospective randomized study. *J Vasc Surg* 18**:** 841–852, 1993
7. Bonelli FS, McKuisick M, Textor SC *et al.*: Renal artery angioplasty: Technical results and outcome in 320 patients. *Mayo Clin Proc* **70**: 1041–1052, 1995
8. Pickering TG, Mann SJ: Renovascular hypertension: medical evaluation and non-surgical treatment. In : Laragh JH, Brenner BM (Eds) *Hypertension: Pathophysiology, Diagnosis and Management* (2nd edn) pp. 2039–2054. New York: Raven Press, 1995
9. Novick AC: Options for therapy of ischaemic nephropathy: Role of angioplasty and surgery. *Semin Nephrol* **16**: 53–60, 1996
10. Beart AL, Wilms G, Amery A *et al.*: Percutaneous transluminal renal angioplasty: Initial results and long-term follow-up in 202 patients. *Cardiovasc Intervent Radiol* **13**: 22–28, 1990
11. Tegtmeyer TC, Matsumoto AH, Angle JF: Percutaneous transluminal angioplasty in fibrous dysplasia and children. In: Novick A, Scoble J, Hamilton G (Eds) *Renal Vascular Disease* pp. 363–383. London: WB Saunders, 1996
12. Jensen G, Zachrisson BF, Delin K *et al.*: Treatment of renovascular hypertension: One year results of renal angioplasty . *Kidney Int* **48**: 1936–1945, 1995
13. Von Knorring J, Edgren J, Lepantalo M: Long-term results of percutaneous transluminal angioplasty in renovascular hypertension. *Acta Radiologica* **37**: 36–40, 1996

14. Canzanello VJ, Millan VG, Spiegel JE *et al.*: Percutaneous transluminal renal angioplasty in management of atherosclerotic renovascular hypertension: Results in 100 patients. *Hypertension* **13**: 163–172, 1989
15. O'Donovan RM, Gutierrez OH, Izzo JL Jr: Preservation of renal function by percutaneous renal angioplasty in high risk elderly patients: short-term outcome. *Nephron* **60**: 187–192, 1992
16. Geroulakos G, Homer-Vanniasinkam S, Wilkinson A, Galloway I: Cholesterol embolisation. A lethal complication of instrumentation of an aneurysmal aorta: a case report. *Int Angiol* **16**: 69–71, 1997
17. Rees CR, Palmaz JC, Becker GJ *et al.*: Palmaz stent in atherosclerotic stenoses involving the ostia of the renal arteries: preliminary report of a multicentre study. *Radiology* **181**: 507–514, 1991
18. Tullis MJ, Zierler RE, Glickerman *et al.*: Results of percutaneous transluminal angioplasty for atherosclerotic renal artery stenosis: A follow up study with duplex ultrasonography. *J Vasc Surg* **25**: 46–54, 1997
19. Baumgartner I, Triller J, Mahler F: Patency of percutaneous transluminal renal angioplasty: A prospective sonographic study. *Kidney Int* **51**: 798–803, 1997
20. Plouin PF, Darne B, Chatellier G *et al.*: Restenosis after a first percutaneous transluminal renal angioplasty. *Hypertension* **21**: 89–96, 1993
21. Ramsay LE, Waller PC: Blood pressure response to percutaneous transluminal angioplasty for renovascular hypertension : an overview of published series. *Br Med J* **300**: 569–572, 1990
22. Tullis MJ, Zierler RE, Caps MT *et al.*: Clinical evidence of contralateral renal parenchymal injury in patients with unilateral atherosclerotic renal artery stenosis. *Ann Vasc Surg* **12**: 122–127, 1998
23. Weibull H, Bergqvist D, Jonsson K *et al.*: Long-term results after percutaneous transluminal angioplasty of atherosclerotic renal artery stenosis. The importance of intensive follow-up. *Eur J Vasc Surg* **5**: 291–301, 1991
24. Tegtmeyer CJ, Selby JB, Hartwell GD *et al.*: Results and complications of angioplasty in fibromuscular disease. *Circulation* **13** (Suppl I): 155–161, 1991
25. Sos TA, Pickering TG, Sniderman K *et al.*: Percutaneous transluminal renal angioplasty in renovascular hypertension due to atheroma or fibromuscular dysplasia. *New Engl J Med* **309**: 274–279, 1983
26. Zierler RE, Bergelin RO, Isaacson JA, Strandness DE Jr: Natural history of atherosclerotic renal artery stenosis: A prospective study with Duplex ultrasonography. *J Vasc Surg* **19**: 250–258, 1994
27. Geroulakos G, Wright JG, Tober JC *et al.*: Use of splenic and hepatic artery for renal revascularization in patients with atherosclerotic renal artery disease. *Ann Vasc Surg* **11**: 85–89, 1997
28. Ames R: Angioplasty for renal artery stenosis. *J Am Med Assoc* **275**: 1476, 1996
29. Novick AC: Percutaneous transluminal angioplasty and surgery of the renal artery. *Eur J Vasc Surg* **8**: 1–9, 1994
30. Harden PN, MacLeod MJ, Rodger RSC *et al.*: Effect of renal artery stenting on progression of renovascular renal failure. *Lancet* **349**: 1133–1136, 1997
31. Fiala LA, Jackson MR, Gillespie DL *et al.*: Primary stenting of atherosclerosic renal artery ostial stenosis. *Ann Vasc Surg* **12**: 128–133, 1998

Commentary

The role of percutaneous transluminal angioplasty of the renal artery is summarized here and one is struck once again by the difficulty in comparing this technique with the surgical alternative. It seems that most will prefer angioplasty in one situation and arterial reconstruction in another and so it is not easy to set up a random controlled trial to settle the matter. The view seems to emerge that if angioplasty is durable and satisfactory, then it is preferable to surgical reconstruction in patients suitable for angioplasty. Once this bias is established, it is very difficult to recommend a random controlled trial. Consequently, any information we can acquire on the durability of renal artery angioplasty is of very great value. *RMG*

The durability of carotid angioplasty and stenting

PA Gaines

INTRODUCTION

Stroke is the third most common cause of death in the Western World and is the principle cause of prolonged neurological morbidity.[1] In the UK 125 000 patients suffer their first stroke each year and this reflects on a 10% usage of NHS bed days and 5% of the annual healthcare expenditure.[2,3] Stroke principally affects the older population and because of the relative increase in this part of the population the overall instances of stroke could increase by 30% by the year 2033.[4]

Not surprisingly stroke prevention is important for the health of the nation, and must be both cheap and accessible to the elderly. The major single cause of carotid territory infarction is thromboembolic disease but unfortunately only 20% of major stokes are heralded by more minor neurological embolic symptoms (transient ischaemic attack (TIA), amaurosis fugax, recovered stroke). A purely haemodynamic stroke accounts for only 1–2% of all strokes.[5] Patients with a TIA have seven times the risk of stroke over the next 7 years compared with a person with no TIAs. The actuarial risk of stroke is approximately 11.6% during the first year after TIA and approximately 5.9% per year of the first 5 years. With increasing stenosis of the ipsilateral internal carotid artery the risk increases by up to 28 ± 8 % over 2 years.[6] Medical therapy directed towards limiting thromboemboli from the unstable carotid plaque, principally using anti-platelet agents, has reduced the risk of stroke in the cohort of patients. Two large multicentre surgical trials have demonstrated a significant reduction in the risk of stroke following carotid endarterectomy in medically fit patients with recent symptoms and an ipsilateral severe carotid stenosis.[6,7] The overall benefit from carotid endarterectomy balances the risk of stroke at the time of surgery (7.5% in the European Carotid Surgery Trial (ECST), 5.8% in North American Symptomatic Carotid Endarterectomy Trial (NASCET)) against the stroke prophylaxis derived from removing the atherosclerotic material. In NASCET, after 2 years, the risk of any stroke was reduced from 27.6% in the medically treated patients to 12.6% in the carotid endarterectomy group. Any major stroke or death was reduced from 18.1% in the medical group to 8% in the surgical group. Similarly, in ECST, after 3 years, the risk of any disabling or fatal stroke (including surgically related death) was reduced from 11% in the medical group to 6% in the surgical group. In the same trial any stroke lasting longer than 7 days (or surgical death) was reduced from 22% to 12% after 3 years.

WHY BOTHER WITH ENDOVASCULAR TECHNIQUES?

The value of carotid endarterectomy relies on the balance between the eventual stroke prophylaxis and the major events surrounding surgery. Symptomatic patients with a tight carotid stenosis (greater than 70%) had a 3.7% risk of disabling stroke and death within 30 days of surgery in ECST. This rose to 7.5% if all strokes of more than 7 days were included. Similarly within NASCET there was a 2.1% risk of major stroke and death related to surgery and a 5.8% risk of all perioperative stroke and death.

In addition NASCET detailed further surgical complications including cranial nerve injury (7.6%), wound haematoma (5.5%), wound infection (3.4%), myocardial infarction (0.9%), congestive heart failure (0.6%) and other cardiovascular problems (1.2%). Whilst it may be that performing endarterectomy under local anaesthesia may remove some of these risks of surgery, as yet data has not yet been provided to substantiate this claim.

Clearly any new therapeutic intervention that is not associated with the risks of general anaesthesia, or neck incision, be they endovascular or pharmaceutical, would be worth pursuing, so long as they had a good risk benefit ratio and was financially prudent. Carotid angioplasty and stenting has the potential to achieve these aims and theoretically it is capable of converting high-risk unstable plaque into a smooth, non-embologenic lesion. The end-point of most damage to vessel wall is the production of a smooth area of myointimal hyperplasia. This has been demonstrated both following surgical intervention and endovascular intervention in the arterial system. The ability to convert carotid plaque into a smooth lesion is clearly there with simple balloon angioplasty. Stents offer the additional potential to reduce carotid dissection, increase the initial lumen gain, and probably restrict distal embolization. The 30-day safety of endovascular manoeuvres on symptomatic and asymptomatic carotid plaque has been demonstrated in the literature.[8] Of particular interest may be the application of endovascular techniques to those patients thought to be at high risk of stroke and death following carotid endarterectomy. The relevant risk factors have been identified by Rothwell and colleagues[9] as cerebral TIAs (rather than monocular), the presence of peripheral vascular disease, occlusion of the contralateral internal carotid artery, hypertension (systolic blood pressure greater than 180 mm Hg), stenosis of the ipsilateral external carotid artery, stenosis of distal ipsilateral internal carotid artery, female sex and age greater than 75 years. It should be noted that some of these high risk groups were specifically excluded from NASCET.

The 30-day major stroke and death rates of endovascular techniques have been presented in the literature. The question raised by this article is whether endovascular intervention on carotid arteries is durable.

THE DURABILITY OF ANGIOPLASTY OR STENTING OF THE INTERNAL CAROTID ARTERY

Durability refers to the quality of lasting, or permanence. The endovascular management of symptomatic carotid disease is a prophylactic procedure performed with the intention of preventing stroke and death. Clearly, if it is to have any place, it should be an improvement upon the best medical therapy, and compare favourably with if not better than conventional carotid endarterectomy.

Comparison against medical therapy

The long-term data published in peer reviewed literature regarding the long-term prophylaxis following endovascular management of carotid disease are very limited. Eckert[10] performed angioplasty on 58 patients with symptomatic internal carotid stenosis greater than 70% and had a procedural major stroke rate of 1.6% (with no deaths); 53 patients were followed up between 3 and 48 months with a mean of 16 months. In this time interval there were two cardiac deaths, one stroke death in a patient who had failed angioplasty and refused endarterectomy, and one stroke in a patient who had undergone what appeared to be a successful angioplasty. Unfortunately these data are not presented as any form of survival analysis (life table or Kaplan-Meier).

Gil-Peralta[11] (Table 1) attempted carotid angioplasty on 82 patients with symptomatic carotid disease greater than 70%. Duplex and clinical examination obtained close follow-up. The team failed in five cases (6%). The 30-day complication rate was zero mortality and four patients with disabling stroke (4.9%). Subsequent follow-up data using Kaplan-Meier survival curves report freedom from ipsilateral disabling ischaemic stroke in 95%, freedom from ipsilateral disabling stroke or death in 91.5%, and freedom from any ipsilateral stroke or death in 86.7%. It should be noted that numbers of patients followed up for 4 years are small and unfortunately the authors do not present tables from which to deduce the success of the procedure at other time intervals.

The group working out of University of Alabama, Birmingham report on 228 patients with stenoses greater than 60% treated with carotid stents; they found a cumulative survival, free of any stroke or neurological death, of 94 ± 2% at 1 year and 91 ± 3% at 2 years (Table 1).[12] Unfortunately these data combine patients with symptomatic and asymptomatic (132 patients) disease.

To make a meaningful comparison of these data the medical limbs of the ECST and NASCET were interrogated since they have reviewed a group of patients with similar clinical and stenotic profiles. Unfortunately, such a comparison is very difficult because the two trials do not use similar definitions of major stroke or

Table 1.

Gil-Peralta, Freedom from, at 4 years	%
Ipsilateral disabling ischaemic stroke	95.0
Ipsilateral disabling stroke or vascular death	91.5
Any ipsilateral stroke or death	86.7
University of Alabama, Birmingham	%
Freedom from any stroke or neurological death at 1 year	94±2
Freedom from any stroke or neurological death at 2 years	91±3

outcome definitions. Clearly a serious attempt at standardizing outcomes of carotid intervention are required.

Against the Gil-Peralta data (Table 1) within NASCET the rate for freedom from major or fatal ipsilateral stroke of 2 years was 86.9%, and freedom from any ipsilateral ischaemic stroke at 2 years was 74%. In ECST patients on best medical therapy had a rate for freedom from major stroke at 3 years of 83% and freedom from any ipsilateral disabling or fatal stroke of 91.6%.

To compare data against that of the Birmingham Group (Table 1), 2-year data in both NASCET and ECST were used. In the medical group of NASCET freedom from any major or fatal stroke was 86.9%, any stroke or death 67.7%, and any major stroke or death 81.9%. Within ECST, freedom from any stroke lasting more than 7 days in the medical group was 81% and freedom from any disabling or fatal stroke was 90%.

Any comparison is necessarily crude but it would appear that on the available published data to date endovascular therapy offers an advantage over the best medical therapy.

Comparison against surgery

Comparison against surgery is fraught with the same issues. Again, the data from the two major surgical trials have been used.

Against the Gil-Peralta data (Table 1), in the surgical group of NASCET, freedom from major or fatal ipsilateral stroke at 2 years was 96.3% and freedom from any ipsilateral ischaemic stroke was 91%. Within the ECST, freedom from any stroke lasting greater than 7 days at 3 years was 97.2%.

For comparison against the Birmingham Group (Table 1), 2-year data from NASCET and ECST was again chosen. In NASCET, freedom from any major or fatal stroke was 96.3%, any stroke or death 84.2%, and any major stroke or death 81.9%. In the ECST, freedom from any stroke lasting more than 7 days or surgical death was 89%, or any disabling or fatal stroke or surgical death was 95%.

Again, any comparison will be necessarily crude but the outcome data between surgery and endovascular techniques do appear to be comparable.

Restenosis

A less clinically useful assessment of durability is the restenosis rate following endovascular intervention compared with that of carotid endarterectomy. Once again, any meaningful comparison is bedevilled by the lack of uniformity of reporting standards. Eckert reported a 6% re-stenosis rate. Neither a definition nor a time interval were provided. Munari reported a 16% re-stenosis rate where re-stenosis was defined as a greater than 30% stenosis.[13] Unfortunately, the time interval is not defined. Yadav and colleagues reported a re-stenosis rate following stent placement of 4.9% where re-stenosis was defined as a stenosis greater than 50%.[14] All patients were asymptomatic, but so were 41% of their patients before treatment. Gil-Peralta reported a 7.4% asymptomatic re-stenosis rate (re-stenosis defined as greater than 70% stenosis) 90% of which occurred between 3 and 6 months.

Retrospective study designs, limited ultrasound or angiographic follow-up and variable definitions similarly bedevil the surgical series addressing re-stenosis. The

Mayo clinic, using serial intravenous digital subtraction angiography found a mild to moderate stenosis in 10% of patients and a severe lesion (> 70%) in 3%.[15] Other series report re-stenosis using serial ultrasound follow-up in up to 14% of cases.[16, 17] It would appear then that using very crude comparative data the re-stenosis rates are between endovascular intervention and surgery are similar.

CAVATAS

This well publicised trial has randomized 504 patients with symptomatic high- grade carotid stenosis between surgery and angioplasty. This trial, as a prospective randomized study, will provide the only meaningful data to date comparing the durability of endovascular intervention and surgery. The study has not yet been published in a peer reviewed medical journal.

REFERENCES

1. Warlow CP: Disorders of the cerebral circulation. In: Walton J (Ed) *Brains Diseases of the Nervous System* pp.197–210. Oxford: Oxford University Press, 1993
2. Bamford J, Sandercock P, Dennid M *et al.*: A prospective study of acute cerebrovascular disease in the community. The Oxfordshire Community Stroke Project 1981–1986. *J Neurol Neurosurg Psychiat* **51**: 1373, 1988
3. Dunbabin D, Sandercock P: Stroke prevention. *Hospital Update* July: 540–545, 1992
4. Malmgren R, Bamford J, Warlow CP *et al.*: Projecting the number of patients with first ever strokes and patients newly handicapped by stroke in England and Wales. *Br Med J* **298**: 656–660, 1989
5. Ringlestein EB, Sievers C, Echer S *et al.*: Non-invasive assessment of CO2 induced cerebral vasomotor response in the normal individual and patients with internal carotid artery occlusions. *Stroke* **19**: 963–969, 1988
6. North American Symptomatic Carotid Endarterectomy Trial Collaborators: Beneficial effect of carotid endarterectomy in symptomatic patients with high-grade carotid stenoses. *New Eng J Med* **325**: 445–453, 1991
7. European Carotid Surgery Trialists Collaborative Group: MRC European Carotid Surgery Trial: interim results for symptomatic patients with severe (70–99%) or with mild (0–29%) carotid stenosis. *Lancet* **337**: 1235–1241, 1991
8. Gaines PA: The endovascular management of symptomatic atherosclerotic carotid disease. *Eur J Vasc Endovasc Surg* **16**: 94–97, 1998
9. Rothwell PM, Slattery J, Warlow CP: A systematic review of the risks of stroke and death due to endarterectomy for symptomatic carotid stenosis. *Stroke* **27**: 260–265, 1996
10. Eckert B, Zanella FE, Thie A *et al.*: Angioplasty of the internal carotid artery: Results, complications and follow-up in 61 cases. *Cerebrovasc Dis* **6**: 97–105, 1996
11. Gil-Peralta A, Mayol A, Marcos *et al.*: Percutaneous transluminal angioplasty of the symptomatic atherosclerotic carotid arteries. Results, complications and follow-up. *Stroke.* **27**: 2271–2273, 1996
12. Lou MW, Roubin GS, Mather A *et al.*: Neurological events after successful carotid stenting. *J Am Coll Cardiol* Feb 1998
13. Munari LM, Belloni G, Perretti A *et al.*: Carotid percutaneous angioplasty, *Neurological Reasearch* **14**: 156–158, 1992
14. Yadav JS, Roubin GS, Iyer S, *et al.*: Elective stenting of the Extracranial Carotid Arteries. *Circulation* **95**: 376–381, 1997

15. Sundt TM, Whisnant JP, Houiser OW *et al.*: Prospective study of the effectiveness and durability of carotid endarterectomy. *Mayo Clin Proc* **65**: 625–635, 1990
16. Cook JM, Thompson BW, Barnes RW: Is routine duplex examination after carotid endarterectomy justified? *J Vasc Surg* **12**: 334–340, 1990
17. Mattos MA, Hodgson KJ, Londrey GL:Carotid endarterectomy: operative risks, recurrent stenosis, long term stroke rates in a modern series. *J Cardiovasc Surg* **33**: 387–400, 1992

Commentary

It is regrettable that the so-called 'Cavatas' trial is scarcely mentioned in this chapter because the results have been presented and are therefore in the public domain although apparently not yet published in a period journal. This is a randomized controlled trial for symptomatic high grade carotid stenosis between surgery and angioplasty. I am sure that the author is right, that data from such a trial will certainly be the most powerful. The word is that the operative mortality for surgery is in the region of 10% and that a similar morbidity has been found for carotid angioplasty. Inevitably, this has produced whispers that a number of large series of carotid surgery have produced stroke rates of much less than this figure and there is great surprise. For any multicentre trial, one can expect a little surprise for overall results of average surgical or angioplasty performance. Some were surprised at the 30-day mortality of the UK Small Aneurysm Trial which is modelled on an expectation of a surgical mortality of 2% at 30 days where 5.8% was found in the event. We must wait for the published results, but speculation is rife. *RMG*

Carotid surgery: Is saphenous vein graft as durable as endarterectomy?

Jean-Pierre Becquemin, Alexandre d'Audiffret, Guillem Seban, Pascal Desgranges and Eric Allaire

INTRODUCTION

Carotid endarterectomy (CEA) has long been established as the technique of choice for the surgical repair of carotid bifurcation stenoses. In centres of excellence the mortality and complication rates of this procedure are often lower than those established by the Stroke Council of the American Heart Association.[1] Thus, it appears difficult to improve the results of this technique. However, this procedure may be technically demanding in unfavourable anatomical conditions with the risk of leaving residual plaques, intimal flaps, or too extensive thrombogenic surface that may result in a catastrophic outcome. Furthermore, significant recurrent stenosis at the endarterectomized site occurs in 6.7–19% of the cases, depending on the imaging technique used.[2–6] In an effort to limit these complications, Cormier *et al.* proposed the systematic use of a saphenous vein graft to bypass the carotid bifurcation.[7]

In most centres carotid bypass (CB) is only considered for selected situations where a conventional CEA is not possible, including severe recurrent stenoses not amenable to simple patching. Good results have been reported with CB techniques. However, this has never been compared in a prospective randomized fashion with CEA in terms of safety, effectiveness, and long-term outcome.[8] Fabiani *et al.* reported their experience with 51 patients suffering from bilateral high-grade stenoses, who underwent a CEA on one side and a saphenous vein bypass on the other.[9] The purpose of their study was to determine the incidence of recurrent carotid stenosis associated with each surgical technique. While this study indicated an equivalent recurrence rate, the investigation design and small sample size were inadequate to fully assess the role of saphenous vein bypass for the management of primary carotid stenosis. As a result, we decided to conduct our own prospective randomized trial using a larger patient population, and to submit saphenous vein bypass of the carotid bifurcation to the same rigorous analysis as CEA, in order to fully determine its effectiveness.

METHOD

Patients

Between January 1984 and December 1992, 183 patients (48 women and 135 men) with carotid high-grade stenosis (>70%) were identified and randomized to either

CEA with Dacron patch closure or saphenous vein bypass of the carotid bifurcation. One-third of the patients were asymptomatic. Indications for CEA are presented in Table 1. Demographic and risk factors were similar in both groups (Table 2). The degree of carotid stenosis was determined preoperatively by duplex and by arteriography. The state of the contralateral carotid artery was also noted in both groups in order to assess its significance in the overall outcome.

Table 1. Indications for carotid interventions

	Procedure			
	Bypass (n = 101)		*CEA (n = 95)*	
	n	*(%)*	*n*	*(%)*
Asymptomatic carotid stenosis	34	(33.8)	32	(33.7)
Transient ischaemic attacks	36	(35.6)	30	(31.2)
Reversible ischaemic neurological deficit	8	(7.9)	10	(10.5)
Minor cerebrovascular accident	10	(9.9)	13	(13.5)
Major cerebrovascular accident	1	(1)	0	(0)
Vertebrobasilar insufficiency	12	(11.8)		(10.5)

Table 2. Demographics and risk factors

	Procedure			
	Bypass (n = 101)		*CEA (n = 95)*	
	n	*(%)*	*n*	*(%)*
Men	79	(78)	80	(84)
Women	2	(22)	15	(16)
Symptomatic	67	(66.2)	63	(66.3)
Asymptomatic	34	(33.8)	32	(33.7)
Active smokers	38	(37.6)	27	(28.4)
Hyperlipidemia	21	(20.7)	24	(25.2)
Hypertension	75	(74.2)	71	(74.7)
Diabetes mellitus	17	(16.8)	15	(15.7)
Coronary artery disease	29	(28.7)	26	(27.3)
Renal insufficiency	6	(5.9)	4	(4.2)
Congestive heart failure	15	(14.8)	14	(14.7)
Peripheral vascular disease	25	(24.7)	26	(27.3)

Surgical technique

The type of anaesthesia used followed a common agreement between the anaesthesiologist, the surgeon and the patient. As a rule, we preferred the use of a regional block, especially in cases of severe coronary disease or severed contralateral carotid disease. General anaesthesia was reserved for difficult necks, high internal carotid stenosis and in anxious or poorly cooperative patients. All patients were

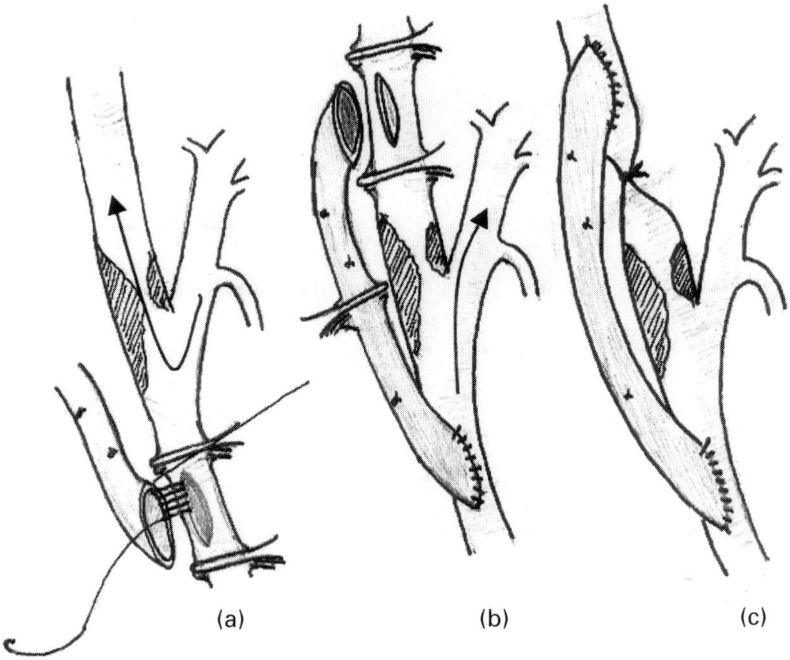

Fig. 1. Surgical technique of saphenous vein bypass. (a) Proximal anastomosis with retrograde flow from the external carotid to the cerebral circulation (Arrow). (b) Distal anastomosis with prograde flow to the cerebral circulation via external carotid collaterals (Arrow). (c) Ligation of internal carotid proximal to the distal anastomosis.

placed in the usual supine position with head hyperextension and one thigh included in the operative field, as the randomization process was done in the operating room. Prior to carotid clamping, 0.5mg/kg of heparin was administrated intravenously. A Pruitt-Tahara shunt was inserted when neurological deficit or loss of consciousness occurred after carotid clamping under loco-regional block. Under general anaesthesia a shunt was used in patients with high-grade contralateral stenoses or occlusion. The endarterectomy was performed in the usual fashion and the arteriotomy was closed using a Dacron patch with 6-0 polypropylene running sutures. The technique of saphenous vein bypass is demonstrated in Fig. 1. The saphenous vein was harvested from the proximal thigh under local or general anaesthesia. If the saphenous vein was estimated to be of poor quality (diameter < 4 mm, or sclerotic) a polytetrafluoroethylene (PTFE) graft was used. Postoperatively, all patients were maintained on heparin with a partial thromboplastin time (PTT) one and a half times normal until discharge when it was substituted for aspirin (250 mg/day).

Follow-up

Prior to discharge, all patients underwent a carotid angiogram (Fig. 2). Follow-up clinical examinations and duplex studies were scheduled every 6 months for the first

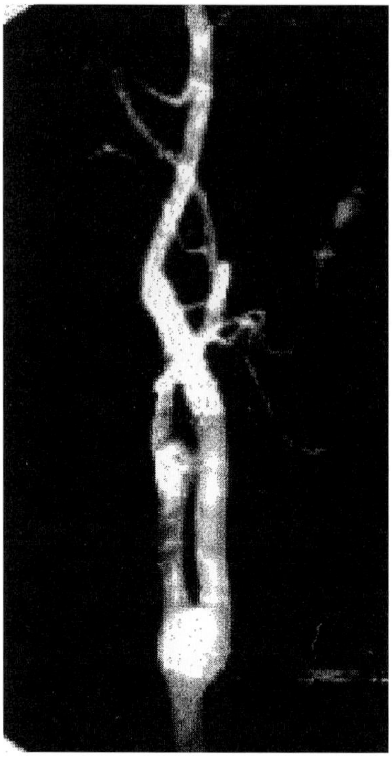

Fig. 2. Postoperative angiographic control following saphenous vein bypass of the carotid bifurcation.

year then annually. If an increased velocity in the bypass or at the endarterectomized site was detected, an angiogram was obtained to assess the degree of stenosis. All deaths, cerebrovascular events, recurrent stenoses and appearance of other pathologies were recorded.

RESULTS

Overall, 101 bypasses and 95 endarterectomies were performed. Thirteen patients underwent bilateral staged procedures consisting of CEA and bypass (n = 3), bilateral bypass (n = 4), and bilateral CEA (n = 6).

Operative variables

Shunt use, anaesthesia type, and clamping times are presented in Table 3. In the bypass group the total clamping time represent the period necessary to perform the proximal and distal anastomosis. Statistically significant differences between the two groups were the clamping time that was longer for the bypass group (30 ± 9 min vs

Table 3. Anaesthesia type, shunt use, and clamping time

	Procedure			
	Bypass (n = 101)		*CEA (n = 95)*	
	n	*(%)*	*n*	*(%)*
Anaesthesia				
general	41	(40.6)	42	(44.2)
locoregional	60	(59.4)	53	(55.8)
Shunted	4	(3.9)	16	(16.8)*
Average total clamping time	30 ± 9 min		25 ± 11 min**	

* $p < 0.001$
** $p = 0.008$

25 ± 11 min, p = 0.008), and the incidence of shunt use that was higher in the CEA group (16.8% vs 3.9%, p< 0.001). In 22 cases, the saphenous vein was deemed of poor quality by the operative surgeon and substituted with a 6-mm thin-wall PTFE graft.

Perioperative events

The perioperative (30-day) mortality and morbidity are shown in Table 4. There was no statistically significant difference among the two groups in the incidence of transient ischaemic attacks (TIA), minor cerebrovascular accident (CVA), major CVA and death. The overall mortality for both procedures was 0.5% and stroke 1.02%. The two patients who suffered a minor stroke postoperatively recovered without sequelae at 30 days. One patient suffered an acute thrombosis of the saphenous vein graft and subsequently expired on postoperative day 8. No acute thrombosis occurred in the CEA group. All strokes and TIAs were noted in the immediate postoperative period and no angiographic anomalies were detected in either group

Table 4. Perioperative complications

	Procedure	
	Bypass (n = 101)	*CEA (n = 95)*
Transient ischaemic attacks	3 (2.97%)	1(1.04%)
Minor cerebrovascular accident	1	1
Major cerebrovascular accident	0	0
Death	1[a]	0
Acute thrombosis	1[a]	0

[a]Patient who suffered an acute postoperative graft thrombosis and died on postoperative day 8.

Follow-up events

The average follow-up was 51.9 (± 29) months, ranging from 8 days to 129 months. Only one patient was lost to follow-up at 10 months with a patent bypass. Events occurring during this period are shown in Table 5. The incidence of saphenous vein graft occlusion was significantly higher than internal carotid artery thrombosis following CEA (4.9% vs 0%, p = 0.011). Interestingly, only one of these late occlusions was symptomatic and occurred at 22 months postoperatively in a patient with a previous CVA in the same cerebrovascular distribution. None of the patients who suffered a late occlusion were reoperated. Two recurrent stenoses of greater than 50% were identified in each group within 24 months following the procedure. One of the patients in the bypass group with a 60% asymptomatic stenosis and followed by

Table 5. Follow-up events

	Procedure	
	Bypass (n = 101)	*CEA (n = 95)*
Mean follow-up time (months)	52 ± 29	52 ± 29
Recurrent stenosis (< 24 months)	2	2
Recurrent disease (> 24 months)	1	3
Late graft occlusion / ICA thrombosis	5 (4.9%)	0*
Ipsilateral transient ischaemic attack	1	2
Ipsilateral cerebrovascular accident	0	1
Contralateral transient ischaemic attack	1	2
Contralateral cerebrovascular accident	1	1
Stroke death	1	0
Non-stroke death	21	24

*p = 0.01

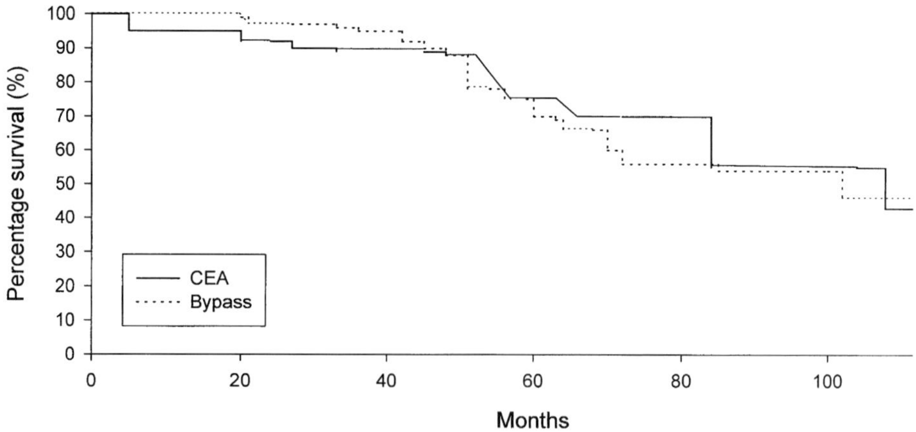

Fig. 3. Life-table plot of survival rates in patients with carotid endarterectomy and carotid bypass.

serial duplex subsequently developed an asymptomatic occlusion 5 months later. The incidence of late recurrent stenoses (> 24months) appeared to be lower in the bypass group, but did not reach statistical significance. The incidence of all ipsilateral and contralateral neurological events, stroke death, and non-stroke death were similar in both groups. A life-table analysis of survival following CEA and CB showed no significant differences (Fig. 3).

DISCUSSION

The main conclusion of our study is that bypasses of the carotid bifurcation have a relatively high incidence of late occlusion (4.9%), predated by a significant stenosis in only 30% of the cases. Despite a comparable mortality and morbidity due to the high number of asymptomatic bypass occlusions, CEA should remain the procedure of choice for the management of carotid artery stenosis. In this study, the perioperative stroke incidence for all procedures was 1.5% and only one perioperative death occurred, which followed an acute graft thrombosis. These results compare favourably with previous reports.[10–12] Few studies comparing CB and CEA are currently available in the literature. Cormier *et al.*, were the first authors to compare CB using the greater saphenous vein to CEA.[7] They reported a comparable morbidity and mortality with no restenosis at a mean follow-up of 29 months in the CB group, and concluded that saphenous vein bypass was an alternative to CEA in patients undergoing primary carotid surgery.

More recently, Branchereau *et al.* reported a 96.4% 10-year patency rate for saphenous vein bypass of the carotid bifurcation.[8] Fabiani *et al.* studied in a prospective fashion 51 patients with bilateral high-grade carotid stenosis who underwent a CEA on one side and a CB on the other.[9] The purpose of their study design was to limit individual variables that would restrict the comparison between the treatment groups. Despite the elegance of this study, it is important to notice that the CEA was the primary procedure in all but four cases. As a result, the CB was performed when the contralateral side was free of stenosis. This may have introduced a certain bias and underestimated the results associated with CEA weighed against CB. They reported an asymptomatic recurrent stenosis rate of 4% with equal incidence and no permanent neurological morbidity in both the CEA and CB groups.

In contrast, our study, designed in a prospective randomized fashion, was aimed at the evaluation of CB as a treatment for primary carotid stenosis. The state of the contralateral carotid was noted in all cases and was comparable in both groups. While our incidence of recurrent stenosis was similar in both groups and comparable to Fabiani's study, the graft occluded in six patients. Interestingly, only one patient suffered a symptomatic occlusion at 22 months. The relatively benign nature of saphenous vein graft thrombosis in this study relates most likely to chance and by no means should we conclude that late graft thrombosis is an innocuous event.

It is our practice, when the greater saphenous vein is of poor quality, to proceed with a PTFE (6-mm, thin-walled) bypass. The quality of such prosthetic bypasses was investigated by Sise *et al.*, in 1992. They reported a 12% significant stenosis rate and a stenosis-free rate of 89% at 39 months.[13] These results are comparable with our recent series with an 89% 4-year patency rate.[14] In this current report, the subgroup of 22 patients who underwent a prosthetic bypass suffered no recurrent stenosis during the follow-up period and only one PTFE graft occlusion occurred. This confirmed the fact that PTFE grafts are a very useful alternative to saphenous vein conduits with acceptable long-term patency. The short length of the graft and the high flow at the carotid bifurcation probably contribute to the favourable results of PTFE bypasses in this location. In contrast, the endothelial surface of a venous graft may be subjected to multiple injuries during the harvesting process. Furthermore, if a shunt is necessary, the added technical complexity of performing a bypass with shunt may result in an intimal injury that could lead to restenosis or premature thrombosis.

The five other graft thromboses occurred in the saphenous vein bypass group. In the case of the acute postoperative graft thrombosis, the procedure had to be performed with a shunt, which led to a laceration of the intimal surface and resulted in an immediate occlusion despite full heparinization. Another thrombosis resulted from a vein of marginal quality with a rather small diameter that led to a 60% recurrent stenosis at 6 months and occluded 1 month later. This experience emphasizes the necessity for a saphenous vein of large diameter, free of sclerotic thickening, harvested in an atraumatic fashion, in order to limit these complications.

As mentioned previously, the overall recurrent stenosis rate was 4.1% (CB 3% vs CEA 5.2%, $p>0.05$). Half of these stenoses occurred within 24 months postoperatively. In the bypass group, the lesions were more commonly at the distal anastomosis, a common finding in bypass procedures. Despite the usual distinction between early and late restenosis, Clagett *et al.* have demonstrated that late restenoses are a continuum of early intimal hyperplasia where atherosclerotic features dominate.[15] With time, the neointimal fibromuscular hyperplasia decreases as it undergoes atherosclerotic degeneration. In a similar fashion, recurrent stenosis in the endarterectomized carotid occurred more commonly in the proximal internal carotid artery and appeared to be associated with a long suture line. The details of local and systemic factors involved in recurrent stenosis and its management are beyond the scope of this chapter.

One of the potential advantages of performing a vein bypass is the maintenance of cerebral perfusion via ophthalmic collaterals during the procedure. Interestingly, shunts were most commonly used in the CEA group (16.8% vs 3.9%, $p<0.05$). Thus, continuous flow through the external carotid while performing the distal anastomosis (Fig. 1.) may indeed be sufficient to decrease shunt use. However, the clinical implications of this collateral flow remains to be defined. The most important aspect of this study remains the number of graft thromboses (six patients), which were clinically significant in two cases. However, as previously mentioned, the relatively high incidence of asymptomatic vein graft thrombosis is most probably fortuitous. Of particular concern is the relative unpredictability of these thromboses, as we demonstrated an asymptomatic medium-grade stenosis (50–60%) in only two patients prior to the occlusion. The other patients did not appear to have any identifiable lesions on serial duplex imaging. The reason for these failures remains unclear, yet possible explanations may be haemodynamic or local compressive forces associated with neck rotation.

In our study, the combined recurrent stenosis and occlusion rate of 7.9% for saphenous vein bypasses does not appear to compare favourably with the combined rate of 11.5% for PTFE bypasses reported by Sise.[13] The choice of conduit for bypass of the carotid bifurcation remains to be determined.

In conclusion, we have demonstrated that bypass of the carotid bifurcation and CEA have a similar clinical outcome. Nevertheless, we remain concerned about the relatively high rate of graft failure and we believe that CEA should remain the procedure of choice for the management of primary carotid bifurcation stenosis. The use of saphenous vein should be limited to selected cases when an endarterectomy is technically not possible, severe kinks are present, or for redo-carotid surgery. While the number of PTFE bypasses in this study is low, the fact that no recurrent stenoses were demonstrated tends to favour its use over autologous conduit.

REFERENCES

1. Moore WS, Mohr JP, Hassan N *et al.*: Carotid endarterectomy: Practice guidelines. Report of the Ad Hoc Committee to the Joint Council of the Society for Vascular Surgery and the North American Chapter of the International society for Cardiovascular Surgery. *J Vasc Surg* **3**: 469–479, 1992
2. Atnip RG, Wengrovitz M, Gifford RR *et al.*: A rational approach to recurrent carotid stenosis. *J Vasc Surg* **11**: 511–516, 1990
3. Zierler RE, Bandyk DF, Thiele BL, Strandness DE: Carotid artery stenosis following endarterectomy. *Arch Surg* **117**: 1408–1412, 1982
4. Thomas M, Otis SM, Rush M *et al.*: Recurrent carotid stenosis following endarterectomy. *Ann Surg* **200**: 74–79, 1984
5. Nicholls SC, Phillips DJ, Bergelin RO *et al.*: Carotid endarterectomy. Relationship of outcome to early stenosis. *J Vasc Surg* **2**: 375–380, 1985
6. O'Donnell TF Jr, Callow AD, Scott G *et al.*: Ultrasound characteristics of recurrent carotid stenosis: Hypothesis explaining the low incidence of symptomatic recurrence. *J Vasc Surg* **2**: 26–41, 1985
7. Cormier JM, Laurian C, Gigou F *et al.*: Greffe veineuse contre thromboendarterectomie carotidienne. *J Mal Vasc* **7**: 25–31, 1982
8. Branchereau A, Pietri P, Magnan PE, Rosset E: Saphenous vein bypass: an alternative to internal carotid reconstruction. *Eur J Vasc Endovasc Surg* **12**: 26–30, 1996
9. Fabiani JN, Julia P, Chemla E *et al.*: Is the incidence of recurrent carotid artery stenosis influenced by the choice of the surgical technique? Carotid endarterectomy versus vein bypass. *J Vasc Surg* **20**: 821–825, 1994
10. North American Symptomatic Carotid Endarterectomy Trial Collaborators: Beneficial effect of carotid endarterectomy in symptomatic patients with high grade carotid stenosis. *New Engl J Med* **325**: 445–453, 1991
11. MRC European Carotid Surgery Trial: Interim results for symptomatic patients with severe (70–99%) or mild (0–29%) carotid stenosis. *Lancet* **337**: 1235–1243, 1991
12. Hobson RW, Weiss DG, Fields WS *et al.*: Efficacy of carotid endarterectomy for asymptomatic carotid stenosis. *New Engl J Med* **328**: 221–227, 1993
13. Sise JM, Ivy ME, Malanche R, Ranbarger KR: Polytetrafluoroethylene interposition grafts for carotid reconstruction. *J Vasc Surg* **16**: 601–608, 1992
14. Becquemin JP, Cavillon A, Desgranges P, Melliere D: Polytetrafluoroethylene grafts for carotid repair. *Cardiovasc Surg* **4**: 740–745, 1996
15. Clagett GP, Robinowitz M, Youkey JR *et al.*: Morphogenesis and clinicopathologic characteristics of recurrent carotid disease. *J Vasc Surg* **3**: 10–23, 1986

Commentary

It is good to see data on carotid vein bypass with some comparison against standard carotid endarterectomy. As the author mentions, Cormier (Ref. 7 in text) stressed the low restenosis rate associated with high vein bypass. Having heard Cormier myself, I used vein bypass as first choice in patients who had already suffered restenosis from conventional carotid endarterectomy and with regret I found that the vein bypasses restenosed as well. Therefore my own personal information is exactly in line with Jean-Pierre Becquemin. It seems therefore that as far as restenosis is concerned, that there could be something in the patient, rather than the technique which predicts the restenosis phenomenon. The randomized controlled trial described here was aimed at the evaluation of carotid vein bypass as a treatment for primary carotid stenosis and as Jean-Pierre Becquemin says, the incidence of recurrent stenosis was similar in both groups. The data would indeed seem to indicate that standard carotid endarterectomy remains the treatment of first choice and that bypass should be used for a subset of patients. The problem is that the nature of that subset is not absolutely clear and there is a risk of vein bypass being used for the more difficult patterns which would be unfair on the procedure. *RMG*

Does bovine pericardial patching improve the durability of carotid endarterectomy?

GM Biasi, P Mingazzini, S Sternjakob, A Sampaolo and SA Ferrari

INTRODUCTION

The beneficial effect of patch angioplasty in improving the results of carotid endarterectomy (CEA) and reducing the risk of early thrombosis, thus lowering the stroke and morbidity rate of the procedure, has been advocated by extensive reviews and prospective studies. Moreover, the carotid patch is proposed in order to reduce the incidence of restenosis, thus contributing also to the durability of endarterectomy results in the long term.

The Report of the Ad Hoc Committee on Clinical Research of the Society for Vascular Surgery (SVS), published in 1992, identified the choice of an appropriate patch material for CEA as one of the unanswered questions facing the speciality. Saphenous, jugular and facial veins, Dacron and expanded polytetrafluoroethylene (PTFE), have all been proposed as potential solutions.

The aim of CEA is to provide long-term freedom from the risk of stroke with a minimal operative stroke/mortality rate. We previously reported on our initial experience using a gluteraldehyde treated bovine pericardial patch. In this report, our 7-year period follow-up data on CEA repair, using the Vascu-Guard® bovine pericardium patch, are reviewed with special emphasis on efficacy and durability.

BACKGROUND

The prevention of stroke through the use of CEA has been one of the most widely studied topics in the field of vascular surgery. Initially discussions were centred on the safety and efficacy of surgical intervention. The superior benefits of CEA over medical therapy have since been defined by a number of large, well controlled studies. The North American Symptomatic Carotid Endarterectomy Study (NASCET),[1] the European Carotid Surgery Trial (ECST),[2] the Asymptomatic Carotid Atherosclerosis Study (ACAS)[3] and the Veterans' Affairs Co-operative Study Group,[4] have demonstrated that favourable results are obtained in both symptomatic and asymptomatic patients. Practice guidelines for CEA have been published in this regard by Ad Hoc Committees of both the American Heart Association (AHA) and the NA-ISCVS.[5,6] The guidelines set by the AHA recommended that the upper levels of risk for combined stroke and/or death, associated with carotid endarterectomy, be set at 3% for asymptomatic patients, 5% for patients with previous transient ischaemic attacks (TIA), 7% for patients with a prior stroke history and 10% for patients undergoing recurrent stenosis surgery. The NA-ISCVS, while agreeing with these 'upper' limit parameters, felt that there was substantial evidence that far lower complication rates were attainable. Based on the reports from the NASCET and the ECST Studies, the Society further recommended that the patient population be limited to those with defined severe stenosis of 70–99%. A review of 51 studies on CEA, reporting mortality and morbidity from 1980 to 1995 by Rothwell *et al.*[7] demonstrated an overall 5.6% risk of stroke and/or death, well in accordance with the established guidelines. These results, from a review of over 15 000 procedures, are in spite of the inherent heterogenicity of the multiple studies. Although patients older than 79 years were excluded from the NASCET and the ACAS studies, O'Hara and his co-workers provided excellent results in a study of 182 CEA procedures performed on octogenarians between 1989 and 1995.[8]

All these data collected by large multicentre studies have shown the benefit of CEA over medical therapy for both symptomatic and asymptomatic patients, provided that the combined perioperative stroke and death rate can be maintained at low levels in the follow-up. The stroke prevention in the long-term outcome is heralded by the possible development of a recurrent carotid stenosis after endarterectomy.

Carotid restenosis is a recognized postoperative complication with a reported incidence ranging between 1 and 36%.[9–12] Certainly one of the main reasons for such a variability in the incidence of this complication is the lack of a unique criterion for the evaluation of restenosis. Furthermore, the reported incidences frequently included residual stenoses, due to incomplete or inappropriate endarterectomy, with true, new stenoses.[12]

Nevertheless, good late results of carotid endarterectomy, in terms of prevention from strokes, have also been reported[13,14] notwithstanding the possibility of restenosis, proving that it is a durable operation.

The great majority of restenoses are not accompanied by symptoms because most of the early recurrences are seen in the first 6–24 months and are due to intimal hyperplasia, which is a benign process with very low tendency to embolize, while late recurrences reproduce the features of atherosclerotic primary lesions, with calcification, ulceration and intraplaque haemorrhage and are more prone to cause cerebral ischemia.[15]

In the attempt to achieve the best postoperative results and to maintain a low stroke and death rate, after CEA, we considered patch reconstruction as a way of improving immediate and long-term outcome after surgery. A certain degree of narrowing (from 15 to 20%) cannot be avoided distal to the carotid bulb when an arteriotomy is primarily closed[16] and the effectiveness of patch angioplasty in preventing carotid restenosis, by widening the arterial lumen to the proper size, in order to avoid accelerated or turbulent flow, has been advocated by several prospective and non-prospective studies.

Nevertheless, primary closure versus patch angioplasty remains for many surgeons a controversial issue. Proponents of primary closure feel that patching prolongs the clamping and operative time, may put patients at risk of infection, may produce bleeding and makes the operation technically more difficult. It is worthwhile mentioning that patch angioplasty was described[17] at about the same time as the CEA procedure.

In a canine study measuring haemodynamic effects, Fietsam *et al.*[18] demonstrated significant increases in peak systolic gradient across the closure associated with primary closure, while there were no significant changes noted with patch angioplasty. The recent prospective studies reported by AbuRahma[19] demonstrated clear superiority of patching over primary closure in both perioperative outcomes and in long-term clinical outcomes and incidence of recurrent stenosis.[20] Archie,[21] in a review article pooled data from six prospective randomized studies comparing CEA primary closure with patch angioplasty, considering three major outcomes: early carotid thrombosis, perioperative (30-day) stroke and ≥ 50% residual or restenosis in the first year. This author observed 3- to 4-fold advantage of patching over primary closure (thrombosis 0.8% vs 4.3%; stroke 1.2% vs 3.9%; ≥ 50% restenosis 2.1% vs 7.4%), reaching the conclusion that future prospective randomized trials may be difficult to accomplish, if not unnecessary.[21]

A review of 3062 carotid endarterectomies by Riles *et al.*[22] concluded that the majority of peri-operative strokes during carotid artery reconstructions were preventable technical errors. Hertzer in his 1994 Editorial in the *Journal of Vascular Surgery*[23] perhaps put this issue into a clearer perspective in discussing surgeon-related factors concerning the closure of CEAs: 'Primary closure of an internal carotid arteriotomy can be a demanding exercise and it is not a prohibitive leap of faith to speculate that postoperative thrombosis, which would be less likely to occur in literally thousands of patients, if surgeons who perform only one or two carotid endarterectomies a year, would instead use patch angioplasty. It is worth noting that all authors who discourage the routine use of carotid patching have had excellent results with primary arteriotomy closure. Unfortunately their experience is not universal and it probably never will be'.

The next question is: What kind of material should we use for patch reconstruction after CEA?

In 1992 the Ad Hoc Committee on Clinical Research of the SVS, published a special article in which they identified the issue of the choice of material for use in patch angioplasty as an area requiring further study.[24] Proponents of vein as the material of choice cite the availability, ease of handling, haemostatic qualities and endothelial surface. Those who prefer synthetics cite the advantage of an off-the-shelf product, the elimination of the co-morbidities associated with the harvest site and the preservation of a potential conduit for future cardiac or vascular procedures. The most common vein used in CEA repair is the great saphenous vein (GSV), although some authors[25,26] have reported good results with the use of external jugular and cervical veins. The mechanical integrity of a specific section of vein is directly related to the site of harvest. Progressive dilatation of the CEA, following vein patch closure, has been reported by Lord and defined as present when the diameter of the common carotid artery (CCA) or the bifurcation was increased to twice the intraoperative measured diameter.[27]

In a review article in 1992, Bergamini and his associates[28] found that while the overall incidence of vein patch aneurysm formation was low, patients with recurrent carotid artery stenosis associated with aneurysmal degeneration, were at high risk for TIAs and stroke.

Rupture of a vein patch following CEA angioplasty is a rare occurrence with various reports placing the incidence at between 0.4 and 0.7%. However, the mortality rate is 30% and the severe morbidity rate approaches 70% in these patients.[29–31] Several recent studies have reported good results using an eversion technique rather than a patched longitudinal endarterectomy.[32,33] In our experience we have reserved this technique in case of elongation and kinking of the internal carotid artery when associated with a stenosis. For those who believe that the risks of aneurysmal degeneration or patch rupture are too great, or who wish to avoid a second wound site or to spare the GSV for other potential revascularization procedures, synthetic, polytetrafluroethylene or Dacron patches should be the choice.

The most widely reported-on synthetic material is PTFE. Prolonged intraoperative bleeding from needle holes has been identified as a complication arising from PTFE use.[34] Although reduction of this type of blood loss is associated with specifically designed PTFE suture with 1:1 needle/suture ratios, AbuRahma reported that his mean haemostasis time was still significantly longer than for primary closure or vein patching.[19] Dacron, especially in the modern very thin and 'preclotted' configurations, has good handling and haemostatic qualities and like PTFE has the great advantage that it can be taken from the shelf – although also like PTFE it presents the problem of the foreign-body reaction from the host, and presumably exposes to a higher risk of infection.

Looking at the pertinent literature and taking into consideration studies giving comparable data, we tried to draw possible conclusions about the patch material of choice. The primary criteria for the evaluation of the efficacy of CEA, established by the SVS guidelines, is that of stroke/mortality rates. Table 1 gives the stroke mortality rates for procedures done with primary closure, PTFE, Dacron, jugular vein, saphenous vein and homologous saphenous vein, as reported in literature in the 1990s.[35–48]

Restenosis of greater than 50% has been used as a benchmark for determining the efficacy of a procedure. The reported restenosis rates are illustrated in Table 2.

It is interesting to note that the heterogenicity of the reports is evidenced by the ranges reported between studies. The rate of restenosis reported for primary closure ranged from 0% in one study to 24% in another. Dacron studies had a range of 0.7–7.9%, while saphenous vein was reported in a 0–13% range.

The third and perhaps most important aspect in the evaluation of a patch material is the freedom from stroke over long periods of time. If the patients, regardless of their 'apparent' levels of restenosis, fail to have untoward events relating to their

Table 1. Stroke mortality rates

Procedure	*No. of studies*	*Cases*	*30-Day stroke mortality*
Primary closure	5	580	2.5
PTFE	6	1442	1.7
Dacron	3	488	1.8
Jugular vein	3	252	1.2
Saphenous vein	8	952	1.8
Homologous saphenous vein	1	1006	2.0
Bovine	1	204	2.0

Table 2. Restenosis rates

Procedure	*No. of studies*	*Cases*	*Restenoses > 50%*
Primary closure	6	830	11.7
PTFE	7	1692	3.7
Dacron	4	738	3.3
Jugular vein	3	252	11.7
Saphenous vein	9	1202	3.6
Homologous saphenous vein	1	1006	6.0
Bovine	1	204	6.8

surgery, then we can conclude that with carotid patching we have provided a more successful operation than by simple endarterectomy with primary closure for the prevention of stroke.[9,49,50]

This was the scenario, with several different materials being used at the beginning of the 1990s, when we were offered the opportunity to use a heterologous stabilized graft, made from bovine pericardium for patch angioplasty in the carotid bifurcation position.

Bovine pericardium patch (Vascu-Guard® Bio-Vascular Inc. Saint Paul, MN, USA) was introduced by us in 1991 and our preliminary experience using this patch for carotid angioplasty with a 30-month follow-up was published in 1996.[48] Vascu-Guard is a processed bovine pericardium stabilized with glutaraldeyde, then stored and shipped in sterile water and 1% propylene oxide. Bovine pericardium has been used as a patch in cardiac procedures with satisfactory results for many years. It was initially proposed as a patch for closure of the patient's pericardium[51,52] and the satisfactory performance of this bioprosthesis, with no significant immunological reaction, good incorporation from host tissue and reduction of adhesion formation, encouraged the increasing use of this material in cardiac, vascular and also general surgery.[53–56] In a more recent publication which appeared in 1998 by Tirone,[57] a series of patients operated on for acquired heart defects, in which reconstructions were performed using glutaraldehyde-fixed bovine pericardium and followed for up to 10 years, very good late results were reported and no calcifications were observed. Implantable glutaraldehyde cross-linked natural tissue products have reported a limited durability due to an accumulation of mineral deposits, resulting in marked calcification.[58–60] In accordance with Tirone's report, we also never experienced any calcification. The thick threshold of collagen fibres (Fig. 1) gives good tensile strength and high suture retention; sterilization and stabilization of collagen tissue is obtained through glutaraldehyde, which creates cross-links between adjacent collagen chains, giving more resistance to collagenase enzymes and increasing physical strength.

The eventual formation of high molecular weight polymers during processing with aldehydes, even after pre-implant rinsing procedure, can cause continuous release of aldehydes into surrounding tissues following implantation, with tissue toxicity and increased inflammatory response from the host. Moreover, residual aldehyde levels with toxic cellular effects may inhibit tissue ingrowth, which is desirable to increase mechanical stability and also stimulate extensive calcification. For these reasons we decided to use the Vascu-Guard bovine pericardium, which is

(a)

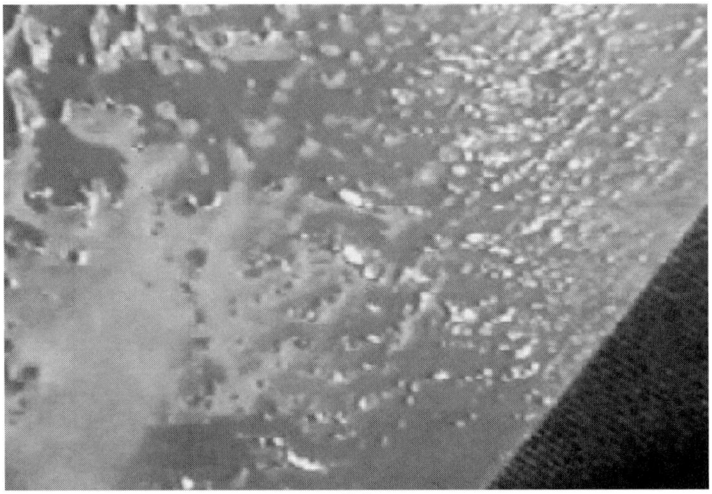

(b)

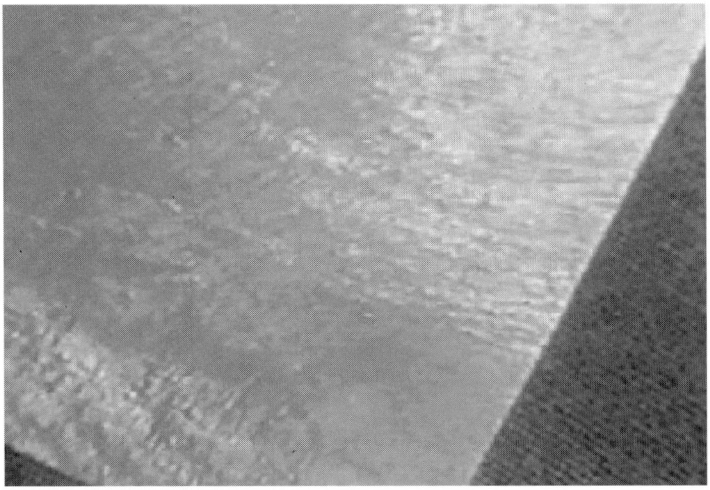

(c)

Fig. 1. Macroscopic aspect of pericardium patch (a). The rough side (b) and the smooth side (c) are identified. The smooth side is positioned towards the blood flow.

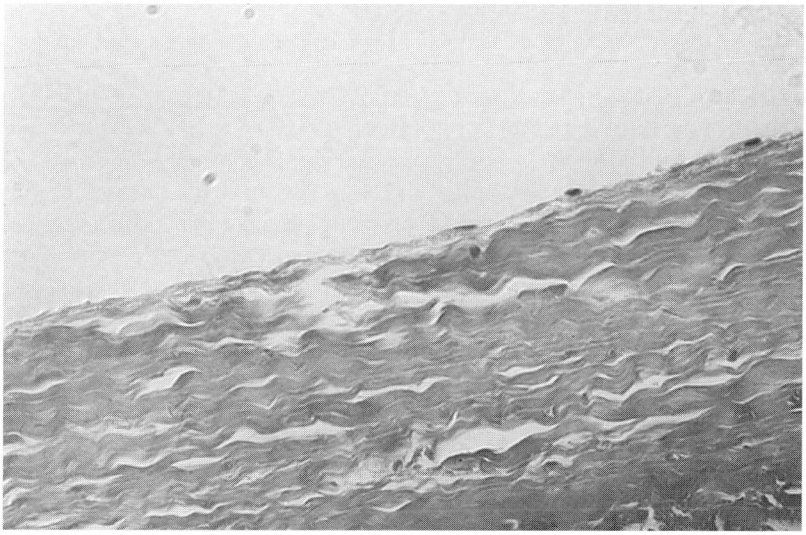

Fig. 2. Microscopic aspect of the biological patch. The well preserved collagen structure is covered by a thin endothelial layer.

cross-linked with glutaraldehyde, but is preserved in propylene oxide and water and necessitates only a 3-minute rinsing in sterile physical saline solution which is able to remove almost completely residual glutaraldehyde and to allow tissue ingrowth and endothelization (Fig. 2).

Particular attention has been dedicated by the manufacturer to the control of the source of pericardium to ensure protection against bovine spongiform encephalopathy (BSE). All pericardia to be used for Vascu-Guard are collected from US slaughterhouses, inspected by the US Department of Agriculture (USDA). No cases of BSE have been reported in the USA.[61] In addition, it is known that the BSE agent is closely associated with neural tissue,[62] to which the pericardium is not exposed.

In 1993 we conducted an animal study on 12 sheep in which we performed a bilateral longitudinal arteriotomy on the common carotid artery, which was sutured in all cases on one side with interposition of a bovine pericardium patch, and on the other side with an autologous jugular vein patch (in three cases) a PTFE patch (seven cases) and direct suture (two cases). All the animals were sacrificed at 3, 12 and 24 weeks after implantation and all specimens explanted were processed by means of scanning electron microscope (SEM) and histologic examination. The result of the study was that none of the materials used demonstrated a perfect integration with the carotid artery but no major differences among the three different materials could be demonstrated. Endothelial cells were found to be present on both the PTFE and Vascu-Guard materials.

PERSONAL EXPERIENCE

From May 1991 to April 1998 at the Division of Vascular Surgery of the University of Milan, Bassini Teaching Hospital, a total of 465 CEAs were performed on 425 patients, 307 male and 118 female. In 176 cases (38.1%) [Group A] a direct suture and in 275 cases (59.1%) a patch angioplasty was performed for closure of the carotid arteriotomy. In the remaining 13 cases a different surgical procedure was adopted.

Patch angioplasty was performed using bovine pericardium (Vascu-Guard) in 204 cases (43.9%), [Group B]; other patch materials (PTFE and Dacron) were used in the remaining 71 cases (15.2%). The mean age of the patients who underwent the 381 CEA procedures in Groups A and B was 71.9 years (ranging from 48 to 87 years) with no statistically significative difference between the two groups. In Group A the male/female ratio was approximately 2/1 (119/58) while in Group B it was 3/1 (147/57). The symptomatic patients were 191 (50%) with no statistically significant difference in the two groups and were divided into: (1) complete stroke: eight (2.1%), (2) Amaurosis fugax: 32 (8.4%) and (3) transient hemispheric symptoms: 151 (39.6%).

There were 16 patients with non-hemispheric symptoms while 174 (45.7%) were symptom-free. The majority of patients were affected by a stenosis of the internal carotid artery ≥70% and identified by real-time B-mode imaging, using a colour duplex scan. Digital subtraction angiography (DSA) was performed in 91.1% of the cases with equal distribution in the two groups. In 16 cases in Group A and 18 in Group B, for a total of 8.9%, the percentage of stenosis was <70% but the lesions were represented by ulcerated plaques or by soft low echogenic plaques with or without necrotic or haemorrhagic core, which in our experience resulted at high risk.[63] The main preoperative risk factors were also evaluated and no statistically significant difference was recorded in the two groups. All patients underwent preoperative electroencephalogram (EEG) and cerebral computed tomography (CT scan).

All patients were operated on under general anaesthesia, with EEC continuing monitoring and systemic heparinization (2500 units, iv) at the time of carotid cross-clamping. Arteriotomy was carried out on the common carotid artery (mean length 3.5 cm) and prolonged on the internal carotid artery (mean length 2.6 cm.). A Pruitt-Inahara shunt was inserted selectively on the basis of the appearance of EEG tracing abnormalities after carotid clamping: 36 patients (20.3%) in Group A and 73 (35.8%) in Group B. A prolene 6/0 continuous suture was applied in both groups. The mean carotid occlusion time of total CEAs was 40.5 ± 16.1 min and in particular: 30.0 ± 12.5 min in Group A and 47.7 ± 15.1 min in Group B. The intraoperative assessment of the haemodynamic result after CEA was obtained by means of Doppler spectral analysis. In the postoperative course, antiplatelet therapy was administered to all patients. Control carotid duplex scans (Fig. 3) were performed at 1, 3, 6 and 12 months postoperatively and yearly thereafter, to check the incidence of carotid restenosis. For the restenosis classification, we used the criteria suggested by Bernstein *et al.*[16] but only recurrent stenoses ≥50% were considered clinically significant. Restenoses ≥80% were included in a closer follow-up control programme and considered for redo surgery.

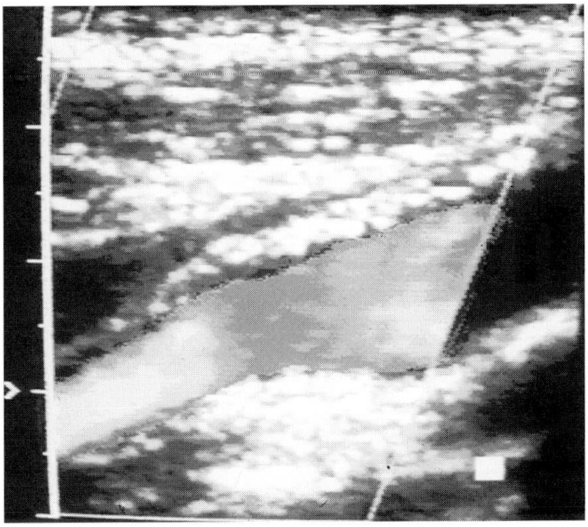

Fig. 3. Duplex scan image in the follow-up shows good integration of the patch without thickening or stenosis.

RESULTS

The major (stroke and death) early postoperative complications were 11 (2.9%) in all patients, being eight strokes (2.1%) and three deaths (0.8%). Nevertheless, the three deaths occurred from stroke and therefore eight patients presented with major postoperative complications (2.1%).

There were six strokes (3.4%) and one death (0.6%) in Group A with a total of six (3.4%) patients and two strokes (1.0%) and two deaths (1.0%) with a total of two (1.0%) patients in Group B. Nerve palsy occurred in 19 cases (5.0%): seven facial, one glossopharingeal, nine hypoglossus and two laringeal. No infection, rupture or dilation was recorded in the two groups.

The adaptability of the pericardium patch to vascular suture and its plasticity allow better configuration especially in the critical point of the distal arteriotomy in the internal carotid artery (Figs 4,5).

All the patients were evaluated in postoperative controls from 0 to 84 months (mean 44.7 months): 29 patients (7.6%) were lost to follow-up. The total number of restenosis ≥50% was 32 (8.4%) and ≥75% was 15 (3.9%). There were nine occlusions (2.4%).

The corresponding numbers for the patients in Group B were: 12 (6.8%) for restenosis ≥50% and five (2.8%) for restenosis ≥75%; the occlusions were three (1.7%). None of the patients presenting with carotid restenosis were symptomatic. Eight patients (2.0%) were re-operated on for restenosis ≥80%. There were no deaths following redo-operations nor strokes or TIAs. One patient presented with a tight new restenosis (70%) after 7 months. The patient is still under observation after 49 months and is symptom-free. Three of the eight redo-operations had a primary bovine pericardium patch angioplasty. In two cases we performed a new bovine pericardium patch angioplasty and in one case a carotid stenting.

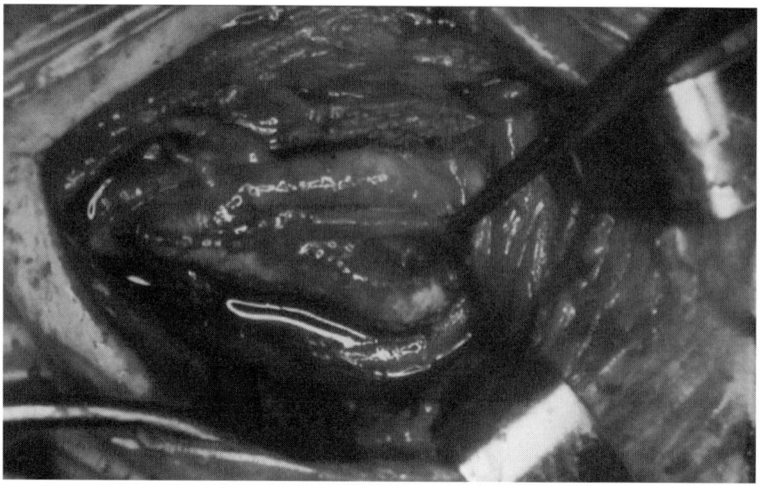

Fig. 4. Intraoperative photograph. The patch adapts well to the shape of the carotid bifurcation.

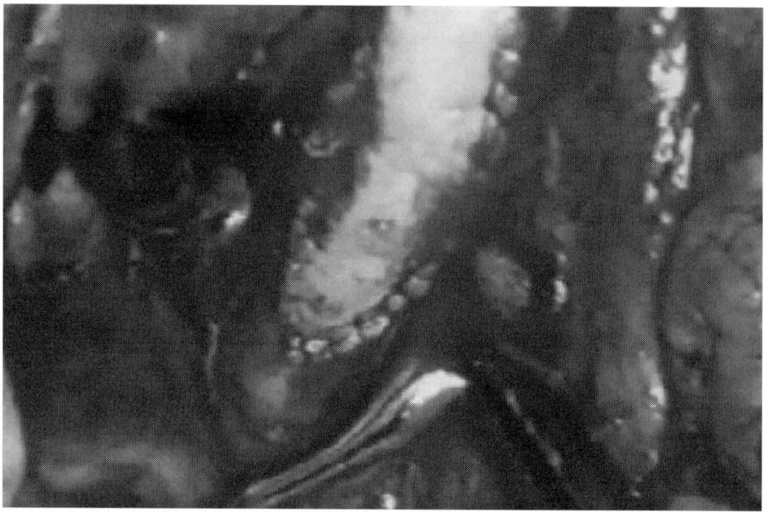

Fig. 5. Closer view of the distal endpoint of the anastomosis showing a smooth continuity with the internal carotid artery without minimal stenosis.

CONCLUSION

In our experience the early and late postoperative results of carotid patch angioplasty, using the Vascu-Guard bovine pericardium patch, compare favourably with the direct suture and other patch materials. In addition the patch is easy to handle and suture and very adaptable to suture line. No infection, rupture or dilation were observed. In one of the redo-operations performed for restenosis of the carotid patch angioplasty, the bovine pericardium patch was removed and examined by means of gross, SEM and histological analysis. The patch appeared intact with no degradation, good incorporation from the host surrounding tissues and no signs of inflammation. The bovine pericardium patch represents, in our opinion, a good alternative to other biological and synthetic material for carotid patch angioplasty.

ACKNOWLEDGEMENTS

The contribution of Dr Håkan Pårsson and Professor Lars Norgren from the University of Lund, Sweden, who performed all the SEM and histological analysis, is gratefully acknowledged.

REFERENCES

1. North American Symptomatic Carotid Endarterectomy Trial Collaborators: Beneficial effect of carotid endarterectomy in symptomatic patients with high-grade carotid stenosis. *New Engl J Med* **325**: 445–453, 1991
2. Dehaene L *et al.*: MRC European Carotid Surgery Trial: Interim results for symptomatic patients with severe (70–99%) carotid stenosis. *Lancet* **337**: 1235–1243, 1991
3. Toole JF: Endarterectomy for asymptomatic carotid artery stenosis. *J Am Med Assoc* **273**: 1421–1428, 1995
4. Mayberg MR *et al.*: Carotid endarterectomy and prevention of cerebral ischemia in symptomatic carotid stenosis. *J Am Med Assoc* **266**: 3289–3294, 1991
5. Moore WS: Guidelines for carotid endarterectomy: A multidisciplinary consensus statement from the ad hoc committee. American Heart Association. *Stroke* **26**: 188–201, 1995
6. Moore WS: Carotid endarterectomy: Practice guidelines. *J Vasc Surg* **15**: 469–479, 1992
7. Rothwell PM *et al.*: A systematic comparison of the risks of stroke and death due to carotid endarterectomy for symptomatic and asymptomatic stenosis. *Stroke* **27**: 266–269, 1996
8. O'Hara PJ *et al.*: Carotid endarterectomy in octogenarians: Early results and late outcome. *J Vasc Surg* **27**: 860–871, 1998
9. Mansour MA: Recurrent carotid stenosis. *Semin Vasc Surg* **11**: 30–35, 1998
10. Raithel D: Recurrent carotid disease: optimum technique for redo surgery. *J Endovasc Surg* **3**: 69–75, 1996
11. Toursarkissian B, Rubin BG, Sicard GA: Recurrent carotid artery stenosis. *J Am Coll Surg* **184**: 93–98, 1997
12. Barnes RW, Nix ML, Nichols BT *et al.*: Recurrent versus residual carotid stenosis. *Ann Surg* **203**: 652–660, 1986
13. Bernstein EF, Humber PB, Collins GM *et al.*: Life expectancy and late stroke following carotid endarterectomy. *Ann Surg* **198**: 80–86, 1983
14. Moore WS, Kempezinski RF, Nelson JJ, Toole JF: Recurrent carotid stenosis; results of the ACAS. *Stroke* **29**: 2018–2025, 1998
15. Sterpetti AV, Schultz RD, Feldhans RJ *et al.*: Natural history of recurrent carotid artery disease. *Surg Gyn Obstet* **168**: 217–223, 1989
16. Bernstein EF, Torem S, Dillet RB: Clinical significance of carotid restenosis. In: Veith F (Ed) *Current Critical Problems in Vascular Surgery* Vol 66, pp. 421–425. New York: Montefiore Medical Center, 1991
17. DeBakey ME *et al.*: Patch graft angioplasty in vascular surgery. *J Cardiovasc Surg* **3**:106–111, 1962

18. Fietsam R, Ranval T, Cohn S *et al.*: Hemodynamic effects of primary closure versus vein patch angioplasty of the carotid artery. *Ann Vasc Surg* **65**: 443–449, 1992
19. AbuRahma AF *et al.*: Prospective randomized trial of carotid endarterectomy with primary closure and patch angioplasty with saphenous vein, jugular vein and polytetraflouroethylene: Perioperative (30-day) results. *J Vasc Surg* **24**: 998–1007, 1996
20. AbuRahma AF *et al.*: Prospective randomized trail of carotid endarterectomy with primary closure and patch angioplasty with saphenous vein, jugular vein and polytetraflouroethylene: Long-term follow-up. *J Vasc Surg* **27**: 222–234, 1998
21. Archie JP: Carotid endarterectomy with reconstruction tailored to operative findings. *J Vasc Surg* **17**: 141–151, 1993
22. Riles TS *et al.*: The cause of perioperative stroke after carotid endarterectomy. *J Vasc Surg* **19**: 206–216, 1994
23. Hertzer NR: The hidden statistics of carotid patch angioplasty. *J Vasc Surg* **19**: 555–556, 1994
24. Bernstein EF: Saphenous versus prosthetic patch materials for carotid endarterectomy. Special article: Clinical research and vascular surgery. *J Vasc Surg* **15**: 867–870, 1992
25. Yu A *et al.*: Everted cervical vein for carotid patch angioplasty. *J Vasc Surg* **12**: 523–526, 1990
26. Dardik H *et al.*: Clinical experience with everted cervical vein as patch material after carotid endarterectomy. *J Vasc Surg* **25**: 545–553, 1997
27. Lord SA *et al.*: Comparison of saphenous vein patch, polytetrafluroethylene patch and direct closure after carotid endarterectomy. Part 1. Perioperative results. *J Vasc Surg* **9**: 521–529, 1989
28. Bergamini TM *et al.*: Symptomatic recurrent carotid stenosis and aneurysmal degeneration after endarterectomy. *Surgery* **113**: 580–586, 1993
29. Tawes RL, Treiman RL: Vein patch rupture after carotid endarterectomy: A survey of the Western Vascular Society *Ann Vasc Surg* **5**: 71–73, 1991
30. Van Damme H *et al.*: Blowout of carotid venous patch angioplasty. *Ann Vasc Surg* **5**: 542–545, 1991
31. O'Hara PJ *et al.*: Saphenous vein patch rupture after carotid endarterectomy. *J Vasc Surg* **15**: 504–509, 1992
32. Darling RC *et al.*: Eversion endarterectomy of the internal carptid artery: Technique and results in 449 patients. *Surgery* **120**: 635–640, 1996
33. Cao P *et al.*: A randomized study on eversion versus standard carotid endarterectomy: Study design and preliminary results: The Everest Trial. *J Vasc Surg* **27**: 595–605, 1998
34. McCready RA *et al.*: Delayed postoperative bleeding from polytetrafluroethylene carotid artery patches. *J Vasc Surg* **15**: 661–663, 1992
35. Gelabert HA *et al.*: Carotid endarterectomy with primary closure does not adversely affect the rate of recurrent stenosis. *Arch Surg* **129**: 648–654, 1994
36. Rhodes V: Expanded polytetrafluoroethylene patch angioplasty in carotid endarterectomy. *J Vasc Surg* **22**: 724–731, 1995
37. Goldman KA *et al.*: A comparative study of saphenous vein, internal jugular vein and knitted Dacron patches for carotid artery endarterectomy. *Ann Vasc Surg* **9**: 71–79, 1995
38. LeGrand DR, Linehan RL: The suitability of expanded PTFE for carotid patch angioplasty. *Ann Vasc Surg* **4**: 209–212, 1990
39. Rosenthal D *et al.*: Carotid patch angioplasty: Immediate and long-term results. *J Vasc Surg* **12**: 326–333, 1990
40. De Letter JA *et al.*: Benefits of carotid patching: A prospective randomized study with long-term follow up. *Ann Vasc Surg* **8**: 54–58, 1993
41. Katz SG, Kohl RD: Does the choice of material influence early morbidity in patients undergoing carotid patch angioplasty? *Surgery* **119**: 297–301, 1996
42. Katz D *et al.*: Long-term follow up for recurrent stenosis: A prospective randomized study of expanded polytetrafluroethylene patch angioplasty versus primary closure after carotid endarterectomy. *J Vasc Surg* **19**: 198–205, 1994
43. Allen PJ *et al.*: Saphenous vein versus polytetrafluroethylene carotid patch angioplasty. *Am J Surg* **174**: 115–117, 1997
44. Gonzalez-Fajardo JA *et al.*: Saphenous vein patch versus polytetrafluroethylene patch after carotid endarterectomy. *J Cardiovasc Surg* **35**: 523–526, 1994

45. Plestis KA *et al.*: Carotid endarterectomy with homologous vein patch angioplasty: A review of 1006 cases. *J Vasc Surg* **24**: 109–119, 1996
46. Meyers SI *et al.*: Saphenous vein patch versus primary closure for carotid endarterectomy: Long-term assessment of a randomized prospective study *J Vasc Surg* **19**: 15–22, 1994
47. Meyer FB, Windschitl WL: Repair of carotid endarterectomy with a collagen-impregnated fabric graft. *J Neurosurg* **88**: 647–649, 1998
48. Biasi GM, Mingazzini P, Baronio L, Sampaolo A: Processed bovine pericardium as a patch angioplasty for carotid endarterectomy: A preliminary report. *Cardiovasc Surg* **4**: 848–852, 1996
49. Archie JP Jr: Patching with carotid endarterectomy: When to do it and what to use. *Semin Vasc Surg* **11**: 24–29, 1988
50. Conusell CE, Salinas R, Naylor R, Varlow CP: A systemic review of the randomized trials of carotid patch angioplasty in carotid endarterectomy. *Eur J Vasc Endovasc Surg* **13**: 345–354, 1997
51. Dietzman RH, Holter AR, Linch MF *et al.*: Protection of the heart during reoperation using bovine pericardial shield. *Contemp Surg* **24**: 4, 1984
52. Crawford FA Jr, Sade RM, Spinale F: Bovine pericardium for correction of congenital heart defects. *Ann Thorac Surg* **41**: 602–605, 1986
53. Randas JVB, Dobrianskij A, Comazzi M *et al.*: Clinical experience with stentless pericardial aortic monopatch for aortic valve replacement. *J Thorac Cardiovasc Surg* **93**: 19–26, 1987
54. Sultan AA, Silverton RN, Yakirevich VS, Ionescu MI: Right ventricular outflow tract reconstruction with a bovine pericardial monocusp patch. *J Thorac Cardiovasc Surg* **89**: 764–771, 1985
55. Salles CA, Puig LB, Casagrande IS *et al.*: Early experience with crimped bovine pericardial conduit for arterial reconstruction. *Eur J Cardio-Thorac Surg* **5**: 273–279, 1991
56. Ionescu M, Tandona MD: Heart valve replacement with the Ionescu-Shiley pericardial xenograft. *J Thorac Cardiovasc Surg* **73**: 31, 1977
57. Tirone ED: The use of pericardium acquired heart disease: A review article. *J Heart Valve Dis* **7**: 13–18, 1998
58. Golomb G, Schoen FJ, Smith M *et al.*: The role of glutaraldehyde-induced cross-links in calcification of bovine pericardium used in cardiac valve bioprostheses. *Am J Pathol* **127**: 122–130, 1987
59. Schoen FJ, Levy R, Nelson A *et al.*: Onset and progression of experimental bio-prosthetic heart valve calcification. *Lab Invest* **52**: 523, 1985
60. Schoen FJ, Levy RJ, Hilbert SL, Bianco R: Antimineralization treatments for bioprosthetic heart valves. *J Thorac Cardiovasc Surg* **104**: 1285–1288, 1992
61. US Department of Agriculture, Animal and Plant Health Inspection Service: Fact-Sheet, Veterinary Services, *Bovine Spongiform Encephalopathy*, 1995
62. Lassrock ME III, Jackson GC, Knox GW: Can acquired immunodeficiency syndrome and Creutzfeldt-Jakob disease be transmitted via otologic homografts? *Arch Otolaryngol Head Neck Surg* **114**: 1252–1255, 1988
63. Biasi GM, Mingazzini M, Baronio L *et al.*: Carotid plaque characterization using digital image processing and its potential in future studies of carotid endarterectomy and angioplasty. *J Endovasc Surg* **5**: 240–246, 1998

Commentary

This centre has a longstanding interest in the use of bovine pericardial patching and here reports that 275 of their described series required patch angioplasty for carotid arteriotomy closure. The bovine pericardium was used in 204 patients which is 44% of the series. The authors describe outcome in terms of the follow-up ranging for up to 84 months with a mean of 44.7 months. No aneurysmal dilatation is reported and the authors concentrate on the development of restenosis and say that three of eight had primary bovine pericardium. Two of these three were operated upon with new bovine pericardium and in a third, carotid stenting was performed. We do not have life-table analysis of the outcome of bovine pericardium in terms of mortality or restenosis or development of aneurysmal dilatation. The absence of comment on aneurysmal dilatation implies that there has been no problem. Surgeons have a healthy concern whenever a heterograft is introduced into the body for any purpose, particularly when there are inert alternatives. It would seem vital that this group follows the outcome of bovine pericardium for patching carotid endarterectomy and the careful plotting of outcome could be a great service to vascular surgery. *RMG*

Do the long-term results of carotid endarterectomy for asymptomatic patients justify the hazards of surgery?

Alison W Halliday

INTRODUCTION

Carotid endarterectomy (CEA) is probably the most closely scrutinized operation in the world. The operation is conceptually simple, but poor operative judgement and technique cause stroke and death. The most acceptable indication for CEA is tight carotid stenosis with recent symptoms. A more controversial indication may be in patients without symptoms who are 'good-risk patients' with operation 'performed by a surgeon whose surgical morbidity and mortality rate is less than 3%'.[1] The criterion for justifying CEA in all these patients is the long-term prevention of stroke.

Long-term stroke prevention in asymptomatic carotid stenosis – the available evidence

The natural history of stroke in asymptomatic carotid stenosis (ACS) is not easily determined, but, in a recent study from Bristol, Irvine[2] found that overall 5-year survival was about 60% and was unrelated to severity of stenosis. Half of all deaths were cardiovascular and only 15% were due to stroke. In this study less than half of all strokes (fatal or otherwise), were ipsilateral to the stenosis.

Large natural history studies of severe ACS are now almost impossible to undertake, as surgery is commonly carried out when severe stenosis is found. Within the context of a randomized controlled trial it may still be possible to measure stroke rates in tight ACS and compare these with surgical intervention after 3–5 years.

Reports in the literature on surgery for asymptomatic carotid stenosis usually consist of

1. Anecdotal selections of patients from one centre, often chosen at a time when the short-term (30-day or inhospital stay only) results reflect favourably on the individual or institution.
2. Surveys by groups of interested surgeons who contribute some (but not necessarily all) cases for 30-day audit or short follow-up.
3. American (usually) reports of state registries or Medicare surveys on utilization of CEA (short-term follow-up with deaths accurately reported, but strokes only included if fatal).

4. A complete (or nearly complete) country register of CEAs with follow-up for 1 or 2 years (e.g. Swedevasc).[3]
5. Randomized clinical trials comparing CEA with normal medical care alone (using Kaplan–Meier survival curves, providing 3-year or more follow-up).
6. Meta-analysis. See Commentary.

Recent long-term series worth considering

1. The Cleveland Clinic reported a series of 182 CEAs undertaken between 1989 and 1995. Patients were all over 80 years (range 80–92, mean 83 years) and 55% were asymptomatic. All but two patients were followed for a mean period of 2.7 years (identical to ACAS, see Point 4 below), and the Kaplan–Meier estimated 5-year rate of freedom from stroke was 85%, survival was 45% and stroke-free survival was 42%.[4]
2. Campron reported an institutional series from Montreal of 75 patients, all with ACS, whose actuarial survival at 5 years was 75%. Patients' mean age was 66 ± 7 years (typical age range for CEA) and at 5 years 74% were stroke free.[5]
3. The Veterans Administration Cooperative Asymptomatic Carotid Artery Stenosis Study Group[6] was the first clinical trial to show benefit for patients who had CEA, but was limited by being performed on only 440 men with >50% carotid stenosis. There was a significant reduction in combined neurological events (amaurosis fugax, transient ischaemic attack and stroke) in the operated group, but this failed to reach significance when stroke only was considered ($p=0.056$). The mean follow-up was 47.9 months and 5 years after CEA 90% survivors were stroke-free on the operated side, with an overall survival free of any stroke or death of 60%.
4. The Asymptomatic Carotid Atherosclerosis Study (ACAS) enrolled 1662 patients who were equally randomized to surgery and risk factor treatment and to risk factor treatment alone.[7] The long-term results estimated from Kaplan–Meier analysis show that about 70% patients were alive at 5 years, free of any stroke or death. The validity of these figures has been questioned by Marcinczyk[8] who looked at the risk factors in patients entered into ACAS from one institution. By comparison with other patients operated on but not entered into ACAS, they had significantly less pulmonary, renal and cardiac disease. Although the 30-day results of surgery were similar, this selection process favoured longer-term survival in ACAS patients. By the use of prophylactic CEA, ACAS achieved a statistically significant reduction in stroke (but not disabling stroke), but at the same time created a clinical dilemma. The number of patients who 'needed' to have CEA was found to be enormous, but the clinical benefit from operation was small.

MEASURING BENEFIT – THE USE OF NUMBERS NEEDED TO TREAT (NNT)

The NNT is the measure of the impact of a treatment or intervention, stating how many patients need to be treated in order to prevent an event which would otherwise occur. The risk of stroke with the 'new' treatment (CEA and medical risk factor

Table 1. Number of operations needed to prevent one stroke over 5 years

	Operative risk (%)	*5-year risk after surgery (%)*	*Total 5-year risk with surgery (%)*	*5-year risk without surgery (%)*	*Absolute 5-year risk reduction of surgery (%)*	*NNT*	*Notes*
ACAS figures	2.3	2.8	5.1	11.0	5.9	17	Original ACAS result
ACAS figures (angiography for all)	2.8	2.8	5.6	11.0	5.4	19	Figures from ACAS paper, projected assuming that all surgical patients have angiography
4% Operative risk	4.0	2.8	6.8	11.0	4.2	24	Assuming higher operative risk, other risks equal
5% Operative risk	5.0	2.8	7.8	11.0	3.2	32	Assuming even higher operative risk, other risks equal
High risk, low effect surgery	5.0	4.0	9.0	11.0	2.0	50	Assuming high operative risk, and lower surgical benefit
High stroke risk patients	3.7	2.8	6.5	25.0	18.5	6	Unoperated patients at high risk of stroke (e.g. symptomatic patients)

Numbers Needed to Treat to prevent one event (NNT) is 1/(absolute risk reduction).
'Risk' is risk of any stroke and death, as per ACAS final result.

management) (R1) and in patients given standard (medical risk factor management) (R2) needs to be known. In ACS the NNT = 1/.R1–R2 = 1/absolute difference in risks. For potentially harmful treatments there is also the possibility of expressing the Number Needed to Harm (NNH). The NNT and NNH can then be used when making clinical and policy decisions. An illustration of the use of NNT from the ACAS and with patients at higher operative or higher stroke risk is shown in Table 1.

THE IMPORTANCE OF LONG-TERM FOLLOW-UP

Surgery for ACS is attractive because there is a lower morbidity than in symptomatic disease and following publication of the ACAS trial the American Heart Association has now endorsed CEA. Between 1989 and 1996 the number of CEAs in the USA more than doubled from 46571 to 108276 and overall mortality and the cost per procedure has gradually fallen.[9] Although operation results are generally considered to be better in large-volume institutions, reported 30-day morbidity may be twice that found in the carefully selected patients in ACAS. Analyses of 12 academic US centres and of Canadian centres found the perioperative stroke and death rates to be much higher than in ACAS (about 2.6–2.8%) and the Canadian Stroke Consortium has therefore decided not to recommend CEA for ACS.[10–12]

Cost-benefit analyses have been carried out assuming the cost of one quality-adjusted life year to be around $50 000. Although symptomatic carotid disease is cost-effectively treated by CEA, ACS is not.[13] Methods of 'improving' cost-effectiveness include reducing length of stay in hospital, and performing CEA without angiography, but these also depend on CEA having a low short-term morbidity.

The issues of cost-benefit, differing morbidity figures and operating for ACS outside the ACAS recommendations have all clouded clinicians' minds, and it is no longer clear whether there really is a place for CEA in the treatment of ACS. There is a 'gut feeling' that some patients must be better treated by operation, but these must be easily identifiable and not a subgroup of such complexity that the overall impact of operation is negligible. There is a need for a real-life trial which has long-term results that can clarify this important problem. In the USA approximately $1.5 billion is currently being spent on CEA for ACS. There is still no evidence that CEA prevents disabling stroke, is indicated for women, or can be more effective targeted on groups with really severe stenosis or soft plaque, but one trial is currently being undertaken which may help answer these questions.

THE ASYMPTOMATIC CAROTID SURGERY TRIAL

The Asymptomatic Carotid Surgery Trial (ACST) began in 1993 and now has more than 2000 patients. A final target number of 3200 has been set (Table 2), and it is hoped that this will be achieved by recruiting and following up patients until there is a mean follow-up of over 3 years. The ACST has collaborators from 26 countries including the USA and Canada, and patients are entered using the principle that if

Table 2. Current and projected long-term follow-up in ACST patients

	Total no. of patients entered	*Patients with up to 3 years follow-up*	*Patients with up to 5 years follow-up*
October 1998 (current)	1980	601	43
April 2003 (projected)	3200	2400	1575

Projecting an even rate of follow-up October 1998–April 2003

the clinician feels that the patient and stenosis are appropriate to operate on, but is uncertain whether operation is necessary, then the patient may be randomized to ACST. All patients receive appropriate best medical treatment for risk factors such as hypertension, and 50% are randomized to receive CEA. The trial protocol has been published[14] and ACST welcomes new collaborators. Because there is a heterogeneous population of collaborators, with differing views on when operation should be carried out, this lends statistical strength to the study. For example, in the UK, many patients are entered with stenoses of more than 90%. The standard of surgery must be acceptable to the Data Monitoring Committee, who perform interim analyses. At present for the first 2000 patients the mean follow-up is 1.9 years (although some patients have now reached 5 years).

The ACST is the largest randomized controlled trial of surgery for ACS in the world. It is unlikely that further trials of this magnitude will take place as they are expensive and require considerable planning and organization. Many collaborators from 26 countries have contributed effort and enthusiasm to answer the question 'Do the long-term results of carotid endarterectomy for asymptomatic patients justify the hazards of surgery?' The trial is still open and more collaborators are invited to help enter the 1200 patients still needed.

REFERENCES

1. Biller J *et al.*: Guidelines for carotid endarterectomy: a statement for healthcare professionals from a special writing group of the Stroke Council, American Heart Association. *Stroke* **29**: 554–562, 1998
2. Irvine CD *et al.*: Unilateral asymptomatic carotid disease does not require surgery. *Eur J Vasc Endovasc Surg* **16**: 245–253, 1998
3. The steering committee of SWEDVASC: Auditing surgical outcome. Ten years with The Swedish Vascular Registry – Swedvasc. *Eur J Surg* **164** (Suppl 581): 3–48, 1998
4. O'Hara, Hertzer NR, Mascha EJ *et al.*: Carotid endarterectomy in octagenarians: early results and late outcome. *J Vasc Surg* **27**: 860–869, 1998
5. Campron H, Cartier R, Fontaine AF: Prophylactic carotid endarterectomy without arteriography in patients without hemispheric symptoms: surgical morbidity and long-term follow-up. *Ann Vasc Surg* **12**: 10–16, 1998
6. Hobson RW *et al.*: Efficacy of carotid endarterectomy for asymptomatic carotid stenosis. *New Engl J Med* **328**: 221–227, 1993
7. Executive Committee for the Asymptomatic Carotid Atherosclerosis Study: Endarterectomy for asymptomatic carotid artery stenosis. *J Am Med Assoc* **273**: 1421–1428, 1995

8. Marcinczyk MJ, Nicholas GG, Reed JF, Nastasee SA: Asymptomatic carotid endarterectomy. Patient and surgeon selection. *Stroke* **28**: 291–296, 1997
9. Hsia DC, Moscoe LM, Krushat WM: Epidemiology of carotid endarterectomy among medicare beneficiaries: 1985–96 update. *Stroke* **29**: 346–350, 1998
10. Goldstein LB, Samsa GP, Matchar DB, Oddone EL: Multicenter review of preoperative risk factors for endarterectomy for asymptomatic carotid stenosis. *Stroke* **29**: 750–753, 1998
11. Smurawska LT, Bowyer B, Rowed D *et al.*: Changing practice and costs of carotid endarterectomy in Toronto, Canada. *Stroke* **29**: 2014–2017, 1998
12. Perry JR, Szilai JP, Norris JW for the Canadian Stroke Consortium: Consensus against both endarterectomy and routine screening for asymptomatic carotid artery stenosis. *Arch Neurol* **54**: 25–28, 1997
13. Kuntz KM, Kent KC: Is carotid endarterectomy cost-effective? An analysis of symptomatic and asymptomatic patients. *Circulation* **94** (Suppl II): 194–198, 1995
14. Halliday AW, Thomas D, Mansfield AO: The asymptomatic carotid surgery trial (ACST): rationale and design. *Eur J Vasc Surg* **8**: 703–710, 1994

Commentary

A meta-analysis of carotid endarterectomy for asymptomatic carotid stenosis has been reported by Benavente *et al.*[1] The authors performed a systematic review and meta-analysis of randomized controlled trials in patients with asymptomatic carotid stenosis in which subjects were allocated to carotid endarterectomy or to medical treatment alone. Five trials, enrolling 2440 patients with stenoses of greater than 50% were considered. Main outcome measures were stroke, ipsilateral to the stenosis, all strokes and perioperative complications such as stroke and death. The authors concluded that in patients who underwent carotid endarterectomy (1215) there was a significant reduction in the odds of ipsilateral stroke plus perioperative stroke or death (odds ratio 0.62:95% confidence interval 0.44–0.86) corresponding to a 2% absolute risk reduction over about 3.1 years. The prevalence of stroke in any location was also reduced (0.68:0.51–0.9) in patients undergoing carotid endarterectomy. During the immediate postoperative period, there was an increased prevalence of stroke or death among such patients (4.51:2.36–8.64).

The authors concluded that carotid endarterectomy in patients with asymptomatic carotid stenosis unequivocally reduces the incidence of ipsilateral stroke, though the absolute benefit is relatively small. Given the modest benefit of surgery for unselected patients with asymptomatic carotid stenosis, carotid endarterectomy cannot be routinely recommended for those patients pending reliable identification of high risk subgroups and the authors concluded that medical management is presently a sensible alternative for most patients. So, once again, there is a call for a search for a subgroup and not to operate upon asymptomatic carotid surgical patients in a blanket way. The authors refer to the ongoing asymptomatic carotid surgical trial mentioned in this chapter and there can be little doubt that those surgeons who believe that they should be operating upon asymptomatic carotid stenosis should submit the patients to this random controlled trial. An editorial in the *New England Journal of Medicine* recently entitled, 'Appropriate use of carotid endarterectomy', draws attention to the recent rise or carotid endarterectomy procedures. The author, Chassin,[2] concludes that data on the efficacy of carotid endarterectomy for asymptomatic patients are less clear and comments that there is only a single large randomized controlled trial, the ACAS trial mentioned above. He stresses the extraordinarily low (2.3%) rate of surgical complications (stroke and death within 30 days of surgery), with about half that rate attributable to the effects of cerebral angiography. This author implies that if there is to be any benefit for asymptomatic carotid stenosis patients from having carotid endarterectomy, then it will be critical that the complication rate of the operation is very low. This implies that any benefit could be stated with provisos that a surgeon's complication rate is less than a certain figure. *RMG*

References

1. Benavente O, Moher D, Ba Pham: Carotid endarterectomy for asymptomatic carotid stenosis: A meta-analysis. *Br Med J* **317**: 1477–1480, 1998
2. Chassin MR: Appropriate use of carotid endarterectomy. *New Engl J Med* **12**: 1468–1471, 1998

DO POPULATION STUDIES AND NATIONAL REGISTRIES PROVIDE EVIDENCE OF DURABILITY IN OUR PATIENTS?

Life expectancy after surgical repair of non-ruptured abdominal aortic aneurysm

K Wayne Johnston

INTRODUCTION

The purpose of this chapter is to summarize the early and late results after surgical repair of a non-ruptured infrarenal abdominal aortic aneurysm (AAA). Specifically, using the data from the Canadian Aneurysm Study, this chapter will document the variables that are predictive of perioperative morbidity and those associated with 5-year survival. Detailed knowledge of the results of surgical repair of AAA will permit identification of high-risk patients, evaluation of the indications for surgical repair based on the balance between the size and growth of the AAA and the patients comorbidity, and establishment of a standard for comparing the results of endovascular treatment. The data presented in this chapter are a summary of some of the analyses from our previous publications.[1–4]

THE CANADIAN ANEURYSM STUDY DATABASE

The Canadian Aneurysm Study overcomes the problems associated with many previous studies that were limited by being retrospective, having referral or selection bias because patients were included from only a single referral centre and undergoing operation by only a few surgeons, analysing results from patients undergoing operation over a very long time interval, and/or having inadequate follow-up.

During a 9-month period in 1986, 72 members of the Canadian Society for Vascular Surgery participated in a prospective study of 680 consecutive patients who had either asymptomatic or symptomatic non-ruptured AAA and undergone elective or urgent (within 3 days of diagnosis) surgery. A total of 116 variables were completely recorded in 96.8% of cases and included patient demographics, surgeon data, atherosclerosis and AAA risk factors, associated diseases and operative risk factors, diagnostic tests, anaesthesia, operative details, intraoperative complications, intensive care management, vascular and general postoperative complications, and mortality. Regular follow-up was maintained by contact with the surgeon, family doctor, and/or patient at 6- to 9-month intervals to determine the patient's status, cause of death, and complications. Of note, 87% of the surgeons had either a vascular surgery or cardiovascular and thoracic certification and devoted an average of 70% of their time to the practice of vascular surgery.

Patient characteristics

The average age of the patients was 69.2 ± 7.7 years (mean ± 1 SD) and 80.0% were male. Details of the risk factors of the study population are given in Table 1. The average diameter of the aortic aneurysms measured by ultrasound was 60.3 ± 13.9 mm: 6.4% were 4.5 cm or less, 13.9% were 5.0 cm or less, and 35.7% were 5.5 cm or less. A positive family history of AAA was documented in 6.1% of cases and was more common if the patient was female (p=0.03) and less than 65 years of age (p=0.04). Inflammatory aneurysms were observed in 4.5%, significant venous anomalies in 1.4%, aneurysms of the iliac, femoral and/or popliteal arteries in 9.9%, and arterial occlusive disease involving the aortoiliac and/or femoral popliteal segments in 33.0% of cases.

Table 1. Details of the study population for non-ruptured AAA

Variable	*% (unless indicated)*
Age	*(average 68.2 ± 7.6 years)*
< 65	25.0
65–75	56.9
> 75	18.2
Sex, male	80.3
Smoking (pack-years)	(average 38.2 ± 26.4)
never	14.3
1–37	31.4
> 37	54.3
Taking antihypertensive drugs	38.2
Diabetes	6.7
Family history AAA	6.3
History of cerebrovascular disease	14.7
Valvular heart disease	4.1
History of previous MI	
> 6 months	23.0
within 6 months	1.5
Previous coronary artery bypass	6.8
Congestive heart failure	
within 1 week preop	0.4
remote episode	8.0
Angina	
with maximum exertion	13.6
when walks 1–2 blocks or 1 flight stairs at normal pace	6.1
angina, unstable	0.7
ECG	
evidence ischaemia	13.5
old infarct	26.2
LVH, strain	9.0
bundle branch block	13.3
rhythm other than sinus or atrial premature beats	7.2
more than 5 VPBs per min	2.6
Clinical evidence of chronic obstructive lung disease	28.0
BUN > 7.0	34.4
Creatinine > 1.3	18.3

AAA: Abdominal aortic aneurysm. MI: myocardial infarction; LVH: left ventricular hypertrophy; BUN: blood urea nitrogen.

Statistical analysis

Statistical significance between groups ($p<0.05$) was determined by a two-tailed *t*-test for continuous variables and chi-square test for categorical variables. The logistic multiple regression model was fit to binary variables (i.e. those categorized as 0 or 1) or categorical dependent variables. This determined those variables associated with a dependent variable and eliminated those with a significant confounding effect. To determine the late survival rates and the potentially important predictive variables associated with late survival, the Kaplan–Meier method was used to calculate the cumulative percent survival rate versus time of follow-up for individual variables; the statistical difference between survival curves was determined using the log-rank test. Variables were not considered significant if $p>0.05$. The Cox proportional hazards model was used for multivariate analysis of the factors associated with late survival.

EARLY MORTALITY RATE

For the 680 patients with non-ruptured aneurysms, the overall 30-day mortality rate was 4.7% (32/680). There was no statistical difference ($p<0.05$) in the mortality rate based on indication (asymptomatic 3.9%, asymptomatic with evidence of enlargement 4.9%, and symptomatic 7.2%) or the urgency of operation (elective 4.5% and urgent 7.1%) and consequently all patients with non-ruptured AAA were grouped together in our analysis. This observation is in contrast to other studies that reported a higher mortality among symptomatic patients having urgent surgery.[5]

The overall mortality for non-ruptured AAA in this study of 4.7% compares with the mortality rate for other series that reported results from multiple surgeons: The Cleveland Vascular Society[6] 6.5%, Norwegian multicentre study 7.5%,[7] State of Michigan 5.6% in 1990.[8–9]

Atherosclerotic risk factors

None of the assessed atherosclerotic risk factors had a relationship with mortality including current or past smoking or the amount smoked, hypertension, diabetes, or obesity (body weight greater than 120% of ideal). Lipid abnormalities were not assessed.

Comorbidity risk factors

As listed in Table 2, mortality rates were higher if patients were older, had a remote episode of congestive heart failure, higher angina grade, ECG evidence of ischaemia, evidence of cerebrovascular disease, clinical evidence of chronic obstructive lung disease, and/or elevated serum creatinine. These factors were also noted by Diehl *et al.*[10]

Table 2. Risk factors and associated operative mortality

Variable	*Mortality (%)*	*p-Value*
Age (years)		
<60	0.0	
60–79	5.3	
≥80	10.9	0.04
Congestive heart failure (remote)		
no	4.2	
yes	18.2	0.0003
Angina		
grade 0 (nil)	3.7	
grade 1 (with maximum exertion)	4.8	
grade 2 (1–2 blocks or 1 flight)	17.6	
grade 3 (with any activity; at rest)	33.3	
grade 4 (not classifiable)	16.7	0.003
ECG evidence ischaemia		
no	3.7	
yes	15.4	0.00007
COLD		
no	3.3	
yes	8.9	0.006
Creatinine		
<110	2.9	
110–199	8.2	
≥200	27.8	0.00006
Cerebrovascular disease		
no	3.9	
yes	10.3	0.003

COLD: Clinical evidence of chronic obstructive lung disease

Predictors of early mortality – the high risk patient

Logistic regression analysis identified the multiple variables that, together, were predictive of early mortality: ECG evidence of ischaemia, clinical evidence of chronic obstructive lung disease, and creatinine >160. Table 3 lists the predicted early mortality based on these three significant variables. Table 4 shows an alternative model that includes the patient's age in addition to these three variables.

Table 3. First model predicting early mortality rate: predicted mortality rate based on results of logistic regression analysis

ECG ischaemia	*Chronic lung disease*	*Creatinine >160*	*Mortality rate (%)*
No	No	No	1.9
No	No	Yes	11.5
No	Yes	No	4.8
No	Yes	Yes	25.0
Yes	No	No	5.7
Yes	No	Yes	28.4
Yes	Yes	No	13.5
Yes	Yes	Yes	50.4

Reproduced from Ref. 2, with permission from Mosby Publishers, St Louis, MO, USA

Table 4. Second model predicting early mortality rate: predicted mortality rate based on results of logistic regression analysis

Age <65												
ECG ischaemia	No	No	No	No	No	No	Yes	Yes	Yes	Yes	Yes	Yes
COLD	No	No	No	Yes	Yes	Yes	No	No	No	Yes	Yes	Yes
Creatinine	<110	110–160	>160	<110	110–160	>160	<110	110–160	>160	<110	110–160	>160
Mortality rate %	1	2	4	1	4	9	2	4	11	4	10	23
Ages 65–80												
ECG ischaemia	No	No	No	No	No	No	Yes	Yes	Yes	Yes	Yes	Yes
COLD	No	No	No	Yes	Yes	Yes	No	No	No	Yes	Yes	Yes
Creatinine	<110	110–160	>160	<110	110–160	>160	<110	110–160	>160	<110	110–160	>160
Mortality rate %	2	4	11	4	10	22	5	12	26	10	24	46
Age >80												
ECG ischaemia	No	No	No	No	No	No	Yes	Yes	Yes	Yes	Yes	Yes
COLD	No	No	No	Yes	Yes	Yes	No	No	No	Yes	Yes	Yes
Creatinine	<110	110–160	>160	<110	110–160	>160	<110	110–160	>160	<110	110–160	>160
Mortality rate %	4	11	25	10	23	45	12	27	49	24	46	30

COLD: Clinical evidence of chronic obstructive lung disease.

EARLY CARDIAC MORTALITY

Cardiac complications accounted for 68.8% (22/32) of the inhospital deaths (i.e. a mortality rate of 3.2%). However, the approach to preoperative assessment remains a challenge. Preoperative evidence of coronary artery disease or its sequelae (i.e. history of myocardial infarction, angina, or congestive heart failure and/or ECG evidence of ischaemia or old infarction) were present in 44.7% of cases. However, patients without clinical evidence of coronary artery disease (i.e. asymptomatic and with an ECG that did not show evidence of ischaemia) had a 0.8% cardiac mortality compared with 6.2% if any stigmata of coronary disease were present ($p<0.001$). These data support the selective investigation of those patients with clinical or ECG evidence of coronary artery disease to determine the subgroup that may benefit from maximum medical and anaesthetic management or aortocoronary bypass or angioplasty before AAA repair as also suggested by Golden *et al.*[11]

LATE MORTALITY RATE

The late survival rate at 1 month was 94.6 ± 0.8%, at 1 year 90.7 ± 1.2%, at 2 years 87.1 ± 1.3%, at 3 years 81.0 ± 1.6%, at 4 years 74.0 ± 1.8%, and at 5 years 67.7 ± 1.9%. These prospective data are in close agreement with the retrospective 5-year survival data reported in other series.[12–16] It appears that late survival has not improved significantly over the past two decades perhaps because improvements in surgical, medical and anaesthetic management have been offset by selecting higher risk patients.

The 5-year survival rate for patients undergoing AAA repair is 67.7% and is significantly less than that for the age- and sex-matched data for the Canadian population (83.1%). A lower survival rate after AAA repair has also been documented in other studies.[8,12,16–19]

Variables that are predictive of late survival

Table 5 lists the individual preoperative variables that were predictive of late survival as determined by Kaplan–Meier analysis.

Cox regression analysis was used to determine the combination of the multiple variables that are predictive of late survival. The significant predictors were age, preoperative ECG indicating a previous myocardial infarction, and serum creatinine. Table 6 lists the predicted 5-year survival for various combinations of these variables. Note that in the original publication,[3] two other Cox models are given as possible alternatives.

Using retrospective data and multivariate analysis, Roger *et al.*[17] noted that age, history of coronary artery disease, and stroke were important predictors of late survival. Nachbur *et al.*,[12] for 204 cases evaluated retrospectively in a Swiss study of patients undergoing operation between 1978 and 1984, reported an operative mortality rate of 3.3% and a 5-year actuarial survival of 68%. They noted reduced survival with increasing age (47.0% for ages 70–79, 76.2% for ages 60–69, and 96.4% for ages 50–59) and concomitant heart disease (59.1% vs 74.5%). In a prospective multicentre observational study in Norway, the significant preoperative factors were age, impaired renal function and the presence of angina.[20] In a follow-up of 95% of 834 patients undergoing operation in France in 1989, the following variables were associated with survival by univariate analysis: age, coronary heart disease (arrhythmia, ECG evidence of ischaemia, or left ventricular insufficiency), carotid occlusion, and renal insufficiency.[16] In their classic study, Crawford *et al.*[13] reported an inhospital mortality rate of 4.8% for 860 patients operated on between 1955 and 1980 and a 5-year actuarial survival of 63%. Multiple regression analysis was not

Table 5. Variables that are associated with 5-year survival heart failure.

Variable	*Kaplan–Meier % 5-year survival*	*Statistical significance*
Age		
<65	82.4	
65–75	66.4	
>75	54.6	p=0.000
History CHF		
no	69.7	
yes	48.2	p=0.000
Angina		
no	69.6	
only with maximal exertion when walks	67.9	
1–2 blocks or 1 flight of stairs at normal pace	47.6	p=0.000
ECG evidence of ischaemia		
no	70.2	
yes	51.5	p=0.000
ECG old infarct		
no	72.8	
yes	54.4	p=0.000
ECG LVH or strain		
no	70.7	
yes	41.8	p=0.000
EGK rhythm other than sinus or atrial premature beats		
no	70.5	
yes	40.2	p=0.000
Clinical evidence of chronic obstructive lung disease or abnormal pO_2, pCO_2, or FEV_1		
no	71.3	
yes	59.0	p=0.003
Creatinine ≥1.5		
no	71.8	
yes	40.4	p=0.000

CHF: Congestive heart failure
LVH: Left ventricular hypertrophy
Reproduced from Ref. 3, with permission from Mosby Publishers, St Louis, MO, USA.

Table 6. Predicted 5-year survival based on Cox regression model

Age	*Preoperative ECG showing old myocardial infarction*	*Creatinine*	*Predicted % 5-year survival*
<65	No	<1.5	85.7
<65	Yes	<1.5	76.8
<65	No	≥1.5	67.7
<65	Yes	≥1.5	51.3
65–75	No	<1.5	75.4
65–75	Yes	<1.5	61.8
65–75	No	≥1.5	49.0
65–75	Yes	≥1.5	29.6
>75	No	<1.5	59.8
>75	Yes	<1.5	41.5
>75	No	≥1.5	27.2
>75	Yes	≥1.5	10.8

For this model, the coefficients are age=0.582, ECG=0.475, and creatinine=0.867, log-likelihood ratio=-1191.20, and p=0.000. Codes for the variables: age (1 is for <65 years; 2 for 65–75 years; 3 for >75 years), preoperative ECG showing old myocardial infarction (0 is for no, and 1 for yes), and creatinine (1 is for value < 1.5, and 2 for ≥1.5).
Reproduced from Ref. 3, with permission from Mosby Publishers, St Louis, MO, USA.

performed, but the following individual variables were found to be related to survival (5-year survival rates are listed): age (for ages <61 years 71%, for ages 61–71 66%, and for ages >71 43%), hypertension (absent 84%, present 59%), arteriosclerotic heart disease (absent 84%, present 54%). Reigel *et al.*[15] retrospectively reviewed 499 cases of elective AAA repair at the Mayo Clinic between 1980 and 1985. The 5-year actuarial survival rate was reduced if there was evidence of coronary artery disease (66% vs 83%) and advancing age (46% if age 80–89, 71% if age 70–79, 76% if age 60–69, and 70% if age 50–59). White *et al.*[18] found that the 5-year actuarial survival rate reduced by advancing age (67% for 60–70 years, 50% for ages 71–80 years, and 35% for >80 years), Goldman classification, cerebrovascular disease, history of cardiac disease, and creatinine level >3 mg/100 ml.

LATE CARDIAC MORTALITY

The causes of late mortality after AAA repair could be determined in 98.5% of the cases and are listed in Table 7 along with the causes for an age- and sex-matched Canadian population.

Cardiac complications accounted for 44.4% (91/205) during 5-year follow-up. Thus, if a patient survives the AAA repair, the chance of dying from a cardiac event

Table 7. Causes of late death (%)

	Elective AAA repair (n=205)	*Age- and sex-matched population*
Cardiac	44.4	34.1
Cancer	28.3	32.6
Cerebrovascular	8.3	5.8
Pulmonary	6.8	8.9
Renal failure	5.4	
Atherosclerosis		0.6
Liver failure	0.5	1.2
Diabetes		2.2
Ruptured thoracic aneurysm	1.5	
Ruptured abdominal aneurysm	1.5	
Gastrointestinal bleeding	1.0	
Other	1.0	14.5
Unknown	1.5	

If a cause of death was not recorded, entry is left blank
Reproduced from Ref. 3, with permission from Mosby Publishers, St Louis, MO, USA

in the next 5 years is 14.3%. Since the cardiac mortality rate for the age- and sex-matched population is 6.4% during a 5-year follow-up period, the increased risk of cardiac death after aneurysm repair is 1.6% per year over the first 5 years. With this relatively small difference between patients having AAA surgery and the general population, it is doubtful that a general preoperative screening and treatment programme can be developed that will be cost-effective. However, a cardiac screening programme may be justified in high-risk groups as discussed below.

Variables that are predictive of late cardiac mortality

Cox regression analysis determined that the significant predictors of late cardiac mortality included age, preoperative angina grade (0: asymptomatic; 1: angina only with maximum exertion; 2: angina when walks 1–2 blocks or 1 flight of stairs at a normal pace) and preoperative ECG indicating a previous myocardial infarction. Table 8 gives the predicted 5-year cardiac mortality rates based on these variables. In developing a strategy to reduce late mortality by selective preoperative cardiac investigation, these data provide a basis for this decision.

DISCUSSION AND CONCLUSIONS

Identification of high risk patient

In this study, as summarized in Table 2, patients with advanced age, abnormal creatinine, or evidence of cerebrovascular or chronic obstructive disease have above-average operative risk. Tables 3 and 4 summarize the results of two alternative models that predict the early mortality rate based on the most significant variables as

Table 8. Predicted 5-year cardiac mortality rate based on Cox regression model

Age	*Preoperative EKG showing old myocardial infarction*	*Angina grade*	*% 5-year cardiac mortality*
1	0	0	8.2
1	1	0	20.0
1	0	1	11.4
1	1	1	27.1
1	0	2	15.8
1	1	2	36.1
2	0	0	11.2
2	1	0	26.6
2	0	1	15.4
2	1	1	35.5
2	0	2	21.1
2	1	2	46.3
3	0	0	15.1
3	1	0	34.8
3	0	1	20.7
3	1	1	45.5
3	0	2	28.0
3	1	2	57.7

Cox regression model include age (1: <65 years; 2: 65–75 years; 3: >75 years), preoperative angina grade (0: asymptomatic, 1: angina only with maximum exertion, 2: angina when walks 1–2 blocks or 1 flight of stairs at a normal pace) and preoperative ECG indicating a previous myocardial infarction (0: no, 1: yes). For this model, the coefficients are age=0.325, angina=0.348, and EGK-MI=0.867, log-likelihood ratio: 609.89 and p=0.000.

determined by logistic regression analysis. In selecting patients for non-operative treatment or endovascular repair and describing the patient population in future studies, it is important to define high risk patients by comparison with these or other clearly defined risk factors.

Indications for repair of AAA

For each patient, it is necessary to balance the potential benefits of surgical repair of an AAA against continued follow-up. Late mortality of a patient who does not undergo repair of an AAA is determined by the mortality caused by their comorbid conditions over time plus the additional mortality as a result of rupture. The predicted mortality attributed to the patient's comorbid conditions can be estimated using clinical judgment or actuarial tables. The risk of rupture is estimated by considering the absolute size and change in size of the AAA and perhaps the presence or absence of diastolic hypertension.[21] Of the available studies, the Kingston experience provides a basis for current practice: AAA less than 5 cm in diameter rarely rupture and follow-up is justified;[22] however, because the authors demonstrated that the aneurysms between 5.0 and 5.4 cm had a definite risk of rupture and showed a progressive increase in expansion rate, repair may be justified for selected patients who are in good general health when the AAA is between 4.5 and 5.0 cm.[23] After AAA repair, overall mortality depends on the operative mortality and late mortality rate. The mortality rate in this study was 4.7% and depended on the risk factors identified above (Table 2, Table 3, and Table 4). Late survival rate can be predicted by considering age, preoperative ECG, and serum creatinine (Table 6).

Standard for comparison of results of endovascular treatment

Observations from this prospective multicentre study can be generalized to reflect current surgical practice and standards of AAA surgery on a national level. It is recognized that some individuals and/or institutions may have outstanding surgical or endovascular results that can only be duplicated by a few others because of their special skills or facilities. These outstanding results should be published to establish safety of the procedure and act as a bench mark for others; eventually, however, results obtained by multiple surgeons and from a broad population of patients must be presented before it is possible to determine if the new technology has generalized application. The Canadian Aneurysm Study provides data from a population of 72 surgeons and patients and because the risk factors have been identified, the results can form a basis for comparison with the results of new interventions.

REFERENCES

1. Johnston KW, Scobie TK: Multicenter prospective study of nonruptured abdominal aortic aneurysms. I. Population and operative management. *J Vasc Surg* **7:** 69–81, 1988
2. Johnston KW: Multicenter prospective study of nonruptured abdominal aortic aneurysm. Part II. Variables predicting morbidity and mortality. *J Vasc Surg* **9:** 437–447, 1989
3. Johnston KW: Nonruptured abdominal aortic aneurysm: six-year follow-up results from the multicenter prospective Canadian aneurysm study. Canadian Society for Vascular Surgery Aneurysm Study Group. *J Vasc Surg* **20:** 163–170, 1994
4. Johnston KW: Influence of sex on the results of abdominal aortic aneurysm repair. Canadian Society for Vascular Surgery Aneurysm Study Group. *J Vasc Surg* **20:** 914–926, 1994
5. Fielding JW, Black J, Ashton F *et al.*: Diagnosis and management of 528 abdominal aortic aneurysms. *Br Med J (Clin Res Ed)* **283:** 355–359, 1981
6. Hertzer NR, Avellone JC, Farrell CJ *et al.*: The risk of vascular surgery in a metropolitan community. With observations on surgeon experience and hospital size. *J Vasc Surg* **1:** 13–21, 1984
7. Amundsen S, Trippestad A, Viste A et al.: Abdominal aortic aneurysms – a national multicentre study. *Eur J Vasc Surg* **1:** 239–243, 1987
8. Hallett JW Jr, Naessens JM, Ballard DJ: Early and late outcome of surgical repair for small abdominal aortic aneurysms: a population-based analysis. *J Vasc Surg* **18:** 684–691, 1993
9. Katz DJ, Stanley JC, Zelenock GB: Operative mortality rates for intact and ruptured abdominal aortic aneurysms in Michigan: an eleven-year statewide experience. *J Vasc Surg* **19:** 804–817, 1994
10. Diehl JT, Cali RF, Hertzer NR et al.: Complications of abdominal aortic reconstruction. An analysis of perioperative risk factors in 557 patients. *Ann Surg* **197:** 49–56, 1983

11. Golden MA, Whittemore AD, Donaldson MC *et al.*: Selective evaluation and management of coronary artery disease in patients undergoing repair of abdominal aortic aneurysms. A 16-year experience. *Ann Surg* **212**: 415–420, 1990
12. Nachbur B, Gut A, Sigrist S: Prognostic factors in the surgical treatment of aorto-iliac aneurysmal disease. Factors affecting survival and long-term results. *J Cardiovasc Surg (Torino)* **28:** 469–478, 1987
13. Crawford ES, Saleh SA, Babb JW *et al.*: Infrarenal abdominal aortic aneurysm: factors influencing survival after operation performed over a 25-year period. *Ann Surg* **194**: 180–188, 1981
14. Vohra R, Reid D, Groome J *et al.*: Long-term survival in patients undergoing resection of abdominal aortic aneurysm. *Ann Vasc Surg* **4:** 460–465, 1990
15. Reigel MM, Hollier LH, Kazmier FJ *et al.*: Late survival in abdominal aortic aneurysm patients: the role of selective myocardial revascularization on the basis of clinical symptoms. *J Vasc Surg* **5**: 222–227, 1987
16. Koskas F, Kieffer E: Long-term survival after elective repair of infrarenal abdominal aortic aneurysm: results of a prospective multicentric study. Association for Academic Research in Vascular Surgery (AURC). *Ann Vasc Surg* **11:** 473–481, 1997
17. Roger VL, Ballard DJ, Hallett JWJ *et al.*: Influence of coronary artery disease on morbidity and mortality after abdominal aortic aneurysmectomy: a population-based study, 1971–1987. *J Am Coll Cardiol* **14:** 1245–1252, 1989
18. White GH, Advani SM, Williams RA *et al.*: Cardiac risk index as a predictor of long-term survival after repair of abdominal aortic aneurysm. *Am J Surg* **156:** 103–107, 1988
19. Aune S, Amundsen SR, Evjensvold J et al.: Operative mortality and long-term relative survival of patients operated on for asymptomatic abdominal aortic aneurysm. *Eur J Vasc Endovasc Surg* **9:** 293–298, 1995
20. Amundsen S, Skjaerven R, Trippestad A *et al.*: Abdominal aortic aneurysms – a study of factors influencing postoperative mortality. Norwegian Aortic Aneurysm Trial. *Eur J Vasc Endovasc Surg* **3:** 405–409, 1989
21. Cronenwett JL, Sargent SK, Wall MH *et al.*: Variables that affect the expansion rate and outcome of small abdominal aortic aneurysms. *J Vasc Surg* **11:** 260–269, 1990
22. Brown PM, Pattenden R, Gutelius JR: The selective management of small abdominal aortic aneurysms: the Kingston study. *J Vasc Surg* **15:** 21–27, 1992
23. Brown PM, Pattenden R, Vernooy C *et al.*: Selective management of abdominal aortic aneurysms in a prospective measurement program. *J Vasc Surg* **23:** 213–222, 1996

Commentary

This chapter and many previous studies have suggested that life expectancy after elective repair of an abdominal aortic aneurysm is less than the life expectancy in an age- and sex-matched population. Recently this viewpoint has been challenged with new evidence from Western Australia. Norman and colleagues[1] in a meticulous study of a stable geographically confined population have shown that for men the 5-year survival following aneurysm repair was 95% of the survival for an age-matched cohort. In contrast, women faired considerably worse after aneurysm repair and their 5-year survival was only 88% of the survival for an age-matched cohort.[1] However, the population of Western Australia must be very healthy since the average 5-year survival following aneurysm repair was 79%. In almost every other study, from Western Europe or North America, the 5-year survival has been reported at about 65%. Recently, we have shown that the 6-year survival following elective repair of a small abdominal aortic aneurysm was 64%.[2] There also is general agreement that cardiovascular disease caused the majority of deaths.[1,2]

During the time period in which these studies have been conducted, life expectancy has continued to increase. Therefore, we cannot use these past studies to compare with the results of newer treatments, including endovascular repair. *JTP*

References

1. Norman PE, Semmens JB, Lawrence-Brown MHD, Holman DJ: Long-term relative survival after surgery for abdominal aortic aneurysm in Western Australia: population based study. *Br Med J* **317:** 852–856, 1998
2. UK Small Aneurysm Trial Participants: Mortality results for randomised controlled trial of early elective surgery or ultrasonographic surveillance for small abdominal aortic aneurysms. *Lancet* **352:** 1649–1655, 1998

Life expectancy for intermittent claudicants (peripheral vascular disease)

Felicity Barbara Smith and Francis Gerald Reid Fowkes

INTRODUCTION

Atherosclerotic peripheral vascular disease (PVD) has become one of the most significant health problems in developed countries in recent times. Intermittent claudication (exercise-induced leg pain) is the most common early symptom and is primarily due to occlusion of the main arteries of the lower limb. By late middle age, approximately 5% of men and women in the UK will demonstrate symptoms of intermittent claudication[1,2] and about 50 000 patients in England and Wales are admitted to hospital each year because of severely disabling disease.[3] In addition, for every claudicant in the community, at least two individuals have asymptomatic disease significant enough to cause a reduction in ankle pressure.[2]

Despite apparent symptomatic improvement in many patients, PVD is a progressive disease. About a quarter of patients referred to a peripheral vascular clinic will deteriorate significantly and progress to rest pain, ulceration and gangrene, and the majority of these will ultimately require vascular surgery of some description.[4] There is also increasing awareness that individuals with PVD have substantially increased risks of premature death, mainly from ischaemic heart disease and stroke.[1,5–10] Hence the diagnosis of PVD itself is a marker for widespread systemic atherosclerosis, which may have important prognostic implications for the patient. The aim of this chapter is to assess the critical role of ischaemic heart disease and stroke in patients with limb ischaemia. The prevalence of coronary and cerebrovascular disease in PVD and the risk of mortality will be described. Factors affecting mortality will also be discussed.

PREVALENCE OF ISCHAEMIC HEART DISEASE

The reported prevalence of ischaemic heart disease in individuals with intermittent claudication varies widely and is dependent on the method of assessing coronary disease and type of population studied. Table 1 is adapted from a review by Dormandy *et al.*[4] summarizing the prevalence of concomitant heart disease in patients with PVD. While between 30% and 50% of hospital claudicants have ischaemic heart disease diagnosed by resting ECG or by clinical history, the prevalence of heart disease is increased to more than 60% if a stress test is used. Newer non-invasive imaging techniques, such as dipyridamole-thallium scanning have also detected evidence of ischaemic heart disease in a similar proportion of patients. However, as many as 90% of patients have been identified as having heart

Table 1. Prevalence of coronary heart disease in selected series of surgical patients with lower limb arterial disease

First author (year)	*No. of patients*	*Method of detection*	*Prevalence of coronary heart disease (%)*
Szilagyi (1979)	531	History + ECG	39
Malone (1977)	180	History + ECG	58
DeWeese (1977)	103	History + ECG	34
Crawford (1981)	949	History + ECG	38
Hertzer (1981)	256	History + ECG	47
Szilagyi (1986)	1748	Not specified	47
Vecht (1982)	100	Treadmill stress ECG	62
Brewster (1985)	54	Dipyridamole - stress thallium imaging	63
Hertzer (1984)	381	Angiography	90

Adapted from Ref. 4. The references cited in the first column may be found in Ref. 4, but are not listed at the end of this chapter.

disease if examined by coronary angiography, with stenosis > 70% found in 57% of the patients in one study.[11] Hence, it can be deduced from these results that the reported prevalence of coronary disease in PVD is dependent on the particular measurement technique used to detect coronary lesions and that the true extent of concomitant coronary disease is likely to be underestimated in most studies.

The prevalence of ischaemic heart disease in population studies has been reported to vary between 20 and 52% and to be between two and four times higher among persons with PVD than those without PVD.[1,2,12–14] In most of the studies, the presence of intermittent claudication has been identified by the World Health Organization (WHO) claudication questionnaire[15] and evidence of ischaemic heart disease using diagnostic criteria such as a history of previous myocardial infarction or the WHO angina questionnaire.[15] These methods undoubtably underestimate the true prevalence of both coronary and lower limb disease and may as a result decrease the overlap between reported frequencies of PVD and concomitant ischaemic heart disease. Underestimation of the true prevalences can occur because the presence of PVD can mask the symptoms of ischaemic heart disease by limiting exercise and also because both the WHO angina and claudication questionnaires have been shown to be only moderately sensitive in detecting those with true disease.[16]

Ankle brachial pressure index and asymptomatic disease

The ankle brachial pressure index (ABPI) test is perhaps the most common non-invasive method of assessing the severity of lower limb atherosclerosis in population surveys. Based on results from clinical studies on selected hospital patients, an ABPI of < 0.9 is considered a highly sensitive marker of PVD, and an index of 1.0 is almost 100% specific in identifying subjects without apparent disease.[17,18] Although the optimal level for an abnormal ABPI in epidemiological surveys has not been determined, it is thought that the true prevalence of asymptomatic PVD in the population may be four times higher than the prevalence of intermittent claudication.[2]

Table 2. Number and percent of participants with cardiovascular disease in subgroups with decreasing ankle-arm index : Cardiovascular Health study

Ankle brachial pressure index	*≥1.0–<1.5* *n=3835*	*≥0.9–<1.0* *n=566*	*≥0.8–<0.9* *n=252*	*<0.8* *n=371*	*p* *(trend)*
Myocardial infarction					
n (%)	264 (7.3)	49 (9.4)	35 (15.0)	74 (21.8)	
RR	1	1.3	2.0	2.7	<0.0001
Angina					
n (%)	416 (11.5)	76 (14.6)	41 (17.4)	88 (26.5)	
RR	1	1.3	1.4	2.1	<0.0001
CHF					
n (%)	60 (1.6)	8 (1.4)	10 (4.0)	22 (6.0)	
RR	1	0.9	2.1	3.1	<0.0001

From Ref. 21.
RR : Relative risk. CHF : Congestive heart failure.

A low ABPI has consistently been associated with an increased prevalence of co-existing ischaemic heart disease in individuals with lower limb disease. For example, in the prospective cohort 'Men born in 1914' study of 60 men with an ABPI< 0.9, 20 (33%) had evidence of angina or previous myocardial infarction and a further 11 (18%) had silent ST-segment depression of ≥ 1mm on electrocardiogram (ECG) recording.[19] Another population study in Holland[20] showed that there was a negative correlation between the prevalence of reported ischaemic heart disease and the ABPI level. Among subjects with an ABPI≥ 0.95, the prevalence of heart disease was only 9% compared with 30% in those with an ABPI< 0.95. In individuals with an ABPI< 0.75, the prevalence rose to 50%. Similarly, the Cardiovascular Health Study of men and women over 65 years in the USA[21] demonstrated a clear graded relationship between decreasing levels of ABPI (indicating greater severity of PVD) and the increasing frequency of myocardial infarction, angina and congestive heart failure (Table 2) This finding was also confirmed in the Atherosclerosis Risk In Communities (ARIC) study.[22] Furthermore, subjects with an ABPI< 0.90 were twice as likely to have prevalent ischaemic heart disease as subjects with an ABPI> 0.90. The association was of similar magnitude in black and white men, but weaker in white women.[22] The ABPI therefore appears to correlate with the occurrence of ischaemic heart disease in individuals diagnosed as having PVD by this test.

PREVALENCE OF CEREBROVASCULAR DISEASE

The percentage of hospital claudicants with a clinical history of cerebrovascular disease appears to be lower overall, with a typical prevalence of 0.5–15.0%, but angiography or duplex scanning was rarely performed to assess the presence of asymptomatic disease in the earlier studies (Table 3). However, in the study of 160

Table 3. Prevalence of cerebrovascular disease in selected series of surgical patients with lower limb disease

First author (year)	*No. of patients*	*Method of detection*	*Prevalence of cerebrovascular disease (%)*
Begg (1962)	198	Clinical history	0.5
Malone (1977)	180	Clinical history and examination	45
DeWeese (1977)	103	Clinical history	4
Hughson (1978)	54	Clinical history	15
Szilagyi (1986)	1748	Unknown	19
Szilagi (1979)	531	Clinical history and angiography	13
Turnipseed (1980)	160	Cervical bruit	44
		Doppler	52

Adapted from Ref. 4. The references cited in the first column may be found in Ref. 4, but are not listed at the end of this chapter.

claudicants, where the presence of cervical bruits (as an indicator of carotid disease) was assessed, the prevalence of cerebrovascular disease was found to be much higher at 44%, with a further 8% diagnosed as having disease on Doppler ultrasonography. As is the case with ischaemic heart disease, variation in prevalence is undoubtably due to differing definitions of disease, methods of assessment and the type of population studied.

Even less information is available on the prevalence of cerebrovascular disease in subjects with PVD in the general population. However, community-based surveys have found an increased history of cerebrovascular disease in those with PVD compared with normals. For example, a higher prevalence of cerebrovascular disease has been noted in subjects with lower limb disease (11%) relative to those without PVD (3%).[20] Furthermore, the frequency of both stroke and transient ischaemic attacks was demonstrated to increase across subgroups with defined categories of decreasing levels of ABPI in the Cardiovascular Health study.[21] In the ARIC study, men with an ABPI< 0.90 had a four-fold risk of stroke/TIA compared with men with a higher index. As with clinical heart disease, the relationship between cerebrovascular disease and a low ABPI was weaker in women and statistically non-significant.[22]

Prevalence of carotid stenosis

In the last 15–20 years, the introduction of non-invasive diagnostic methods, particularly duplex scanning has permitted detection of asymptomatic cerebrovascular disease, as well as determining the site and severity of carotid lesions in those with a history of stroke or transient ischaemic attacks. From the limited data available, selected patients with PVD appear to have a higher prevalence of carotid stenosis than patients with heart disease or apparently healthy subjects. For example, in one large screening study, the proportion of patients who had a carotid stenosis > 50% was 32.8% in patients with PVD, 6.8% in those with coronary disease and 5.9% in those with raised levels of cardiovascular risk factors.[23] Klop *et al.*[24] confirmed that the overall prevalence of > 50% carotid stenosis was significantly raised (26.6% of study patients) in those with lower limb disease.

Prevalence studies of asymptomatic carotid disease have rarely been undertaken in community surveys. However, the Cardiovascular Health study[20] showed that the occurrence of carotid plaques detected by B-mode ultrascan correlated with decreasing ABPI. Among those with an ABPI≥ 1.0, the prevalence of carotid plaques was 60%, which increased to 88% in those with an ABPI≤ 0.8. Furthermore, a level of ABPI between 0.8 and 0.9 was associated with a ten-fold increase in risk in subjects having a stenosis > 75% relative to an ABPI of 1.0–1.5.

Relationship between carotid intimal medial thickness and peripheral vascular disease

Measurement of carotid wall thickness is increasingly being assessed in epidemiological surveys as an indicator of early atherosclerosis, and has been shown to be a valid and accurate marker of subclinical disease.[25–27] A relationship between carotid intimal-medial thickness (IMT) and the ABPI has already been demonstrated in two population studies. In the Rotterdam study of 7983 subjects aged 55 years or over, the ABPI including levels indicative of asymptomatic PVD, decreased with increasing levels of carotid IMT, especially in males.[28] This association has also been shown in the Edinburgh Artery study.[29] Furthermore, carotid IMT levels were significantly higher in subjects with claudication in this study compared with those with no evidence of claudication.[28] A strong and highly consistent inverse relationship between the ABPI and carotid atherosclerosis, assessed by either pre-clinical carotid plaque or carotid IMT was also demonstrated across both racial and gender subgroups in the ARIC study.[22] Interestingly, the inverse correlation between ABPI and IMT was shown as a quadratic curve rather than a straight-line relationship. Overall, these associations between the IMT and ABPI suggest that subjects predisposed to atherosclerosis in the lower limb may also exhibit a tendency to disease in other peripheral arteries.

RISK OF MORTALITY

A major concern in individuals with intermittent claudication or asymptomatic PVD is that they are at significantly increased risk of dying prematurely, primarily from ischaemic heart disease and stroke. This has become apparent not only from earlier studies of hospital referrals[8,9,30–34] but from observations from several population surveys, including Framingham,[35] Basle,[36] London Whitehall,[7] Lipid Research Clinics study,[5] Malmo,[19] Edinburgh Artery study,[6] and studies in Belgium[37] and Finland.[38]

One of the most recent large cohort studies of patients with intermittent claudication referred to hospital, reported an all-cause mortality rate of 35% after 6 years of follow-up.[39] This finding is in keeping with the majority of studies of hospital patients followed for 5 years or more, regardless of differences in patient selection in respect to age, severity of disease and stage of presentation. In general, the culmulative 5-year mortality rate among hospital claudicants is between 20% and

Table 4. 5-Year cumulative mortality rates among subjects with intermittent claudication and age-matched comparison groups

	Age of subjects (years)	5-Year mortality: Intermittent claudication (%)	5-Year mortality: Comparison group (%)	Relative risk
Population studies				
Kannel and Shurtleff (1971)[10]	30–74	17	11	1.5
Reunanen *et al.* (1982)[38]	40–59	12.7	5.7	2.2
Leng *et al.* (1996)[6]	55–74	19	10	1.6
Hospital studies				
(a) Prior to reconstructive surgery				
Juergens *et al.* (1960)[70]	60	23	8	2.9
Bloor (1961)[32]	65–74	42	33	1.3
Begg and Richards (1962)[8]	21–76	25	11	2.3
(b) Surgery not required				
Mathieson *et al.* (1970)[71]	age not stated	52	27	1.9
Kallero (1981)[34]	40–69	28	8	3.5
Jelnes *et al.* (1986)[9]	36–85	31	15	2.0

50%. Claudicants at the time of presentation are three times more likely to die during the following 10 years than the general population matched for age and sex (Table 4).

In prospective epidemiological studies, the 5-year culmulative mortality rates in subjects with intermittent claudication based on the WHO questionnaire are lower overall than in selected hospital series, and range between 10 and 20% (Table 4) although this may be partly due to the greater age of hospital claudicants. Higher levels of risk factors which may predispose to a faster rate of progression of atherosclerotic disease or the severity of concomitant vascular disease at the time of presentation may also be relevant in patients. There is also evidence of an increasing trend in mortality across successive age groups; for example the Edinburgh Artery study reported that the proportion of deaths rose from 10% in the 55–59 year age group to approximately 40% in those aged 70–74 years.[6]

However, the relative mortality risks for claudicants in the general population are not appreciably different from those of patients attending peripheral vascular clinics. Relative risk estimates have varied between 1.3 and 3.5 for all-cause mortality in both patient and population studies when compared with age-matched normals. Most of the excess in mortality was due to cardiovascular disease, particularly ischaemic heart disease. For example, in the Lipids Research Clinics study, the 10-year risk of mortality due to coronary disease among patients with large-vessel PVD was 6.6, whereas all-cause mortality was associated with a relative risk of 3.1.[5] Exclusion of subjects with evidence of cardiovascular disease at baseline, or adjustment for cardiovascular risk factors had little effect on the risk of coronary death. Similar findings were reported in the Framingham study over 10 years[14] and in subjects who were followed-up over 17 years in the London Whitehall study.[7]

One recent study has examined the relationship between incident intermittent claudication (i.e. newly developed cases) and cause-specific mortality in a population sample of male government employees aged between 40 and 65 years over a 21-year period of follow-up. Subjects with symptoms of PVD or cardiovascular disease at baseline were excluded.[40] The findings indicated that incident PVD was more strongly related to stroke deaths than mortality due to ischaemic heart disease. The relative risk for stroke in new onset claudication was more than twice (2.76) that of the risk of coronary death (1.31) relative to men with no claudication. This is in contrast to reports from both hospital and community surveys of prevalent cases of claudication, where a stronger association has been found with future mortality from heart disease in most instances. However, the difference in results may be due to the use of prevalent cases of PVD in previous studies which may introduce selection and survival biases. Also, it is likely that these men with newly diagnosed claudication will have less severe and widespread atherosclerosis than either prevalent cases of PVD in the community or hospital referrals.

CAUSES OF MORTALITY

Because many individuals with PVD have a significant degree of concomitant vascular disease, particularly coronary disease, it is not surprising that between 30% and 60% of deaths among those with symptomatic PVD have been reported to be due to ischaemic heart disease. The proportion of patients dying of cerebrovascular disease is lower, at approximately 10–15%, although the recent Prevention of Atherosclerotic Complications by Ketanserin (PACK) study reported that the percentage of deaths due to stroke was twice as high at 28%.[41] In all, 10% of patients will die from causes related to visceral ischaemia or rupture of an abdominal aneurysm, and the remainder die from non-cardiovascular causes, primarily smoking-related cancers and respiratory disease.[4] Very few deaths, in fact, are due to PVD itself with the exception of operative mortality due to limb amputation.[8]

It also appears that mortality rates may be higher in males than in females. For example, the Prognostic Study of Intermittent Claudication[38] showed that the mortality rate in males for all causes of death was higher than in women, with the exception of stroke. Figure 1 shows the survival curves for men and women separately. A comparison of the survival experience between the sexes was highly statistically significant, with the men dying at a faster rate than the women.

In addition to the prognostic significance of symptomatic PVD, asymptomatic PVD as measured by a low ABPI has also been consistently associated with increased mortality in cohort studies, regardless of the length of follow-up. Most studies have found that an ABPI cut-off point of < 0.9 relative to an index > 0.9 is an independent predictor of future cardiovascular death.[6,19,37,41,46] Relative risks of vascular-related mortality in both men and women with no evidence of baseline cardiovascular disease but an ABPI< 0.9, range between 2 and 5 compared with control groups with an ABPI within the normal range.[5,6,19,37] The relevance of an ABPI cut-off point of < 0.9 to detect subclinical disease in more elderly subjects is less clear however. Two studies based on women with a mean age > 66 years[47] and > 85 years[48] respectively, have reported that the relative risk of mortality was only significant at a lower level of ABPI of either 0.7 or 0.8.

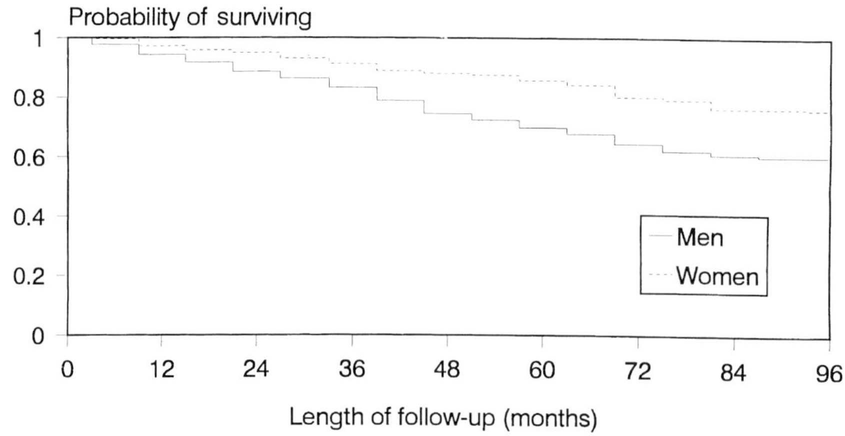

Fig. 1. Survival curves for men and women from the Prognostic Study of Intermittent Claudication.

RISK OF NON-FATAL CARDIOVASCULAR EVENTS

There are comparatively few data on the incidence of non-fatal ischaemic heart disease and stroke events in subjects with intermittent claudication. Most information is derived from population studies in which there are relatively few subjects with claudication. Given that coronary atherosclerosis may co-exist in at least 90% of hospital patients, it is not surprising that there is a high incidence of coronary events in persons with PVD. Among claudicants referred to hospital, around 10–15% have been shown to have a non-fatal coronary event within 6 years[38] and the incidence of coronary events is comparable with that of claudicants derived from the general population. For example, in the Northwick Park study, which followed up 400 claudicants for over 5 years, 14% of subjects had a non-fatal coronary event.[49] Similarly, the Basle study, based on a population of workers in the pharmaceutical industry found that 17% of the surviving cases with PVD developed angina pectoris and 15.0% developed a non-fatal myocardial infarction.[50] Another cohort study, found that approximately 8% of claudicants had a non-fatal infarction, with a similar proportion (9.6%) developing new angina.[6] Interestingly, the risk of future infarction (but not angina) was even higher in subjects with both major and minor categories of asymptomatic PVD than for those with intermittent claudication in this study. Also of note, was the finding that in a Swedish survey, men with PVD only had a cardiac event rate of 21.2 per 1000 person years, but for men with PVD and disease in the carotid and coronary arteries, the event rate was almost twice as great at 38.5 per 1000 person years.[19]

Non-fatal stroke occurs more frequently in individuals with PVD than in non-claudicants, but the incidence is less than for ischaemic heart disease events. The Edinburgh Artery study found that in claudicants, there was a raised relative risk of combined stroke and transient ischaemic attack of 2.0 over 5 years, which was slightly higher than the risk of myocardial infarction (1.2), but both estimates had wide confidence intervals reflecting the relatively low number of new events.[6] The cerebrovascular event rate (stroke and TIA) was three times greater in those who had an ABPI< 0.9 than in those with a higher index in the Malmo study,[19] but surprisingly a low ABPI in conjunction with carotid stenosis was not associated with an increased stroke rate over the 10-year follow-up period.

RISK FACTORS AND OUTCOME

The reason why individuals with lower limb disease are at increased risk of acute cardiovascular events is not fully understood. Since increased mortality is only partly explained by co-existent coronary and cerebrovascular disease associated with claudication[5,7,19,51] attempts have been made to identify factors which might contribute to the increased risk of both fatal and non-fatal cardiovascular events in persons with PVD.

What are the factors which influence outcome in the subjects with intermittent claudication ? Certain traditional risk factors have been associated with increased mortality, notably cigarette smoking, blood pressure, serum lipids and diabetes mellitus. Thrombotic risk factors may also be important in determining cardiovascular outcome in subjects with intermittent claudication which is compatible with results showing that anti-platelet therapy can reduce the incidence of events in claudicants.[52] Evidence relating these factors to adverse outcome in PVD is examined below.

Cigarette smoking

Cigarette smoking is one of the most important risk factors both in the onset and worsening of PVD.[53,54] Patients with claudication who smoke have a faster rate of progression to rest pain, decreased patency of bypass grafting and an increased risk of losing a limb after surgical reconstruction.[55–57] In terms of decreased survival, mortality rates for claudicants who continue to smoke are higher than for those who abstain and most die from myocardial infarction. Survival rates even at 1 year are better in non-smokers than smokers.[58] The effect of cessation of smoking on vascular complications are substantial. In one study, 53% of claudicants who continued to smoke suffered a myocardial infarction and over half had died at 10 years.[59] Conversely, only 11% of patients who had stopped smoking had a myocardial infarction and a much lower proportion of patients (18%) died.[59]

Serum lipids

Numerous clinical and epidemiological studies have found that elevated serum cholesterol and triglyceride levels, and reduced levels of HDL cholesterol are important risk factors in the development of PVD.[60] In longitudinal studies, the association between total cholesterol and the onset of intermittent claudication, or disease estimated by the ABPI is weak, but statistically significant on multivariate analysis.[35,61] At present, there are few data on the predictive value of serum lipid levels in either the progression of PVD or in the development of cardiovascular events. However, one hospital study has identified hypertriglyceridaemia as the most important factor in the onset of critical limb ischaemia in patients with mild to moderate claudication.[62] Lipid-lowering treatments have been shown to have favourable effects on the progression of PVD, primarily reducing the rate of progression in the femoral arteries.[63,64] In addition, a number of randomized controlled trials have shown that lipid-lowering therapy reduces mortality in patients with PVD, although these findings were based on relatively few events.[65]

Blood pressure

Elevated blood pressure is considered a relatively weak risk factor for intermittent claudication. Systolic blood pressure is on the whole, however, thought to be more closely related to the risk of claudication than diastolic pressure, but it is not known whether the relationship is causal or not.[35] Evidence relating blood pressure to clinical outcome in claudication is sparse. In the PACK study, 3899 patients with intermittent claudication were randomized either to ketanserin (which has partly antihypertensive effects) or placebo. Almost half these subjects had hypertension, defined as systolic pressure ≥160 mmHg or diastolic pressure ≥ 95 mmHg. The incidence of lower limb amputation was signifcantly lower in the ketanserin group than in those allocated to placebo. However, as ketanserin also inhibits platelet activation, it is not clear whether the observed effect was due to its anti-thrombotic properties, or because of a reduction in hypertension.[41]

Diabetes mellitus

Diabetes mellitus has long been recognized as associated with vascular disease in the distal arteries and with a poor prognosis in terms of development of critical limb ischaemia, graft failure and amputation, although peripheral neuropathy may also contribute.[66] The risk of non-fatal myocardial infarction and stroke are also elevated in diabetic PVD patients,[41] as is vascular mortality.[67]

Hypercoagulability

There is some evidence that thrombotic risk factors may be important in determining cardiovascular outcome in symptomatic PVD. Banerjee *et al.*[68] studied the association between mortality and fibrinogen levels in stable claudicants and found that there was a two-fold increase in the odds of dying associated with an increase in fibrinogen of 1g/litre. Conversely, in the ADEP (Atherosclerotic Disease Evolution by Picotamide) study, high plasma fibrinogen significantly increased the risk of cerebrovascular events (but not mortality) occurring in patients with PVD over 18 months of follow-up.[69] In a more recent study of hospital claudicants, levels of fibrinogen, t-PA antigen, vWF and fibrin D-dimer were higher in claudicants who developed an ischaemic heart disease or stroke event, but all the relationships became weaker and no longer statistically significant after adjusting for common cardiovascular risk factors.[39] These results suggest that the associations between haemostatic factors and vascular outcome are partly due to inter-relationships with confounding risk factors. However, since the claudicants who experienced coronary events and stroke had higher levels of haemostatic factors at baseline than claudicants who had no events, the elevations in these factors, regardless of their origin are likely to be of pathological importance and may have contributed to the development of these thrombotic events.

CONCLUSION

Peripheral vascular disease, ischaemic heart disease and cerebrovascular disease are clinical manifestations of the same pathological process, and not surprisingly, the three conditions frequently co-exist. The prevalence of clinical ischaemic heart disease is two to three times more common in individuals with intermittent claudication than non-claudicants. Indeed, in patients referred to hospital with leg ischaemia, investigation of the coronary arteries will invariably reveal some degree of atherosclerotic disease. Also, around 15% have a history of stroke, and the prevalence of carotid stenosis, carotid bruits and the degree of intimal-medial thickness in the carotid arteries is greater in those with lower limb disease than in the general population.

For patients with symptomatic or asymptomatic PVD, the natural history of the condition is variable and deterioration to critical limb ischaemia (rest pain, ulceration, gangrene) and amputation is relatively uncommon. Patients are, however, at a greatly increased risk of death (two to three times the relative risk of normals) mostly due to ischaemic heart disease and, to a lesser extent, stroke. This increased risk occurs irrespective of the presence of concomitant heart disease. The magnitude of risk is similar for non-fatal coronary events and stroke. These risk estimates are influenced by the presence of cardiovascular risk factors, particularly smoking, but even when account is taken of risk factors and of the presence of ischaemic heart disease and stroke, patients with PVD are still at increased risk of death.

REFERENCES

1. Hughson WG, Mann JI, Garrod A: Intermittent claudication: prevalence and risk factors. *Br Med J* **1**: 1379–1381, 1978
2. Fowkes FGR, Housley E, Cawood EHH *et al.*: Edinburgh Artery Study: prevalence of asymptomatic and symptomatic peripheral arterial disease in the general population. *Int J Epidemiol* **20**: 384–391, 1991
3. Department of Health and Social Security of Population, Censuses and Surveys: *Hospital In-Patient Enquiry*. Main tables, London: Her Majesty's Stationary Office, 1986
4. Dormandy J, Mahir M, Ascady G *et al.*: Fate of the patient with chronic leg ischaemia. *J Cardiovasc Surg* **30**: 50–57, 1989
5. Criqui MH, Langer RD, Fronek A *et al.*: Mortality over a period of 10 years in patients with peripheral vascular disease. *New Engl J Med* **326**: 381–386, 1992
6. Leng GC, Lee AJ, Fowkes FGR *et al.*: Incidence, natural history and cardiovascular events in symptomatic and asymptomatic peripheral vascular disease in the general population. *Int J Epidemiol* **25**: 1172–1181, 1996

7. Davey Smith G, Shipley MJ, Rose G: Intermittent claudication, heart disease risk factors, and mortality: the Whitehall Study. *Circulation* **82**: 1925–1931, 1990
8. Begg TB, Richards RL: The prognosis of intermittent claudication. *Scot Med J* **7**: 341–352, 1962
9. Jelnes R, Gaardsting O, Hougaard Jensen K *et al.*: Fate in intermittent claudication – outcome and risk factors. *Br Med J* **293**: 1137–1140, 1986
10. Kannel WB, Shurtleff D: The natural history of arteriosclerosis obliterans. *Cardiovasc Clin* **3**: 37–52, 1971
11. Hertzer NR, Beven EG, Young JR *et al.*: Coronary artery disease in peripheral vascular patients: A classification of 1000 angiograms and results of surgical management. *Ann Surg* **199**: 223–233, 1984
12. Reid DD, Holland WW, Hummerfelt S, Rose G: A cardiovascular survey of British postal workers. *Lancet* **i**: 614–618, 1966
13. Bothig S, Metelitsa VI, Barth W *et al.*: Prevalence of ischaemic heart disease, arterial hypertension and intermittent claudication and distribution of risk factors among middle aged men in Moscow and Berlin. *Cor Vasa* **18**: 104–118, 1976
14. Criqui MH, Denenberg JO, Langer RD, Fronek A: The epidemiology of peripheral arterial disease: importance of identifying the population at risk. *Vasc Med* **2**: 221–226, 1997
15. Rose GA: The diagnosis of ischaemic heart pain and intermittent claudication in field surveys. *Bull WHO* **27**: 645–658, 1962
16. Richard JL, Ducimetiere P, Elgrishi I *et al.*: Depistage par questionnaire de l'insuffisance coronarienne et de la claudication intermittente. *Rev Epidemiol Med Soc Sante Publ* **20**: 735–755, 1972
17. Berstein EF, Fronek A: Current status of non-invasive tests in the diagnosis of peripheral arterial disease. *Surg Clin North Am* **62**: 475–487, 1982
18. Laing S, Greenhalgh RM: The detection and progression of asymptomatic peripheral arterial disease. *Br J Surg* **70**: 628–630, 1983
19. Ogren M, Hedblad B, Isacsson S-O *et al.*: Non-invasively detected carotid stenosis and ischaemic heart disease in men with leg arteriosclerosis. *Lancet* **342**: 1138–1141, 1993
20. Stoffers HEJH, Rinkens PELM, Kester ADM *et al.*: The prevalence of asymptomatic and unrecognised peripheral arterial occlusive disease. *Int J Epidemiol* **25**: 282–290, 1996
21. Newman AB, Siscovick DS, Manolio TA *et al.*: Ankle-arm index as a marker of atherosclerosis in the Cardiovascular Health Study. *Circulation* **88**: 837–845, 1993
22. Zheng Z-J, Sharett AR, Chambless LE *et al.*: Associations of ankle-brachial index with clinical coronary heart disease, stroke and preclinical carotid and popliteal atherosclerosis: the Atherosclerosis Risk in Communities (ARIC) Study. *Atherosclerosis* **131**: 115–125, 1997
23. Hennerici M, Aulich A, Sandeman W, Freund H-J: Incidence of asymptomatic extracranial arterial disease. *Stroke* **12**: 750–758, 1981
24. Klop RBJ, Eikelboom BC, Taks ACJM: Screening of the internal carotid arteries in patients with peripheral vascular disease by colour-flow duplex scanning. *Eur J Vasc Surg* **5**: 41–45, 1991
25. Howard G, Sharrett AR, Heiss G *et al.*: Carotid artery intima-media thickness in general populations as evaluated by B-mode ultrasound. *Stroke* **24**: 1297–1304, 1993
26. Kanters SDJM, Algra A, van Leeuwen MS, Banja J: Reproducibility of *in vivo* carotid intima-media thickness measurements: a review. *Stroke* **28**: 665–671, 1997
27. O'Leary DH, Polak JF, Kronmal RA *et al.*: Distribution and correlates of sonographically detected carotid artery disease in the Cardiovascular Health Study. *Stroke* **23**: 1752–1760, 1992
28. Bots ML, Hofman A, Grobbee DE: Common carotid intimal medial thickness and lower extremity arterial atherosclerosis – The Rotterdam Study. *Arterioscler Thromb* **14**: 1885–1891, 1994
29. Allan PL, Mowbray PI, Lee AJ, Fowkes FGR: Relation between carotid intima-media thickness and symptomatic and asymptomatic peripheral arterial disease: the Edinburgh Artery Study. *Stroke* **28**: 348–353, 1997
30. Silbert S, Zazeela H: Prognosis in arteriosclerotic peripheral vascular disease. *J Am Med Assoc* **166**: 1816–1821, 1958
31. Singer A, Rob C: The fate of the claudicator. *Br Med J* **27**: 633–636, 1960

32. Bloor K: Natural history of arteriosclerosis of the lower extremities. *Ann Roy Coll Surg Engl* **28**: 36–52, 1961
33. Taylor GW, Calo AR: Atherosclerosis of arteries of lower limbs. *Br Med J* **1**: 507–510, 1962
34. Kallero KS: Mortality and morbidity in patients with intermittent claudication as defined by venous occlusion plethysmography. A ten year follow-up study. *J Chron Dis* **34**: 455–462, 1981
35. Kannel WB, McGhee DL: Update on some epidemiological features of intermittent claudication: The Framingham Study. *J Am Ger Soc* **33**: 13–18, 1985
36. Widmer LK, Biland L, Da Silva A: Risk profile and occlusive peripheral artery disease (OPAD). In: *Proceedings of 13th International Congress of Angiology*, Athens 9–14th June, 1985
37. Kornitzer M, Dramaix M, Sobolski J *et al.*: Ankle/arm pressure index in asymptomatic middle-aged males: an independent predictor of ten-year coronary heart disease mortality. *Angiography* **46**: 211–219, 1995
38. Reunanen A, Takkunen H, Aromaa A: Prevalence of intermittent claudication and its effect on mortality. *Acta Med Scand* **211**: 249–256, 1982
39. Smith FB, Rumley A, Lee AJ *et al.*: Haemostatic factors and prediction of ischaemic heart disease and stroke in claudicants. *Br J Haematol* **100**: 758–763, 1998
40. Bowlin SJ, Medalie JH, Flocke SA *et al.*: Intermittent claudication in 8343 men and 21-year specific mortality follow-up. *Ann Epidemiol* **7**: 180–187, 1997
41. Dormandy JA, Murray GD: The fate of the claudicant – a prospective study of 1969 claudicants. *Eur J Vasc Surg* **5**: 131–133, 1991
42. Vogt MT, McKenna M, Anderson SJ *et al.*: The relationship between ankle-arm index and mortality in older men and women. *J Am Geriat Soc* **41**: 523–530, 1993
43. Ouriel K, McDonnell AE, Metz CE, Zarins CK: A critical evaluation of stress testing in the diagnosis of peripheral vascular disease. *Surgery* **91**: 686–693, 1982
44. Yao ST, Hobbs JT, Irvine WT: Ankle systolic pressure measurements in arterial disease affecting the lower extremities. *Br J Surg* **56**: 676–679, 1969
45. McKenna M, Wolfson S, Kuller L: The ratio of ankle and arm arterial pressure as an independent predictor of mortality. *Atherosclerosis* **87**: 119–128, 1991
46. Ogren M, Hedblad B, Jungquist G *et al.*: Low ankle-brachial pressure index in 68-year-old men: prevalence, risk factors and prognosis. Results from prospective population study 'Men Born in 1914', Malmo, Sweden. *Eur J Vasc Surg* **7**: 500–506, 1993
47. Vogt MT, Cauley JA, Newman AB *et al.*: Decreased ankle/arm blood pressure index and mortality in elderly women. *J Am Med Assoc* **270**: 465–469, 1993
48. Cammer Paris BE, Libow LS, Halperin JL, Mulvihill MN: The prevalence and one-year outcome of limb arterial disease obstructive disease in a nursing home population. *J Am Geriat Soc* **36**: 607–612, 1988
49. Gilliland EL, Llewellyn CD, Goss DE, Lewis JD: The morbidity and mortality of stable claudicants – results of five year follow-up. Presented at 2nd International Vascular Symposium, London, September, 1986
50. Widmer LK, Da Silva A: Historical perspectives and the Basle study. In: Fowkes FGR (Ed) *Epidemiology of Peripheral Arterial Disease*, pp. 69–83. London: Springer-Verlag, 1991
51. Bainton D, Sweetnam P, Baker I, Elwood P: Peripheral vascular disease: consequences for survival and association with risk factors in the Speedwell prospective heart disease study. *Br Heart J* **72**: 128–132, 1994
52. Antiplatelet Trialists' Collaboration: Collaborative overview of randomised trials of antiplatelet therapy. *Br Med J* **308**: 81–106, 1994
53. Kannel WB, Shurtleff D: The Framingham Study. Cigarettes and the development of intermittent claudication. *Geriatrics* **28**: 61–68, 1973
54. Fowkes FGR, Housley E, Riemersma RA *et al.*: Smoking, lipids, glucose intolerance, and blood pressure as risk factors for peripheral atherosclerosis compared to ischaemic heart disease in the Edinburgh Artery Study. *Am J Epidemiol* **135**: 331–340, 1992
55. Jonason T, Ringquist I: Factors of prognostic importance for subsequent rest pain in patients with intermittent claudication. *Acta Med Scand* **218**: 27–33, 1985
56. Sayers RD, Thompson MM, Dunlop P *et al.*: The fate of infrainguinal PTFE grafts and an analysis of factors affecting outcome. *Eur J Vasc Surg* **8**: 607–610, 1994

57. Ameli FM, Stein M, Provan JL, Prosser R: The effect of postoperative smoking on femoropopliteal bypass grafts. *Ann Vasc Surg* **3**: 20–25, 1989
58. Lassila R, Lepantalo M: Cigarette smoking and the outcome after lower limb arterial surgery. *Acta Chir Scand* **154**: 635–640, 1988
59. Jonason T, Bergstrom R: Cessation of smoking in patients with intermittent claudication: effects on the risk of peripheral vascular complications, myocardial infarction and mortality. *Acta Med Scand* **221**: 253–260, 1987
60. Leng GC, Fowkes FGR: Lipids: Epidemiology. In: Fowkes FGR (Ed) *Epidemiology of Peripheral Arterial Disease* pp. 165–179. London: Springer-Verlag, 1991
61. Schroll M, Munck O: Estimation of peripheral arteriosclerotic disease by ankle blood pressure measurements in a population study of 60 year-old men and women. *J Chron Dis* **34**: 261–269, 1981
62. Smith I, Franks PJ, Greenhalgh RM *et al.*: The influence of smoking cessation and hypertriglyceridaemia on the progression of peripheral arterial disease and the onset of critical ischaemia. *Eur J Vasc Endovasc Surg* **11**: 402–408, 1996
63. Ost CR, Stenson S: Regression of peripheral atherosclerosis during therapy with high doses of nicotinic acid. *Scand J Clin Lab Invest* (Suppl) **93**: 241–245, 1967
64. Duffield RGM, Miller NE, Brunt JNH *et al.*: Treatment of hyperlipidaemia retards progression of symptomatic femoral atherosclerosis. A randomized controlled trial. *Lancet* **ii**: 639–642, 1983
65. Leng GC, Price JF, Jepson RG: Lipid-lowering therapy in lower limb atherosclerosis (Cochrane review). In: *Cochrane library* issue 3. Oxford: Update software, 1988
66. Jarrett RJ: Diabetes mellitus. In: Fowkes FGR (Ed) *Epidemiology of Peripheral Arterial Disease* pp. 187–193. London: Springer-Verlag, 1991
67. Cimminiello C, Milani M: Diabetes mellitus and perpheral vascular disease: is aspirin effective in preventing vascular events? *Diabetologia* **39**: 1402–1404, 1996
68. Banerjee AK, Pearson J, Gilliland EL *et al.*: A six year prospective study of fibrinogen and other risk factors associated with mortality in stable claudicants. *Thromb Haemost* **68**: 261–263, 1992
69. Violi F, Criqui M, Longoni A, Castiglioni C for the ADEP Group: Relation between risk factors and cardiovascular complications in patients with peripheral arterial disease. *Atherosclerosis* **120**: 25–35, 1996
70. Juergens JL, Barker WW, Hines EA: Arteriosclerosis obliterans: a review of 520 cases with special reference to pathogenic and prognostic factors. *Circulation* **21**: 188–195, 1960.
71. Mathieson FR, Larsen EE, Wulff M: Some factors influencing the spontaneous course of arterial vascular insufficiency. *Acta Chir Scand* **136**: 303–308, 1970.

Commentary

This chapter underscores the significance of the onset of intermittent claudication: both coronary and carotid arteries may also be heavily diseased with athersclerosis. Vascular surgeons should remember these associations when they care for the patient with intermittent claudication. Life expectancy, after the onset of intermittent claudication is much better than the life expectancy of patients who present with critical limb ischaemia (see following chapter, pp. 163–173). Interestingly the sex differences are reversed. Women claudicants have a longer life expectancy than male claudicants, whereas women with critical limb ischaemia have a much poorer diagnosis than their male counterparts. Why is this? Does the undervalued exercise provided by housework, shopping and gardening improve the cardiovascular fitness and longevity of women claudicants? Will the beneficial effects of female sex become more prominent as hormone replacement therapy become more widespread. Good news for women, but not for men. *JTP*

Life expectancy for critical ischaemia

Lars Norgren

INTRODUCTION

Compared with patients with abdominal aortic aneurysms or intermittent claudication, those suffering from critical limb ischaemia have the worst prognosis for survival. In general, 1 year after the diagnosis has been established, the mortality rate is about 20%. Another common finding is that only about half of the patients have both their legs after a year. Death is usually not related to the leg ischaemia *per se* but to the concomitant severe coronary disease and occasionally to a stroke. There are data to support a close correlation between severe atherosclerotic changes of the crural arteries and the coronary arteries.[1] Although there is good agreement between mortality figures reported from various studies, differences do exist, which may be attributed to variations in the definition of critical limb ischaemia (CLI).

Several attempts have been made to define CLI more appropriately than just using the Fontaine classification, in which stage III is equal to rest pain and stage IV to tissue loss, either ulceration or necrosis. The European consensus document of the early 1990s[2] required either an ankle or toe pressure of ≤50mmHg or ≤30mmHg, respectively, in addition to rest pain or tissue loss. Although this definition has been used in recent reports, it has been criticized, not least since the pressure limits have been found questionable.[3,4] Possibly, different pressure limits should be used for patients with rest pain only in comparison with the more severe ischaemia, which gives rise to tissue loss.

Recent knowledge of the natural history of CLI is lacking because most patients with such severe ischaemia are candidates for intervention. However, there are data from earlier studies on CLI when reconstruction policy was less active and angioplasty less frequently used. Whether life expectancy can be improved after a successful revascularization or after effective pharmacotherapy is a question of great concern. Another question is whether the quality of life is improved for patients undergoing vascular reconstruction.

SURVIVAL IN UNRECONSTRUCTED CRITICAL LIMB ISCHAEMIA

In a study from the 1970s and 1980s in patients with rest pain and/or necrosis and contraindications for revascularization, it was found that 50% of non-diabetic and 60% of diabetic patients died within 5 years.[5] The prognosis was slightly worse for patients with tissue loss and of the surviving patients about 50% had undergone an amputation. In a Danish study, 8% of patients referred for an infrapopliteal reconstruction due to CLI, were found to be inoperable.[6] After 28 months 74% of them had an amputation and the cumulative survival rate at 2 years was 60%. A Finnish study utilizing the European consensus document definition of CLI found that 46% of patients were alive after 1 year if no vascular reconstruction had been performed. Of these only 28% had kept the leg at 1 year.[7]

Amputations are often the natural consequence of a non-reconstructable CLI. Spontaneous improvement has, however, been seen in a considerable group of patients with rest pain and minor tissue loss. In a report from 1962, 28% of 84 patients improved spontaneously.[8] At present, as stricter definitions of the ischaemic stage are probably used, it is reasonable to assume that the chance of spontaneous recovery is more limited. On the other hand, there are patients who may develop rest pain during a phase of cardiac insufficiency or any other concomitant disorder. After general treatment these patients may improve, returning to a more benign stage of leg ischaemia.

Most amputations are performed on elderly patients. In a Swedish study from 1983 it was found that 45% of the amputees were at least 80 years of age.[9] In a Danish survey[10] comparing patients under the age of 40 with those over 80 years, the amputation rates were 0.3 and 226 per 100 000 patients respectively. Not unexpectedly, the risk of amputation increases, the more severe is the ischaemic condition. The Joint Vascular Research Group in Britain found that patients with gangrene or ulceration were twice as likely to require a major amputation as those with rest pain alone.[11]

Amputees have a particularly short life expectancy, and 30-day mortality of about 15% is commonly described after a below-knee amputation, and about 25% after an above-knee procedure. After 2 years, mortality rates of 25–45% are reported. Dormandy and Ray[12] in their analysis found that after 2 years, 15% of those with a below-knee amputation had undergone an extended above-knee amputation, 15% had a contralateral amputation, and 30% were dead.

There are several reasons why vascular reconstruction may not be attempted. Attitudes may vary, e.g. a reluctance to perform extremely distal bypasses to foot arteries. This should be reflected in the proportion of non-operated cases, but this is seldom reported. Also the attitude to angioplasty differs, and there is a considerable variation between different institutions in the proportion of patients found suitable for an angioplasty due to CLI. As a consequence, several factors limit the possibility of estimating the true death rate today of CLI patients.

THE EFFECT OF REVASCULARIZATION ON SURVIVAL

In the British JVRG study from the 1980s[11] including more than 400 ischaemic legs, 61% had undergone arterial reconstruction, while 17% had undergone primary major amputation. The overall 1-year mortality was 18%. The post-reconstruction mortality was about half of that achieved after primary amputation. In the Danish study reported above[6] there was an 18% difference in survival rates (60% vs 78%) between patients with reconstructed and non-reconstructed distal arteries. In a more recent discussion on the definition of CLI it was found that whatever definition was used, the mortality rate for CLI patients is high. However, arterial reconstructions diminished the mortality rate considerably.[13]

Although recent series point to a short-term benefit of revascularization, measured as an increased survival rate after 1 year, the long-term prognosis for CLI patients is still poor. In a Norwegian study of 1400 patients operated on for chronic lower limb ischaemia, the 10-year survival rate was only 26%. The expected survival in an age- and sex-matched population was 49%. It was also found that the patient's age at the time of operation significantly influenced the survival.[14] Any effect of the revascularization on mortality was not discussed in this report.

In his careful analysis of the outcome of surgical treatment for CLI in the Vaasa region of Finland, Luther[15] came to the following conclusions regarding survival. The 30-day mortality was 8% after vascular reconstruction and 24% after a primary amputation. The median survival was 51 months after vascular reconstruction. For those undergoing an amputation as a secondary procedure, the median survival was 31 months and for those with a successful reconstruction 53 months. Moreover, 1 year after an amputation 43% of the patients were dead, while the corresponding figure for patients after vascular reconstruction was 20%. After 5 years these figures were 84% and 57%, respectively. The severity of ischaemia influenced the results, as there were shorter survival rates for patients with more severe ischaemia.

The fact that mortality following an amputation is high and that even after a successful revascularization, the remaining life span is short, prompts the need for a cost analysis. All studies agree that amputation is more expensive than vascular reconstruction, particularly when the costs for institutionalization of disabled patients are included. As an example, Myhre calculated for Norway that the cost for a successful bypass procedure was $5700 while a primary amputation implied a cost of $13 000 and amputation after a failing reconstruction cost $25 000.[16] Hunink and coworkers analysed the cost-effectiveness of revascularization of femoropopliteal disease and found that for a 65-year-old man with CLI and a femoropopliteal stenosis, an initial angioplasty increased quality adjusted life expectancy by 2-13 months, while the one with a femoropopliteal occlusion had the benefit of an increased quality adjusted life expectancy by 1–4 months after bypass surgery.[17]

Data from the Swedish Vascular Registry

Most reports on the outcome of patients with CLI appear from single centres. An exception is the British study presented above.[11] The Swedish Vascular Registry has enabled compilation of data from vascular centres all over Sweden, including county hospitals and university hospitals. The registry includes data from follow-up at 30 days and at 1 year. Long-term results of revascularization procedures are not available. However, the registry is connected to the Swedish Population Registry, which gives the opportunity to follow the survival of the patients for an indefinite time. In a study on the influence of age on the outcome after infrainguinal revascularization in patients suffering CLI,[18] all infrainguinal procedures performed between 1987 and 1995 were analysed. There were 3730 surgical (bypass) procedures and 1199 endovascular angioplasty procedures. Patients were classified as alive/improved; alive/not improved; alive/amputated and dead at 30 days and at 1 year, respectively. At the 1-year evaluation, there was a further classification according to the following: procedure occluded/limb amputated; procedure occluded/limb not amputated, and patent vessel. For this analysis patients were divided into two age groups, those 75 years or younger, and those 76 years or older.

The 30-day mortality rate was 5.3% and the 1-year mortality rate 22.9%, without any differences between patients treated with surgery and those undergoing angioplasty. On the other hand, there were significantly more patients who were alive and improved after surgery than after angioplasty at 1 month (82.3% vs 77.7%) and at 1 year (49.6% vs 44.3%). The amputation rate was 5.6% at 1 month and 14.4% at 1 year. Diabetic patients had the highest mortality rate of 17%.

The cumulative mortality rate after surgery did not differ between patients with a patent or a non-patent reconstruction as long as the limb was salvaged (Fig. 1). However, the mortality rate was significantly higher after an amputation. After an endovascular procedure, a patent reconstruction was associated with a more favourable survival rate (Fig. 2).

There was a significant difference between the mortality rates in the older (>75 years) and the younger patient groups (at 1 month 6.4% vs 3.8% and at 1 year 26.4% vs 17.6%). The amputation rate did not differ according to age.

The role of repeated surgery in this group of patients with severe peripheral arterial disease has also to be evaluated. In a survey of reoperations and redo-surgery in patients registered in the Swedish Vascular Registry,[19] 2828 procedures for critical limb ischaemia were included between 1987 and 1991. Further arterial procedures were identified until the end of 1995. Of the primary procedures, 22.8% were endovascular while 77.2% were open surgery. Reoperations within 30 days were performed in 11.4%, redo-procedures later than 30 days in 12.4% and other site

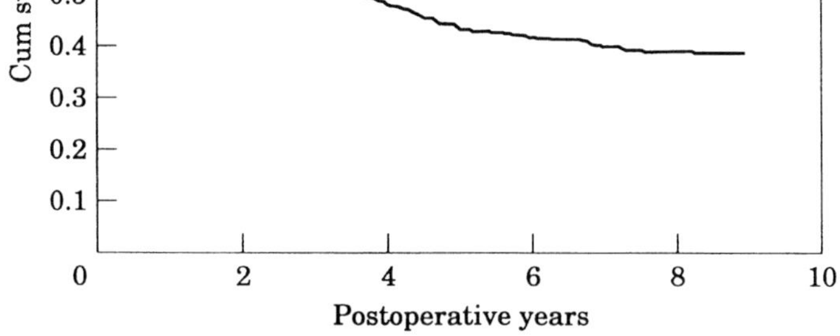

Fig. 1. Cumulative survival of three patient groups, those with a patent surgical reconstruction at 1 year (thin line); those with an occlusion but no amputation (interrupted line) and those with amputation following an occluded reconstruction (thick line). (From Ref. 18 with permission.)

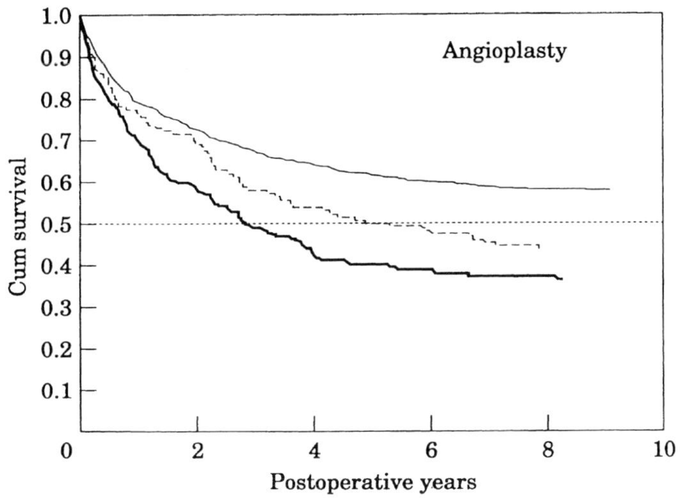

Fig. 2. Cumulative survival after angioplasty (cf Fig. 1). (From Ref. 18 with permission.)

interventions in 16.3%. Corresponding figures after angioplasty were 3.4%, 9.8% and 9.5%, respectively. Figures 3 and 4 depict survival curves, showing the proportion without repeated surgery. These two curves have been combined into a curve for 'event-free survival', which was about 25% after 5 years. It was found that the cumulative mortality rate was not higher for patients undergoing repeated surgery than for patients who just had the primary operation (40.2% vs 53%).

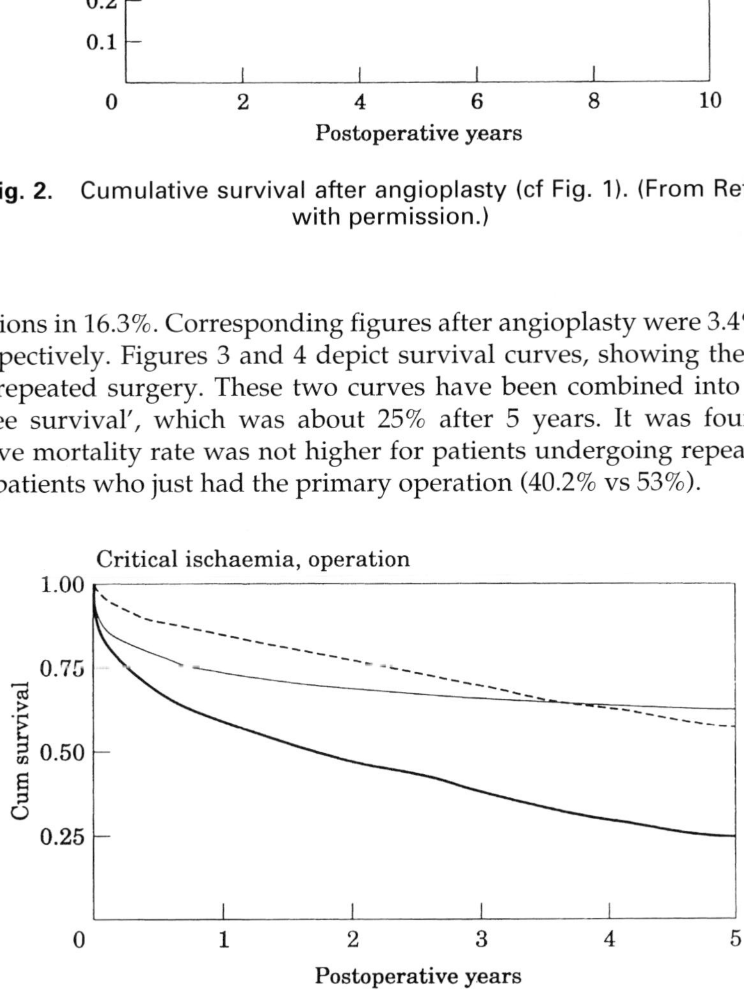

Fig. 3. Cumulative survival for patients with critical limb ischaemia after surgical reconstruction, showing the proportion without repeated surgery (thin line); patient survival (broken line) and a combination of these two curves into the event-free survival (thick line). (From Ref. 19 with permission.)

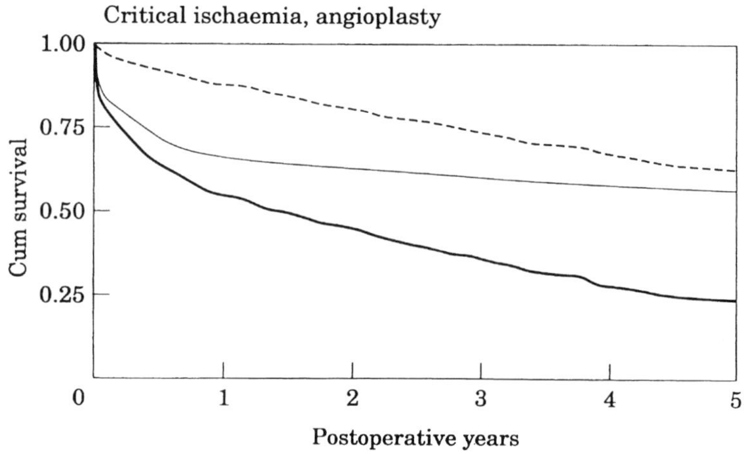

Fig. 4. Cumulative survival for patients with critical limb ischaemia after angioplasty, showing the proportion without repeated angioplasty (thin line); patient survival (broken line) and a combination of these two curves into the event-free survival (thick line). (From Ref. 19 with permission.)

The conclusions from the Swedvasc data are therefore that in this non-selected, large group of patients, a successful surgical revascularization might increase the chance of long-term survival. Also, patients where the reconstruction had occluded had a similar outcome, which may be attributed to a short-term benefit of an open bypass to improve collaterals in the ischaemic limb. This latter finding did not hold true for the endovascular group, in which only a patent reconstruction was associated with an improved survival rate. The other finding, that secondary reconstructions did not decrease the long-term survival is more difficult to interpret. Perhaps this only reflects that such patients are survivors.

THE INFLUENCE OF RISK FACTORS

It is well known that diabetes, smoking and high age are crucial factors in the progression of vascular disease to critical limb ischaemia. To what extent these factors also are responsible for the short expected survival in this group of patients is less well known. As diabetics constitute 30–40% of all patients with CLI, the outcome for diabetics and non-diabetics can be separated, while smoking is less easy to use as a predicting parameter. Usually, about 30% of CLI patients are smokers, far less than the proportion among claudicants. Data on smoking are also less reliable, and former smokers are often classified as non-smokers. For these reasons, it is uncommon to find that smokers and non-smokers among CLI patients are different groups with a different life expectancy.

Separation between age groups is possible but few studies have validated which age should be the cut-off point. In the Finnish study reported above,[15] age did not influence survival rates while diabetes did. Also from other sources it is evident that survival rates are lower for diabetics than for non-diabetics.[7,20] In the Swedvasc survey, the risk of amputation was 14.4% at 1 year for the whole population, for diabetic patients it was 17%.[18] Diabetes was also a significant risk factor for repeated vascular surgery.[19] However, as foot care for diabetic patients improves, the incidence of major amputations is likely to decrease. This is shown by a study from southern Sweden, where the incidence of major amputation decreased from 19.1 to 9.4 per 100 000 inhabitants between 1982 and 1993.[21] Survival rates for diabetics who have undergone an amputation are extremely poor; only about 50% survived 3 years.[22]

End-stage renal disease is not uncommon in patients with CLI. Although reconstruction should be attempted on the same indications as for other CLI patients, the morbidity is higher and so is the operative mortality.[23] Limb loss is also more common in this group of patients.[23,24]

Female sex may be an additional risk factor. In a study from 1982 to 1990 Enzler and coworkers found a relative risk of failure in women compared with men of 1.30.[25] Redo-surgery, diabetes and crural procedures further increased the risk of failure. This is of importance, not least as women constitute a greater proportion of those operated on than previously thought. In the Swedvasc material[18] 53% of those patients operated on with an infrainguinal procedure were women.

Critical ischaemia in one leg often is a warning for the other leg. In patients who had a unilateral surgical or percutaneous intervention between 1990 and 1995, the annual occurrence of contralateral critical ischaemia was 3.3–8.3% during the first 4 years.[26]

THE EFFECT OF PHARMACOTHERAPY ON SURVIVAL

If vascular reconstruction cannot be performed, due to an unsuitable vascular morphology or other contraindications, few possibilities exist to treat the patient. Various kinds of pharmacotherapy have been tried, unfortunately in many cases without formal trials and with only short follow-up. Prostanoids have been studied in randomized controlled trials, enabling interpretation of results at medium-term follow-up, 6 months. Six randomized control studies of the prostacyclin analogue Iloprost have used two endpoints, major amputation and death.[27–32] In a meta-analysis of these studies,[33] the interpretation was that a better outcome was achieved in the treatment group than in the placebo group with respect to both major amputation and death. In two of the studies it was possible to evaluate death subsequent to a major amputation. In the Iloprost group 35% had a major amputation or died during the follow-up, while the corresponding figure for the placebo group was 55%. In conclusion, it was found that there was a significant beneficial effect of the prostanoid treatment with regard to the probability of being alive with both legs after 6 months follow-up.

QUALITY OF LIFE

Although the remaining life time for patients once developing CLI is restricted, it is important to find out whether this life is acceptable in terms of freedom from pain, sleep and social life. From recent studies it is evident that if the ischaemia can be turned to a pain-free situation, the life quality might be significantly improved.[34] Many questions remain to be answered, e.g. the effect of various reconstructive procedures, the negative influence of delayed wound healing, extended hospitalization, remaining postoperative pain and swelling etc. There is some evidence that reoperations to keep a graft patent, implying a long-lasting hospital stay and further pain, may deteriorate the patient's general condition, and even though this kind of procedure may end with a patent graft the situation can be devastating for the patient.

WHAT CAN THE PATIENT WITH CRITICAL LIMB ISCHAEMIA EXPECT?

The mortality rates discussed in this chapter point to an even higher death risk at 1 year than the average figure of 20% which frequently is presented. This is, however, only true for CLI as a group. It is not possible to separate patients who were not revascularized but could avoid an amputation from those who needed an amputation and estimate any difference in their natural history. There is certainly a variation in the severity of ischaemia in these groups, and one would expect a better chance of survival for those who do not need an amputation during the follow-up time. This is, however, not possible to claim. On the other hand, a well working below-knee amputation without need for re-amputation and after which the patient can walk on his prosthesis, seems to predict a better outcome than for other unreconstructed patients. The great difference between those who have undergone an above-knee and a below-knee amputation regarding their life expectancy may be attributed to the severity of the disease.

For revascularized patients both the 1-year and 2-year mortality rate is considerably lower, ranging from 18 to 23% in the studies reported. In most studies there is little information on the difference between successful and failing reconstructions regarding the risk of death. The Swedvasc material points at the same outcome concerning survival for patients who can avoid an amputation whether the reconstruction is open or not. This holds true only for open surgery, and not for the PTA group. Again, there may be differences in the severity of ischaemia as a factor in the decision on which treatment to select.

The fact that diabetics constitute a group with higher risk of mortality as well as the fact that in some studies older patients are at a higher risk cannot be taken as a reason not to revascularize them. There are even studies which cannot find any difference between the outcome for older and younger patients.

Pharmacotherapy should theoretically be of great value as it is the only treatment which has a more general mode of action. Provided there is an effect not only on the limb circulation but in the coronary circulation as well, there should possibly be a greater chance of survival. As most of the drugs which are being used are rather ineffective it is difficult to draw a firm conclusion, but from studies on prostanoids one may conclude that at least the combination amputation and death is reduced after treatment compared with the outcome in the placebo groups.

It seems that the outcome for patients with critical limb ischaemia is better if a reconstruction can be performed. On the other hand, many questions remain to be answered, specifically on the quality of the remaining life correlated to the burden of a surgical procedure. This is most important in case there is a delayed healing after surgery or an immediate thrombotic occlusion which can imply one or more reoperations. There are cases in which a primary amputation might be the better solution. Whether this is positive or negative concerning the life expectancy is impossible to predict. On the other hand, reluctancy to treat patients with critical limb ischaemia has no place. For the future, it is hoped that better predictors of the outcome of various treatments can be available. There is good reason to make every effort to improve the quality of the remaining life for these patients, and keeping the leg is an important factor – albeit at not too high a price from the patient´s point of view.

REFERENCES

1. Källerö KS, Bergqvist D, Cederholm C *et al.*: Arteriosclerosis in popliteal artery trifurcation as a predictor for myocardial infarction after arterial reconstructive operation. *Surg Gyn Obstet* **159**: 133–138, 1984
2. Second European Consensus Document on chronic critical leg ischemia: *Circulation 1991* **84**: No. 4, 1991
3. Thompson MM, Sayers RD, Varty K *et al.*: Chronic critical leg ischaemia must be redefined. *Eur J Vasc Surg* **7**: 420–426, 1993
4. Belch JJ, Diehm C, Sohngen M *et al.*: Critical limb ischaemia: a case against Consensus II. *Int Angiol* **14**: 353–356, 1995
5. Bolin T, Aldman Å, Gustafsson PO *et al.*: Hur går det för patienter med viloischemi som ej opereras? *Läkartidningen* **85**: 2398–2399, 1988
6. Sørensen S, Lorentzen J, Schroeder T: Prognosen for den kritisk iskæmiske underekstremitet som ikke kan revaskulariseres karkirurgisk. *Ugeskr Læger* **155/18**: 1379–1382, 1993
7. Lepantalo M, Matzke S: Outcome of unreconstructed chronic critical leg ischaemia. *Eur J Vasc Endovasc Surg* **11**: 153–157, 1996
8. Taylor MS, Calo MR: Atherosclerosis of arteries of lower limbs. *Br Med J* **24**: 507–519, 1962
9. Liedberg E, Persson BM: Age, diabetes and smoking in lower limb amputation for arterial occlusive disease. *Acta Orthop Scand* **54**: 383–388, 1983
10. Eickhoff JH, Buchardt Hansen HJ, Lorentzen JE: The effect of arterial reconstruction on lower limb amputation rate. *Acta Chir Scand* **502**: 181–187, 1980
11. Wolfe JHN: Defining the outcome of critical ischaemia: a one year prospective study. *Br J Surg* **73**: 321, 1986
12. Dormandy JA, Ray S: The natural history of peripheral arterial disease. In: Tooke JE, Lowe GD (Eds). *A Textbook of Vascular Medicine* pp. 162–175. London: Arnold, 1996
13. Tyrrell MR, Wolfe JH: Critical leg ischaemia: an appraisal of clinical definitions: Joint Vascular Research Group. *Br J Surg* **80**: 177–180, 1993
14. Aune S, Amundsen SR, Trippestad A: The influence of age on long-term survival pattern of patients operated on for lower limb ischaemia. *Eur J Vasc Endovasc Surg* **12**: 214–217, 1996
15. Luther M: Treatment of chronic critical leg ischaemia – a cost benefit analysis. *Ann Chir Gyn* **86**: (Suppl) 213, 1997
16. Myhre H, Fosby B, Witsoe E *et al.*: Cost-effectiveness of therapeutic options for critical limb ischaemia. *Crit Ischaem* **6**: 37–41, 1996
17. Hunink MG, Wong JB, Donaldson MC *et al.*: Revascularization for femoro-popliteal disease. A decision and cost-effectiveness analysis. *J Am Med Assoc* **274**: 165–171, 1995

18. Zdanowski Z, Troeng T, Norgren L on behalf of The Swedish Vascular Registry: Outcome and influence of age after infrainguinal revascularisation in critical limb ischaemia. *Eur J Vasc Endovasc Surg* **16**: 137–141, 1998
19. SWEDVASC: Reoperations, redo surgery and other interventions constitute more than one-third of vascular surgery. A study from Swedvasc (The Swedish Vascular Registry). *Eur J Vasc Endovasc Surg* **14**: 244–251, 1997
20. Fratezi AC, Albers M, De Luccia N *et al.*: Outcome and quality of life of patients with severe chronic limb ischaemia: a cohort study on the influence of diabetes: *Eur J Vasc Endovasc Surg* **10**: 459–465, 1995
21. Larsson J, Apelqvist J, Agardh CD *et al.*: Decreasing incidence of major amputation in diabetic patients: a consequence of a multidisciplinary foot care team approach? *Diabet Med* **12**: 770–776, 1995
22. Bild DE, Selby JV, Sinnock P *et al.*: Lower-extremity amputation in people with diabetes mellitus. Epidemiology and prevention. *Diabetes Care* **12**: 24–31, 1989
23. Simsir SA, Cabellon A, Kohlman-Trigoboff D *et al.*: Factors influencing limb salvage and survival after amputation and revascularization in patients with end-stage renal disease. *Am J Surg* **170**: 113–117, 1995
24. Taylor LM, Hamre D, Dalman RL *et al.*: Limb salvage vs amputation for critical ischemia. The role of vascular surgery. *Arch Surg* **126**: 1251–1258, 1991
25. Enzler MA, Ruoss M, Seifert B *et al.*: The influence of gender on the outcome of arterial procedures in the lower extremity. *Eur J Vasc Endovasc Surg* **11**: 446–452, 1996
26. de Vries SO, Donaldson MC, Hunink MG: Contralateral symptoms after unilateral intervention for peripheral occlusive disease. *J Vasc Surg* **27**: 414–421, 1998
27. Brock FE, Abri O, Baitsch G *et al.*: Iloprost in der behondlung ischaemischer Gewebslaesionen bei Diabetikern. *Schweiz Med Wschr* **120**: 1477–1482, 1990
28. Diehm C, Abri O, Baitsch G *et al.*: Iloprost, ein stabiles Prostacyclin derivat bei arterieller Verschlüsskrankheil im Stadium IV. *Dtsch Med Wschr* **114**: 783–788, 1989
29. Bliss B, Wilkins D, Campbell WB *et al.*: Treatment of limb threatening ischaemia with intravenous Iloprost: a randomised double-blind placebo controlled study. *Eur J Vasc Surg* **5**: 511–516, 1991
30. Norgren L, Alwmark A, Angqvist KA *et al.*: A stable prostacyclin analogue [Iloprost] in the treatment of ischaemic ulcers of the lower limb. A Scandinavian–Polish placebo-controlled, randomised multicentre study. *Eur J Vasc Surg* **4**: 463–467, 1990
31. Guilmot JL, Diot E: Treatment of lower limb ischaemia due to atherosclerosis in diabetic and non-diabetic patients with Iloprost, a stable analogue of prostacyclin: results of the French multicentre trial. *Drug Invest* **3**: 351–359, 1991
32. Balzer K, Bechara G, Bisler H *et al.*: Reduction of ischaemic rest pain in advanced peripheral arterial occlusive disease – a double blind placebo controlled trial with Iloprost. *Int Angiol* **10**: 229–232, 1991
33. Loosemore TM, Chalmers TC, Dormandy JA: A meta-analysis of randomized placebo control trials in Fontaine stages III and IV peripheral occlusive arterial disease. *Int Angiol* **13**: 133–142, 1994
34. Chetter IC, Spark JI, Scott DJ *et al.*: Prospectived analysis of quality of life in patients following infrainguinal reconstruction for chronic critical ischaemia. *Br J Surg* **85**: 951–955, 1998

Commentary

The patients with critical limb ischaemia need help even though their life span may be short. The quality of their remaining life span is paramount and few studies have paid proper attention to this. From the evidence presented in this chapter and elsewhere, the vascular surgeon should be convinced of the benefits of searching hard for patent distal vessels to enable vascular reconstruction with a bypass procedure. Sometimes angioplasty will 'buy time' for the ischaemic leg, although the failure rate after angioplasty in the context of critical ischaemia is very high (see Golledge chapter, pp. 37–48).

This chapter has focused on life expectancy. The role of Iloprost is discussed. Iloprost is an expensive drug and perhaps other trials are needed to confirm the role of Iloprost in critical limb ischaemia. Vascular surgeons should be willing to cooperate in such trials.

What has not been mentioned in this chapter are the novel approaches based on a knowledge of vascular biology, which are being developed to treat critical limb ischaemia. Foremost amongst these is the use of vascular endothelial growth factor (VEGF) – a growth factor which encourages endothelial cell proliferation, capillary sprouting and development of collateral circulation. Isner and colleagues have pioneered this approach. Injection of plasmids encoding VEGF have been injected directly into the leg muscle of patients with critical limb ischaemia, to improve collateral blood supply within 4 weeks.[1] This is exciting news for vascular surgeons. In the future such treatment may permit a vascular reconstruction, where previously this had been impossible. Such an approach is likely to increase life expectancy in patients with critical limb ischaemia. *JTP*

Reference

1. Isner JM, Piecze KA, Schainfeld R *et al.* Clinical evidence of angiogensis after gene transfer of phVEGF-165 in patient with ischaemic limb. *Lancet* **348**: 370–374, 1996

Major amputation in England and Wales

T Coddington

INTRODUCTION

Major amputation of the leg because of vascular disease in a modern industrial society, is an end-stage surgical procedure. It is a destructive operation removing tissue, disease and symptoms. It is also an enabling process by restoring function if a prosthesis (artificial limb) is used. It is usually undertaken after multiple procedures and reconstructive surgical attempts. The planning of amputation surgery for function begins at its decision point.[1–3]

SCIENTIFIC SURGICAL APPROACH

The scientific surgical approach to amputation surgery includes a reasoned level of selection, a flap muscle closure designed for function, adequate and precise handling of bone section and shaping, clean handling of nerve section, and good functional plastic surgical closure.

Modern prostheses which complement these surgical approaches use modern materials to maximize the benefit. These materials include modern thermoplastics, carbon fibre, titanium and silicones. The joint componentry in the ankle and knee mechanisms incorporate scientifically and engineered designs to enable normal gait function. This includes modern hydraulics, computer technology and electronics with energy storing and release componentry with a damping function. Ambrose Paré (1510–1590) was the 'father' of this amputation surgical practice as, clearly, he was a surgeon with vision and practice, and his amputations were made with the prosthesis in mind.[1]

Major amputation in vascular disease is an end-stage event and may be an indicator of previous successes or failures of other surgical techniques. The various statistics which are available are not co-ordinated to give an easy picture. The national statistics which were kept in the past by the Department of Health for the Artificial Limb Service, from 1957 to 1990, were fragmented and devolved to the individual NHS Trusts with an interest in amputation and artificial limb supply. The co-ordinated and consistent nature of these statistics became fragmented. No central co-ordinating body was charged with the responsibility for collating the information. The Department of Health keeps hospital episode statistics (HES) and these record completed episodes of primary amputation operations and include information relating to age and sex of patients involved. Aetiology, morbidity, rehabilitation and mortality are not routinely kept in these statistics. However, some individual regions have kept some of these required categories for Public Health surveillance.[4] The patchy nature of this data requires assumptions and extrapolations to obtain a national view of vascular major leg amputation; however, even with this limitation of incomplete data, useful trends can be seen and if viewed with past reliable data, a consistency is observed.[5,6]

THE AMPUTEE POPULATION

The amputee population in England, Wales and Northern Ireland remains in the order of some 65 000 people.[5,6] Major leg amputations for the last recorded year 1997, showed 5626 new cases.[6] If young and early middle-aged people are excluded from these figures, 5319 new cases are seen representing a population from the age of 45 onwards. Vascular leg pathology predominantly occurs in this age group. Vascular disease is the major cause of amputation. It accounts for 64% of major amputations of the leg and if diabetes mellitus is included, an extra 20% is added; the total is then 84%.[4,6,7]

Amputations of the leg in the younger age group are mainly a result of trauma and malignancy. These account for 9% and 4% respectively. Road traffic accidents and osteosarcoma are the predominant causes here. Infection, including gas gangrene, deformities, both congenital and neurogenic, comprise some 3% of the total. The principle pathology in vascular disease leading to major amputation is atherosclerosis, and accounts for 88%.[4,5,7] Embolism, thromboangiitis, and varicose ulcerations total 8.4% of vascular disease pathology.[4,5,7] Thus the principle indication for major amputation of the leg is peripheral vascular disease and the major amputation levels of the leg for this group are predominantly transfemoral (mid-femur, distal femur): 50% of cases, knee disarticulation: 4% of cases, transtibial (proximal tibia, mid-tibia, distal tibia): 46%.[3,4,7]

The population age group 65 years and above show the predominant proportion of major amputations. This indicates that it is the elderly who have major amputations of the leg, and indeed looking in detail at the over 65-year age group, the peak incidence is in the 75–84-years age group, and a substantial number of amputations takes place after the age of 65 (Table 1).[6] The male to female ratio is in the order of 1.5 until the over 75-year age group which equates for men and women. Women who are over the age of 85 show as a higher proportion, and this indicates their survival over men which is borne out by death rate figures (Table 2).[6] The trend over the last decade is that major lower limb amputation is thus in the more elderly group. If information is combined with past statistics, a 3% increase can be seen in the trend in vascular disease.[3,4,7] The trend in new patients with primary leg amputation is shown in Fig. 1, and over the last decade and a half remains relatively constant.[1–4]

The population figures of Britain have steadily increased until 1991 and then steadied and now there is a slight rise to 59 008 634 (53 million people for England) Fig. 2.[3,8,9] However, when the age structure is examined, it can be seen that a change has occurred. There is a lower proportion of children under 15 and a higher proportion of people over the age of 60. The change in the population in the over 60-year age group is shown in Fig. 3.[3,5] The population statistics also show an increase in people over 85 years of age. The death rate has fallen over the past decade, giving a

Table 1. Number of primary major amputations of the leg in England by age

Year	*All ages*	*45–64*	*65–74*	*75–84*	*85+*
1990–91	5465	1041	1581	1910	643
1991–92	5735	1106	1662	1969	700
1992–93	5848	1104	1708	2014	748
1993–94	6014	1122	1843	1958	786
1994–95	5879	1089	1882	1888	732
1995–96	5661	1131	1696	1774	737
1996–97	5626	1087	1677	1796	759

Table 2. Male to female ratio of primary amputation in England by age

Year	*All ages*	*45–64*	*65–74*	*75–84*	*85+*
1990–91	1.5	2.6	1.9	1.0	0.6
1991–92	1.5	3.4	2.0	1.1	0.5
1992–93	1.4	2.5	1.9	1.2	0.5
1993–94	1.4	2.5	2.0	1.1	0.5
1994–95	1.5	2.6	2.1	1.1	0.6
1995–96	1.5	3.0	2.0	1.1	0.6
1996–97	1.4	2.6	1.8	1.1	0.6

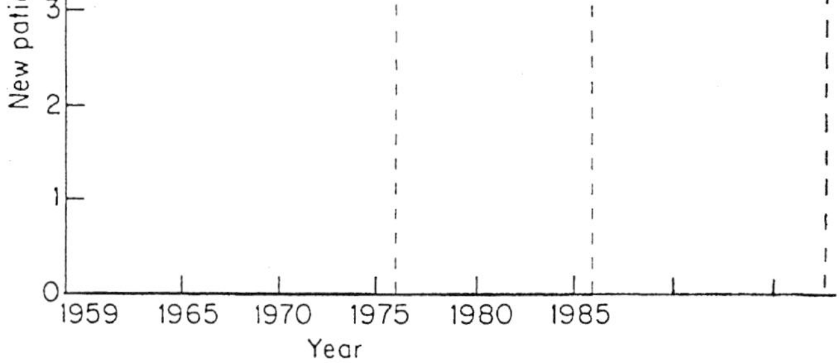

Fig. 1. The total number of new patients in England, Wales and Northern Ireland.

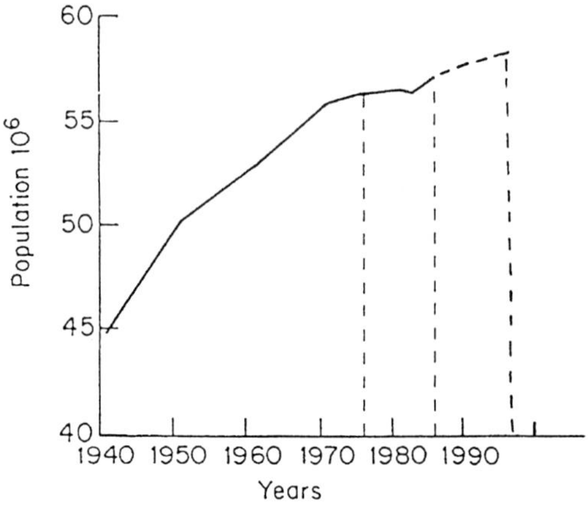

Fig. 2. The population of the United Kingdom of both sexes and all ages from 1940 to 1997.

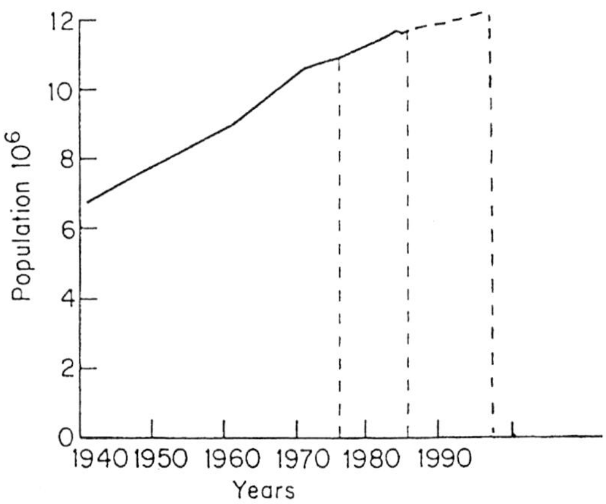

Fig. 3. The population of the United Kingdom of both sexes over the age of 60 years from 1940 to 1997.

survival trend, which if related to the major leg amputation population, is clearly seen to be in the more elderly age group.[3,5] Therefore, using these population figures with the primary amputation data, it can be seen that major amputations per head of population for vascular disease have fallen over the last decade. It must be concluded that surgical techniques and interventions are aiding reduction of this incidence and are maintaining effectiveness. Vascular surgery is thus shown indirectly from these figures to be durable and effective to date. The influence of the newer techniques and endovascular approaches are in their early stages and would not be expected to show currently in these figures.

END-STAGE DATA

A better means of co-ordinating the end-stage data is needed, and I am pleased to report this has been addressed and data will be collected from this year onwards. The Amputee Medical Rehabilitation Society in the UK has formed a National Amputee Statistical (UK) Database.[10] Here, all NHS Trusts with an involvement in amputee care will be involved in data collection and there will be a central co-ordinating body who analyse and keep the data. The database will include patient identity in the form of:

1. Patient's number
2. Date of birth
3. Purchaser code
4. Centre code
5. Gender
6. Category of patient: (i) new patient, (ii) revision, (iii) transfer from another centre
7. Ethnic origin
8. Date of referral relating to level and side of amputation
9. Level of amputation, and for the lower limb these levels will be:
   (a) Hemipelvectomy
   (b) Hip disarticulation
   (c) Transfemoral
   (d) Knee disarticulation
   (e) Transtibial
   (f) Ankle disarticulation (Symes)
   (g) Partial foot
   (h) Digits
10. Cause of amputation (aetiology) and for the dysvascular group:
    (a) Diabetes mellitus
    (b) Non-diabetic arteriosclerosis
    (c) Embolism
    (d) Vasospastic conditions (including Raynaud's)
    (e) Disseminated intravascular coagulation
    (f) Endovascular chemical trauma (= substance abuse)
    (g) Buerger's disease
    (h) Iatrogenic vascular trauma
    (i) Arteritis (including rheumatoid arthritis, autoimmune disease)
    (j) Venous disease.

This information will be available annually and should correspond in detail with other information held by professional societies and will help to complete a register for monitoring events for vascular surgery, surgical rehabilitation and planning services, practices and research.

REFERENCES

1. Vitali M *et al.*: *Amputation and Prostheses*. London: Baillière Tindall, 1978
2. Coddington T *et al.*: How can we improve amputation practices? In: Greenhalgh RGM (Ed) *Vascular Surgical Issues in Current Practice* Vol. 12 pp. 301–308. London: Grune and Stratton, 1986
3. Coddington T: Why are legs amputated in Britain? *Limb Salvage and Amputation for Vascular Disease* p. 180. London: W B Saunders Co, 1988
4. NHS: *Amputation Rates Statistics* West Midlands: NHS Executive, 1991–1995
5. DHSS Statistics and Research Division: *Amputation Statistics for England, Wales and Northern Ireland*. DHSS, 1976–1986
6. Department of Health: *Hospital Episode Statistics* 1990–1997
7. RRC: *Regional Rehabilitation Centre Statistics*: Birmingham: RRC 1990–1997
8. Common Services Agency: Information and Statistics Division, Edinburgh, Scotland, Personal communication, November 1987
9. HMSO: *Social Trends* Ch.1, pp. 29–36. London: Central Statistical Office, 1987
10. National Amputee Statistical (UK) Database Guidelines: Scotland: ISD, November 1997

Commentary

Vascular surgeons with their skills in vascular reconstruction have made a substantial contribution to reducing the number of major amputations per head of population. As an increasing proportion of the population gains access to a specialist vascular surgeon, we can hope that the number of amputations per head of population will be reduced further. In this context it should be remembered that the costs involved in vascular reconstruction of a critically ischaemic limb are less than the costs relating to amputation and long-term support of the amputee.[1,2] *JTP*

References

1. Singh S, Evans L, Datta D *et al.*: The costs of managing lower limb-threatening ischaemia. *Eur J Vasc Endovasc Surg* **12**: 359–362, 1996
2. Panayiotopoulos YP, Tyrrell MR, Arnold FJ *et al.*: Results and cost analysis of distal (crural/pedal) arterial revascularisation for limb salvage in diabetic and non-diabetic patients. *Diabet Med* **14**: 214–220, 1997

Is a national vascular registry worth the effort?

D Bergqvist, T Troëng, J Elfström, B Hedberg, K-G Ljungström,
L Norgren and P Örtenwall on behalf of Swedvasc

INTRODUCTION

During the last two decades there have been attempts to develop vascular surgical registries, with the aim of analysing the outcome of vascular procedures within well defined populations.[1,2] In Sweden this process started some 10 years ago in the Southern health care region, and since 1994 it has become a national vascular registry, in that all hospitals performing vascular operations report their procedures and 30-day as well as 1-year results.[3] Currently, national vascular registries have also been established in Finland, Norway, Denmark, New Zealand and Northern Ireland.

The aim of this chapter is to discuss the problems, efforts and costs which are involved in the creation and maintenance of a registry, and also the benefits and advantages. The question posed in the title will not be analysed from a health economics point of view but rather the problems and advantages will be discussed.

REASONS FOR CREATING A VASCULAR REGISTRY

The general aim of a vascular registry is to cover all procedures used on the whole population, not just reports from specialized centres where bias is likely. The specific aims are:

1. To monitor the outcome of routine care.
2. To obtain a basis for optimal planning of health care resources such as number of beds, number of vascular surgeons and educational resources.
3. To create an instrument for quality measurement and assurance. Each department should be able to compare its own results with those of the whole registry. These data are important in documenting the vascular surgical care provided to the inhabitants living in the catchment area of the different centres. It should be possible to identify suboptimal results and by feedback mechanisms correct them. This is important for the patients and will probably also influence health care costs.
4. To follow trends in new technologies and possible changes in results over time.
5. To elucidate the relationship between volume and outcome of vascular surgery.
6. To establish a basis for research. To serve this function the registry may be used in several ways:
   - to study results of vascular surgical procedures on a population basis;
   - to collect data on rare diseases and events;
   - to study how various treatment procedures function on a 1-year basis;

- to study long-term survival;
- to identify patients and procedures for more detailed studies with specific aims;
- to create a basis for prospective trials with addition of trial-specific protocols.

7. To serve educational purposes. Surgeons training in vascular surgery can check their results against the collective results.

THE DEVELOPMENT OF THE SWEDISH VASCULAR REGISTRY (SWEDVASC)

Planning for the regional vascular registry in Southern Sweden (VRISS) started in late 1985. The aims were to monitor practice, changes and outcome of vascular surgery in routine care on a population basis; to maintain a high standard of data; to establish a basis for scientific studies; and to develop techniques to enable quality to be monitored. An additional aim was to compare the results of vascular surgical treatment at county hospitals with results from established centres in the University Hospitals.

Table 1. Variables recorded in Swedvasc

Preoperative	
1.	Level of care
2.	Responsible surgeon
3.	Risk factors
4.	Operation code number (official by Board of Health and Welfare)
5.	Surgical classification (primary, secondary, elective, emergency)
6.	Indication
7.	Ankle pressure
Peroperative	
8.	Anatomy of inflow/outflow
9.	Reconstructive procedure
10.	Graft material including manufacturer
Outcome at 30 days	
11.	Surgical complications
12.	General complications
13.	Vascular reoperations
14.	Non-vascular reoperations
15.	Level of care
16.	Function/patency
17.	Ankle pressure
18.	Death
Outcome at 1 year	
19.	Date of any reoperation
20.	Date of any amputation
21.	Date of any occlusion
22.	Level of care
23.	Function/patency
24.	Ankle pressure
25.	Death

After a year of preparation, and 30 days of pilot testing, VRISS started in 1987, covering 1.9 million inhabitants. The number of participants increased continuously and since 1994 the whole population of Sweden – 8.5 million – has been covered. Data are mostly acquired by mailed questionnaires but an increasing number of centres are developing computer programs for direct data input. Patients' data are fed into the main computer of the Regional Cancer Registry in Southern Sweden, which is connected to the Swedish population registry, where the date of death of every Swedish inhabitant is registered within 3 weeks. Apart from the 30-day and 1-year patient survival, long-term survival data are available.

The variables in the Swedvasc have remained unchanged over the years (Table 1). At present, however, the registry is under revision, primarily to fulfil the needs emerging from new endovascular procedures. The organization is simple with a steering committee representing university, county and district hospitals. Every hospital has appointed one surgeon responsible for the registry. The representatives meet once-yearly. Since 1995 the registry has been part of the Swedish Society for Vascular Surgery with specific by-laws.

CRITERIA FOR A REGISTRY

Certain minimum criteria must be considered, a registry always being a compromise between wishes and practicalities:

1. There must be sufficient information for a meaningful database.
2. The registry must be sufficiently simple to keep a high level of compliance. This is a key factor for success.[1,4]
3. All hospitals within the geographical area of the registry should participate.
4. The registry must supply participants with data and feedback on a regular basis.
5. Data must be readily available for participants and there must be rules on how to handle those data.
6. There must be agreement on how to use the data in scientific publications.

THE EFFORT NEEDED

Needless to say running a registry covering a whole country is not achieved without considerable effort and a few problems, even in a small country like Sweden. The creation of a protocol took about 2 years to achieve. However, this must not be a hasty procedure, because if participants are not satisfied to start with the compliance will certainly decrease. Over time more hospitals have joined the scheme voluntarily but a few have probably been 'forced' by group pressure and it takes some effort to make all feel real participants.

Although the administration of the scheme has been kept to a minimum, considerable effort has been made by those starting the registry and much has depended on their enthusiasm. All data are fed into the main computer from the secretariat of one hospital. This has been quite an extensive job, which hopefully will decrease when more centres use computer programs for inputting data. To this end, a common standard has been agreed upon for file exchange.

Another effort has been made to create an economic basis for the registry. During the first years of the registry, secretarial and analysis work was financed by various research grants. From 1991 national agencies promoting quality development in health care have supported clinical registries, among them Swedvasc. The grants so far correspond to approximately £230 000, the cost per case being around £3.1. Also when adding participants and secretarial work at the local level, the cost is only a small fraction of the overall costs for this type of surgery (0.25–0.4%). Although official financing is important, participating surgeons' volunteer work and sponsor support for the yearly meetings have been essential prerequisites for proper function of the registry. Hopefully this will continue, but responsibility for participation in various registries must devolve to the hospital administration, giving defined working hours for these activities.

It has also been an effort to maintain continuity in the scheme over the years when the leading surgeons have changed. So far every hospital has created its special routines to enable the registry to function and this has been reasonably successful in allowing the whole country to be covered.

The registry has also had to overcome various problems and difficulties:

1. *Registration of all procedures.* To evaluate how successful registration has been, the registry is compared with other sources of information, although there is no 'gold standard'. In Sweden there are three ways to gather information on this subject. The first is to use computer-based registries of operative procedures from the anaesthesia departments. Because their focus is on operative procedures this is probably the most relevant comparison, provided anaesthesia was used. The second way is to use data from discharge abstracts mainly concerning hospital admissions and diagnoses, but here information on operative procedures is not emphasized. These files are annually reported to the National Board of Health and Social Welfare, nationwide. The third way is to compare the registry data with lists and files obtained manually from operating departments. Despite drawbacks, all validation systems show that patients are missed. The true frequency of missing cases is difficult to estimate, but 10–20% seems to be a reasonable assumption. This figure is not acceptable and our objective is to attain a >95% reporting rate. Hospital routines must contain a second survey to collect cases missed at the primary report.

2. *Follow-up of all patients.* The aim is to follow all patients for 1 year. People who die within 1 year are identified with the help of the Swedish National Population Registry and date of death is added to the Swedvasc file. Reports on living patients are requested at 30 days and at 1 year. To minimize the number of cases lost to follow-up, a list of patients pending for 1-year follow-up are sent to each centre on a monthly basis. Still patients are lost. In a study on femorodistal bypass operations 12% were lost to follow-up.[5] The follow-up rate in Swedvasc has improved somewhat over the years and, if vascular access is excluded, now exceeds 90%.

3. *Inclusion of all data.* The registration form is the basis for data collection and contains more than 40 variables. All data relevant for the various procedures are compulsory but not all data are complete. Information on risk factors are less often

reported than type and outcome of the procedure. Ankle pressure data are frequently missing as are data on patient independence at home which is not reported in 18% of cases. Half of the hospitals have organized their own computer-based routines with electronic transfer to the main computer system at regular intervals. With this system it is possible to compel the surgeons to feed all data into the computer before the whole entry is accepted. There is, however, the possibility of escaping this demand by reporting 'unknown'.

4. *Accuracy of data.* Information on the accuracy of data can be obtained by reproducibility studies performed by repeatedly filling out a random sample of protocols. An overall agreement of about 90% is usually achieved.

5. *Definition of variables and factors.* There are difficulties defining risk factors and postoperative complications. Definitions must be as clear and as simple as possible, and sophisticated evaluations should not be necessary. Similar criteria must be used in all participating departments. There is a special hand-book for completing the protocols.

6. *Alterations of the protocol over time.* Alterations should be made as rarely as possible and only if there are really good reasons. Otherwise there will be difficulties following changes in outcome over time. A recent revision of the protocol deals with all new endovascular procedures.

7. *Long-term follow-up.* Again there has to be a compromise between various aims. Although a follow-up for several years would be optimal, the 1-year follow-up has been practical and possible. However, by the linkage of Swedvasc to the population registry, survival follow-up has no time limit.

8. *Comparability between centres.* Although this is one of the aims of this type of registry, interpretations must be made cautiously. Besides real differences in results between centres, other factors which may explain differences in outcome are: different indications for surgery, different types of interventions for one single indication, differences in background population, differences in patient compliance etc. Epidemiological variations are not considered in the registry. In addition, primary amputations are performed by orthopaedic surgeons and not included in Swedvasc. A wish for the future would be to include all patients with the same diagnosis, treated invasively and conservatively.

9. *Quality of outcome.* This is only superficially dealt with in the present registry. It is, however, important as is the relationship between the patency of the reconstruction and the patient's experience of the result, concerning both relief of symptoms and expectations. More detailed analyses will be of importance in the future when choosing methods to treat and indications for treatment. However, quality of outcome has so far been considered too difficult, not least methodologically, to include in the present registry.

10. *Publications from the registry.* Publications from the registry may cause problems. To avoid this there have been publication rules from the very start of the registry, with one recent revision. The rules are agreed upon by all participants. One problem, which has not been fully tested, is how participants can use the publications from the registry as academic qualifications.

11. *Coding aspects.* A problem with all long-term registries is the possibility of changes in coding systems, both for diagnosis and procedures. This has recently occurred when the Swedish health care system changed the codes for surgical procedures to the very detailed 'Classification of surgical procedures' in 1997. This needs a very delicate translation process. As a check the Swedvasc itself registers both symptoms and interventional procedures on the basis of techniques and anatomy.

12. *Data access.* Data belong to the registry. The collective data are distributed yearly to the responsible surgeon in each hospital together with similar data on his/her own hospital. The collective data are official, the individual hospital data are not (it is up to the hospital to decide how to handle that information). Data on certain topics could be distributed after application to the Swedvasc registry steering committee, for example data on the use of a specific type of graft.

ADVANTAGES

The main advantages can be summarized as:

1. *Overview.* The information on all the vascular surgery undertaken in a country gives an overall view of our speciality. In time it will also provide information on results of vascular surgery in that country.

2. *Survival analysis.* With linkage to the population registry, survival analysis is possible without time limits.

3. *Research activities.* The registry can be used as a basis for research activities. There are several possibilities:

- to use data from the registry to analyse time trends and variations between hospitals and regions;
- to extend the protocol for a defined period with a specific aim;
- to identify patients in the registry for more detailed analysis such as in case control studies;
- to study the outcome and effectiveness of vascular surgery on a population basis;
- to study unusual diseases and events;
- to identify patients and procedures for more detailed analysis with specific aims;
- to initiate prospective studies using more comprehensive protocols, i.e. efficacy, randomized trials.

Data from Swedvasc have been presented at more than 50 national and international meetings. There are by now a number of publications concerning the organization and early experiences of the whole registry, using data to analyse various problems. using data as part of or as a starting point for a variety of studies, and using data as a part of prospective studies. (See the ADDITIONAL READING section at the end of this chapter.)

4. *Common problems.* The present structure makes it possible for vascular surgeons to meet and discuss common problems and to analyse their own results in comparison

with the collective results. Although difficult to quantify, this is a basis for improvement of quality. It can also allow the development of standards of quality.

5. *Quality development*. There are no common standards of quality control and development agreed upon by vascular surgeons. A number of measures have been suggested. *Sentinel events* are events that normally should not occur, are easily identified from data files and, if increasing, should prompt an investigation. In Swedvasc this concept is tested using four different events.

These are early reoperation for occlusion in femoropopliteal bypass surgery (possible technical error); amputation within 30 days of operation for claudication; stroke within 30 days of carotid endarterectomy for transient ischaemic attacks; and graft infection after elective procedures. These serious complications have shown a low and constant frequency of 1–2%.

Treatment outcome, in general, compares favourably with published results from specialized centres using parameters such as survival after aneurysm surgery, clinical outcome of procedures for leg ischaemia, and complications of carotid surgery. In critical limb ischaemia, clinical success is in excess of 80% after 1 month, but after 1 year both amputation and death occur in 20% of cases. The individual that benefits from surgery for less than 1 year may represent a valuable outcome of medical care but modest 1-year results may also indicate that the selection of patients for active treatment could be improved.

6. *Linkage to other registries*. This is a current concern for carotid artery disease, where all patients coming to a duplex examination are registered and where there are more preoperative details than in the Swedvasc. The aim is to identify and analyse in detail patients with serious outcome, i.e., permanent stroke and/or death. In this way it is possible to discuss the individual cases and analyse the most probable cause of failure. In this process there are technical/surgical causes, problems with care etc. but the majority of patients develop a complication, which is the price of surgery in this high risk group of patient.[6]

FOR WHOM IS THE REGISTRY OF VALUE?

There are many groups of individuals who will hopefully benefit from a national vascular registry:

- *The patient*. The ultimate aim with the registry is to be able to improve the quality of vascular surgery. Although difficult to quantitate, there is for instance a tendency to better results over time when treating severe lower limb ischaemia.
- *The surgeon*. The individual surgeon can compare his/her results on a per year basis with the collective results and thereby have a basis for educational discussion.
- *The researcher*. The registry can be used in various ways to form the basis for research projects. For many clinical questions and issues, it may simply be impossible to organize a randomized controlled trial. Other approaches may be necessary. Examples are treatment outcome in clinical practice, differences and their possible causes between hospitals, geographic areas and different groups of

patients. Other applications include development over time of treatment options and results, unusual conditions and complications, late complications and long-term treatment outcome. Basic data for studies in decision-making and health economy are mostly generated in outcome studies. It can be argued that outcome studies, reflecting routine care, can be considered general, as neither patients nor doctors are selected and are representative.[7,8] A randomized controlled trial can demonstrate the effect of a treatment method under optimal conditions (efficacy) while the effect in routine care under average conditions (effectiveness) demands a population-based clinical registry for evaluation. Studies based on clinical registry data are often called observational studies or outcome research.[9–11] Randomized controlled trials and registry research should be complemetary rather than conflicting and contradictory.

- *The health care system.* As has already been indicated there is an increasing need to register procedures and results and to evaluate the outcome and also to analyse the cause of potential differences. It is important that these characteristics are registered but equally important that the analysis is made within the profession and not by administrators or politicians who do not have the necessary competence and possibility to evaluate correctly the background influences. Collecting population based data can form the basis of optimal planning. With the registry in the hands of the vascular surgical profession with its competence to analyse and interpret data it is important to distribute the results both to health care consumers and health care authorities.

IS A NATIONAL VASCULAR REGISTRY WORTH THE EFFORT?

The answer to that question can hardly be given on the basis of a health economic analysis such as by monetary costs per life year or limbs saved. There are so many subjective steps in the analysis of value and effort. Although there are problems with a nationwide registry, the benefits and outcome are of such magnitude that it seems reasonable to continue. The prerequisites, however, are that the outcome is continuously reported and discussed and, if necessary, leads to internal changes as a result of feedback; and that the registry *per se* or through additional protocols is used for research purposes. Just registering tens of thousands of surgical procedures has no value in itself.

To conclude somewhat provocatively, but also – I believe – fairly realistically, the total 1-year registration cost of £31 000 (10 000 procedures at £3.1 each) in Sweden may be compared with the cost of the first year for one patient after amputation (around £140 000).

REFERENCES

1. Plecha FR, Avellone JC, Beven EG *et al.*: A computerised vascular registry: experience of the Cleveland Vascular Society. *Surgery* **86**: 826–835, 1979
2. Karmody AM, Fitzgerald K, Branagh M, Leather RP: Development of a computerized vascular registry for large scale use. *J Vasc Surg* **1**: 594–600, 1984

3. Bergqvist D, Troëng T, Elfström J *et al.*: Auditing surgical outcome. Ten years with the Swedish Vascular registry – Swedvasc. *Eur J Surg* (Suppl) **581**: 1–48, 1998
4. Gruer R, Gordon DS, Gunn AA, Ruckley V: Audit of surgical audit. *Lancet* **i**: 23–25, 1986
5. Elfström J, Stubberöd A, Troëng T: Patients not included in medical audit have a worse outcome than those included. *Int J Quality Assurance* **8**: 153–157, 1996
6. Troëng T, Bergqvist D, Norrving B, Ahari A: Complications of carotid endarterectomy are related to surgical errors in less than one fifth of cases. *Eur J Surg Endovasc Surg* 1999 (in press)
7. Ellwood PM: Outcome management – A technology of patient experience. *New Engl J Med* **318**: 1549–1556, 1998
8. Hu X, Wright JG, McLeod RS *et al.*: Observational studies as alternatives to randomized clinical trials in surgical clinical research. *Surgery* **19**: 473–475, 1996
9. Feinstein AR: An additional basic science for clinical medicine: II. The limitations of randomized trials. *Ann Int Med* **99**: 544–550, 1983
10. Moses LE: The series of consecutive cases as a device for assessing outcomes of interventions. In Bailar JC and Mosteller F (Eds), *Medical Uses of Statistics* pp. 111–127. Mass. USA: NEJM Books, 1986
11. Schroeder SA: Outcome assessment 70 years later : Are we ready? *New Engl J Med* **316**: 160–162, 1987

ADDITIONAL READING

Publications based on vascular registries

The Swedish and Finnish vascular registries (Swedvasc, Finnvasc) are very similar in their design and below are listed the scientific articles, which are based on the registries. This is at least one important way to measure if registry of vascular surgery is worth the effort and to increase our knowledge on problems related to clinical vascular surgery. Discussions have started on the possibility of cooperation between countries with similar registries. The volume of interventions in Swedvasc and Finnvasc together is by now around 100 000.

Bergqvist D, Bengtsson H, Sternby NH: Associated atherosclerotic manifestations. In: Greenhalgh RM, Mannick JA (Eds) *The Cause and Management of Aneurysms*. London: WB Saunders Co., 1990

Bergqvist D, Einarsson E, Norgren L, Troëng T: A comprehensive regional vascular registry. How is the population served ? In Greenhalgh RM, Hollier L (Eds) *The Maintenance of Arterial Reconstruction*. London: WB Saunders Co., 1991

Bergqvist D, Einarsson E, Elfström J *et al.*: Experiences with the Swedvasc registry. *Vasc Med Rev* **5**: 92–101, 1994

Bergqvist D, Troëng T, Elfström J *et al.*: Auditing surgical outcome. Ten years with the Swedish vascular registry – Swedvasc. *Eur J Surg* (Suppl) **581**: 1–48, 1998

Björck M, Bergqvist D, Troëng T: Incidence and clinical presentation of bowel ischaemia after 2930 aortoiliac operations in Sweden. *Eur J Vasc Endovasc Surg* **12**: 139–144, 1996

Björck M, Bergqvist D,Troëng T: Risk-factors for postoperative intestinal ischaemia after aortoiliac surgery. A combined cohort and case-control study of 2824 operations. *Eur J Vasc Endovasc Surg* **13**: 531–539, 1997

Elfström J, Stubberöd A, Troëng T: Patients not included in medical audit have a worse outcome than those included. *Int J Quality Ass* **8**: 153–157, 1996

Elfström J, Stubberöd A, Troëng T: Adjusting outcome measurements for casemix in vascular registry – is it possible and desirable?. *Eur J Vasc Endovasc Surg* **12**: 459–463, 1996

Eneroth M, Apelqvist J, Troëng T, Persson BM: Operations, inhospital length of stay and costs in 321 patients with critical leg ischaemia.A population-based longitudinal outcome study. *Acta Ortop Scand* **67**: 459–465, 1996

Kantonen I, Lepäntalo M, Salenius J-P *et al.*: Auditing a nationwide vascular registry – the 4-year Finnvasc experience. *Eur J Vasc Endovasc Surg* **14**: 468–474, 1997
Kantonen I, Lepäntalo M, Salenius J-P *et al.*: Mortality in abdominal aortic aneurysm surgery. The effect of hospital volume, patient mix and surgeon's case load. *Eur J Vasc Endovasc Surg* **14**: 375–379, 1997
Kantonen I, Lepäntalo M, Luther M *et al.* and the Finnvasc Study Group: Factors affecting the results of surgery for chronic critical leg ischemia – a nationwide survey. *J Vasc Surg* **27**: 940–947, 1998
Kantonen I, Lepäntalo M, Salenius J-P *et al.* and the Finnvasc Study Group: Influence of surgical experience on the results of carotid surgery. *Eur J Vasc Endovasc Surg* **15**: 155–160, 1998
Karlström L, Bergqvist D: Effects of vascular surgery on amputation rates and mortality. *Eur J Vasc Endovasc Surg* **14**: 273–283, 1997
Kuukasjärvi P, Salenius J-P and the Finnvasc Study Group: Perioperative outcome of acute lower limb ischaemia on the basis of the national vascular registry. *Eur J Vasc Surg* **8**: 578–583, 1994
Lepäntalo M, Salenius J-P, Luther M, Ylönen K for the Finnvasc Study Group: Introduction of a population-based vascular registry: validity of data and limitations of registration. *Br J Surg* **81**: 797–981, 1994
Lepäntalo M, Salenius J-P, Albäck A *et al.*: Frequency of repeated vascular surgery. *Eur J Surg* **162**: 279–285, 1996
Lepäntalo M, Salenius J-P, Harjola P-T: Trends in vascular surgery – an evaluation of operative activity in Finland 1976–1992. *Ann Chir Gyn* **85**: 225–229, 1996
Logason K: Low-molecular weight heparin versus dextran in the prevention of early occlusion following arterial bypass surgery distal to the groin. *Eur J Surg* **164** (Suppl) **581**: 40–41, 1998
Salenius J-P and The Finnvasc Study Group: National vascular registry in Finland – Finnvasc. *Ann Chir Gyn* **81**: 257–260, 1992
Salenius J-P, Lepäntalo M, Loponen, Luther M *et al.*: Do vascular registries affect decision-making? *Ann Chir Gyn* **87**: 131–134, 1998
Salenius J-P, Lepäntalo M, Ylönen K, Luther M and the Finnvasc Study Group: Treatment of peripheral vascular disease – basic data from the nationwide vascular registry FINNVASC. *Ann Chir Gyn* **82**: 235–240, 1993
Swedvasc: Vascular surgical audit during a five year period. Changing patterns of vascular surgery 1987–1991. *Eur J Vasc Surg* **8**: 472–477, 1994
Troëng T: Is it possible to predict outcome in an individual patient? *Ann Chir Gyn* **87**: 126–127, 1998
Troëng T, Bergqvist D, Einarsson E *et al.*: Experiences from Swedvasc/VRISS – a vascular registry. *Ann Chir Gyn* **81**,2: 248–252, 1992
Troëng T, Janzon L, Bergqvist D: Adverse outcomes in surgery for chronic leg ischaemia – risk factors and risk prediction when using different statistical methods. *Eur J Vasc Surg* **6**: 628–635, 1992
Troëng T, Bergqvist D, Janzon L *et al.*: The choice of strategy in the treatment of intermittent claudication – a decision tree approach. *Eur J Vasc Surg* **7**: 438–443, 1993
Troëng T, Bergqvist D, Janzon L: The incidence and causes of adverse outcomes of operation for chronic ischemia of the leg. *Eur J Surg* **160**: 17–25, 1994
Troëng T, Bergqvist D, Elfström J *et al.*: Reoperations, redo surgery and other site interventions constitute more than one third of vascular surgery. A study from Swedvasc – the Swedish vascular registry. *Eur J Vasc Endovasc Surg* **14**: 244–251, 1997
Troëng T, Bergqvist D, Norrving B, Ahari A: Complications of carotid endarterectomy are related to surgical errors in less than one fifth of cases. *Eur J Surg Endovasc Surg* 1999 (in press)
VRISS (Vascular Registry in Southern Sweden): The Vascular Registry – a responsibility for all vascular surgeons? *Eur J Vasc Surg* **1**: 219–226, 1987
VRISS (Vascular Registry in Southern Sweden): Vascular surgery in southern Sweden – the first year experience of a vascular registry. *Eur J Vasc Surg* **3**: 563–569, 1989
Zdanowski Z, Troëng T, Norgren L: Outcome and influence of age after infrainguinal revascularisation in critical limb ischaemia. *Eur J Vasc Endovasc Surg* **16**: 137–141, 1998

Commentary

The Swedish vascular surgeons must be congratulated on the establishment of Swedvasc. It provides an invaluable resource for maintaining good standards of clinical practice and planning future healthcare resources. However, audit and research are separate. Audit can be used to generate hypotheses which need to be tested prospectively, whereas the registry itself cannot be used to evaluate hypotheses. For instance, if the registry indicates that women fare worse than men after bypass surgery (see Norgren chapter, p. 163), this needs to be assessed prospectively to ensure equivalence of baseline risk factors associated with graft occlusion e.g. ankle brachial pressure index (ABPI) or plasma fibrinogen. Similarly, if the registry indicates that 30-day mortality for aneurysm repair is higher when bifurcated (trouser) grafts are used than when tube grafts are used, a randomized controlled trial is needed. Perhaps all the registry patients who received bifurcated grafts had more extensive aneurysmal disease and athersclerosis than the patients who recved tube grafts.

In the future, registries will find ways to record all procedures so that mistakes cannot be forgotten. I hope too that Swedvasc will collaborate with orthopaediac surgeons to monitor all amputations. This would add enormously to the value of Swedvasc. Swedvasc is but young and I am sure that these changes will be effected in the near future. *JTP*

WHAT IS THE INFLUENCE OF PHARMACOLOGICAL AGENTS?

The effect of antiplatelet therapy on peripheral vascular disease

Dominic Slade and Charles McCollum

INTRODUCTION

Maintaining arterial patency involves a complex equilibrium between vascular endothelium and flowing blood. The endothelium resists platelet adhesion by secreting a mixture of highly potent platelet inhibiting agents. Of these, nitric oxide (NO) and prostacyclin (PGI_2) are perhaps the best known. Not only do these agents inhibit platelets through increasing the concentration of intraplatelet inhibitory molecules such as cyclic guanosine monophosphate (cGMP) by NO and cyclic adenosine monophosphate (cAMP) by PGI_2, but they also relax vascular tone ensuring optimal blood flow.[1] Usually platelets are efficiently inhibited from adhering to healthy endothelium by these mechanisms and thrombus forms only when this inhibitory lining is disrupted or diseased.

PLATELET ACTIVATION AND ADHESION

A breach in the endothelium activates platelets through the exposure of subendothelial prothrombotic elements such as collagen. Platelets adhere to the subendothelium or the constituents of a ruptured atherosclerotic plaque through interactions involving endothelium-derived von Willebrand factor (vWf), released following injury, and a specific platelet receptor, glycoprotein Ib (GpIb).[2] Following adhesion, platelets release a number of factors, including adenosine diphosphate (ADP) and thromboxane (TxA_2) which bind to platelet receptors amplifying platelet activation and lead to aggregation.

Once degranulated, the platelet, stimulated by the presence of ADP, expresses a surface glycoprotein complex, GPIIb/GPIIIa, which can bind either vessel wall (via vWf) or neighbouring platelets (via fibrinogen). Coagulation pathways are then stimulated to produce thrombin, which stabilizes the platelet thrombus by generation of a fibrin lattice. Thrombin is also the most potent stimulus for further platelet activation.

THE CONTRIBUTION OF DISTURBED BLOOD FLOW

Shear stress between flowing blood and diseased artery or prosthetic graft may lead to the aggregation of platelets by disrupting cellular elements from laminar flow.

Under these conditions, vWf may assume greater importance than fibrinogen in platelet aggregation;[3] TxA_2 also contributes significantly to platelet adhesion under these conditions.[4] In the presence of peripheral vascular disease (PVD), platelets are exposed to both shear stress and disrupted endothelium, substantially increasing the likelihood of platelet of activation and thrombus formation.

ANTIPLATELET DRUGS AND THEIR MODES OF ACTION

The multiple steps involved in platelet–endothelial and platelet–platelet interactions have been the targets of a number of therapeutic strategies. They can be classified by their mode of action (Fig. 1).

Aspirin

Aspirin exerts most of its antithrombotic effect through the irreversible acetylation of cyclooxygenase, which in turn inhibits platelet TxA_2 production. Being anucleate, platelets lack the cellular machinery to generate further cyclooxygenase. The effect is

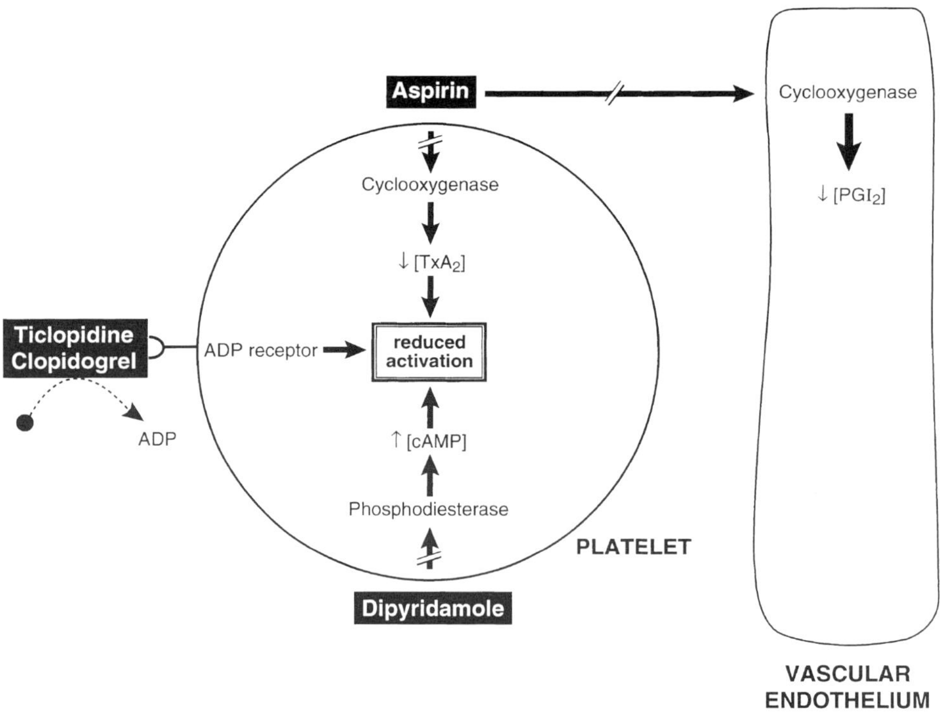

Fig. 1. Mechanisms of action of four antiplatelet drugs: aspirin, dipyridamole, ticlopidine and clopidogrel. PGI_2: prostacyclin. cAMP: cyclic adenosine monophosphate. TxA_2: thromboxane. ADP: adenosine diphosphate.

both dose- and time-dependent, and is identical in healthy controls and in patients with atherosclerosis.[5] The sustained pharmacological effects of aspirin are therefore related to platelet survival and turnover.

Endothelial prostacyclin (PGI_2), crucial to the thromboresistant properties of blood vessels, is a vasodilator and a powerful inhibitor of platelet aggregation. Aspirin inhibits PGI_2 production, although the effect is offset partially by endothelial cells generating further cyclooxygenase between aspirin doses. Inhibition of PGI_2 production is also responsible for the gastrointestinal side-effects of aspirin. PGI_2 synthesis is enhanced in patients with severe atherosclerosis, probably because of increased platelet–endothelial interactions and may reduce the tendency to thrombosis associated with advanced vascular disease.[5]

Considerable research and debate has focused on the apparent dilemma that aspirin is beneficial through its inhibition of TxA_2 production but at the same time potentially detrimental in its reduction of PGI_2 synthesis. A number of clinical trials have attempted to identify the optimum dosage of aspirin required to block platelet TxA_2 whilst retaining endothelial PGI_2 levels. Interestingly, even at doses of more than 1g/day, aspirin still exerts beneficial antithrombotic effects, and conversely, is only thrombogenic in doses exceeding 200mg/kg.[6] These findings suggest that the thrombogenic effects of aspirin are independent of PGI_2 blockade, (PGI_2 production is inhibited even by 30mg aspirin/day) but raise the possibility that aspirin can prevent thrombosis by mechanisms independent of prostaglandin inhibition.[7] Prostaglandin-independent effects of aspirin include inhibition of platelet aggregation by shear stress and fibrinolysis.[4]

Dipyridamole

Dipyridamole is thought to directly stimulate PGI_2 synthesis, potentiating its antiplatelet action, whilst also raising intraplatelet concentrations of cAMP through inhibition of phosphodiesterase activity. It is unclear, however, which of these effects accounts for its antiplatelet activity.[8] Dipyridamole is at best a weak platelet-inhibitory drug of doubtful value.

The thienopyridine derivatives: ticlopidine and clopidogrel

The thienopyridines exert their antiplatelet effects through the inhibition of ADP binding to its platelet receptor. This prevents the subsequent activation of the GP IIb/IIIa complex, and leads to reduced platelet activation and impaired thrombus formation.[9] Neither agent appears to modify GP IIb/IIIa directly, suggesting that the reduction of fibrinogen binding by this protein is an indirect effect.[10] Both drugs are inactive *in vitro*, requiring metabolic activation by the liver before mediating their antiplatelet effects. ADP-receptor blockade is independent of circulating drug levels of the agent, and like aspirin is irreversible, lasting for the lifetime of the platelet.[11,12]

Inhibition of platelet aggregation by both agents is concentration-dependent and requires four to seven repeated daily doses to achieve a maximal effect, after which point, subsequent dosing does not inhibit platelet function further.[12] These drugs may also blunt platelet responses to other stimuli, the actions of which are mediated by ADP release. Both drugs inhibit platelet aggregation in response to high shear stress with the effect being greatest for clopidogrel.

Ticlopidine

Ticlopidine was the first thienopyridine approved by the FDA, its development a byproduct of a search for a new anti-inflammatory agent. Despite its effective use in a large number of clinical trials, ticlopidine carries a 1% risk of profound, life-threatening neutropenia.[9] It can also predispose to thrombotic thrombocytopenic purpura, which whilst rare, carries a 33% mortality rate. For these reasons, ticlopidine was never licensed for use in the UK.

Clopidogrel

Clopidogrel, the newest agent in this class, differs structurally from ticlopidine by just a carboxymethyl side chain but is 100 times more active than ticlopidine. It has a considerably safer side-effect profile, with gastrointestinal disturbance (nausea, vomiting and indigestion) and rash being the most common complaints. During long-term therapy, the risk of bone marrow depression is less than that with aspirin.[13]

THE EFFECT OF ANTIPLATELET DRUGS ON PERIPHERAL VASCULAR DISEASE

Interpreting the effect of individual platelet-modifying drugs from the many studies that have been conducted is difficult. Early trials compared novel drugs only against placebo. However, as aspirin is cheap, generally well tolerated and a highly effective antiplatelet drug, it would be inappropriate to study the benefits of any newer therapy without comparing these with aspirin.

Aspirin

As early as 1953, an American Ear Nose and Throat surgeon reported that in an uncontrolled clinical trial involving over 8000 patients treated with aspirin none had suffered a myocardial infarction.[1]

It was later shown that aspirin delayed the progression of atherosclerosis, with the addition of dipyridamole enhancing this effect.[14] A meta-analysis of 25 separate clinical trials, including some 29 000 patients who had undergone treatment with antiplatelet therapy for transient ischaemic attack (TIA), occlusive stroke, unstable angina, or myocardial infarction (MI) was published in 1988.[15] The therapies used centred mainly on varying doses of aspirin, or combinations of aspirin with dipyridamole.

Overall vascular mortality was reduced by 15% (SD 4%), which approximates to the benefit expected from β-blockade following a recent MI, or long-term diuretic therapy in a patient with hypertension.[15]

At the time platelet-inhibitory therapy in patients with PVD was prescribed mainly to prevent thrombosis in aortocoronary and peripheral arterial bypass grafts. Platelet deposition, as a continuing process, already had been implicated in prosthetic graft failure.[16] With this in mind, the multicentre femoropopliteal bypass trial was initiated in 1984.[17] Where the saphenous vein was adequate for bypass, 549 patients were randomized in a double-blind trial of aspirin 300mg + dipyridamole 150mg or placebo twice-daily started just before surgery. Although the aim was to investigate the effects of antiplatelet therapy on graft patency, the most important outcome was that antiplatelet therapy had a dramatic influence on subsequent rates of MI and stroke in patients with PVD (Table 1).

At a mean follow-up of 34 months, there were only 35 (73/1000 patient-years) cardiovascular events (MI or stroke) on aspirin + dipyridamole, compared with 53 (132/1000 patient-years) with placebo ($p=0.004$).

By the time the Antiplatelet Trialists' Collaboration published their second meta-analyses of antiplatelet studies there had been an explosion of trials investigating their effects in all types of vascular disease, including PVD. Sub-analysis of the 'other high risk patient' groups, including over 20 000 patients with an increased risk of 'vascular events', demonstrated a reduction in the risk of suffering any vascular event of 23 per 1000 ($2p<0.00001$).[18]

Studies investigating the effect of antiplatelet therapy in aortocoronary and peripheral arterial bypass grafting demonstrated a reduction in the odds of suffering a vascular event (non-fatal MI, non-fatal stroke or vascular death) by one-quarter.[19] These findings suggest that a common disease process may underlie all vascular events, be they cerebrovascular, cardiac or peripheral occlusive. In these studies, the duration of treatment for patients undergoing arterial bypass was only half that in the major studies in patients following MI or stroke, but a statistical benefit from therapy was still evident. Secondly, there was no important difference in outcome across the patients undergoing different vascular procedures. The overall reduction in mortality for all patients should therefore translate into benefit for each individual disease type.

Dipyridamole

Dipyridamole alone has failed to demonstrate any antithrombotic efficacy when exposed to scrutiny by clinical trial. Although it may add to the aspirin effect in prevention of PVD progression, dipyridamole's variable absorption, cost, significant

Table 1. Cardiovascular events (rate/1000 patient-years of therapy)

	Placebo (n=263)		*ASA + DPM (n=286)*		
	n	*rate*	*n*	*rate*	*p*
Myocardial infarction	34	84.4	19	39.7	0.006
Stroke	19	47.1	16	33.5	0.30
Total	53	131.5	35	73.2	0.003

ASA: aspirin. DPM: dipyridamole.

side-effects and absence of proven clinical benefit, have caused it to fall from favour as an antiplatelet agent.[8,14]

Ticlopidine

Whilst ticlopidine has demonstrated superior efficacy over other antiplatelet drugs in prevention of vascular events in patients suffering TIA, stroke or following coronary stenting, its position in PVD is less clear.[9,20] A meta-analysis of a number of short-term studies of ticlopidine vs placebo in PVD showed a 6% reduction of fatal or non-fatal vascular events ($p=0.006$).[21] Despite this there is no convincing evidence that it is any more effective than aspirin.[20]

Clopidogrel

In 1996, *The Lancet* reported the results of the largest phase III randomized, blinded, international, placebo-controlled trial ever conducted – the CAPRIE study.[13] Over 19 000 patients were recruited into one of three subgroups (recent stroke, recent MI, or symptomatic PVD), randomized to treatment with clopidogrel 75mg once-daily or aspirin 325mg once-daily and followed for an average of 1.91 years. It was the first study of an antiplatelet drug to include patients from cerebrovascular, cardiac and PVD groups in a common protocol. The assumption was that cardiovascular events such as MI and stroke were caused by thrombosis at sites of arterial disease mediated by platelets.

The study showed a relative-risk reduction of 8.7% in favour of clopidogrel ($p=0.043$) over aspirin. For PVD, subgroup analysis suggested an estimated relative-risk reduction of 23.8% by clopidogrel over aspirin compared with no additional benefit for MI patients. However, CAPRIE was only powered to detect a realistic treatment effect over the whole study cohort and not in the clinical subgroups.

The findings of the CAPRIE trial confront the clinician with further dilemma. Does the expected prevention of a further five major clinical events per 1000 patient-years by clopidogrel over and above the 19 events already prevented by aspirin justify the increased treatment cost (clopidogrel is 30 times more expensive than aspirin)?[12]

Thienopyridines block ADP receptor-dependent platelet activation whilst aspirin inhibits cyclooxygenase blocks TxA_2 production: as TxA_2 and ADP contribute about equally to thrombogenesis, the next step must surely be to study combination therapy in a randomized controlled trial.[22]

We should not exclude the possibility that there may be other important differences between the clinical subgroups of CAPRIE and that patients with PVD may be at particular risk due to chronic low-grade ischaemia-reperfusion injury related to intermittent claudication.

PERIPHERAL VASCULAR DISEASE AND ITS MORTALITY

The risk to patients with intermittent claudication is not to their limb but to their life. Claudicants carry a three-fold increased risk of all-cause mortality when compared with an age-matched population; most (75%) of these deaths will be cardiovascular, of which 50% will be cardiac and 15% cerebrovascular.[23] This risk is related to the severity of disease at presentation and is greater in men under the age of 60, who show four times the expected mortality.[24,25] In the Speedwell heart disease study, the relative odds risk of death in men with PVD was 3.8, even after correction for age and smoking habit.[23]

THE SYSTEMIC EFFECTS OF CLAUDICATION

These data suggest that the effects of PVD on life expectancy cannot be explained simply in terms of generalized atherosclerosis or standard risk factors. There is mounting evidence that the increased risk of myocardial infarction (MI) and stroke in

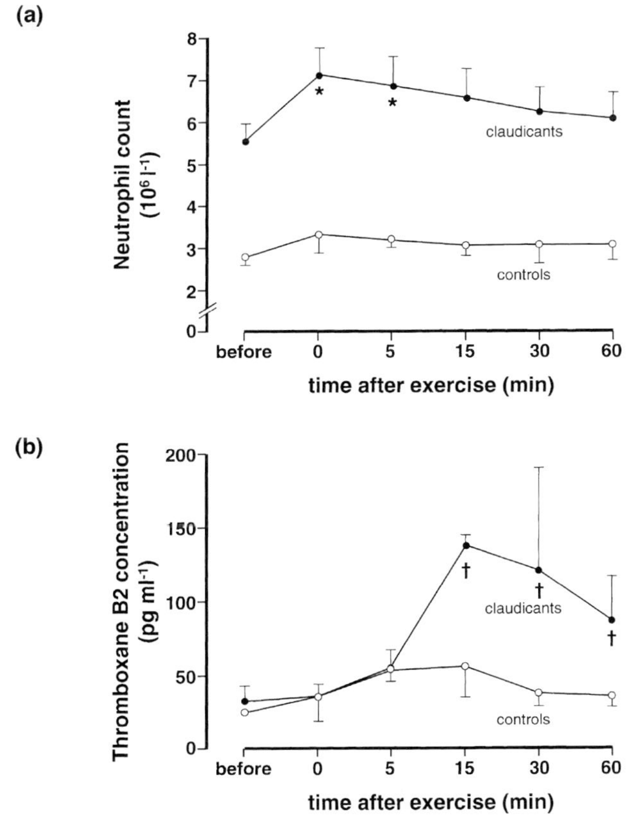

Fig. 2. Median neutrophil counts (a), plasma thromboxane B_2 concentrations (b), (interquartile range) demonstrate a higher initial neutrophil count which rises significantly on exercise in claudicants but not in healthy controls. There is a subsequent dramatic rise in thromboxane which again occurs only in claudicants; * $p<0.05$ compared with pre-exercise value (Wilcoxon signed rank test), † $p<0.05$ compared with control value (Mann-Whitney *U* Test).

claudicants may in part be due to activation of inflammatory cells and platelets during recurrent low-grade ischaemia-reperfusion caused by claudication.

When claudicants exercise, the increased metabolic requirements of their muscles are not matched by an increase in tissue perfusion, creating muscle ischaemia and pain. On resting, reperfusion of the ischaemic muscle with oxygenated blood stimulates a burst of free radical production. This effect stimulates activation of platelets and leukocytes and may damage vascular endothelium.

Evidence for these events comes from a number of studies investigating changes in serum inflammatory markers in claudicants at rest and following exercise. We first investigated the effect of 5-minute treadmill exercise in claudicants and healthy controls.[27] Neutrophil count and plasma thromboxane levels both significantly increased immediately after exercise in claudicants but not in controls (Fig. 2). These findings suggest platelet activation and release reactions stimulated through the inflammation of ischaemia-reperfusion. Plasma soluble P-selectin, an adhesion molecule crucial for initiating platelet–endothelial interactions, rises following cumulative exercise suggesting progressive platelet activation (Fig. 3).[28] Raised plasma neutrophil elastase levels measured concomitantly imply neutrophil activation.[29] There is a suggestion that these effects may be ameliorated by surgical intervention.[30]

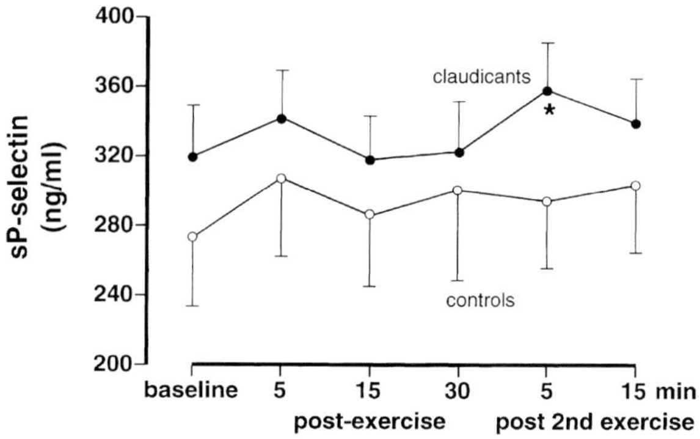

Fig. 3. Mean plasma levels of soluble P-selectin (standard deviation) demonstrate the effect of repeated exercise in claudicants and healthy controls. A significant rise in soluble P-selectin 5 minutes following the second period of exercise in claudicants demonstrates progressive platelet activation and adhesion reactions; * $p<0.05$ compared with control value (repeated measures of analysis variance).

PRIMARY OR SECONDARY PREVENTION?

The role of antiplatelet drugs in secondary prevention of cardiovascular events in patients with symptomatic vascular disease is assured. The logical question now, is whether they should be used in primary prevention. The American Physicians'

Health study, which randomized 22 071 participants to low-dose aspirin (325mg/day) in a double-blind trial vs placebo, demonstrated an overall reduction in myocardial infarction of 44% (relative risk 0.56, p=0.00001).[31] The benefit was only apparent in those over 50 years of age and was coupled with a slight increase in the risk of haemorrhagic stroke (which failed to reach statistical significance).

The results of trials involving 28 000 patients, considered low risk 'primary prevention' subjects, were analysed in the second cycle of the Antiplatelet Trialists' Collaboration.[18] Five years of continued antiplatelet therapy produced a small but significant decrease in the number of non-fatal myocardial infarctions (5/1000, 2p<0.0005). No significant benefits were seen in reducing the risk of fatal or non-fatal stroke and though not statistically significant, there was a suggestion of an increase in mortality from haemorrhagic stroke.

CONCLUSION

Platelet-inhibitory therapy is clearly indicated for all patients with vascular grafts and for all patients with symptomatic cardiovascular disease. There is mounting evidence that low-dose aspirin is appropriate for high-risk individuals over the age of 50. Where there is aspirin intolerance, then clopidogrel seems to be the drug of choice but it is doubtful that we have sufficient evidence to justify prescribing this as a prophylactic therapy in asymptomatic patients.

ACKNOWLEDGEMENT

We would like to acknowledge the kind and considerable help of Helen Carruthers, Department of Medical Illustration, South Manchester University Hospital, UK.

REFERENCES

1. Schafer A: Antiplatelet therapy. *Am J Med* **101**: 199–209, 1996
2. Blann A, McCollum C: von Willebrand factor, endothelial cell damage and atherosclerosis. *Eur J Vasc Surg* **8**: 10–15, 1994
3. Peterson D, Sthopoulos N, Giorgio T *et al.*: Shear-induced platelet aggregation requires von Willebrand factor and platelet membrane glycoproteins Ib and IIb-IIIa. *Blood* **69**: 625–628, 1987
4. Folts J, Crowell E, Rowe G: Platelet aggregation in partially obstructed vessels and its elimination with aspirin. *Circulation* **54**: 365–370, 1976
5. Patrono C, Ciabattoni G, Patrignani P: Clinical pharmacology of platelet cyclooxygenase inhibition. *Circulation* **72**: 1177–1184, 1985
6. Marcus A: Aspirin as an antithrombotic medication. *New Engl J Med* **309**: 1515–1516, 1983
7. Hirsh J, Dalen J, Fuster V *et al.*: Aspirin and other platelet-active drugs. The relationship among dose, effectiveness, and side effects. *Chest* (Suppl) **108**: 247–257, 1995
8. Fitzgerald G: Dipyridamole. *New Engl J Med* **316**: 1247–1257, 1987
9. Sharis P, Cannon C, Loscalzo J: The antiplatelet effects of ticlopidine and clopidogrel. *Ann Int Med* **129**: 394–404, 1998

10. Mills D, Puri R, Hu C-J: Clopidogrel inhibits the binding of ADP analogues to the receptor mediating inhibition of platelet adenylate cyclase. *Arterioscler Thromb* **12**: 430–436, 1992
11. Harker L, Bruno J: Ticlopidine's mechanism of action on human platelets. In: Hass W, Easton J (Eds) *Ticlopidine, Platelets and Vascular Disease* pp. 41–59. New York: Springer, 1993
12. Coukell A, Markham A: Clopidogrel. *Drugs* **54**: 745–750, 1997
13. CAPRIE Steering Committee: A randomised, blinded, trial of clopidogrel versus aspirin in patients at risk of ischaemic events (CAPRIE). *Lancet* **348**: 1329–1339, 1996
14. Hess H, Mietaschk A, Deichsel G: Drug-induced inhibition of platelet function delays progression of peripheral occlusive arterial disease. A prospective double-blind arteriographically controlled trial. *Lancet* 415–419, 1985
15. Antiplatelet Trialist's Collaboration: Secondary prevention of vascular disease by prolonged antiplatelet treatment. *Br Med J* **296**: 320–331, 1988
16. Goldman M, Hall C, Dykes J *et al.*: Does III Indium-platelet deposition predict patency in prosthetic arterial grafts? *Br J Surg* **70**: 635-638, 1983
17. McCollum C, Alexander C, Dip N: Antiplatelet drugs in femoropopliteal vein bypasses: A multicenter trial. *J Vasc Surg* **13**: 150–162, 1991
18. Antiplatelet Trialist's Collaboration: Collaborative overview of randomised trials of antiplatelet therapy-I: Prevention of death, myocardial infarction, and stroke by prolonged antiplatelet therapy in various categories of patients. *Br Med J* **308**: 81–106, 1994
19. Antiplatelet Trialist's Collaboration: Collaborative overview of randomised trials of antiplatelet therapy-II: Maintenance of vascular graft or arterial patency by antiplatelet therapy. *Br Med J* **308**: 159–167, 1994
20. Gent M: A systematic overview of randomized trials of antiplatelet agents for the prevention of stroke, myocardial infarction and vascular death. In: Hass W, Easton J (Eds) *Ticlopidine, Platelets and Vascular Disease*, pp. 99–116. New York: Springer, 1993
21. Boissel J, Peyrieux J, Destors J: Is it possible to reduce the risk of cardiovascular events in subjects suffering from intermittent claudication of the lower limbs? *Thromb Haem* **62**: 681–685, 1989
22. Lowe G, Fowkes F, Dawes J, Donnan P: Blood viscosity, fibrinogen, and activation of coagulation and leukocytes in peripheral arterial disease and the normal population in the Edinburgh artery study. *Circulation* **87**: 1915–1920, 1993
23. Dormandy J: Natural history of intermittent claudication. *Hosp Update* (April): 314–320, 1991
24. Jelnes R, Gaardsting O, Jensen KH, Baekgaard N: Fate in intermittent claudication: outcome and risk factors. *Br Med J* **293**: 1137–1140, 1986
25. O'Riordain D, O'Donnell J: Realistic expectations for the patient with intermittent claudication. *Br J Surg* **78**: 861–863, 1991
26. Bainton D, Sweetnam P, Baker I, Elwood P: Peripheral vascular disease: consequences for survival and association with risk factors in the Speedwell prospective heart disease study. *Br Heart J* **72**: 128–132, 1994
27. Edwards A, Blann A, Suarez-Mendez V *et al.*: Systemic responses in patients with intermittent claudication after treadmill exercise. *Br J Surg* **81**: 1738–1741, 1994
28. Kirkpatrick U, Mossa M, Blann A, McCollum C: Repeated exercise induces release of soluble P-selectin in patients with intermittent claudication. *Thromb Haem* **78**: 1338–1342, 1997
29. Turton E, Spark J, Mercer K *et al.*: Exercise-induced neutrophil activation in claudicants: a physiological or pathological response to exhaustive exercise? *Eur J Vasc Endovasc Surg* **16**: 192–196, 1998
30. Hickey N, Gosling P, Baar S, Shearman C: Effect of surgery on the systemic inflammatory response to intermittent claudication. *Br J Surg* **77**: 1121–1124, 1990
31. Physicians Health Study: Final report on the aspirin component of the ongoing physicians' health study. *New Engl J Med* **321**: 129–135, 1989

Commentary

For many years we have assumed that the beneficial effects of low dose aspirin can be attributed to the inhibition of cyclooxygenase in platelets. Very new evidence indicates that aspirin has additional effects on the cellular machinery which regulates the inflammatory response. This inflammatory response in the vessel wall is likely to aggravate most forms of cardiovascular disease.

The cellular genes which regulate the inflammatory response are switched on by a family of cellular transcription factors known as NF-κB. Aspirin and salicylate have direct effects to inhibit the 'switching on' of inflammatory response by NF-κB.[1]

Whatever the mechanisms involved, no vascular patient should be denied the benefit of aspirin therapy. *JTP*

Reference

1. Yin M-J, Yamamoto Y, Gaynor RB: The anti-inflammatory agents aspirin and salicylate inhibit the activity of 1κB-kinase-β. *Nature* **396**: 77–80, 1998

Anticoagulation to prolong lower limb bypass graft patency

Jonathan B Towne

INTRODUCTION

It is logical to conclude that if a patient is anticoagulated the patency of lower extremity bypass grafts could be prolonged. Although this simplistic concept is rational, the determinants of patency of lower extremity bypass grafts are multifactorial. The chief discriminating factor is the type of conduit. Autogenous vein is generally considered to be superior to prosthetic grafts at all sites. Although there is still some disagreement in the literature about the patency of above-knee femoral popliteal bypasses, long-term data with below-knee and tibial bypasses demonstrate the superiority of autogenous grafts. Because of the vastly different nature of the conduit, those factors which prolong patency in autogenous veins are different from those which affect prosthetic grafts, and in any discussion these conduits must be considered separately.

In prosthetic grafts, factors which affect patency fall into several areas. First is the perioperative period when the graft is subjected to all the changes that tend to promote thrombosis, e.g., injured endothelium at the anastomosis and at sites of placement of vascular clamps. Also there seems to be a time period of up to 4 weeks where grafts can occlude without an obvious anatomic reason, presumably with platelet aggregation being the initiating factor. Long-term prosthetic grafts usually do not develop lesions within the conduit but are principally affected by the development of fibrointimal hyperplasia which is more commonly marked at the distal anastomosis. Later in the follow-up, the progression of atherosclerosis in inflow and outflow arteries will also affect the patency of the conduit.

The autogenous vein representing living tissue also has several phases which vary somewhat from the prosthetic graft. In the perioperative period trauma to the arterial endothelium can endanger the endothelium. There can be endothelial injury of the conduit which can take up to 3 weeks to totally reverse, which is more common in reverse vein grafts than in *in situ* grafts. During the follow-up period the graft is subject to development of lesions. In the first 24 months these are often fibrointimal hyperplasia in type and can occur at either anastomosis or more commonly at sites of value.[1] Beyond 24 months the autogenous grafts are prone to develop atherosclerosis which becomes more prominent when follow-up exceeds 5 years.[2]

As with prosthetic grafts, progression of atherosclerosis in inflow and outflow vessels can adversely affect graft patency. It is not unusual for vein grafts to develop obstructive type lesions at sites of a previous defect in the vein graft, in particular, sites where venovenous anastomosis were made or sites where venotomies were required because of injury to the vein. Long-term graft patency is affected by postoperative revisions. In a study by the author, 53% of grafts that came to revisions in the follow-up period were conduits that had previously been modified in the early follow-up period.[1]

The other causes of bypass graft failure are common to all types of arterial grafting, i.e., inadequate inflow or inadequate outflow and technical problems with the construction or tunnelling of the conduit. Anticoagulation would not be expected to make up for these technical and judgmental errors.

The appeal of anticoagulation in autogenous grafts is to allow healing and re-endothelialization of the autogenous conduit and the artery in the perianastomotic region. A secondary benefit is that, in grafts that are doomed to failure there is the potential that an anticoagulated patient will resist propagation of thrombus following the development of graft occlusion. This could minimize the ischaemic effects of the limb prior to potential reinterventions. There has been significant work done determining the affect of antiplatelet treatment on overall patient survival and its effect on the risk of the development of myocardial infarction and stroke. The Antiplatelet Trialists' Collaboration in an exhaustive review of the world literature determined that in each of the four main high-risk categories of patients, antiplatelet therapy was protective.[3] There was a reduction of 33% in non-fatal myocardial infarction, 33% in non-fatal stroke, and about 17% in vascular death in high-risk patients taking antiplatelet therapy. The most widely tested antiplatelet regimen was a medium dose of 75–325 mg of aspirin per day. Among low risk patients, a significant reduction of one-third in non-fatal myocardial infarctions was accompanied by a non-significant increase in stroke. The absolute reduction of vascular events was much smaller than for high-risk patients despite a longer treatment period. A 5-year benefit of about four per 100 000 was noted. The effect of aspirin as an antiplatelet agent in reducing the incidence of occlusion of vein grafts to coronary arteries has been well established.[4] Because of these findings there has been considerable interest in evaluating lower leg bypass graft patency and the effect of anticoagulation on improving results.

ANTIPLATELET AGENTS

There are a variety of antiplatelet agents that can be used in an attempt to increase patency of bypass grafts. Dextran is a high molecular weight polysaccharide produced from sucrose by the action of *Leuconostoc mesenteroides* (a species of blue green algae). Fractionation and hydrolysis produce a product with a mean molecular weight of 40 000.[5] Dextran decreases platelet adhesiveness, reduces factor 8 activity, and increases clot lysability. It also decreases the viscosity of blood and reduces the surface thrombogenicity.

Rutherford and associates demonstrated in a randomized, multicentre trial the efficacy of intravenous dextran 40 in preventing early postoperative thrombosis.[5] The experimental group received dextran given at 100 cc per hour for 5 hours followed by 75 cc per hour in the first postoperative day. On postoperative days 2, 3, and 4 the patients were give 500 cc per day at 75 ml per hour. Heparin was only used intraoperatively. The categories included: femoropopliteal bypass using autogenous vein with poor runoff, femoropopliteal bypass grafts using prosthetic grafts, single or sequential bypass to infrapopliteal arteries and bypasses to popliteal or infrapopliteal arteries associated with adjunctive procedures, e.g., endarterectomy, thrombectomy, angioplasty and transluminal dilatation.

The authors noted no difference in the femoral popliteal autogenous vein graft since there were no occlusions in either group. However, in all other groups a significant difference was noted in prosthetic grafts and inframalleolar tibial bypass reconstructions. The favourable effect on patency had disappeared by the first postoperative month. The critical point to determine is demonstrated in the fact that the median day of occlusion in the control group was 3 days compared with 8 days in the treated group. Since there is no statistically significant difference in the 30-day patency rates, one wonders what ultimate effect the dextran has. It does delay thrombosis but more importantly it is hard to determine from this study if there are grafts that remain patent with dextran that would not have if it had not been used.

The use of aspirin as an antiplatelet medication is also a therapeutic option. Aspirin inhibits platelet aggregation by irreversibly affecting platelet cyclooxygenase in blocking the production of thromboxane A2.[6] Higher doses of aspirin may be harmful as the synthesis of prostacyclin, a potent inhibitor of platelet aggregation, is blocked in the vascular endothelium. Aspirin does not prevent platelet adherence to collagen, adenosine diphosphate (ADP)-induced platelet aggregation, or platelet release.

The role of platelet aggregation on the graft surface as the cause of graft failure was suggested by work done by Saad and colleagues.[7] These authors developed a numerically derived platelet aggregation score based on the aggregation pattern and platelet count in patients who had femoropopliteal bypass using an externally supported knitted Dacron graft. With a mean follow-up time of 50 months they were able to show that patients with a high platelet aggregation score had an increased incidence of graft thrombosis. In their study, 15 of 16 grafts remained patent in patients with a platelet aggregation score of 15 or less but only two of 17 remained patent in patients with a platelet aggregation score of 30 or more.

Several studies have been done on both prosthetic and autogenous vein grafts with mixed results. Green and associates performed a randomized, double-blind clinical trial to assess the effect of aspirin alone or in combination with dipyridamole on the patency rates of expanded polytetrafluoroethylene (PTFE) grafts placed in the infrainguinal position.[8] In above-knee prosthetic grafts the aspirin and dipyridamole group did better than the placebo group. However, in the below-knee graft there is no statistically significant difference between the groups.

Kohler and associates in a prospective study evaluated the use of aspirin and dipyridamole and its effect on patency rates in patients with infrainguinal PTFE grafts as well as autogenous vein infrainguinal bypass grafts.[9] They studied 100 patients with 102 grafts. At 24 months the cumulative patency was not significantly different for treatment vs the control group or for any of the subgroups. They concluded that aspirin and dipyridamole administered postoperatively in doses did not improve the overall patency of prosthetic grafts.

McCollum and associates reported a prospective randomized multicentre clinical trial which evaluated the effect of aspirin and dipyridamole on the patency of femoral popliteal vein bypass grafts.[10] This study included patients who had bypasses to the above-knee or below-knee popliteal artery or to the tibial peroneal trunk. Patients were randomized to 300 mg of aspirin plus 150 mg of dipyridamole given twice-daily; 549 patients undergoing saphenous vein bypass were randomized with 286 taking aspirin and dipyridamole and 263 taking placebo capsules. The mean follow-up was 35 months. There was no statistical difference in patency when life-table patency was evaluated over 36 months. Graft patency was not significantly influenced by placement of the distal anastomosis above or below the knee nor did aspirin or dipyridamole have an effect on the patency in the above-knee or below-knee bypasses.

One of the factors noted in these types of trials is the high incidence of patients who have very poor compliance with taking the drugs. In this trial, 31% of the patients in the experimental group taking aspirin and persantine and 27% of the placebo group had poor drug compliance or did not take the trial medication because of an adverse event or reaction. However, when one looks at the cardiovascular events and mortality rate, the total number of cardiovascular events consisting of myocardial infarction or strokes were significantly reduced in the patients taking the aspirin and dipyridamole. The greatest difference was in the number of myocardial infarctions in the placebo group compared with those taking the study medication.

More recently a new antiplatelet drug, ticlopidine, has been developed. In a prospective randomized study involving 243 patients using 250 mg of ticlopidine twice-daily comparing it with placebo in a 2-year study, Becquemin and associates demonstrated a significant improvement in patency rates in infrageniculate autogenous vein bypasses.[11] The patency rate in the study group was 66.4% compared with 51.2% in the placebo group.

It is my recommendation that patients with lower extremity bypass grafts should take 325 mg of aspirin per day. There has been no study demonstrating any additional benefit derived by adding dipyridamole to this regimen.[12] Despite the fact that in autogenous vein bypass grafts the effect of the aspirin on patency is difficult to ascertain, the effect on cardiovascular complications primarily myocardial infarction are improved with the administration of aspirin. In patients who can tolerate aspirin, there are minimal adverse effects, making this an ideal treatment.

ANTICOAGULATION WITH WARFARIN

Warfarin is a vitamin K antagonist and is a potent oral anticoagulant that has been used to prevent thrombotic complications in patients with bypass grafts. Arfvidsson, in a study to evaluate the effect of anticoagulation on vascular reconstruction of the lower extremities, performed a randomized study allocating patients to warfarin or no anticoagulation.[13] The patients were given heparin preoperatively and postoperatively. The postoperative heparin was administered as an infusion of 10 000 to 20 000 international units for 24 hours for 3–5 days. In the study group, warfarin therapy was started on the first or second postoperative day and heparin infusion continued until an adequate therapeutic prothrombin time was obtained. The study had similar groups of autogenous vein and synthetic grafts. The study also contained patients who had undergone thromboendarterectomy. There was no statistically significant difference in the 12-month cumulative patency between the two groups. The patients were then analysed according to the type of vascular reconstruction done, e.g., vein bypass thromboendarterectomy or PTFE, and there were no differences between the treatment and control groups. It is of note that the authors found a serious bleeding complication rate between 4% and 5% in this study.

Contrary to this, results obtained by Kretschmer in a study of 130 patients receiving femoropopliteal vein grafts randomly assigned to treatment with warfarin and a control group demonstrated that the median duration of primary patency and limb salvage were significantly longer for treated patients than for controls.[14] In addition, survival in the anticoagulation group was longer. Following autogenous vein bypass surgery in the treated group, the results were superior in terms of graft patency, limb salvage, and survival. The median duration of primary graft function for the treated patients was 120 months compared with 93 months for the control group. The median duration of limb salvage was more than 120 months in the therapy group whereas it was 100 months in the control group. The median postoperative survival was 120 months in the treated group and only 72.9 months in the control group. All of these were statistically significant. The 18-month patency was 88% in the experimental group vs 60% in the control group. The patients in the study did not start the anticoagulation until the second postoperative week.

Sarac and associates studied the effect of warfarin treatment on the outcome of infrainguinal vein bypass grafting in patients whom they felt were at high risk for failure.[15] The patients in this study were randomly assigned to either long-term anticoagulation therapy with warfarin plus aspirin or aspirin alone. The criteria for enrollment in the study included suboptimal venous conduit, poor arterial runoff, or redo infrainguinal bypass grafting. The venous conduit was considered suboptimal if it was <3.0 mm in diameter with preoperative duplex ultrasound mapping, if the vein was sclerotic with intraoperative angioscopy, or insufficient saphenous vein was available which would necessitate the use of arm vein or a composite saphenous vein graft. Runoff was considered poor if the distal anastomotic site of the bypass graft was in the distal one-third of the tibial vessels, if runoff to the foot was only through collateral vessels, and if the entire runoff bed was diffusely diseased with multiple sites of >50% stenosis, or if selection of the distal target was compromised as a result of inadequate vein length so that the anastomosis could not be placed beyond all significant disease.

Anticoagulation with heparin was given intraoperatively which was not reversed at the completion of the procedure. Patients were given 325 mg of aspirin per day. Those patients randomized to warfarin underwent anticoagulation therapy with heparin 15 units per kg continuous drip between 6 and 24 hours after completion of the bypass procedure. The warfarin anticoagulation was begun on postoperative days 2 or 3 and the dosage was adjusted to maintain an internalized normalized ratio (INR) between 2 and 3. In the warfarin group the incidence of haematoma was significantly higher, 32% in the treatment group compared with only 4% in the aspirin group. Four of the 12 patients who developed a wound haematoma in the experimental group required evacuation of the haematoma. The 3-year primary graft patency rate was significantly higher in the warfarin group than the aspirin group, 74% vs 51%. The 3-year primary assisted graft patency was 77% in the warfarin group compared with 56% in the control group. The limb salvage rate at 3 years was 81% in the warfarin group compared with 31% in the aspirin group. An interesting aspect of this study is that the authors combined aspirin with the use of warfarin. The positive effects of using anticoagulation is counterbalanced by the increased incidence of wound haematomas, several of which required operative evacuation.

It is my feeling that it is not necessary to use heparin in the perioperative period when a patient is to be placed on long-term warfarin therapy. This eliminates the wound problems which are often seen. Warfarin can be initiated when the patient begins taking fluids, often the night of surgery. The short interval between the operation and obtaining an adequate therapeutic level of the warfarin usually does not result in graft thromboses. The determination of the ultimate value of anticoagulation has to be considered in terms of the operative judgement. I also feel that sclerotic veins should not be used for bypass since the results of these are so poor. Alternative vein should be searched for and if not found a prosthetic bypass gives better results. The second aspect is the vigilance with which the various authors conduct postoperative surveillance of the grafts. A vigorous surveillance protocol may help identify those lesions which cause graft failure prior to the thrombosis of the graft allowing for revisions. This is a variable which is hard to elucidate in evaluating the variety of clinical series which have been presented.

The use of the anticoagulant warfarin requires careful monitoring to avoid problems. Lifetime anticoagulation is a therapeutic option for patients at risk for arterial thrombosis due to hypercoaguable states, prosthetic infrainguinal bypasses, or recurrent thrombophlebitis. Patients for whom such therapy is considered contraindicated include those with concurrent medical problems requiring multiple medications, elderly patients, and patients who travel extensively, consume alcohol regularly or are engaged in strenuous physical activity.

To demonstrate that warfarin can be prescribed safely for extended periods of time, we reviewed a protocol administered by a vascular nurse clinician supervised by a physician for monitoring and regulating outpatient anticoagulation therapy on an academic vascular surgery service.[16] Patients maintained on warfarin included those who had a variety of concomitant medical conditions including hypertension, coronary artery disease, and insulin-dependent diabetes mellitus, age in the ninth decade and a habit of regular alcohol consumption. The efficacy and safety of the protocol was reviewed with respect to patient selection and maintenance of optimal intensity of anticoagulation vs the incidence of thrombotic or haemorrahgic complications.

Ninety-three patients were maintained on a long-term oral outpatient anticoagulation therapy programme administered by a nurse clinician. There were 56 men and 37 women whose ages ranged from 18 to 89 years with a median of 63 years. Indications for therapy included hypercoaguable states in which a coagulation defect was documented, prosthetic infrainguinal arterial grafts, venous thrombosis, arterial emboli, and unexpected prosthetic graft thrombosis. At the initiation of the warfarin therapy, a nurse clinician reviewed the patient's medical record for demographic data, concurrent medical problems, medications, current warfarin dose, and coagulation laboratory values to determine if he/she could understand the risk and implications of long-term anticoagulant therapy, report in a systematic fashion for laboratory monitoring of prothrombin time, and be able to adjust the warfarin dose based on telephone instructions.

Patients excluded from participation in the programme included those without a residence or telephone, those with uncontrolled mental illness, or those incapable of understanding the arithmetic necessary to alter warfarin dosage based on verbal instructions. The goal of therapy was to maintain the prothrombin time at 1.5 to 2 times the control resulting in a target prothrombin time between 18 and 24 seconds. With the institution of INRs we try to keep the INR between 2 and 3. This study reviewed 1891 patient months of warfarin therapy. During this time 3479 prothrombin times were measured resulting in a mean of 2.6 prothrombin times per month; 88% of the patients required periodic alteration in the prescribed warfarin dose after establishment of an initial stable dose; 66% of the patients were prescribed a dosing regimen of warfarin alternating between two strengths of the drug from day to day. During the course of therapy, 14% of the 3479 prothrombin times prompted an adjustment in the warfarin dose. Those were evenly distributed between those who were below the therapeutic range and had to have their warfarin dose increased and those who were above the range and had to have it decreased.

There were no deaths related to the anticoagulant therapy. There were no venous thrombotic events during the study period. Four patients received warfarin because antecedent arterial graft occlusion led to prosthetic graft thrombosis while receiving anticoagulation. Three of these patients had therapeutic prothrombin times when their grafts occluded.

Six major haemorrhagic complications (defined as bleeding resulting in a need for hospitalization, blood transfusion, or cessation of anticoagulant therapy) occurred 12 to 42 months from commencement of therapy, resulting in a complication rate of 3.2 per 1000 patient months of treatment. Causes of haemorrhage included retroperitoneal bleeding, diverticulosis, ulcerative colitis, duodenal ulcer and two gastric ulcers. No gastrointestinal malignancies were discovered. The patient with retroperitoneal bleeding was continued on warfarin therapy because of a history of recurrent graft thrombosis caused by a coagulation factor defect. Anticoagulation therapy was discontinued in the other five patients. Eleven minor haemorrhagic complications were identified, including epistaxis, subcutaneous haematoma, haematuria, hyphaema, menorrhagia, and gingival bleeding representing a rate of 5.3 events per 1000 patient months of treatment. Each of these complications was self-limited and resulted in no significant morbidity. There was no evidence of warfarin-related skin necrosis.

Fihn and associates in a cooperative study involving five different clinics over a mix of geographic location and practice settings evaluated the risk of haemorrhage in a large group of patients undergoing warfarin therapy.[17] The study sample included 928 patients who received 1103 doses and distinct courses of therapy resulting in 33 962 clinic visits. The mean duration of their follow-up was 1.9 years ranging from 6 months to 2.8 years. Fifty-four percent of the therapeutic courses exceeded 6 months duration. In the 1950 patient years of follow-up, 510 first-time bleeding events occurred. Incidence of first bleeding events consisted of minor bleeding at a rate of 71.3 events per 100 patient years, serious bleeding rate of 7.5 events per 100 patient years, life threatening bleeding 1.1 event per 100 patient years, and fatal bleeding 0.2 events per 100 patient years. The fatal bleeding consisted of four cerebral haemorrhages. The cumulative incidence of fatal bleeding among patients was 1% at 1 year, 2% at 3 years. Cumulative incidence of the first episodes of life threatening and serious bleeding at 1 year was 1%, 2 years 2%, 4 years 5%, and 8 years 9%. The first episodes of life threatening bleeding was 1% at 1year, 2% at 2years, 5% at 4years, and 9% at 8 years. The incidence of serious bleeding was 12% at 1 year, 20% at 2 years, 28% at 4 years, and 40% at 4 years. More than half of the serious and life threatening haemorrhages originated in the gastrointestinal tract. In all, 32% of the patients having one bleeding event that was serious or life threatening had a second event, the majority of which occurred within 1 year of the initial event. During the first 3 months of therapy serious bleeding occurred at rates of 21 per 100 patient years. Patients who had three or more chronic conditions other than the indication for anticoagulation were significantly more likely to have bleeding complications than those with fewer than three conditions. These data indicate that the administration of warfarin needs to be done carefully because it does have potential complications. Our own experience shows that these complications can be kept to a minimum in a well-run anticoagulation clinic.

CONCLUSION

It is preferred to have all patients taking aspirin 325 mg per day if they can tolerate it. The effect on graft patencies is variable and more likely to be affected with prosthetic grafts than autogenous vein grafts. The positive effect on the decrease in the incidence of cardiovascular events, primarily myocardial infarction make this an easy treatment. I do not recommend warfarin therapy for autogenous vein grafts. The exception is in those patients with high-risk grafts, which include patients with potential hypercoaguable states, those who have had thrombosis of grafts due to unknown causes, or who have disadvantaged runoff. The size of the saphenous vein has not been an indication to use anticoagulation. For prosthetic grafts, however, I recommend warfarin therapy. As indicated in this chapter the data for this are soft. However, the risk of the anticoagulation has been slight which makes its use reasonable. I do not recommend prescribing anticoagulation for patients in the perioperative period, particularly heparin. The incidence of wound complications does not make it a good choice. In my experience, it is rare for grafts to fail in the first 72 hours postoperatively unless there are technical problems or difficulty in selecting patients for distal bypass. I do not feel the heparin has any advantage. We start patients on coumadin as soon as they are ready for oral intake which is often the night of surgery and usually the next day. The exception to this are patients who may have prothrombotic states, or who have previously thrombosed grafts in the perioperative period. I keep these patients taking heparin postoperatively. The risk of further graft thrombosis is so high that it warrants the increased incidence of wound complications.

REFERENCES

1. Reifsnyder T, Towne JB, Seabrook GR, Bandyk DF: Biology of long-term autogenous vein grafts: a dynamic evolution. *J Vasc Surg* **17**: 207–217, 1993

2. Erickson CA, Towne JB, Seabrook GR *et al.*: Ongoing vascular laboratory surveillance is essential to maximize long-term *in situ* saphenous vein bypass patency. *J Vasc Surg* **23**: 18–27, 1996
3. Antiplatelet Trialists' Collaboration: Collaborative overview of randomized trials of antiplatelet therapy-I: Prevention of death, myocardial infarction, and stroke by prolonged antiplatelet therapy in various categories of patients. *Br Med J* **308**: 81–106, 1994
4. Goldman S, Copeland J, Meritz T *et al.*: Improvement inn early saphenous vein patency after coronary artery bypass surgery with antiplatelet therapy: results at a Veterans Administration Co-op Study. *Circulation* **77**: 13–32, 1988
5. Rutherford RB, Jones DN, Bergentz SE *et al.*: The efficacy of dextran 40 in preventing early postoperative thrombosis following difficult lower extremity bypass. *J Vasc Surg* **1**: 765–773, 1984
6. Stein B, Fuster V, Israel DH *et al.*: Platelet inhibitor agents in cardiovascular disease: An update. *J Am Coll Cardiol* **14**: 813–836, 1989
7. Saad EM, Kaplan S, El-Massry S *et al.*: Platelet aggregometry can accurately predict failure of externally supported knitted Dacron femoropopliteal bypass grafts. *J Vasc Surg* **18**: 587–595, 1993
8. Green RM, Roedersheimer LR, DeWeese JA: Effects of aspirin and dipyridamole on expanded polytetrafluorethylene graft patency. *Surgery* **92**: 1016–1026, 1982
9. Kohler TR, Kaufman JL, Kacoyanis G *et al.*: Effect of aspirin and dipyridamole on the patency of lower extremity bypass grafts. *Surgery* **96**: 462–481, 1984
10. McCollum C, Alexander C, Kenchington G *et al.*: Antiplatelet drugs in femoropopliteal vein bypasses: A multicenter trial. *J Vasc Surg* **13**: 150–167, 1991
11. Becquemin JP: Effect of ticlopidine on the long-term patency of saphenous vein bypass grafts in the legs. *New Engl J Med* **337**: 1726–1731, 1997
12. Kraiss LW, Johnsen K: Pharmacologic intervention to prevent graft failure. *Surg Clin North Am* **75**: 761–772, 1995
13. Artvidsson B, Lundgren F, Drott C *et al.*: Influence of Coumadin treatment on patency and limb salvage after peripheral arterial reconstructive surgery. *Am J Surg* **159**: 556–560, 1990
14. Kretschmer G, Wenzl E, Piza F *et al.*: The influence of anticoagulant treatment on the probability of function in femoropopliteal vein bypass surgery: analysis of a clinical series (1970–1985) and interim evaluation of a controlled clinical trial. *Surgery* **102**: 453–459, 1987
15. Sarac TP, Huber TS, Back MR *et al.*: Warfarin improves the outcome of infrainguinal vein bypass grafting at high risk for failure. *J Vasc Surg* **28**: 446–457, 1998
16. Seabrook GS, Karp D, Schmitt D *et al.*: An outpatient anticoagulation protocol managed by a vascular nurse-clinician. *Am J Surg* **160**: 501–505, 1990
17. Fihn SD, McDonell M, Martin D *et al.*: Risk factors for complications of chronic anticoagulation. *Ann Int Med* **118**: 511–520, 1993

Commentary

Thrombosis is the final common pathway of graft occlusion, irrespective of whether the conduit is vein or prosthetic. This thrombosis occurs gradually in a failing graft as the flow diminishes. The sudden thrombotic occlusion of a newly implanted graft is a different problem. In such a situation the patient may have an inherited predisposition to thrombosis, with mutation in any of the proteins involved in coagulation, including protein C, protein S, factor V and other factors. We also have considered that for vein grafts, the pulsatile arterial flow through the graft may alter the anticoagulant properties of the endothelium. We have shown that the anticoagulant protein thrombomodulin is expressed abundantly on saphenous vein endothelium. However, after exposure of this venous endothelium to arterial flow conditions for only 90 minutes, the amount of thrombomodulin is decreased threefold.[1] Changes such as these may precipitate the unexpected, sudden graft thrombosis.

Vigilance and some form of 'blood thinning' can bring major benefits for the patient with a lower limb bypass graft. *JTP*

Reference

1. Gosling M, Golledge J, Turner RJ, Powell JT: Arterial flow conditions down-regulate thrombomodulin on saphenous vein endothelium. *Circulation* 1999 (in press)

The effect of lipid-lowering therapy

Gillian C Leng

INTRODUCTION

Raised serum cholesterol levels are an important risk factor for the development of peripheral arterial disease. Most studies have demonstrated raised cholesterol levels in subjects with intermittent claudication compared with controls, in both the hospital setting[1–9] and in community-based studies.[10–14] In longitudinal studies, which provide the strongest evidence between a risk factor and disease, positive associations between serum cholesterol and the development of peripheral arterial disease have also been demonstrated consistently. After long periods of follow-up, serum cholesterol has been shown to be significantly correlated with the ankle brachial pressure index (ABPI),[10] and with an increasing risk of developing intermittent claudication.[15]

Good evidence, therefore, exists that cholesterol is an independent risk factor for the development of peripheral arterial disease, but it is probably less important in the aetiology of disease than cigarette smoking.[16] In contrast, cholesterol is relatively more important in the development of coronary heart disease, and smoking less so,[17] This suggests that slightly different mechanisms may be operating in the different tissues, and thus the effects of lipid-lowering therapy may also differ in the lower limb compared with the heart.

This chapter focuses on the role of cholesterol in peripheral arterial disease, and does not address in detail other factors related to lipid metabolism including fatty acids, antioxidants and triglycerides. Cholesterol-lowering is known to be effective in reducing the risk of coronary heart disease,[18] but less research has been performed on patients with lower limb disease. This chapter examines the effectiveness of different lipid-lowering regimens, and reviews the evidence from randomized controlled trials of lipid-lowering in peripheral arterial disease. In the light of this evidence, implications for the management of patients with lower limb disease are discussed and future research requirements are highlighted.

LIPID-LOWERING REGIMENS

The two principal methods for lowering cholesterol levels are dietary modification and lipid-lowering drug therapy. Most management strategies for lipid-lowering suggest an initial trial of dietary modification before progressing to drug therapy.

Dietary modification

The effect of a low fat diet depends on how restrictive it is, and how closely it is adhered to. Substantial reductions in cholesterol levels can be achieved with very strict control, such as in a metabolic ward,[19] but in the general population the changes are much smaller.[20] The extent of cholesterol reduction resulting from dietary change has been estimated at only 1–5%, with a non-significant decrease in risk of a cardiovascular event.[21] The generally poor performance of some lipid-lowering diets may be partly explained by the fact that complex carbohydrates are often used to replace fats, which reduce both high density lipoprotein (HDL) as well as low density lipoprotein (LDL) cholesterol.[22] Other dietary interventions include garlic, oats and soy protein. Evidence for the effect of garlic is not reliable,[23] but systematic reviews of consuming oats and soy protein suggest that they can significantly reduce cholesterol levels.[23–25]

Drug therapy

HMG CoA reductase inhibitors (the statins)

These drugs are the most powerful class of cholesterol-lowering drugs, and can reduce LDL cholesterol levels by more than 20%.[18] They act by competitively inhibiting 3-hydroxy-3-methylglutaryl coenzyme A reductase, an enzyme that catalyses the rate-limiting step in cholesterol synthesis in the liver[26] (Fig. 1). Pravastatin and simvastatin appear to be equally effective in reducing coronary

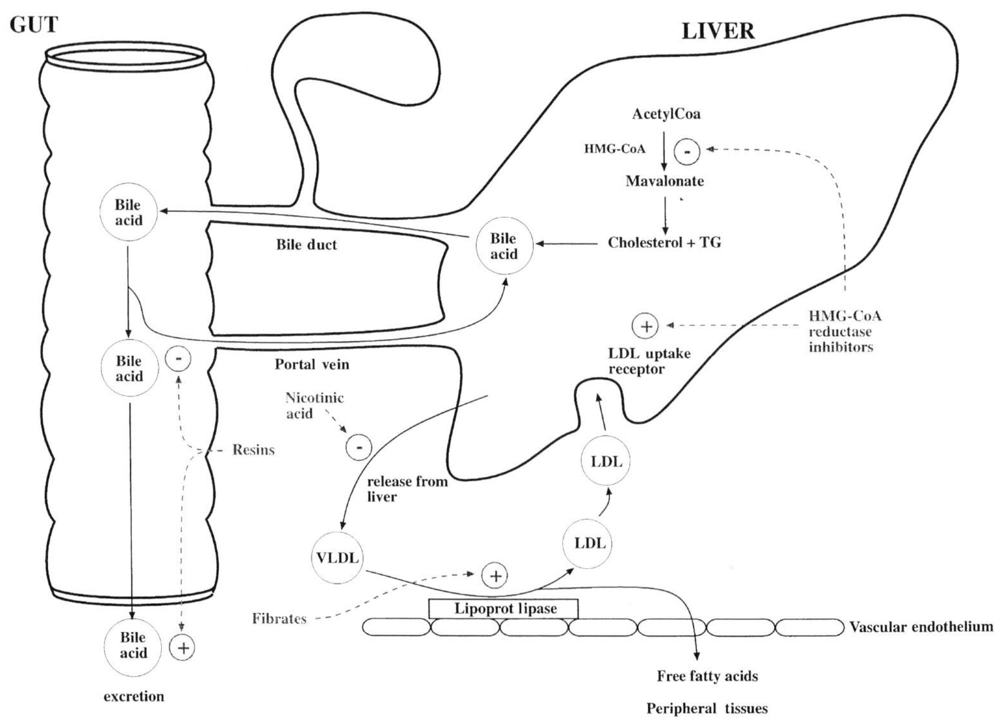

Fig. 1. Mechanism of action of cholesterol-lowering drugs.

events,[18] but data are not available from large scale studies to demonstrate the efficacy of fluvastatin, atorvastatin and cerivastatin, although similar effects might be expected as they lower LDL cholesterol by amounts equivalent to the other statins.

Other cholesterol-lowering drugs

In addition to the statins, there are four other main classes of lipid-lowering agents: 1) fibrates (bezafibrate, fenofibrate and gemfibrozil), which primarily decrease serum triglyceride rather than cholesterol, by stimulating lipoprotein lipase in muscle and adipose tissue capillaries. They also enhance the uptake of LDL by the liver, thus lowering plasma LDL cholesterol; 2) anion exchange resins (cholestryamine and colestipol) which bind bile acids in the gut, thus increasing bile acid excretion and reducing hepatic cholesterol levels; 3) nicotinic acid, which reduces the release of very low density lipoprotein from the liver; and 4) probucol which increases LDL cholesterol catabolism and inhibits LDL oxidation. All these older lipid-lowering agents are less effective than the statins in lowering cholesterol,[18] and are less widely used. Their mechanisms of action are outlined in Fig. 1.

LIPID-LOWERING THERAPY IN PERIPHERAL VASCULAR DISEASE

Identifying evidence of effectiveness

The following criteria were used to identify evidence of lipid-lowering therapy in patients with peripheral atherosclerosis:

- *Study design.* Only randomized controlled trials of lipid-lowering therapy versus control were selected for review. The quality of all potential trials was determined by assessing three key features: method of randomization, including allocation concealment; degree of blinding of patients, physicians and measurement technicians; and the numbers lost to follow-up.
- *Participants.* Trials in any patients with lower limb atherosclerosis were selected, including either intermittent claudication (diagnosed by questionnaire or clinically), or subjects with critical limb ischaemia and asymptomatic disease identified by testing (angiography, ankle pressures etc). Studies of patients with aortic disease and post-bypass grafting were excluded.
- *Intervention.* Any therapeutic regimen aimed at reducing blood lipids was included, for example diet, a hypolipidaemic drug of the five major classes, or any other agent specifically used to treat hyperlipidaemia.
- *Outcomes.* Any of the following outcome measures were eligible for inclusion: all cause mortality; non-fatal events; direct measurement of disease progression (e.g. angiography, duplex ultrasound); indirect tests of disease (e.g. ankle pressure measurements, treadmill testing); and subjective measures (e.g symptom progression, drug side-effects). Lipid-lowering trials reporting only changes in biochemical markers were excluded.

To reduce the possibility of publication bias, an extensive search for trials was performed by hand-searching relevant medical journals, searching on-line electronic database (MEDLINE and EMBASE), cross-referencing lipid-lowering papers, and by direct contact with principal investigators of trials in Europe, and pharmaceutical companies listed as manufacturing lipid-lowering drugs.

Eligible randomized controlled trials

Nine trials were identified which met the inclusion criteria, but two of these were excluded due to poor quality.[27,28] The included trials involved a total of just under 700 participants, and were conducted in seven different countries. The two largest trials were the Cholesterol Lowering Atherosclerosis Study (CLAS) which randomized 188 patients,[29,30] and the Probucol Quantitative Regression Swedish Trial (PQRST) on 303 subjects.[31,32] The remaining trials involved relatively small numbers of patients (Table 1).[29–37] One ongoing study was identified, the LEADER Trial (Lower Extremity Arterial Disease Event Reduction). This is a 4-year randomized placebo-controlled trial of bezafibrate in 1500 men with lower extremity arterial disease, scheduled to report at the turn of the century (Professor TW Meade, personal communication).

Quality

Concealment of allocation was clearly ensured in five of the trials, and in the other two cases 'random' was stated but no further information was available (Nye, St Thomas's).[36,37] All trials were double-blind except the St Thomas's trial which did not use a placebo, probably because of a complicated treatment regimen,[37] and the CLAS trial in which 93% knew to which study group they belonged despite the use of a placebo.[30] Losses to follow-up were common, particularly in the Davis trial of 49 patients where six were lost to follow-up and ten were withdrawn because of adverse effects.[34]

Participants

Four of the trials were in patients with intermittent claudication,[33–35,37] and the remainder were in patients with known peripheral arterial disease: in two of these, disease was defined angiographically (CLAS, PQRST);[29,31] and in a third no clear definition was given (Nye).[36] Trials were generally in middle-aged to elderly subjects and were not restricted by sex, except the CLAS trial which was men only.[30] Four trials did not use hyperlipidaemia as an inclusion criterion, with the exception of the St Thomas's trial[37] and two other trials which randomized only subjects with known response to lipid-lowering therapy (CLAS, PQRST).[29,31] Most trials excluded subjects with concomitant medical conditions.

Interventions

The interventions were varied: CLAS and the St Thomas's trial used combinations of drugs and diet to lower lipids;[29,37] the PQRST Study used both cholestyramine and diet in treatment and control groups, plus probucol in the treatment group only;[31]

Table 1. Characteristics of lipid-lowering trials in patients with peripheral arterial disease (PAD)

Trial	*No. patients randomized/ analysed*	*Description of patients*	*Intervention*	*Duration*	*Outcomes of interest*
CLAS 1991[29,30]	188/162	Men aged 40–59 years PAD on angiogram Hypercholesterolaemia	Colestipol, niacin and diet	2 years	Mortality, non-fatal events, angiographic change, side-effects.
Corsi *et al.* 1985[33]	30/30	Men and women, mean age 68 years Intermittent claudication	Sulodexide and diet	90 days	Walking distance, ABPI, symptoms, side-effects
Davis *et al.* 1975[34]	49/43	Men and women aged 25–78 years Intermittent claudication	Xanthinol nicotinate	2 months	Mortality, side-effects.
Gans *et al.* 1990[35]	37/32	Men and women aged 18–80 years Intermittent claudication	Fish oil	4 months	ABPI, walking distance, side-effects.
Nye *et al.* 1973[36]	68/68	Men and women aged 40–74 years PAD of aorta or lower limb	Betapyridyl carbinol	2 years	Mortality, walking distance, side-effects.
PQRST 1994[31,32]	303/274	Men and women aged <71 years PAD on angiogram Hypercholesterolaemia	Probucol, cholestyramine and diet	3 years	Mortality, non-fatal events, angiographic change, ABPI, walking distance, side-effects
St Thomas's 1983[37]	24/24	Men and women aged <66 years Intermittent claudication Hyperlipidaemia	Cholestyramine and nicotinic acid, or clofibrate, or nicotinic acid (depending on type of hyperlipidaemia)	19 months	Angiographic change

one trial used sulodexide, a glycosaminoglycan with lipid-lowering properties (Corsi);[33] another used polyunsaturated fatty acids derived from fish (Gans);[35] and two trials used drugs related to nicotinic acid (Davis, Nye).[34,37] Duration of treatment also varied: 4 months or less in three trials;[33–35] a mean of 19 months in the St Thomas's Trial;[37] and between 2 and 3 years in the largest trials (CLAS and PQRST).[30,31]

Outcomes

Mortality was reported by three trials (CLAS, PQRST and Nye),[30,31,36] and two of these also reported non-fatal events (CLAS and PQRST). Angiographic endpoints were reported in three trials (CLAS, PQRST and St Thomas's).[30,31,37] The ankle brachial pressure index (ABPI) was reported in several trials, but walking distance was the most commonly reported outcome,[31,33,35,36] determined using a variety of methods. Other outcomes were inconsistently reported.

Effect of lipid-lowering therapy on outcome

The inconsistent reporting of outcome measures in the nine trials restricted the degree of statistical pooling that could be performed. All eligible trials for each outcome were considered sufficiently similar to warrant meta-analysis, however, and statistical homogeneity was confirmed using the chi-squared test.

Cholesterol lowering

Only four trials reported significant falls in cholesterol levels in the treated groups compared with controls (Table 2). This was important, as change in outcome could be ascribed to lipid-lowering therapy only if cholesterol levels were significantly decreased. In the trials by Corsi and Gans, significant reductions in triglyceride levels occurred, but no change in cholesterol.[33,35] In the PQRST study, there was a 24% reduction in HDL cholesterol in those taking probucol.[31]

Table 2. Change in cholesterol levels in trials of patients with lower limb disease

Trial	*Treatment*	*Control*	*Between group difference (p<0.05)*
CLAS 1991[30]	27%↓	4%↓	Yes
Corsi *et al.* 1985[33 a]	5%↓	2%↓	No
Davis *et al.* 1975[34]	Not reported	Not reported	Not reported
Gans *et al.* 1990[35]	3%↑	3%↓	No
Nye *et al.* 1973[36 a]	15%↓	10%↑	Yes
PQRST 1994[31 a]	33%↓	21%↓	Yes
St Thomas's 1982[37]	25%↓	3%↓	Yes

[a] Change estimated from graphical data

Mortality

The three trials which examined mortality (CLAS, PQRST and Nye) all achieved a significant fall in total cholesterol in the treated groups, and were of at least 2 years' duration (chi-squared test for homogeneity 0.51, $p>0.05$).[30,31,36] Treatment produced a small non-significant reduction in mortality in each individual trial, and a small overall reduction in mortality which was also not statistically significant (Mantel-Haenszel odds ratio (OR) 0.21, 95% CI 0.03–1.17). In total, 0.7% of the treated subjects died compared with 2.9% of the controls, a 75% reduction in mortality. This estimate is based on very small numbers, however, and must therefore be treated with caution. In the large coronary prevention trials, treatment with statins is reported to reduce the risk of death from coronary heart disease by about 25%.[18]

Non-fatal cardiovascular events

The two trials reporting non-fatal cardiovascular events (CLAS and PQRST, chi-squared test for homogeneity 0.29, $p>0.05$), both demonstrated slightly more events in the treated than the control subjects.[30,31] The overall difference was not statistically significant (Peto OR 1.21, 95% CI 0.80–1.83, Fig. 2). In total, 26% of the treated subjects had events compared with 22% of the controls.

Angiographic change

Two of the three trials reporting angiographic change (CLAS and St Thomas's) categorized their findings into overall measures of disease progression, no change or regression.[30,37] Both trials used a combination of lipid-lowering agents that significantly reduced cholesterol levels, but the CLAS trial was much larger (188 subjects compared with 24, chi-squared test for homogeneity 0.71, $p>0.05$). Disease progression was reduced in both treated groups, but was statistically significant in only the St Thomas's Trial.[37] Overall, there was a statistically significant reduction in atheroma in those undergoing treatment (Peto OR 0.47, 95% CI 0.29–0.76, Fig. 3). In total, 14% of the treated subjects progressed compared with 25% of the controls.

Study	Expt (n)	Ctrl (n)	Peto odds ratio (95%CI)	Weight (%)
CLAS 1991[30]	94	94		40.3
PQRST[31]	152	151		59.7
Total (95%CI)	246	245		100.0

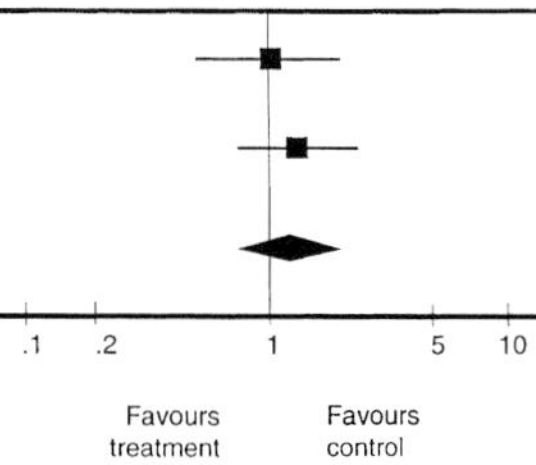

Chi-square 0.29 (df=1) Z=0.92

Fig. 2. Effect of lipid-lowering therapy on non-fatal cardiovascular events in patients with peripheral atherosclerosis (fixed effects model).

Study	Expt (n)	Ctrl (n)	Peto odds ratio (95%CI)	Weight (%)
CLAS 1991[30]	77	76		51.3
St Thomas's[37]	144	156		48.7
Total (95%CI)	221	232		100.0

Chi-square 0.70 (df=1) Z=3.04

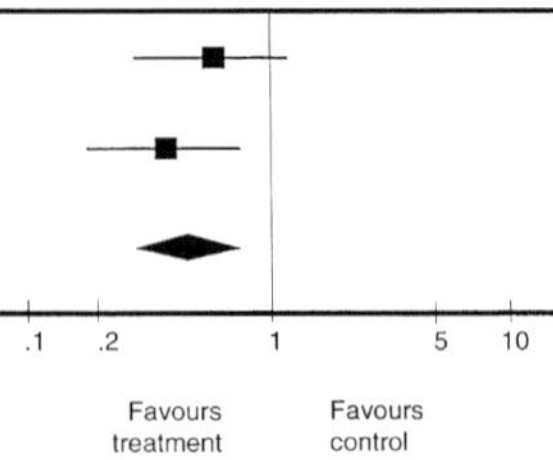

Fig. 3. Effect of lipid-lowering therapy on peripheral atherosclerosis demonstrated on angiogram (fixed effects model).

In the third angiographic trial (PQRST), data could not be obtained in a format suitable for inclusion in the meta-analysis.[31] Change in lumen volume of the femoral artery was the primary end point in this trial, and a 4.2% increase in volume occurred in the control group ($p<0.001$), with an increase of only 0.6% in the treatment group ($p=0.61$). The trial concluded that addition of probucol to diet and cholestyramine did not result in any significant regression of atherosclerosis compared with that found in patients treated with only diet and cholestyramine, and that there was significant evidence of improvement in the control group. This lack of improvement in the probucol group is likely to have been related to the reduction in HDL cholesterol in this arm of the trial.

Ankle brachial pressure index

Information on the ABPI, sufficient to include in a meta-analysis, was recorded in two trials (Corsi and Gans, chi-squared test for homogeneity 2.76).[33,35] Neither of these trials produced a significant drop in cholesterol levels, however, and both were of short duration. In the Corsi trial there was a 28.3% increase in ABPI in the treatment group, significantly greater than in the controls. There was no significant increase in the Gans trial, and there was no significant difference overall (weighted mean difference (WMD) 0.02, 95% CI –0.03 to 0.09, Fig. 4). The ABPI was also measured in the PQRST study, which demonstrated no significant change in either the treatment or control groups.[31]

Walking distance

Information on pain-free walking distance was available from the same trials as those recording the ABPI (Corsi and Gans).[33,35] The Corsi trial showed a significant improvement in walking distance in the treated group compared with controls ($p<0.01$ quoted in original paper), whereas Gans demonstrated no significant difference, and there was no overall improvement (WMD –13.4, 95% CI –55.74 to 28.93, Fig. 5). In two additional trials where data were not suitable for inclusion in a

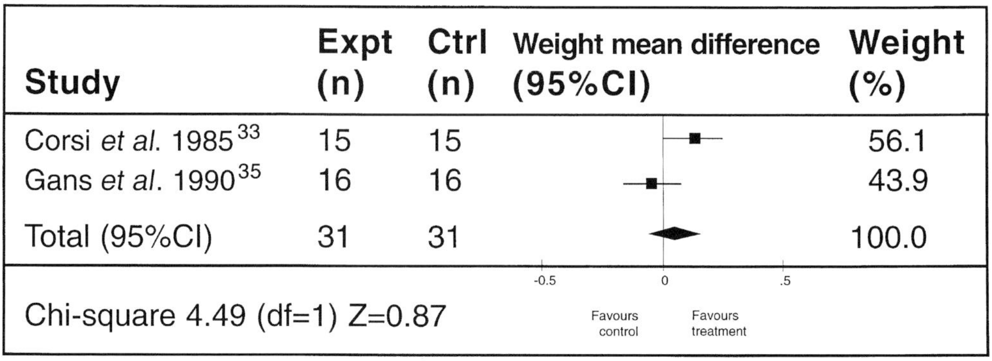

Fig. 4. Effect of lipid-lowering therapy on the ankle brachial pressure index (fixed effects model).

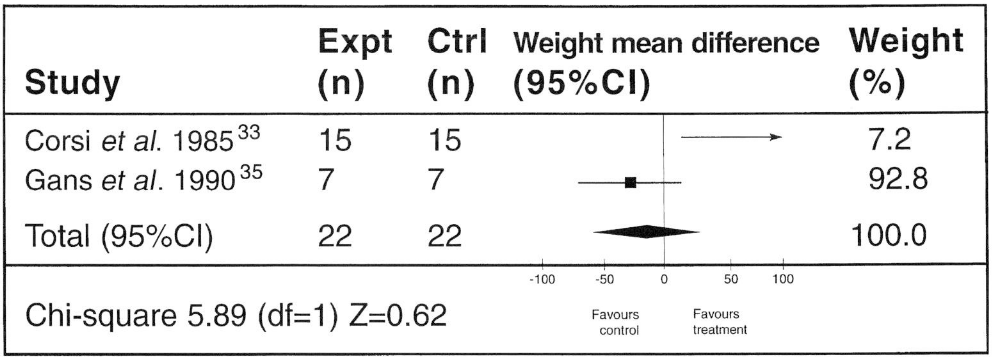

Fig. 5. Effect of lipid-lowering on pain-free walking distance (fixed effects model).

statistical meta-analysis (PQRST, Nye), no significant differences in walking distance were demonstrated at the end of the intervention period.[31,36]

Symptomatic change

The recording of symptoms of intermittent claudication was too variable for the results to be included in a meta-analysis. In three trials, however, treated subjects reported fewer symptoms of claudication: no treated subjects were worse at the end of the Corsi trial compared with 20% of controls;[33] 24% of treated subjects experienced no worthwhile effect compared with 88% of controls ($p<0.001$) at the end of the trial by Davis;[34] and 8% of treated subjects reported worsening of claudication compared with 4% of controls ($p>0.05$) throughout the trial by Nye.[36]

Side-effects

Side-effects were generally mild, with the exception of liver toxicity produced in two men taking betapyridyl carbinol in the Nye study,[36] and the adverse effect on lipoprotein profile in the PQRST study in which the beneficial HDL cholesterol levels were reduced.[31]

CONCLUSIONS

Trials of lipid-lowering therapy in peripheral arterial disease are relatively uncommon, primarily because interest has centred around lipid-lowering in coronary heart disease. The limited trials included in this review varied in the type of drugs used, the degree of lipid-lowering achieved and the reporting of outcome measures. Several trials were small and of short duration, and none used the most potent lipid-lowering agents, the HMG-CoA reductase inhibitors. These factors may explain why there was no clear impact on fatal or non-fatal events, ankle pressures or walking distance. Care must therefore be exercised before generalizing any conclusions to different patient groups and treatment regimens. There were some encouraging effects of lipid-lowering, however, including a significant reduction in femoral atheroma on angiogram, plus some improvement in symptoms.

Implications for research and practice

It is important that future trials in peripheral arterial disease include outcomes specifically relevant to the lower limb, in particular clinically relevant measures such as progression to bypass surgery, angioplasty and amputation, plus tests of underlying disease progression. Follow-up periods of at least 2 years are likely to be required to demonstrate any significant benefits. Further trials are necessary both in patients with intermittent claudication, and in patients with early asymptomatic peripheral arterial disease to establish whether progression to symptomatic disease can be prevented.

Until this evidence is available, however, it would seem reasonable to extrapolate the conclusions from coronary trials that show significant falls in mortality in subjects at high risk. Patients with established intermittent claudication are at an increased risk of death from coronary heart disease, and should therefore be treated with statins, the most effective cholesterol lowering agents. There is currently no evidence that this will improve walking distance, however, and therefore additional strategies for managing disabling symptoms of intermittent claudication are likely to be required.

REFERENCES

1. Schrade W, Boehle E, Biefler R: Humoral changes in arteriosclerosis. Investigations on lipids, fatty acids, ketone bodies, pyruvic acid, lactic acid and glucose in the blood. *Lancet* **ii**: 1409–1416, 1960
2. Greenhalgh RM, Rosengarten DS, Mervart I *et al.*: Serum lipids and lipoproteins in peripehral vascular disease. *Lancet* **ii**: 947–950, 1971
3. Sirtori CR, Biasi G, Vercellio G *et al.*: Diet lipids and lipoproteins in patients with peripheral vascular disease. *Am J Med Sci* **268**: 325–332, 1974

4. Vyden JK, Thorner JK, Nagasawa K *et al.*: Metabolic and cardiovascular abnormalities in patients with peripheral arterial disease. *Am Heart J* **90**: 703–708, 1975
5. Skrede S, Kvarstein B: Hyperlipidaemia in peripheral atherosclerotic arterial disease. *Acta Clin Scand* **141**: 333–341, 1975
6. Angquist KA, Johnson O, Ericsson M, Tollin C: Serum lipoproteins and apolipoproteins A1 and A11 in male patients with arterial insufficiency. *Acta Chir Scand* **148**: 675–678, 1982
7. Jacobsen UK, Dige-Pederseen H, Gyntelberg F, Svendsen UG: 'Risk factors' and manifestations of arteriosclerosis in patients with intermittent claudication compared with normal persons. *Dan Med Bull* **31**: 145–148, 1984
8. Ruhling K, Zabel-Langhenning R, Till U, Thielmenn K: Enhanced net mass transfer of HDL cholesteryl esters to Apo B-containing lipoproteins in patients with peripheral vascular disease. *Clin Chim Acta* **184**: 289–296, 1989
9. Cardia G, Grisorio D, Impedovo G *et al.*: Plasma lipids as a risk factor in peripheral vascular disease. *Angiology* **41**: 19–22, 1990
10. Schroll M, Munck O: Estimation of peripheral arteriosclerotic disease by ankle blood pressure measurements in a population study of 60 year-old men and women. *J Chron Dis* **34**: 261–269, 1981
11. Gofin R, Karic JD, Friedlander Y *et al.*: Peripheral vascular disease in a middle-aged population sample. The Jerusalem Lipid Research Clinic Prevalence Study. *Int J Med Sci* **23**: 157–167, 1987
12. Fowkes FGR, Housley E, Cawood EH *et al.*: Edinburgh Artery Study: prevalence of asymptomatic and symptomatic peripheral vascular disease in the general population. *Int J Epidemiol* **20**: 384–392, 1991
13. Reunanen A, Takkunen H, Aromaa A: Prevalence of intermittent claudication and its effect on mortality. *Acta Med Scand* **211**: 249–256, 1982
14. Davey Smith G, Shipley MJ, Rose G: Intermittent claudication, heart disease risk factors, and mortality. The Whitehall Study. *Circulation* **82**: 1925–1931, 1990
15. Kannel WB, McGhee DL: Update on some epidemiological features of intermittent claudication: the Framingham Study. *J Am Ger Soc* **33**: 13–18, 1985
16. Fowkes FGR: Epidemiology of atherosclerotic disease in the lower limbs. *Eur J Vasc Surg* **2**: 283–291, 1988
17. Leng GC, Lee AJ, Fowkes FGR *et al.*: The relationship between cigarette smoking and cardiovascular risk factors in peripheral arterial disease compared with ischaemic heart disease. The Edinburgh Artery Study. *Eur Heart J* **16**: 1542–1548, 1995
18. NHS Centre for Reviews and Dissemination: Cholesterol and coronary heart disease: screening and treatment. *Effective Health Care* **4**: 1–15, 1998
19. Clarke R, Frost C, Collins R *et al.*: Dietary lipids and blood cholesterol: quantitative meta-analysis of metabolic ward studies. *Br Med J* **314**: 112–117, 1997
20. Neil HAW, Roe L, Godlee RJ *et al.*: Randomised controlled trial of lipid-lowering advice in general practice: the effects on serum lipids, lipoproteins and antioxidants. *Br Med J* **310**: 569–573, 1995
21. Ebrahim S, Davey Smith G: Systematic review of randomised controlled trials of multiple risk factor interventions for preventing coronary heart disease. *Br Med J* **314**: 1666–1674, 1997
22. Durrington PN: Dietary fat and coronary heart disease. In: Poulter N, Sever P, Thom S (Eds) *Cardiovascular Disease. Risk Factors and Interventions* pp. 119–128. Oxford: Radcliffe Medical Press, 1993
23. Rispin C, Keenan J, Jacobs D et al: Oat products and lipid-lowering. A meta-analysis. *J Am Med Assoc* **267**: 3317–3325, 1992
24. Olson BH, Anderson SM, Becker MP *et al.*: Psyllium-enriched cereals lower blood cholesterol and LDL cholesterol, but not HDL cholesterol, in hypercholesterolaemic adults: results of a meta-analysis. *J Nutrit* **127**: 1973–1980, 1997
25. Anderson J, Johnstone B, Cook-Newell M: Meta-analysis of the effects of soy protein intake on serum lipids. *New Engl J Med* **333**: 276–282, 1995
26. Stone BG, Evans CD, Prigge WF *et al.*: Lovastatin treatment inhibits sterol synthesis and

induces HMG-CoA reductase activity in mononuclear leukocytes of normal subjects. *J Lipid Res* **30**: 1943–52, 1989
27. Hutchinson K, Oberle K, Crockford P *et al.*: Effects of dietary manipulation on vascular status of patients with peripheral vascular disease. *J Am Med Assoc* **249**: 3326–3330, 1983
28. Schumer W, Battung VR, Foa PP: A clinical evaluation of diethanolamine salt of p-tolylmethylcarbinol camporic acid (gallogen) in arteriosclerosis obliterans. *Angiology* **14**: 381–382, 1963
29. Blankenhorn DH, Johnson RL, Nessim SA *et al.*: The Cholesterol Lowering Atherosclerosis Study (CLAS): design, methods and baseline results. *Controlled Clin Trials* **8**: 356–387, 1987
30. Blankenhorn DH, Azen SP, Crawford DW *et al.*: Effects of colestipol-niacin therapy on human femoral atherosclerosis. *Circulation* **83**: 438–447, 1991
31. Walldius G, Erikson U, Olsson AG *et al.*: The effect of probucol on femoral atherosclerosis: the Probucol Quantitative Regression Swedish Trial (PQRST). *Am J Cardiol* **74**: 875–883, 1994
32. Erikson U, Nilsson S, Stenport G: Probucol Quantitative Regression Swedish Trial: new angiographic technique to measure atheroma volume of the femoral artery. *Am J Cardiol* **62**: 44B–47B, 1988
33. Corsi C, Bocci L, Cipriani C *et al.*: The effectiveness of glycosaminoglycans in peripheral vascular disease therapy: a clinical and experimental trial. *J Int Med Res* **13**: 40–47, 1985
34. Davis E, Rozov H: Xanthinol nicotinate in peripheral vascular disease. *Practitioner* **215**: 793–798, 1975
35. Gans ROB, Bilo HJG, Weersink EGL *et al.*: Fish oil supplementation in patients with stable claudication. *Am J Surg* **160**: 490–495, 1990
36. Nye ER, Macbeth WAAG: The treatment of intermittent claudication with beta-pyridy carbinol over two years. *Atherosclerosis* **17**: 95–106, 1973
37. Duffield RG, Lewis B, Miller NE *et al.*: Treatment of hyperlipidaemia retards progression of symptomatic femoral atherosclerosis. *Lancet* **ii**: 639–642, 1983

Commentary

Much less attention is focussed on peripheral arterial disease than is focussed on coronary artery disease. In addition, the outcome measure of greatest concern to the patient with intermittent claudication, walking distance, is very difficult to measure objectively and reliably. Taken together, these two factors might explain the paucity of reliable evidence concerning the role of lipid lowering therapy in peripheral arterial disease. Many of the best studies cited in the chapter, predate the introduction of statins to lower plasma cholesterol efficiently. Nevertheless, since so many patients with peripheral arterial disease die from ischaemic heart disease, the use of statins is likely to prolong the life of many of these patients. Many of the recent statin trials indicate that this benefit of prolonging life can be seen 'across the board' and not just in those with high plasma cholesteral concentration. However, as the author comments, smoking is more dominant than hypercholesterolaemia as a risk factor for peripheral arterial disease. Diabetes and hypertriglyceridaemia also are important risk factors for peripheral atherosclerosis. Smoking and the eating habits of smokers may combine to increase plasma concentrations of insulin, triglycerides and fibrinogen. For these reasons fibrates may prove more effective than statins in patients with peripheral arterial disease. The results of the LEADER trial are awaited eagerly. *JTP*

THE DURABILITY OF VENOUS PROCEDURES

Does colour duplex scanning improve the durability of varicose vein surgery?

JJ Smith, AH Davies and RM Greenhalgh

INTRODUCTION

In 1971 Lofgren stated that 'Recurrence of varicose veins continues to be a problem of great magnitude to the patient and physician alike.' [1] It was also stated that the recurrence rate of the time (20–26%) had not changed much over the preceding 10 years despite surgical advances. Varicose veins are one of the most common of all surgical problems with a prevalence of 25% in women and 15% in men.[2] Around 56 000 operations were performed for varicose veins in the United Kingdom alone in 1997, approximately 20% of them for 'recurrence'.[3,4] Patient expectation of outcome is high and 'recurrence' of varicose veins can be considered to be grounds of negligence.[5]

Satisfactory surgical varicose vein results depend upon a number of factors including correct preoperative assessment. We question here if colour duplex is of any adjuvant benefit beyond clinical assessment (and hand-held Doppler if desired) for superficial varicose veins for first-time surgery.

WHY ARE THE RESULTS OF SURGERY SO POOR?

So called 'recurrence' of varicose veins can be veins left behind in the original operative procedure (Fig. 1a).[1,4–7] Reconstitution of the saphenofemoral/popliteal junctions or even the proximal long saphenous vein can lead to clinical reappearance of veins The phenomenon of 'neovascularization' is said to account for a proportion of 'recurrent' varicose veins (Fig. 1b).[8,9] Inadequate or incorrect preoperative evaluation of patients can lead to the wrong operation being performed. A study evaluating colour coded duplex scanning in the preoperative assessment of varicose veins showed that 26% of the planned surgical procedures were changed when colour duplex was added to clinical and hand-held Doppler assessment.[10] Table 1 shows a series of reported 'recurrence rates' ranging from 4 to 36% over a period of 18 months to 10 years. Some authors have reported even higher 'recurrence rates' of up to 77%.[11,12] Around 20% of all varicose vein operations performed are for second-time surgery, [13] which is consistent with the mean 'recurrence rate' in Table 1 of 20.8%. One in five operations on varicose veins results in apparent 'recurrence'.[14,15] In a study examining 267 legs in patients with recurrent varicose vein disease, 45% had an intact saphenofemoral junction and long saphenous vein.[16] A further study of 779 limbs gave very similar figures in

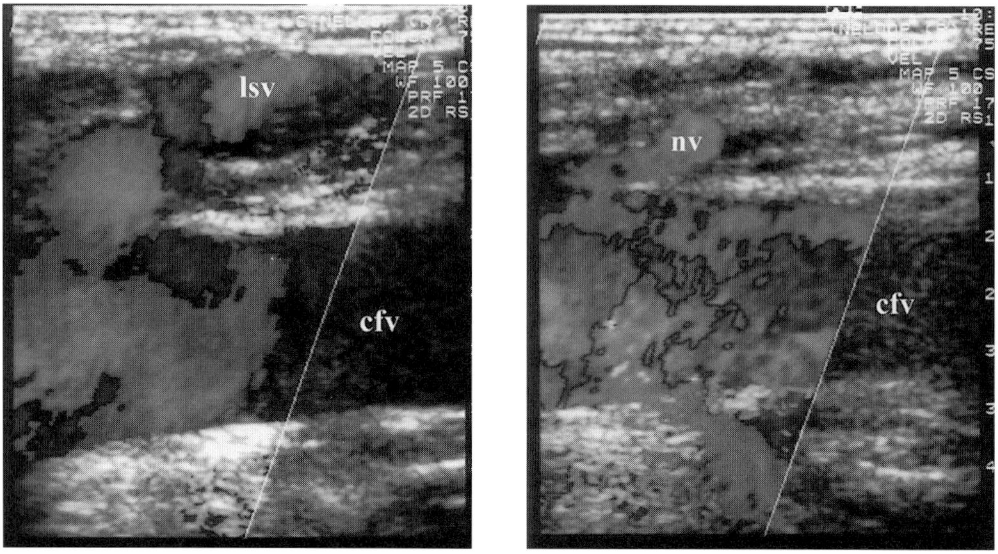

(a) (b)

Fig. 1. Colour duplex demonstration of recurrence at the saphenofemoral junction (a) inadequate surgery; (b) neovascularization. lsv: long saphenous vein; cfv: common femoral vein; nv: neovascularization.

that 46.3% of the recurrent varicose veins were due to a single large connection in the groin.[17] 'Neovascularization' is also cited as the principal cause of 'recurrence' of varicose veins.[8,9] It is claimed that if the cribriform fascia is obliterated by some method, 'recurrence' still occurs in some patients.[18]

Table 1. Reported recurrence rates for varicose vein surgery

Author	*Year*	*Recurrence rate (%)*	*Time period*
McElwee[29]	(1947)	19	18 months
Mathiesen[30]	(1953)	24	4 years
Lofgren[1]	(1971)	24	10 years
Larson[31]	(1974)	13–15	10 years
Jakobsen[32]	(1979)	10.2	3 years
Munn[33]	(1981)	36	3 years
Negus[34]	(1986)	13	4 years
Koyano[35]	(1988)	10.6	3 years
Hammartsen[36]	(1990)	12	5 years
Sarin[14]	(1994)	34	2 years
Laurikka[37]	(1994)	28	10 years
Jones[38]	(1996)	25	2 years

HOW RELIABLE IS COLOUR DUPLEX?

Colour duplex scanning can produce excellent images showing the anatomical distribution of veins and giving some idea of their function.[19–22] Some consider it to be the investigation of choice.[23] Should we accept this view without question?

The sensitivity and specificity of colour duplex in diagnosing reflux in various venous segments was demonstrated in a study by Phillips *et al.*[24] (Table 2) Colour duplex was found to be as accurate as venography in diagnosing saphenofemoral and saphenopopliteal junction reflux (kappa = 0.74 and 0.90 respectively) but not as accurate for deep venous and perforator vein reflux (kappa = 0.42 and 0.21 respectively). It is now widely believed that colour duplex can replace venography as the 'gold standard' in the assessment of varicose veins.[25,26]

Many vascular surgeons consider that patients with saphenopopliteal junction incompetence (Fig. 2) and those with 'recurrent' varicose veins should have a duplex scan performed before the operation, but many argue that primary varicose veins only need clinical and/or continuous wave Doppler,[22,23] but the evidence is lacking to support this viewpoint. Table 3 demonstrates a series of studies comparing hand-held Doppler with colour duplex.

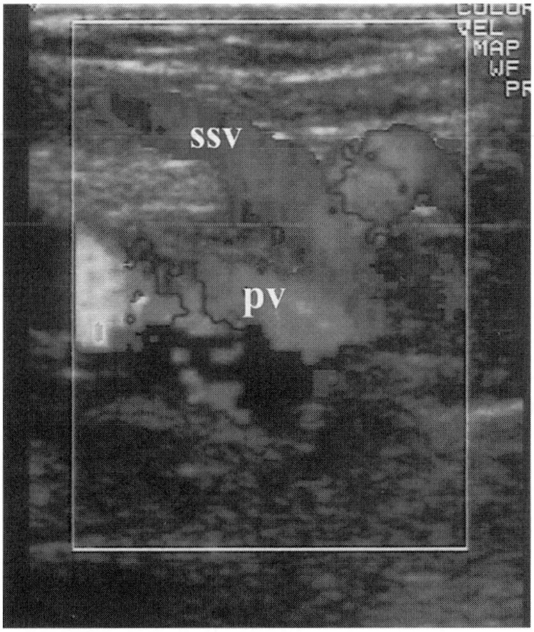

Fig. 2. Duplex demonstrated anatomy of the saphenopopliteal junction. ssv: short saphenous vein; pv: popliteal vein.

Table 2. The ability of colour duplex to diagnose venous reflux

Site	*Sensitivity (%)*	*Specificity (%)*
Saphenofemoral junction incompetence	90.7	83.3
Saphenopopliteal junction incompetence	95.0	96.9
Deep venous incompetence	33.1	98.7
Mid-thigh perforator incompetence	58.8	97.0
Calf perforator incompetence	52.2	17.6

The ability of colour duplex to show the anatomical distribution of veins non-invasively has led some authors to suggest that varicose vein surgery should be tailored to the individual patient's requirements.[27] Whether this improves the results of surgery has not been tested in a randomized controlled trial.

Colour duplex has been shown to be as accurate as venography (accuracy 96%) for marking before operation the positions of the superficial to deep venous connections in the lower leg.[28] The required randomized controlled trial to test duplex scanning is therefore between duplex scan and clinical assessment against hand-held Doppler and clinical assessment (with hand-held Doppler if desired) against clinical assessment and hand-held Doppler alone for non-recurrent varicose veins. Ethical committee approval was obtained for such a trial, which is described below. The groups are referred to as the 'duplex' and 'non-suplex' arms of the study. The purpose of the trial was to check patients of both arms of the trial with colour duplex at 6 weeks and 12 months and to see if colour duplex marking led to a lower 'recurrence' rate of varicose veins.

METHODS AND PATIENT SERIES

A consecutive cohort of patients with superficial varicose veins without venous ulceration was randomized into one of the two groups. In group one the patients underwent clinical assessment with optional hand-held Doppler and in addition the sites of deep to superficial incompetence were marked preoperatively with colour duplex. In group two the only difference in assessment was that the patients did not have a colour duplex scan.

An experienced vascular technologist performed all of the colour duplex scans with the patient standing with the weight taken mainly on the opposite foot. Reflux for this purpose was defined as reverse flow for greater than one second following release of calf pressure. An Acuson 2000 scanner with a 7.5 MHz linear array probe was used for all venous scans. For those patients in the 'non-duplex' group an Imex continuous wave Doppler with an 8MHz probe was used at the discretion of the operating surgeon.

All patients underwent elective surgery under general anaesthetic, the operation being performed by a vascular consultant or a vascular surgical trainee in the Regional Vascular Service. Operative procedures on the long saphenous system comprised flush saphenofemoral transfixion with division of surrounding tributaries

Table 3. Comparison of hand-held Doppler with colour duplex to detect venous incompetence

	Sensitivity %	*Specificity* %
Saphenofemoral junction incompetence (primary varicose veins)[39,40]	70–80	80–85
Saphenofemoral junction incompetence (recurrent varicose veins) [41,42]	47–90	40–80
Saphenopopliteal junction incompetence (primary varicose veins)[39,40]	40–90	50–90

of the femoral vein and removal of the long saphenous vein to the knee. Operative procedures on the short saphenous system comprised flush saphenopopliteal division, transfixion and removal of at least 5cm of the short saphenous vein. The removal of varicosities was performed via tiny stab incisions and the use of the Oesch phlebectomy hooks or a curved mosquito forceps. In both groups these varicosities were marked by the operating surgeon with the patient standing immediately before surgery in both groups. Follow-up was scheduled at 6 weeks and 1 year after surgery when all patients were assessed clinically and by colour duplex scan. The saphenofemoral and short saphenopopliteal junctions were interrogated and any remaining saphenous vein incompetence was noted.

Results are analysed by numbers of limbs and procedures performed in order to compare any difference made by preoperative duplex marking. The median age of the patients was 48 years and 66% were women; 104 limbs were included in the study (55 right legs and 49 left legs) of 109 procedures of which 53 limbs were randomized to preoperative duplex marking and 51 limbs to non-duplex. As described above 92 long saphenous and 17 short saphenous procedures were performed. Statistical analysis was performed using chi-squared tests with continuity correction or Fishers Exact Test as appropriate.

RESULTS

Long saphenous system

Of the 92 long saphenous procedures, five were found to have saphenofemoral reflux at the 6-week duplex scan, but a further 12 had evidence of saphenofemoral reflux at the 12-month scan (18%). Of the five residual problems at 6 weeks, three of 48 were in the duplex group and two of 44 were in the non-duplex group ($p=1.0$). In 15 of 92 patients, the vascular technologists found a saphenous vein in the distal thigh at 6-weeks and the number increased to 22 of 92 at 12 months (24%) of which 12 were in the duplex arm and 10 in the non-duplex arm of the study ($p=0.812$). It is to be presumed that the saphenous veins were certainly left behind in the 15 patients and of the remaining seven, they were probably residual and became more easily detected at 12 months.

Short saphenous system

Of the 17 short saphenous procedures, five had evidence of continuing reflux into a short saphenous vein at 6 weeks and the number rose to eight at 12 months. Of the five at 6-weeks, two were in the duplex arm and three were in the non-duplex arm of the study (p=1.0). Of the eight at 12 months, five were in the duplex arm and three in the clinical arm (p=0.637).

DISCUSSION

The trial has not demonstrated any adjuvant benefit of colour duplex scan over clinical and hand-held Doppler in terms of satisfactory varicose vein surgery performance at 6 weeks or 12 months in these patients with primary varicose veins. The striking finding of the study has been the number of patients with saphenofemoral incompetence that developed between 6 weeks and 12 months. Is this neovascularization? It certainly would be convenient to imagine that new vessels somehow came along automatically and ruined the surgery! This would imply that the surgeon could do no better, but is this true? Can we achieve better results if we divide every single tributary of the femoral vein for 5 cm above and below the saphenofemoral junction? When we are sure that we have done that, should we suture cribriform fascia across the femoral vein to discourage the joining of blood vessels? Are there technical manoeuvres that can reduce this development of new connections between 6 weeks and 12 months? If the answer is no, then we can say that neovascularization is at fault. It could be dangerous to attribute recurrence to neovascularization without trying to achieve better surgical results.

As far as the saphenous vein in the distal thigh is concerned, we presume that greater effort must be made to remove the saphenous vein to the knee level. As far as the short saphenopopliteal is concerned, this study confirms that the anatomy is difficult. The deep fascia has to be opened and the short saphenous vein has to be followed to the popliteal vein and divided flush and also with the relevant medial and lateral popliteal venous tributaries. This has clearly not been done adequately in some of these patients. The question also arises how far the short saphenous vein should be followed down the calf. Presumably it must be removed to at least the point where the mid-calf perforating vein normally joins.

We cannot be complacent in our performance of varicose vein surgery. Regrettably, colour duplex scan is no substitute for meticulous surgical practice. It does not make the surgery more effective.

REFERENCES

1. Lofgren EP, Lofgren KA: Recurrence of varicose veins after the stripping operation. *Arch Surg* **102**: 111–114, 1971
2. Callam MJ: Epidemiology of varicose veins. *Br J Surg* **81**: 167–173, 1994
3. Robbins MA, Frankel MJ, Nanchahal K *et al.*: Varicose veins treatment: Health care needs assessment: *The Epidemiologically Based Needs Assessment Reviews* 1998

4. Lees T, Singh S, Beard J *et al.*: Prospective audit of surgery for varicose veins. *Br J Surg* **84**: 44–46, 1997
5. Tennant WG, Ruckley CV: Medicolegal action following treatment for varicose veins. *Br J Surg* **83**: 291–292, 1996
6. Negus D: Recurrent varicose veins: a national problem. *Br J Surg* 1993 **80**: 823–824, 1993
7. Rivlin S: Recurrent varicose veins. *Med J Aust* **1**: 1097–1102, 1966
8. Glass GM: Neovascularization in recurrence of varices of the great saphenous vein in the groin: phlebography. *Angiology* **39**: 577–582, 1988
9. Glass GM: Neovascularisation in recurrent sapheno-femoral incompetence of varicose veins:surgical anatomy and morphology. *Phlebology* **10**, 136–142, 1995
10. van der Heijden FH, Bruyninckx CM: Preoperative colour-coded duplex scanning in varicose veins of the lower extremity. *Eur J Surg* **159**: 329–333, 1993
11. Royle JP: Recurrent varicose veins. *World J Surg* **10**: 944–953, 1986
12. Rivlin S: The surgical cure of primary varicose veins. *Br J Surg* **62**: 913–917, 1975
13. Bradbury AW, Stonebridge PA, Ruckley CV, Beggs I: Recurrent varicose veins: correlation between pre-operative clinical and hand held Doppler examination and anatomical findings at surgery. *Br J Surg* **80**: 849–851, 1993
14. Sarin S, Scurr JH, Coleridge SP: Stripping of the long saphenous vein in the treatment of primary varicose veins. *Br J Surg* **81**: 1455–1458, 1994
15. McMullin GM, Coleridge, Smith PD, Scurr JH: Objective assessment of high ligation without stripping the long saphenous vein. *Br J Surg* **78**: 1139–1142, 1991
16. Englund R: Duplex scanning for recurrent varicose veins. *Aust N Z J Surg* **66**: 618–620, 1996
17. Myer KA, Zeng GH, Ziegenbein RW, Matthews PG: Duplex ultrasound scanning for chronic venous disease: Recurrent varicose veins in the thigh after surgery to the long saphenous vein. *Phlebology* **11**: 125–131, 1996
18. Glass GM: Prevention of recurrent saphenofemoral incompetence after surgery for varicose veins. *Br J Surg* **76**: 1210, 1989
19. Thibault PK, Lewis WA: Recurrent varicose veins. Part 1: Evaluation utilising duplex venous imaging. *J Dermatol Surg Oncol* **18**: 618–624, 1992
20. Katsamouris AN, Kardoulas DG, Gourtsoyiannis N. The nature of lower extremity venous insufficiency in patients with primary varicose veins. *Eur J Vasc Endovasc Surg* **8**: 464–471, 1994
21. Quigley FG, Raptis S, Cashman M, Faris IB: Duplex ultrasound mapping of sites of deep to superficial incompetence in primary varicose veins. *Aust N Z J Surg* **62**: 276–278, 1992
22. Smith JJ, Davies AH, Greenhalgh RM: Do we know if duplex should be used for varicose vein surgery? In: Greenhalgh RM (Ed) *Indications in Vascular and Edovascular Surgery* pp. 409–421. London: WB Saunders Co, 1997
23. Coleridge SP: Does duplex ultrasonography improve the results of varicose veins surgery? In: Greenhalgh RM, Fowkes FGR (Eds) *Trials and Tribulations of Vascular Surgery* pp. 395–404. London: WB Saunders Co, 1996
24. Phillips GW, Paige J, Molan MP: A comparison of colour duplex ultrasound with venography and varicography in the assessment of varicose veins. *Clin Radiol* **50**: 20–25, 1995
25. Campbell WB, Halim AS, Aertssen A *et al.*: The place of duplex scanning for varicose veins and common venous problems. *Ann Roy Coll Surg Engl* **78**: 490–493, 1996
26. Darke SG, Foy DM: Preoperative assessment for varicose veins. In: Greenhalgh RM (Ed) *Vascular Imaging for Surgeons*, pp. 401–414. London: WB Saunders Co, 1995
27. Hanrahan LM, Kechejian GJ, Cordts PR *et al.*: Patterns of venous insufficiency in patients with varicose veins. *Arch Surg* **126**: 687–690, 1991
28. Vasdekis SN, Clarke GH, Nicolaides AN: Evaluation of invasive and non-invasive methods in the assessment of short saphenous vein termination. *Br J Surg* **76**: 929–932, 1989
29. McElwee RS, Maisel B: A study of the results of surgical treatment of varicose veins. *Ann Surg* **126**: 350–357, 1947
30. Mathiesen FR: Late results following 239 operations for varicose veins. *Acta Chir Scand* **105**: 376–389, 1953
31. Larson RH, Lofgren EP, Myers TT, Lofgren KA: Long term results after vein surgery: Study of 1000 cases after 10 years. *Mayo Clin Proc* **49**: 114–117, 1974

32. Jakobsen BH: The value of different forms of treatment for varicose veins. *Br J Surg* **66**: 182–184, 1979
33. Munn SR, Morton JB, Macbeth WA, McLeish AR: To strip or not to strip the long saphenous vein? A varicose vein trial. *Br J Surg* **68**: 426–428, 1981
34. Negus, D: Should the incompetent varicose vein be stripped to the ankle? *Phlebology* **1**: 33–36, 1986
35. Koyano K, Sakaguchi S: Selective stripping operation based on Doppler ultrasonic findings for primary varicose veins of the lower extremities. *Surgery* **103**, 615–619, 1988
36. Hammartsen J, Pedersen P, Cederlund C, Campanelo M: Long saphenous vein saving surgery for varicose veins. A long term follow up. *Eur J Vasc Surg* **4**: 361–364, 1990
37. Laurikka J, Sisto T, Salenius P *et al.*: Long saphenous vein stripping in the treatment of varicose veins: Self and surgeon assessed results after 10 years. *Phlebology* **9**: 13–16, 1994
38. Jones L, Braithwaite BD, Selwyn D *et al.*: Neovascularisation is the principal cause of varicose vein recurrence: results of a randomised trial of stripping the long saphenous vein. *Eur J Vasc Endovasc Surg* **12**: 442–445, 1996
39. McMullin GM, Coleridge, Smith PD: An evaluation of Doppler ultrasound and photoplethysmography in the investigation of venous insufficiency. *Aust N Z J Surg* **62**, 270–275, 1992
40. Mercer KG, Scott DJ, Berridge DC, Weston MJ: Outpatient varicose vein assessment: Hand held Doppler or duplex scanning? (Abstracts of VSS). *Br J Surg* **83**, 563–564, 1996
41. Bradbury AW, Stonebridge PA, Callam MJ *et al.*: Recurrent varicose veins: assessment of the sapheno-femoral junction. *Br J Surg* **81**: 373–375, 1994
42. DePalma RG, Hart MT, Zanin L, Massarin EH: Physical examination, Doppler ultrasound and colour flow duplex scanning: Guides to therapy for primary varicose veins. *Phlebology* **8**: 7–11, 1993

Commentary

It is not easy to be sure what this study proves other than that the authors have found, as have others, that the careful audit of the results of varicose surgery proves disappointing to the surgeons. Particularly disconcerting is a short saphenous recurrence rate of around 50% at 12 months. No information is provided on late duplex findings in patients with varicose veins who did not have saphenofemoral or saphenopopliteal. As the study was designed it does not evaluate the accuracy of duplex scanning in detecting reflux or guiding surgery, but simply the adequacy of the surgery in achieving its aims.

Not enough information is provided on the scope and technique of the duplex scanning, nor upon the details of surgical techniques employed to enable us to attribute explanations to where they appropriately lie. If venous surgery is hastily performed, indifferently taught and standard texts perpetuate techniques which fail to take account of the real anatomy and its variations, then standards of surgery will be poorer than they need be. For example examination of the anatomy, especially when the common variations are present, tells us that if it is not standard practice to dissect and obliterate saphenofemoral tributaries out at least beyond their first divisions, the pathways connecting perineum, pelvis abdominal wall and gluteal region with the thigh will remain undisturbed to feed recurrences.

Residual saphenous vein was found in the lower thigh in 22 of 92 cases at 12 months. Was the saphenous vein along its length scanned for duplication preoperatively? What was the technique of stripping that was employed? Stripping, particularly inversion stripping is often associated with vein rupture, leaving segments behind – was this technique employed? Whatever technique was used, was the stripped vein checked for completeness?

One can only agree with the authors that it is too easy to attribute recurrence to 'neovascularization' when there are simpler, if less palatable, explanations. *CVR*

The effectiveness of subfascial endoscopic perforator surgery

G Stansby and P Lintott

INTRODUCTION

Subfascial endoscopic division of perforating veins was first reported by Hauer in 1985.[1] He described a new technique whereby a telescope was introduced into the medial subfascial space through a small incision in the upper calf and then passed down the leg dividing incompetent calf perforating veins under direct vision. Hauer's initial report of this technique, in the German language, was not widely disseminated until the first report in English by Fischer in 1989.[2] Since then widespread interest has developed in this new technique for carrying out what is essentially an old operation.

Ever since the pioneering work of Linton in the 1930s,[3] surgery to divide the medial calf perforating veins by open operations had been proposed as useful in some patients with chronic venous insufficiency and leg ulceration.[4–7] However, these operations have been used only very occasionally in recent years because of problems with wound healing (in up to 50% of cases in some series),[8,9] a need for prolonged inhospital stay and lack of any data showing benefit in the context of a randomized controlled trial with long-term follow-up. In addition most of the published series of open perforator surgery are now historical and relied on venography for assessment. Now that duplex scanning is able to non-invasively assess patients with chronic venous insufficiency more patients are being discovered who may potentially benefit from medial perforator interruption and the advent of subfascial endoscopic perforator surgery (SEPS) has rekindled interest and research in this field.

THE ROLE OF THE CALF PERFORATING VEINS

The exact pathophysiology of chronic venous skin changes remains poorly understood but it is widely agreed that the pathological changes are secondary to sustained venous hypertension in the microcirculation. The venous hypertension is in its turn due to the presence of deep or superficial reflux or a mixture of both of these. Large studies based on duplex ultrasonography have investigated the relative contributions of these two components. They reveal that the overwhelming majority of patients presenting to hospital for treatment have either isolated deep or a mixture of deep and superficial venous disease.[10,11] In particular, reflux within the popliteal and crural veins is associated with especially high incidences of chronic venous ulceration[12] and likewise failure to respond to medical intervention.[13] This suggests that the key factor in generating high microcirculatory venous pressures is likely to be incompetence in major veins such as the popliteal vein.

However, one of the features of venous ulceration or its precursor skin changes is that they occur on the medial side of the leg above the medial malleolus in the majority of cases. Ulceration or changes down on the foot or laterally are much rarer. This feature alone suggests that there must be some local factor in addition to global changes in the venous system and for some time it has been recognized that this may well be due to the presence of incompetent perforating veins on the medial aspect of the calf transmitting the increased pressure to the medial gaiter area. This has provided the rationale for medial perforator interruption.

PATIENT SELECTION FOR SUBFASCIAL ENDOSCOPIC PERFORATOR SURGERY

There is considerable disagreement about which patients may be suitable for SEPS, mainly because of a lack of any trials involving randomization, long-term follow-up or stratification for the degree of venous insufficiency. Many of the series reported to date either include patients with simple varicose veins or inadequately describe the severity of disease present. Currently the most appropriate group to consider for a SEPS procedure would appear to be those with class 4,5 or 6 venous insufficiency on clinical examination as described by the CEAP[9] classification (i.e. lipodermatosclerosis, healed ulceration or ulceration.). Hopefully the CEAP classification will be used to standardize reporting in any future trials on SEPS. The role of SEPS in primary varicose veins is much more difficult to justify, even from a theoretical prespective. A large prospective audit on the outcome of incompetent calf perforators following superficial varicose vein procedures involving the long or short saphenous system revealed that the majority, 182 of 226 (80%) in 185 limbs, became competent or were not visible at a follow-up duplex examination.[14] Either they must have been disrupted by surgery, or possibly a reduction of venous hypertension due to ligation of other sites of superficial incompetence had allowed the dilated incompetent perforating veins to narrow and regain competence. This last mechanism was speculated on by the authors, but would be less likely to occur in the presence of deep venous hypertension, perhaps making physical disruption of calf perforators of greater importance in such patients.

Currently it would only seem reasonable to perform a SEPS procedure, or SEPS trials, on CEAP class 4–6 patients who have had the presence of incompetent medial calf perforators demonstrated on duplex scanning, especially if they have failed with conservative treatment or have already had other sites of superficial incompetence ligated. The presence of deep venous incompetence (and again this is best demonstrated by duplex ultrasound) is not a contraindication and may represent the group that will derive the greatest benefit. Certainly it would not seem sensible to exclude such patients from future trials. Deep venous obstruction, however, should be regarded as an absolute contraindication as the perforating veins will be providing a necessary alternate venous drainage route.

EFFECTIVENESS OF SUBFASCIAL ENDOSCOPIC PERFORATOR SURGERY

Many thousands of these procedures have now been described, mostly in the German literature. After Hauer's original report in 1985[1] Fischer[2] in 1989 presented data on a series of 463 legs treated with this procedure with excellent technical results. However any new procedure must prove itself to be both (i) safe and (ii) technically effective as well as providing (iii) a clinical benefit. We will consider the effectiveness of SEPS in these three separate areas.

Is it safe?

As previously stated, open perforator surgery has been associated with an alarmingly high wound-complication rate.[15] A number of studies have therefore focused on the practicality and safety of this newer procedure. The main complications of SEPS appear to be haematomas, wound infections and neuropraxias (usually sensory but occasionally motor).[16] In Fischer's series it was impossible to pass the endoscope in one case; 11 patients developed subfascial haematomas and only one developed a neurological lesion. In 1992 Jugenheimer and Junginger published data on a series of 103 legs in 72 patients undergoing the SEPS procedure.[16] Mean duration of the procedure was 27 minutes (range 20–36). There were no intraoperative complications. The mean number of perforators divided was four (range 2–11). In three patients there was delayed healing at the insertion incision. Sensory loss in the distribution of the sural nerve was found in two patients (1.9%), saphenous nerve distribution in ten patients (9.7%) and significant haematomas in six patients (5.8%). In the invited commentary on this paper the opinion of the commentator is that these complications are likely to be less than for other methods of dealing with the perforating veins. In 1997 the North American SEPS study (NASEPS) published its preliminary data.[17] This was a voluntary register set up to evaluate the feasability and safety of the procedure. They had data on 155 SEPS operations carried out on 148 patients. There were no early deaths or problems with deep venous thrombosis. Wound infection occurred in 5% of the patients, most of whom had an open ulcer at the time of surgery. Stuart *et al.*[18] compared 30 patients who had undergone a SEPS procedure with 37 retrospective controls who had the traditional open Linton's procedure. The two groups were well matched for age and indication for surgery. The open group had a significantly longer stay in hospital and a greater wound infection rate (9/37) compared with none (0/30) in the SEPS group. Pierik *et al.*[19] published results from a prospective randomized trial comparing open with endoscopic perforator surgery for grade 6 disease (CEAP classification). The trial was stopped by the monitoring committee after 39 patients had been entered because of the much greater incidence of wound complications in the open group (10/19 cf 0/20 $p<0.001$). These data would suggest that overall the complications rate for SEPS is certainly much less than that in open surgery and also acceptably low. It would seem that as far as its ability to divide the medial perforator safely, SEPS is an effective procedure.

Is it technically effective?

The number and position of calf perforators has been described by several prominent historical figures including Von Loder (1803), Linton (1938)[19] and Cockett (1955).[20] More recently their anatomy has been revisited and well described by Mozes *et al.*[21] However, despite the tendency of various reports to describe them in fixed anatomical points their number and position vary widely between different individuals. As far as SEPS is concerned this makes preoperative assessment, preferably with duplex ultrasonography, essential. A further anatomical point that has emerged since the advent of SEPS is that many of the perforators are 'paratibial' and thus require the division of the deep fascia to expose them during the SEPS procedure as they cannot be otherwise reached from the medial subfascial approach. This manoeuvre places the posterior tibial vessels at a greater risk, as these relationships are not the same at all levels of the calf. Notably the posterior tibial neurovascular bundle is at greater risk as one approaches the ankle.

Obviously to be effective in eradicating perforator reflux a SEPS procedure must be capable of accessing all the relevant perforators. Essentially this means all the medial calf perforators with reflux greater than an arbitary value (usually 0.5 seconds) as identified on duplex assessment. The mean number of perforators identified in the NASEPS registry[17] was 3.8 but included a wide range from one to ten. There have been a number of studies that have further investigated their technical success rate by using postoperative duplex assessments. Iafrati *et al.*[22] reported on 18 limbs in 15 patients where an average of 4.3 veins was identified. Follow-up revealed four patients (22%) with residual perforators. Pierik *et al.*[23] reported the successfully ligation of all perforators in 17 of 20 patients (85%) and advocated the routine division of the intermuscular septum to ensure a complete exploration. As well as paratibial perforators, perforators near the medial malleolus may be difficult reach and can be missed at operation. There is said to be a learning curve for this procedure with more perforators being successfully identified and clipped the more procedures the surgeon performs.[23] A review of practice amongst UK surgeons showed that only nine of 26 who responded had performed in excess of five procedures, with only four having performed more than ten.[24] Now experience is likely to be increasing and formal training courses are also available. Obviously in some respects SEPS development may still be in the steep part of the learning curve with regards to its technical effectiveness and as such results in studies published to date may not yet be optimal. However, when combined with duplex marking and with a paratibial fasciotomy when necessary it seems capable of obliterating at least the majority of medial calf perforating veins.

Does it provide a clinical benefit?

This is obviously the key question with regard to the SEPS operation. The clinical outcome following venous surgery is not always easy to quantify especially with less severe disease. The initial healing of previous persistent open ulceration (grade 6) is perhaps the most easily assessed and most appropriate measure of effectiveness. Still, however, factors such as size, location and chronicity of the ulcer as well as the time to healing (and not just overall healing) need to be considered when comparing studies. 'Best medical treatment' for chronic venous ulceration is centred on graduated multilayer compression bandaging. Well-trained and motivated medical and nursing staffs have reported healing rates of up to 75% at 12 weeks for small venous ulcers. Community healing rates are lower, though can still be impressive at 50–60% at 6 weeks.[25] It is against these results that surgery must be compared. A further and perhaps more important marker of the efficacy of an intervention is the ulcer recurrence rate. The Lothian and Forth valley study reported on 600 patients with chronic venous ulceration; 67% had ulcers heal and recur with 35% having more than three episodes of recurrence.[26]

Unfortunately, reports rarely document all these data. Follow-up information is particularly scarce, but bearing this in mind there are a number of centres that have published results of their SEPS case series. The first of the large series to emerge from outside Germany came from Pierik *et al.*[27] in 1995. They looked at 40 legs in 38 patients with recurrent or protracted venous ulcers in whom they identified calf perforator veins using duplex scanning. They used a mediastinoscope with no tourniquet on the leg to identify and divide the veins. The results were impressive and included sufficient long-term figures with only one patient developing a recurrent leg ulcer at 3.9 years median follow-up. Of 40 patients, 31 had associated deep venous incompetence. Bergan *et al.*[28] described 31 limbs that underwent a SEPS procedure in 1996. Of these, 13 limbs had a history of chronic (>6 months duration), recurrent ulceration and of these ulcers 11/13 (86%) healed within 8 weeks. Unfortunately no long-term follow-up is yet available. Sparks *et al.*[29] published results of 19 limbs treated with SEPS as day-cases. In his series, 75% (13/19) of limbs had CEAP class 6 changes and the remainder classes 4 and 5. All active ulcers had healed at 90 days, and none had recurred at a mean follow up of 8½ months. Finally NASEPS[16] published healing rates for 85 of the 106 patients included with open ulceration at time of surgery for whom data was available. There was again a high success rate with 88% (75 patients) reportedly healed at follow-up with the probability for healing at 90 days being 67% (95% confidence interval 55–76%). There were, however, also four new or recurrent ulcers in the 120 total patients followed-up.

The data available to date suggest that SEPS is effective in healing active ulceration; however, what is not always clear from these studies is whether the benefit is distinct from that given by other venous reflux surgery performed at the same time as a SEPS procedure. There is no trial to date comparing best surgical treatment with best surgical treatment and SEPS, nor even with best medical treatment. In the large NASEP[16] group, 88 patients (59%) had saphenofemoral junction ligation whilst 38 patients (26%) had only the SEPS procedure performed and a further 16 only had additional calf avulsions or vein excisions. There was, however, no subgroup analysis. In Sparks' study[29] 12 of the 19 cases had additional procedures and in the reports from Bergan[28] and Pierik *et al.*[27] no mention is made of how many patients had further surgery only that any long saphenous incompetence was also dealt with at the time of operation.

There has been one recent study where SEPS was performed in isolation on a group of 40 patients who all had previous stripping or high ligation.[30] Sixteen patients had active ulceration at time of surgery and nine of these healed (57%) within a median of 21 days although there were no data on long-term follow-up.

Although this is suggestive of benefit there was no control group so it is difficult to tell if the benefit is greater than that which could be gained by intensive dressings and strict elevation.

It is thought that one of the most important factors in determining whether an ulcer will heal is the completeness of the control of reflux.[31] One of the major criticisms frequently levelled at the SEPS procedure is that the role of the incompetent perforator is still unproven in the aetiology of venous ulcers; especially in the presence of other major reflux. Indeed there is some evidence that correction of all superficial main stem reflux can render previously incompetent calf perforators competent again, although in the presence of deep venous reflux this may be less likely. In the study from Pierik *et al.*[23] where duplex scans were performed on 20 patients having SEPS procedures, three patients had ulcers that did not heal and of these, two had persistent incompetent perforators on follow-up. In Iafrati's group of 18 patients;[22] 12 had ulceration prior to treatment and four failed to heal after SEPS. All four had incompetent perforators seen on follow-up duplex ultrasound.

CONCLUSION

Venous ulceration places a very heavy burden on the patient and the health service. The prognosis is poor with only 50% healed at 4 months,[32] 20% remaining open after 2 years and 8% still unhealed at 5 years.[33] Duplex has provided us with more information about the dynamics of the venous system in these difficult cases and from this knowledge arises potential for surgical intervention. Endoscopic calf perforator surgery appears now to be a reliable technique; however the extent to which eradication of medial calf perforators will be helpful in these patients in the long-term has yet to be established. Many of the patients operated on in series reported to date have had additional procedures making analysis of the SEPS component of surgery more difficult. However, long-term ulcer healing does appear possible and the incidence of complications is seemingly acceptable and certainly markedly less than for an equivalent open procedure. To become established as a recognized effective treatment SEPS must not only show that it can consistently improve the symptoms of chronic venous insufficiency without significant morbidity, but also that any improvement is greater than that which could have been achieved by current accepted best practice. Properly constructed trials with long follow-up are therefore needed before the technique can be unequivocally endorsed.

REFERENCES

1. Hauer G: Die endoscopische subfasciale diszision der perforansvenen-vorlaufige mitteilung. *VASA* **14**: 59, 1985
2. Fischer R: Surgical treatment of varicose veins; endoscopic treatment of incompetent Cockett veins. *Phlebology* **4**: 1040–1041, 1989
3. Linton RR: The communicating veins of the lower leg and the operative technique for their ligation. *Ann Surg* **107**: 582–593, 1938

4. Silver D, Gleysteen JJ, Rhodes GR *et al.*: Surgical treatment of the refractory postphlebitic ulcer. *Arch Surg* **103**: 554–560, 1971
5. Hyde GL, Litton TC, Hull DA: Long-term results of subfascial vein ligation for venous stasis disease. *Surg Gyn Obstet* **153**: 683–686, 1981
6. Negus D, Friedgood A: The effective management of venous ulceration. *Br J Surg* **70**: 623–627, 1983
7. Jamieson WG, DeRose G, Harris KA: Management of venous stasis ulcer: long-term follow-up. *Can J Surg* **33**: 222–223, 1990
8. Bowen FH: Subfascial ligation (Linton operation) of the perforating leg veins to treat post-thrombophlebitic syndrome. *Am Surg* **41**: 148–151, 1975
9. Beebe HG, Bergan JJ, Bergqvist D *et al.*: Classification and grading of chronic venous disease in the lower limbs – a consensus statement. Organised by Straub Foundation with the cooperation of the American Venous Forum at the 6th Annual General Meeting 22–25 February, 1994, Maui, Hawaii. *VASA* **24**: 313–318, 1995
10. Bradbury AW, Stonebridge PA, Callam MJ *et al.*: Foot volumetry and duplex ultrasonography after saphenous and subfascial perforating vein ligation for recurrent venous ulceration. *Br J Surg* **80**: 845–848, 1993
11. Labropoulos N, Leon M, Nicolaides AN *et al.*: Superficial venous insufficiency: correlation of anatomic extent of reflux with clinical symptoms and signs. *J Vasc Surg* **20**: 953–958, 1994
12. Bradbury AW, Brittenden J, Allan PL, Ruckley CV. Comparison of venous reflux in the affected and non-affected leg in patients with unilateral venous ulceration. *Br J Surg* **83**: 513–515, 1996
13. Brittenden J, Bradbury AW, Allan PL *et al.*: Popliteal vein reflux reduces the healing of chronic venous ulcer. *Br J Surg* **85**: 60–62, 1998
14. Campbell WA, West A: Duplex ultraound audit of operative treatment of primary varicose veins. *Phlebology* **10**(Suppl 1): 407–409, 1995
15. Whiteley MS, Smith JJ, Galland RB: Tibial nerve damage during subfascial endoscopic perforator vein surgery. *Br J Surg* **84**: 512, 1997
16. Jugenheimer M, Junginger T: Endoscopic subfascial sectioning of perforating veins in the treatment of primary varicosities. *World J Surg* **16**: 971–975, 1992
17. Gloviczki P, Bergan JJ, Menawat SS *et al.*: Safety, feasibility, and early efficacy of subfascial endoscopic perforator surgery: a preliminary report from the North American registry. *J Vasc Surg* **25**: 94–105, 1997
18. Stuart WP, Adam DJ, Bradbury AW, Ruckley CV: Subfascial endoscopic perforator surgery is associated with significantly less morbidity and shorter hospital stay than open operation (Linton's procedure). *Br J Surg* **84**: 1364–1365, 1997
19. Pierik EG, van UH, Hop WC, Wittens CH: Endoscopic versus open subfascial division of incompetent perforating veins in the treatment of venous leg ulceration: a randomized trial. *J Vasc Surg* **26**: 1049–1054, 1997
20. Cockett FB: The pathology and treatment of venous ulcers of the leg. *Br J Surg* **34**: 260–278, 1955
21. Mozes G, Gloviczki P, Menawat SS *et al.*: Surgical anatomy for endoscopic subfascial division of perforating veins. *J Vasc Surg* **24**: 800–808, 1996
22. Iafrati MD, Welch HJ, O'Donnell-TF J: Subfascial endoscopic perforator ligation: an analysis of early clinical outcomes and cost. *J Vasc Surg* **25**: 995–1000, 1997
23. Pierik EG, van UH, Wittens CH: Efficacy of subfascial endoscopy in eradicating perforating veins of the lower leg and its relation with venous ulcer healing. *J Vasc Surg* **26**: 255–259, 1997
24. Whiteley MS, Smith JJ, Galland RB: Subfascial endoscopic perforator vein surgery (SEPS): current practice among British surgeons. *Ann Roy Coll Surg Engl* **80**: 104–107, 1998
25. Ruckley CV, Bradbury AW, Stuart W: Chronic venous ulcer. Causes are often multifactorial and a holistic approach is required. *Br Med J* **315**: 189, 1997
26. Callam MJ, Harper DR, Dale JJ, Ruckley CV: Arterial disease in chronic leg ulceration: an underestimated hazard? Lothian and Forth Valley leg ulcer study. *Br Med J Clin Res Ed* **294**: 929–931, 1987
27. Pierik EGJM, Wittens CHA, van Urk H: Subfascial endoscopic ligation in the treatment of incompetent perforating veins. *Eur J Vasc Endovasc Surg* **9**: 38–41, 1995

28. Bergan JJ, Murray J, Greason K: Subfascial endoscopic perforator vein surgery: a preliminary report. *Ann Vasc Surg* **10**: 211–219, 1996
29. Sparks SR, Ballard JL, Bergan JJ, Killeen JD: Early benefits of subfascial endoscopic perforator surgery (SEPS) in healing venous ulcers. *Ann Vasc Surg* **11**: 367–373, 1997
30. Proebstle TM, Weisel G, Paepcke U *et al.*: Light reflection rheography and clinical course of patients with advanced venous disease before and after endoscopic subfascial division of perforating veins. *Dermatol Surg* **24**: 771–776, 1998
31. Nash TP: Venous ulceration: factors influencing recurrence after standard surgical procedures. *Med J Aust* **154**: 48–50, 1991
32. Skene AL, Smith JM, Dore CJ *et al.*: Venous leg ulcers: a prognostic index to predict time to healing. *Br Med J* **305**: 1119–1120, 1992
33. Da Silva A, Widmer LK, Martin H *et al.*: Varicose veins and chronic venous insufficiency – prevalence and risk factors in 4376 subjects in the Basic Study II. *VASA* **3**: 118–125, 1974

Commentary

In commenting on the chapter by Meyer and Burnand (p. 285) on the durability of perforator surgery I have pointed out the difficulty of evaluating the procedure in the face of innumerable variations in surgical technique and a lack of correlation of outcome with haemodynamic tests. The same points can be reiterated *à propos* the subfascial approach. However, a high degree of standardization of technique should be possible. Stansby and Lintott do a valuable service in reminding us of the importance of carrying out paratibial fasciotomy of the deep fascia bounding the superficial posterior compartment posteriorly, without which paratibial perforating veins will be missed. If the endoscope is turned directly towards the tibia at the level of its introduction in the upper calf and the fasciotomy commenced at that level and continued as far as possible down the calf, not only will paratibial perforators come readily into view but also the whole subfascial space will open up more easily.

Thus there should be no doubt as to what the surgeon should do to find perforators and to achieve adequate exposure. However, access to the lowermost (Cockett 1) perforator at the ankle can be very difficult or even impossible in the presence of open ulcer and/or chronic inflammation. Indeed one suspects most surgeons do not usually reach this vessel. Whether it is necessary to do so is unclear.

As far as efficacy and durability are concerned Stansby and Lintott are right to emphasize the prevention of recurrence rather than the achievement of initial healing. They are also right to point out the poverty of adequate information in the literature on late outcome. In order that we can objectively judge the role of this operation in the future we need standardized preoperative information on clinical condition and patterns of reflux, operative information on all concurrent venous surgery together with the number and location of perforators interrupted, objective postoperative duplex information on the extent to which surgical objectives were achieved and late follow-up information on clinical outcome, duplex findings and whether compression therapy was employed. *CVR*

Is venous valve reconstruction durable?

Andries J Kroese, Antonio Rosales and Carl Erik Slagsvold

INTRODUCTION

Although repair of incompetent valves in the great saphenous vein has been attempted,[1] venous valve reconstruction (VVR) is defined as a procedure to restore venous valve function in patients with symptomatic *deep* venous reflux. Bypass operations for patients with obstructive venous disease are not included in the present overview.

There are several reasons why venous surgery has not developed to the same extent as arterial surgery. The patient with chronic venous insufficiency is rarely threatened by amputation. In addition, a better understanding of the pathophysiological basis for venous surgery has only recently evolved, partially due to the development of improved haemodynamic investigations. Finally, the technique of VVR is a challenge which not all surgeons wish to cope with. Among those who have been engaged in this type of surgery, many have given up because their results were not satisfactory.

The indications for VVR are ambiguous, partially due to the uncertainty about anticipated results. Therefore, it is appropriate to regularly assess the durability of the reconstructions.

TYPES OF VENOUS VALVE RECONSTRUCTION

The rationale for VVR is based on improving the venous muscle pump mechanism by restoring competence to one or more venous valves. These anti-reflux operations may be divided into *direct* and *indirect* procedures:

Direct repair (valvuloplasty)

Direct repair can be subdivided into:

1. Reefing of the incompetent edges of the valve cusps by open venotomy using a longitudinal,[2] a transverse[3] or T-shaped incision[4] (Fig. 1).
2. External reefing of the valve commissures,[5] preferably under the guidance of angioscopy[6,7] (Fig. 2).

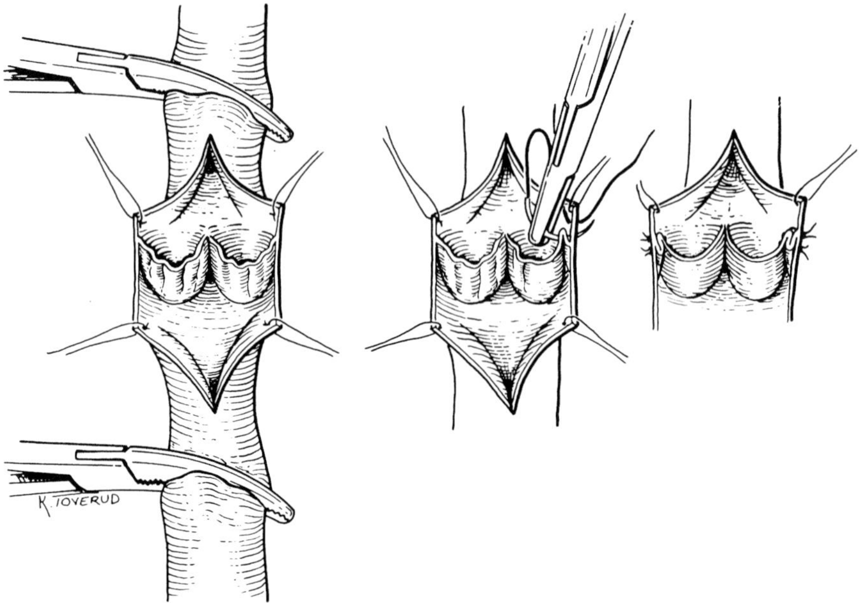

Fig. 1. Internal (open) valvuloplasty. 'Floppy' valve cusps are exposed through a venotomy and repaired by multiple sutures at the commissures.

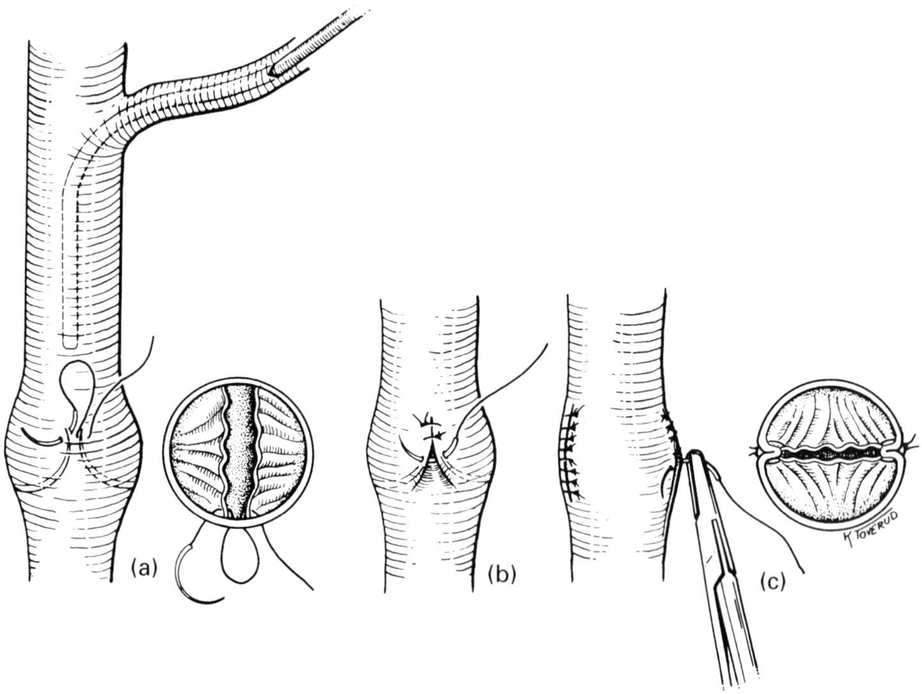

Fig. 2. External (closed) valvuloplasty. Multiple sutures are externally placed in both commissures coapting cusp margins. Competency is obtained by deepening the valve cusps and slightly narrowing the vein.

Indirect repair

Indirect repair can also be subdivided into:

1. Valve autotransplantation,[8] where a competent valve containing segment of the axillary vein is interposed into the incompetent femoral or popliteal vein. Recently patent valves from the contralateral saphenous vein have been used.
2. Transposition of a venous segment[9] with incompetent valves to a competent deep or superficial vein, e.g. by anastomosing the insufficient superficial femoral vein end-to-side to the profunda or great saphenous vein.

Other anti-reflux operations, e.g. application of a Dacron or polytetrafluoroethylene (PTFE) cuff alone,[10] gracilis muscle tendon transfer,[11] venous wall plication[12] and the use of homograft[13] or prosthetic valves[14] have not made any clinical impact and will not be discussed.

PERIOPERATIVE INVESTIGATIONS

Clinical information and indications for surgery

It is generally accepted that inclusion criteria for this type of surgery should be strict, since information concerning individual prognosis after VVR still is not conclusive. Only patients who are very disabled because of chronic venous insufficiency should be considered for surgery.

These patients are usually between 35 and 60 years old, and generally younger than those operated upon for obliterative atherosclerosis. They should have an acceptable potential for compliance during the follow-up period and good prospects for work rehabilitation. Those who are eligible for operation belong to 'classes' IV, V and VI according to the CEAP (Clinical, Etiology, Anatomical, Pathophysiological) classification.[15,16] Symptoms and signs comprise chronic skin ulceration, eczema or cellulitis which is refractory to appropriate compression therapy and local wound care (70%), or disabling symptoms of 'heaviness' and leg swelling.

Coagulopathies

The high incidence of postoperative thrombosis after VVR reported from some centres may be related to the finding that approximately 30–40% of the patients with post-thrombotic syndrome have hereditary thrombophyllia. It is important that patients with secondary chronic venous insufficiency are screened for coagulopathies. This group of patients should receive heparin perioperatively and subsequent life-long anticoagulation.

Previous varicose vein surgery

Incompetent superficial and perforator veins are usually removed before valve surgery to reduce distal venous hypertension which is a major cause of skin ulceration. Without this precaution the effect of a well performed VVR would be significantly reduced.

Functional investigations

Based on physiological investigations 60% of patients with chronic venous insufficiency have primary valve reflux. The remaining patients suffer from either post-thrombotic syndrome or a mixture of primary and secondary valve insufficiency. Modern VVR is impossible without help from a sophisticated vascular laboratory. Indications for VVR and the assessment of its durability are based on the results of functional tests of venous outflow, calf muscle pump function and valve reflux.

Venous outflow

Raju's test is preferred to assess venous outflow by comparing venous pressure in the arm and leg in the supine patient at rest and measuring the pressure gradient before and after reactive hyperaemia induced by a thigh tourniquet.[17] A venous outflow obstruction causing a gradient of more than 8 mm Hg, indicates the need for a venous bypass procedure before VVR is attempted. To visualize venous vessels we still rely on ascending venography. In the future colour duplex scanning may become the method of choice.

Calf muscle pump function

To assess the overall efficacy of the calf muscle pump, ambulatory pressure measurements in a distal vein on the leg are still considered as the gold standard. First it provides information about the efficacy of venous outflow from the leg. Another aspect of this test is refilling time of the leg veins following a period of ambulation; a re-fill time of less than 20 seconds is a sign of overall venous reflux. Alternatively, ambulatory volume changes in the calf measured by plethysmography may be used, but varying correlation with venous pressure measurements have been found.

Venous reflux

Colour duplex scanning is the main tool to evaluate segmental venous reflux.[18] The patient is examined standing with a relaxed lower limb, holding on to a frame. Reflux may be induced by either performing a Valsalva manoeuver or by rapidly deflating a pneumatic cuff applied to the calf, i.e. distal to the actual venous segment. Reflux duration, i.e. valve closure time, should not exceed 0.5 seconds.

Indications for operation are based on clinical symptoms and signs. However, patients who are selected for VVR, usually have a grade III–IV reflux, which extends below the level of the knee.[19] In these patients VVR should include the popliteal level.

If the profunda vein proves to be incompetent, care should be taken to effectively address this problem. Otherwise the result of a technically well-performed VVR in the superficial femoral or popliteal vein will be disappointing.

Ascending and descending video venography

The main reasons for doing ascending venography are to confirm the presence of anatomic outflow obstruction and to visualize the extent of collateral circulation.[7]

Insufficient recanalization combined with a very extensive collateral network will in most cases preclude the performance of VVR.

Descending video venography is used to determine the location of valves which may be amenable for reconstruction,[7] and helps to estimate the grade of reflux.[19]

Intraoperative evaluation

The technical results can be estimated intraoperatively by a simple 'strip test'. Blood is 'milked' digitally towards the reconstructed valve whereby its competency can be assessed by direct inspection.

The quality of external valveplasty is greatly enhanced by performing angioscopy[6,7,20] (Fig. 2). Alternatively, duplex scanning may be used to evaluate the results of valve repair intraoperatively. Furthermore, with improved resolution of the duplex system it may become possible to anatomically assess individual valves and localize the valve commissures, which would be very helpful when doing external valvuloplasties.

Postoperative follow-up

Preferably these patients are evaluated clinically and functionally before discharge from the hospital, after 3 months and subsequently at 1-year intervals.

HOW TO ASSESS THE DURABILITY OF VENOUS VALVE RECONSTRUCTION

Centres which are dedicated to VVR must adhere to standardized reporting if this part of vascular surgery is to achieve generally accepted indications and surgical techniques. The CEAP classifications system comprises valuable data which enables us to evaluate and compare the durability of VVR.[15,16] Its clinical staging is based on symptoms and signs, and on information from functional tests and venography.

Perioperative morbidity and mortality rates are usually low in this category of patients, but obviously need to be reported. For the patient clinical improvement is the most interesting aspect of VVR durability. The surgeon also needs to know patency rates following different types of VVR, assessed functionally and morphologically. To increase the durability of these procedures, the causes of clinical and functional failure should be clarified.

It is relevant to speculate whether the eventual failure of a VVR is primarily due to dysfunction of the repair itself or to progression of the underlying venous disease. Most failures of valvuloplasty occur within 1–2 years in patients who have been suffering from chronic venous insufficiency for many years and who probably have attained a stable measure of venous dilatation. It is doubtful that a progression of venous insufficiency would suddenly occur as the primary cause of VVR failure.

Preferably, clinical and functional results of valve repair should be evaluated in a randomized manner. However, it would be very difficult to establish sufficiently large groups because few patients are suitable for VVR. Furthermore, randomization is almost impossible due to the variety in types and extent of chronic venous insufficiency among patients with leg ulceration. In addition, treatment is individualized in patients with post-thrombotic chronic venous insufficiency, depending on the availability of a competent valve from the axillary or saphenous vein. Either single or multiple transplants may be done, sometime combined with a plasty of a valve which has not been completely destroyed by previous deep vein thrombosis. Finally, a randomized comparison would be complicated by the diversity of strategies for perioperative anticoagulation and patient compliance with compression therapy.

For information concerning the durability of VVR, we have to rely on long-term follow-up studies. There are few relevant reports in the literature; only two centres have presented series of more than 100 cases.

DURABILITY OF VENOUS VALVE RECONSTRUCTION – THE LONGEST FOLLOW-UP STUDY

Kistner is a major pioneer of venous reconstructive surgery and has introduced a number of technical innovations.[21] His group published the results of a follow-up study with a mean observation time of 10 years (range 4–21). What can be learned from their experience is that the best durability of VVR is obtained if:

1. *The patient has primary insufficiency*. The prognosis after direct valvuloplasty for primary insufficiency is almost twice as good as for valve autotransplantation or transposition in patients with secondary insufficiency: 73% and 43% ulcer-free period during the follow-up period, respectively.
2. *The primary operation is successful*. In 17 of 51 limbs ulceration re-occurred due to the following causes: failed primary reconstruction: 10; incompetent profunda femoris vein: 3; lymphoedema: 1.
3. *An ulcer-free period of at least 2 years is achieved.*

DURABILITY OF VENOUS VALVE RECONSTRUCTION – THE LARGEST FOLLOW-UP STUDY

Raju and co-workers reported the results of 423 valve repairs in 256 limbs, with a mean follow-up period of 3.5 years.[22] It was concluded that clinical results following VVR for primary and secondary venous insufficiency were similar; approximately 74% of 211 limbs remained ulcer-free. In contrast, Masuda and Kistner observed a significant difference between the fate of limbs with primary and secondary CVI.[21]

Masuda and Kistner, and also Raju have become increasingly aware that approximately 30% of patients show signs of both primary and secondary CVI.[20,21] As a consequence, patients have more often been treated with multiple level repairs, combining valvuloplasty and valve transplantation. An individualized rather than a standardized approach probably improves the results in patients with secondary or 'mixed' valve insufficiency.

Several other relevant conclusions were drawn. The clinical and functional results were correlated, i.e. in very few patients with patent and competent valves did ulcers re-occur. Second, open, internal repair rendered better functional results than external repair, which confirms Masuda and Kistner's findings.[21] However, external valve repair guided by angioscopy may become the method of choice. It is technically easier and less time consuming, allowing multiple level repairs to a greater extent.[6,7,20] Furthermore, the proximal valve station in the superficial femoral artery rendered superior results compared with other locations. This is surprising because the popliteal site has usually been preferred, due to its 'gate keeper' function at the proximity of the calf muscle pump. Lastly, axillary vein transfer showed the poorest outcome.

VALVULOPLASTY

The majority of valvuloplasties are of the *direct* type where a venotomy is performed to expose the valve cusps. In recent years the closed, external repair has been used. In some instances the reconstruction is wrapped with a Dacron or PTFE cuff to prevent venous dilatation and subsequent incompetency. No available data can adequately elucidate the long-term effect of this additional measure.

Table 1 (below) summarizes information on the largest follow-up series in the literature.[3,22–26] Information is scant compared with that for arterial surgery. Not all reports give the mean time of follow-up, and in most studies many patients were lost to control investigations after a few years, except for one series where complete data were presented for 60 of 61 limbs.[3]

The general results were quite favourable: 70–80% of patients had 'good clinical results', which is defined as ulcer healing or significant relief of symptoms. 'Haemodynamic improvement' is variously defined and usually encompasses the results from a combination of methods, often including duplex scanning. The functional durability of this operation also appears to be satisfactory in 70–85% of cases during a 2- to 4-year follow-up time. These reports confirm the value of valvuloplasty in carefully selected patients.

Table 1. Results after valvuloplasty

Author(s)	*No. of limbs*	*Follow-up (years)*	*% Good clinical results*	*Haemodynamic improvement*
Raju and Fredericks (1988)[3]	61	2–8	76	50/60
Ferris and Kistner (1982)[23]	32	1–13	83	7/8
Cheatle and Perrin (1994)[24]	52	1	85	23/27
Eriksson *et al.* (1985)[25]	27	1–9	70	19/20
Sottiurai (1988)[26]	21	2–8	80	10/10

VALVE AUTOTRANSPLANTATION

Valve transplantation is mostly used for the treatment of secondary chronic venous insufficiency. Most surgeons use the axillary vein as the donor site and the femoral vein as the recipient vein. However, there seems to be a tendency to transplant the competent valve-containing segment to the popliteal vein. Again the reported materials are small, except for one study, and a general problem is the high drop-out rate[24,27–31] (Table 2).

Taheri and co-workers reported 'good' clinical and haemodynamic results for valve transplantation,[27] whereas other series are too small to draw definite conclusions regarding long-term durability. Eriksson's study does not comprise many patients, but all of them were functionally assessed postoperatively and after 1 year.[28] Postoperative results were 'good' in 90% of cases, but after 1 year in only 10%. The disappointing late results may be partially due to secondary venous dilatation or destruction of the valve itself because of long-lasting exposure to a venous pressure higher than at the donor site.

The results of this technique may be improved by the support of a Dacron or PTFE cuff to prevent dilatation. Instead of applying synthetic material, we use an inlay technique (Fig. 3), where the recipient femoral or popliteal vein wall is wrapped around the transplanted vein segment, comparable with how the aortic wall is sutured over the implanted synthetic graft after the resection of an aneurysm.

In conclusion, valve transplantation has its place in the treatment of secondary chronic venous insufficiency. Since this operation aims at ameliorating axial reflux, it cannot be effective in patients with incomplete recanalization of deep vein thrombosis causing venous outflow obstruction. Most patients will still need lifelong compression therapy. Our impression is that in 30–40% of cases the harvested axillary vein is incompetent, needing bench repair. This fact and the tendency of the axillary vein to dilate after implantation into a vein of the lower limb, has inspired us to look for segments with a competent valve in a contralateral saphenous vein, which we find to be available in a surprising 30–40% of cases.

Table 2. Results after valve autotransplantation, by axillofemoral (AF), axillopopliteal (AP), brachiofemoral (BF) and brachiopopliteal (BP) transfers, respectively

Author(s)	*No. of limbs*	*Follow-up (years)*	*% Good clinical results*	*Haemodynamic improvement*
Taheri (1985)[27]	72 (BF)	5	78	18/20
Eriksson and Almgren (1988)[28]	26 (AP) 9 (AF)	2.3	31	90% postop. 10% 1 year
Cheatle and Perrin (1994)[24]	26 (AF)	4	69	–
Nash (1988)[29]	25 (BP)	1.5	31	19/25
Raju and Fredericks (1988)[3]	18 (AF)	2	46	8/18
Bry *et al.* (1995)[30]	15 (AP)	5	92	1/10
Sottiurai (1991)[31]	8 (BF)	2.8	75	2/8

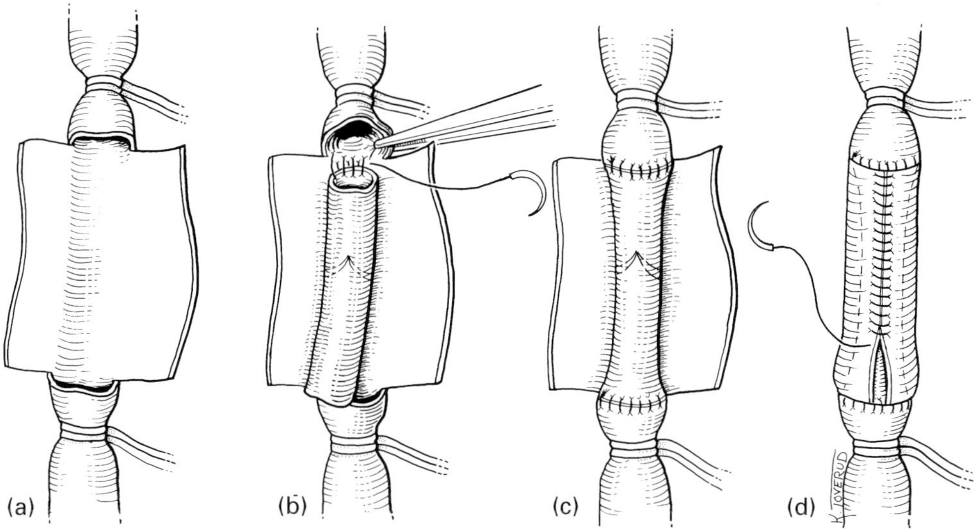

Fig. 3. Illustration of 'in-lay' technique used for valve transplantation. The femoral or popliteal vein is opened longitudinally and transversely (a). A competent valve containing segment of an axillary or saphenous vein is interposed by performing a proximal (b) and distal (c) end-to-end anastomosis. The wall of the femoral or popliteal vein is sutured around the transplanted venous segment (d).

VENOUS TRANSPOSITION

Venous transposition has been used in the treatment of primary and secondary chronic venous insufficiency, provided a neighbouring vein, the profunda or great saphenous vein contains a competent proximal valve. Transposition of a vein is rarely applied, because ideal prerequisites for this type of operation are rarely fulfilled. In addition, if the superficial femoral vein is transposed end-to-side to the profunda vein, the required dissection is extensive.

Most of the patients in the studies listed in Table 3, have been followed-up clinically for approximately 3 years.[23,28,30,31] The haemodynamic results were initially quite satisfactory, but in none of the series were these re-assessed during the follow-up period. The clinical results were 'good' compared with other types of VVR, except for one series.[32]

In conclusion, the concept of venous transposition is ingenious, but its long-term benefit has not been convincingly proved.

THE DURABILITY OF VENOUS VALVE RECONSTRUCTION – A PERSONAL EXPERIENCE

A prospective study from our own clinic, consequently using the CEAP classification, has rendered valuable information on factors influencing the short-term durability of VVR. Forty-three VVRs were performed in 29 patients, of whom 19 had secondary and 10 primary CVI. Twenty-one were men. The predominance of males was unclear. Since almost all of these men were tall, 190 cm, and weighing over 100 kg, the force of gravity may have played a role. The preoperative work-up was usually done by the vascular surgeon himself at the vascular laboratory; he was also present during venographies. Thirteen patients had skin ulceration (class 6), five healed ulcers (class 5), 11 skin changes (class 4). Twenty-six had a grade III or IV reflux, three patients belonged to grade II. Seven patients had hereditary thrombophilia.

Twenty-three external valve plasties were performed and 20 transplantations (14 saphenous and six axillary). In 12 patients, six of whom suffered from secondary chronic venous insufficiency, multilevel VVRs were carried out. This agrees with the experience of Raju's group which found reconstructible valves in 70% of patients with secondary chronic venous insufficiency.[22] Although venous bypass operations are not within the scope of this overview, it seems that many of these patients need an additional valve repair. In five of seven venous bypass operations we performed during the last 2 years, a subsequent VVR was required to relieve symptoms effectively.

The finding that many patients have 'mixed' chronic venous insufficiency, supports the notion that deep vein thrombosis may affect the deep veins segmentally, thereby only destroying veins in certain parts. Second, it seems that proximal thrombotic occlusion can cause non-thrombotic, secondary insufficiency of distal valves, which may be amenable for valvuloplasty.

The mean duration of follow-up was 1.3 years (0.1–4.1). According to CEAP reporting, four patients became asymptomatic, all of whom had primary chronic venous insufficiency. Fifteen patients improved significantly, both clinically and functionally, and in none of them was residual reflux found on duplex examination. Five patients reported only mild improvement and five an unchanged condition associated with persistent reflux. The CEAP classification does not specify the rate of ulcer healing, although this is a crucial end-point. Among our 13 patients with ulceration, nine achieved healing.

In conclusion, we learned to be aware of the relatively high incidence of hereditary thrombophilia in patients with chronic venous insufficiency. Better results were achieved by the multiple level approach than with single reconstructions (Fisher's test, $p < 0.05$). In addition, the use of saphenous valves seemed to improve the results after valve transplantation. We developed an 'inlay technique' for the

Table 3. Results after valve transposition

Author(s)	*No. of limbs*	*Follow-up (years)*	*% Good clinical results*	*Haemodynamic improvement*
Ferris and Kistner (1982)[23]	14	4	78	10/11
Sottiurai (1991)[31]	14	4	86	7/8
Johnson *et al.* (1981)[32]	12	1	25	9/12
Eriksson and Almgren (1988)[28]	4	3	50	–

transplantation of a competent valve-containing segment to avoid venous dilatation (Fig. 3). Color duplex scanning has proved to be useful to locate patent valve segments in the saphenous vein preoperatively, thus avoiding unnecessary dissection.

CONCLUSIONS

From the limited number of reports in the literature and our own experience we conclude that in 70–80% of cases the goals of VVR can be achieved, with healing of skin ulcerations and improvement of the quality of life. If the primary results are good, durability of this success beyond 5 years is rather the rule than the exception. The majority of patients still need elastic stockings, although with a lower grade of compression, to avoid recurrence of symptoms later in life. It is generally known that conservative measures with continuous elevation of the limb and bed rest can relieve even severe symptoms, but most people expect a higher quality of life.

FUTURE IMPROVEMENTS OF VENOUS VALVE RECONSTRUCTION

In order to achieve good primary results appropriate case selection, based on clinical, haemodynamic and venographic findings is paramount. In the near future Doppler ultrasound investigations will probably replace venography. Since treatment has to be individualized, the vascular surgeon should preferably participate in the functional assessment at the vascular laboratory to fully understand the pathophysiology in each patient. Multiple level repairs should be performed wherever possible.

Although in competent hands open valvuloplasty may render good results, this technique is more demanding than external repairs. Preferably, the external repair should be guided by angioscopy. In the near future duplex scanning may become a useful intraoperative aid. High resolution equipment may be able to visualize the valve commisures which would simplify the procedure and possibly improve the results. In addition, secondary insufficiency following successful primary valve plasty may be reduced in a number of cases by applying a synthetic cuff to avoid distension of the involved vein segment.

In our experience approximately 30% of patients have a contralateral saphenous vein segment with a competent valve which is suitable for transplantation. This type of transplant is probably less prone to distend in the course of time. In addition, the 'inlay technique' we developed to reduce dilatation of the transplanted vein segment, may improve the durability of this procedure.

Concerning the durability of VVR, some questions remain unanswered. Is long-term outcome improved by:

1. doing open instead of external valvular plasties?
2. doing multiple segmental VVR?
3. applying external cuffs?

4. using contralateral saphenous vein segments for valve transplantation?
5. earlier surgical interventions to avoid irreversible damage of the muscle pump?
6. endovascular methods, for example the inplantation valve containing vein segments by means of catheter and stent techniques?

To improve the results of VVR, this type of surgery should be centralized to dedicated clinics, where new devices and techniques can be appropriately developed, tested and reported upon.

REFERENCES

1. Jessup G, Lane RJ: Repair of incompetent venous valves: a new technique. *J Vasc Surg* **8**: 569–575, 1988
2. Kistner RL: Surgical repair of the incompetent femoral vein valve. *Arch Surg* **110**: 1336–1351, 1975
3. Raju S, Fredericks R: Valve reconstruction procedures for nonobstructive venous insufficiency: rationale, techniques, and results in 107 procedures with two- to eight-year follow-up. *J Vasc Surg* **7**: 301–310, 1988
4. Sottiurai VS: Technique in direct venous valvuloplasty. *J Vasc Surg* **8**: 646–648, 1988
5. Kistner RL: Surgical technique of external venous valve repair. *The Straub Foundations Proceedings* **55**: 15–16, 1990
6. Gloviczki P, Merrell SW, Bower TC: Femoral vein valve repair under direct vision without venotomy: a modified technique with use of angioscopy. *J Vasc Surg* **14**: 645–648, 1991
7. Kroese AJ, Rosales A, Flørenes T *et al.*: Video venography and angioscopy for reconstructive venous surgery. In Greenhalgh RM (Ed) *Vascular Imaging for Surgeons* pp. 513–521. London: WB Saunders Co, 1995
8. Taheri SA, Lazar L, Elias SM *et al.*: Vein valve transplant. *Surgery* **91**: 28–33, 1982
9. Kistner RL, Sparkuhl MD: Surgery in acute and chronic venous disease. *Surgery* **85**: 31–41, 1979
10. Hallberg D: A method for repairing incompetent valves in deep veins. *Acta Chir Scand* **138**: 143–145, 1972
11. Psathakis ND: Surgical treatment of deep venous insufficiency of the lower limb. *Surg Gyn Obstet* **166**: 131–141, 1988
12. Jones JW, Elliot F, Kerstein MD: Triangular venous valvuloplasty. *Arch Surg* **117**: 1250–1251, 1982
13. Burkhart HM, Steven WF, Dalsing MC *et al.*: Experimental repair of venous valvular insufficiency using a cryopreserved venous valve allograft aided by a distal arteriovenous fistula. *J Vasc Surg* **26**: 817–822, 1997
14. Taheri SA, Rigan D, Wels P *et al.*: Experimental prosthetic vein valve. *Am J Surg* **156**: 111–114, 1988
15. Porter MP, Moneta GL: Reporting standards in venous disease: and update. *J Vasc Surg* **21**: 634–645, 1995
16. Kistner RL, Eklof B, Masuda EM: Diagnosis of chronic venous disease of the lower extremities: the "CEAP" classification. *Mayo Clin Proc* **71**: 338–345, 1996
17. Raju S: New approaches to the diagnosis and treatment of venous obstruction. *J Vasc Surg* **4**: 42–54, 1986
18. Bemmelen P, Bedford G, Beach K *et al.*: Quantitative segmental evaluation of venous valvular reflux with duplex ultrasound scanning. *J Vasc Surg* **10**: 425–431, 1989
19. Masuda EM, Kistner RL: A prospective comparison of duplex scanning and descending venography in the assessment of venous insufficiency. *Am J Surg* **164**: 254–259, 1992
20. Welch HJ, McLaughlin RL, O'Donnell TF: Femoral vein valvuloplasty: Intropoperative angioscopic evaluation and hemodynamic improvement. *J Vasc Surg* **16**: 694–700, 1992

21. Masuda EM, Kistner RL: Long-term results of venous valve reconstruction: a four- to twenty-one-year follow-up. *J Vasc Surg* **19**: 391–403, 1994
22. Raju S, Fredericks RK, Neglén PN *et al.*: Durability of venous valve reconstruction techniques for "primary" and postthrombotic reflux. *J Vasc Surg* **23**: 357–367, 1996
23. Ferris BF, Kistner R: Femoral vein reconstruction in the management of chronic venous insufficiency. *Arch Surg* **117**: 1571–1579, 1982
24. Cheatle TR, Perrin M: Venous valve repair: early results in fifty-two cases. *J Vasc Surg* **19**: 404–413, 1994
25. Eriksson I, Almgren B, Norgren L: Late results after venous valve repair. *J Int Angiol* **4**: 413–417, 1985
26. Sottiurai VS: Technique in direct venous valvuloplasty. *J Vasc Surg* **8**: 646–648, 1988
27. Taheri SA, Prendergast DR, Lazar *et al.*: Vein valve transplantation. *Am J Surg* **150**: 201–202, 1985
28. Eriksson I, Almgren B: Surgical reconstruction of incompetent deep vein valves. *Ups J Med Sci* **93**: 139–143, 1988
29. Nash T: Long term results of vein valve transplants placed in the popliteal vein for intractabel post-phlebiti venous ulcers and pre-ulcer skin changes. *J Cardiovasc Surg* **29**: 712–716, 1988
30. Bry JDL, Muto PA, O'Donnell T *et al.*: The clinical and hemodynamic results after axillary-popliteal vein valve transplantation. *J Vasc Surg* **21**: 110–119, 1995
31. Sottiurai VS: Surgical correction of recurrent venous ulcer. *J Cardiovasc Surg* **32**: 104–109, 1991
32. Johnson ND, Queral LA, Yao ST *et al.*: Late objective assessment of venous valve surgery. *Arch Surg* **116**: 1461–1465, 1981

Commentary

Little effort has been made in the UK to adopt valve repair into the vascular surgical armamentarium. The reasons for international differences are unclear, but probably relate as much to resource constraints as to lack of surgical enterprise. When a review, such as this, of a particular edifice of surgical endeavour shows that it rests on shaky foundations – in terms of evidence-base – the usual response is to emphasize the need for clinical trials. I believe that on this occasion the authors are correct in their view that trials in the field of valve reconstruction are impractical, or at least extremely difficult. The small proportion of the venous population who are suitable, the heterogeneity of the pathology and of the patterns of reflux, with the attendant need to 'individualize' both the surgery and the aftercare, constitute real obstacles. The authors are strongly supported therefore in their plea for standardized reporting and registries, with agreed follow-up and outcome criteria. *CVR*

Durability of the healed venous ulcer

SD Blair and A Hamsho

INTRODUCTION

In the last 10 years the management of venous ulcers has improved enormously although the application of new technology and a consistent approach to the management of venous disease is still patchy worldwide. Before the introduction of multilayer compression bandaging, the 12-week healing rate was consistently around 24%.[1,2] Following the introduction of four-layer bandaging, healing rates have consistently risen to between 50 and 80% depending on the initial size of the ulcer.[3,4] The longer a universal treatment programme is available in a community the better the reported healing rates are.[5] In the Riverside district of London around Charing Cross Hospital the results over a 4-year period were reported. During this time the prevalence dropped 20% per year. Therefore to discuss the durability of the healed venous ulcer one has to look at the setting in which ulcers are being treated.

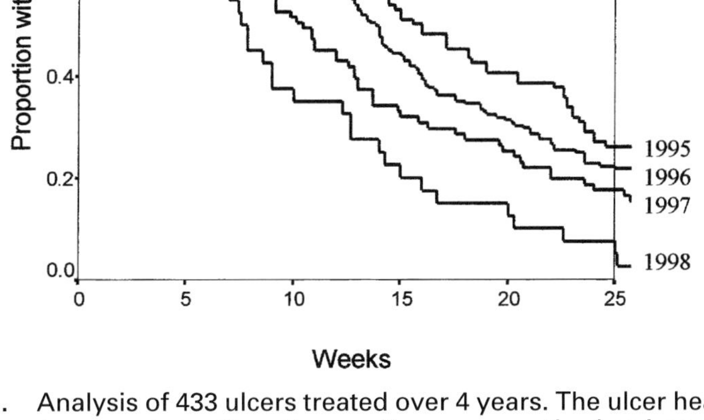

Fig. 1. Analysis of 433 ulcers treated over 4 years. The ulcer healing rate has increased significantly over time as expertise has improved and as the most chronic ulcers have healed. There was no significant change in initial ulcer size over time.

On the Wirral Peninsular in North West England an audit in 1994 showed a 12-week healing rate of 24 %, and the mean time patients had suffered an unhealed ulcer was 1 year. In 1995 we introduced a community-based venous ulcer care programme based on national consensus guidelines. When multilayer compression was introduced in this context the 12-week healing rate improved to 34.4% and then progressively this improved year on year to 65% in 1998. Over the same period the 24-week healing rate improved from 71% to 92.5% (Fig. 1) This improvement was not related to the initial size of the ulcer on presentation; however, the length of time patients had suffered ulcers before presenting did reduce. Clearly if ulcers have not healed initially they cannot recur and therefore recurrence rates in a community are obviously related to how successful we are at getting ulcers to heal in the first place.

PREVALENCE AND INCIDENCE OF RECURRENT VENOUS ULCERS

The prevalence of venous ulcers has been variously reported at between 0.11 and 0.16% of the population but the prevalence rises with age to 2% in those over 80.[6,7] Within this population, recurrent ulcers account for 67–76% of ulcers found giving a prevalence of recurrent ulcers of between 0.07 and 0.11%.[6] However, when a comprehensive ulcer management system is introduced the prevalence of venous ulceration falls. Looking at the figures for Riverside in 1988 they were treating 475 ulcers when they first introduced four-layer bandaging. By 1993 the prevalence had dropped to 144 ulcers in the same population.[5]

While the prevalence of recurrent ulcers is high, studies looking at the incidence of recurrence once an ulcer has healed vary considerably. The reported incidence of recurrence within 1 year varies from 26% to 69%.[8–11]

PREDISPOSING FACTORS FOR RECURRENCE OF VENOUS ULCERATION

In a prospective study in the Riverside district of London, 188 healed ulcers were followed up for 18 months. A 26% recurrence rate at 12 months rising to 31% at 18 months was reported. The main predisposing factors for recurrence were initial ulcer size larger than 10cm, unsuitability for stockings, and previous deep vein thrombosis. Curiously, in hypertensive patients ulcers recurred less commonly.[10] Other factors considered as risk factors for recurrence such as obesity, mobility and the duration of ulceration, showed no correlation.

On the Wirral, 170 ulcers were identified during the year September 1995-August 1996 and these were healed using multilayer compression bandaging. These patients were then prospectively followed up for between 2 and 3 years. The mean age was 73 years and 35% were men. Of the 170 initial ulcers studied, 70 (44%) patients said they had experienced a previous ulcer. During the follow-up period ten patients refused treatment, 30 died (18.75%) and nine moved or were lost from follow-up leaving 121 healed ulcers. With a minimum follow-up of 2 years, 32 (26%) ulcers recurred, 17 underwent superficial venous surgery and only one (6%) of these recurred. In contrast to the previous study we found no correlation between recurrence and a history of deep vein thrombosis or a previously large ulcer. However, looking at those patients whose ulcers did not recur during this follow-up period, 38% had suffered a previous ulcer and 23% were overweight. Of those who did experience recurrence during this follow-up period 65% had suffered a previous ulcer and 41% were overweight ($p < 0.05$). The recurrence rate reported here is lower than the previous studies, even though 37% of our ulcers were more than 10 cm^2 compared with only 27% of those treated in London where the patients were also a mean of 5 years younger. It is therefore difficult to make generalizations about recurrence rates when populations may be so different (Table 1).

Table 1. Wirral leg ulcer study

	Stayed healed	*Recurrent*
Age	72.9+15	73.6+14
Age range	38–93	32–96
Initial ulcer (cm^2)	19.4+37	20.2+39
Mobile	85 (66%)	22 (69%)
Walk with aid	37 (29%)	8 (25%)
Chairbound	6 (5%)	2 (6%)
Previous DVT	27 (21%)	7 (21%)
Previous recurrence	49 (38%)	21 (66%) *
Normal weight	93 (73%)	18 (56%) *
Overweight	30 (23%)	13 (41%) *
Underweight	5 (4%)	1 (3%)
Venous surgery	16	1 *

The difference in risk factors between those patients whose ulcer recurred and those who stayed healed over a follow-up period of 2–3 years.
* Significant difference: $p < 0.05$. DVT: Deep vein thrombosis.

STRATEGIES TO REDUCE RECURRENCE

There are two main methods of reducing venous ulcer recurrence. Corrective venous surgery to abolish venous hypertension, and continued compression. Having shown the benefits of compression to achieve healing, most would use continued compression to reduce recurrence. There is sound logic to this as the benefits of prolonged compression are numerous. At the very least compression should prevent further rapid deterioration in the quality of the skin and at best some have measured quantitatively, improvements in the area of lipodermatoscerosis. The various mechanisms by which compression has its effects are shown in Table 2.

In terms of major vessels, compression improves the venous pump by reducing venous reflux and increasing flow through smaller undilated veins. At the microcirculatory level the capillaries have a reduced diameter with faster flowing blood which reduces white cell trapping as demonstrated by laser Doppler and capillaroscopy. Capillary filtration is reduced and absorption is increased due to the

Table 2. Mechanisms by which compression affects the limb beneficially to reduce the progression of disease and reduce the risk of recurrent ulceration

Benefits of compression	*Investigation*
1. Reduces venous reflux	Duplex, plethysmography
2. Improves venous pumping	Plethysmography, foot volumetry
3. Affects arterial flow	Laser Doppler, xenon clearance
4. Reduces vein diameter	Venography
5. Increases venous flow velocity	Duplex
6. Improvement of microcirculation	Laser Doppler, capillaroscopy
7. Reduces oedema	Measuring tape,volumetry
8. Increases lymphatic drainage	Lymphography
9. Softens lipodermatosclerosis	Ultrasound, CT durometer

increased tissue pressure. Compression also affects mediators of the local inflammatory response, which may be responsible for the pain that is experienced. Similarly lymphatic flow is increased. These many factors may combine to ultimately improve the quality of the skin with softening of lipodermatosclerosis as demonstrated by ultrasound or computed tomography (CT) scanning and using a durometer.[12–15]

Compression stockings

It is widely held that wearing compression stockings after the ulcer has healed should be the main stay of treatment. However, the hard evidence for this is not so easy to find as there do not appear to have been any prospective randomized trials. Looking at people who have or have not chosen to wear the stockings they were prescribed is not very helpful. In one study from Florida, USA, 53 patients with healed ulcers were prescribed zippered stockings applying 30 mmHg pressure. Interestingly all these patients had proven deep vein incompetence shown on duplex scanning and therefore were a subset of venous ulcers. Follow-up was from 6 to 69 months. Twenty-five patients were good compliers with compression and only one developed recurrence (4%). Of the 28 who complied poorly, 22 (79%) had at least one recurrence. The reasons for poor compliance were difficulty in applying or remembering how to apply the stockings and 78% complained at the cost of the stockings.[16] At the other end of the spectrum in a British study 138 healed ulcers were followed up for a minimum of 18 months: 96 patients wore class II compression stockings for at least 75% of the time and 36% of ulcers recurred by 18 months compared with 6% of the 42 patients who did not regularly wear their stockings: $p < 0.06$.[17] However, a 36% recurrence rate in patients at 18 months is still considerably better than the 69% recurrence rate at 1 year reported by Monk *et al.*[11]

There have been two further trials which have tried to compare different types of compression stockings. The first compared two similar below-knee class II stockings which produced a mean of 23 mmHg pressure at the ankle. When 166 patients were followed up for 18 months there was no significant difference between the recurrence rates between the groups. Cumulative recurrence rates were 26% at 1 year and 31%

at 18 months with 81 and 84% compliance rates. In this trial the recurrence rate for the 29 patients not complying with wearing stockings was 38% at 18 months. However, another 17 were deemed unsuitable for stockings and in 65% of those, ulcers recurred.[10]

The second trial compared class II (20–25 mmHg) stockings with class III (35–40 mmHg) stockings. In this trial 300 patients were randomized and then followed up for 3–5 years. At the end of this period, in 32% of those randomized to class II stockings, ulcers had recurred compared with only 21% recurring where class III stockings had been worn $p < 0.034$.[18] Therefore compression stockings continue to be widely held as the basis of preventing ulcer recurrence.

Pharmacological interventions

Stanozolol – anabolic steroid

Stanozolol was introduced in the treatment of venous ulcers because of its ability to enhance deficient fibrinolysis. It was hoped that it would work by reducing the 'fibrin cuff' which had been described outside vessels in venous ulceration. Despite high hopes it proved to be ineffective at preventing recurrence in a double-blind placebo study. Following 6 months treatment ulcers recurred in 7/25 (20%) of patients taking stanozolol and 4/23 (17%) of patients taking placebo. Having been shown to be ineffective but with a high incidence of side-effects and the potential for misuse in athletic activities, stanozolol is no longer available in the UK.[19,20]

Oxerutins

Oxerutins [O-(β-hydroxyethyl)-rutosides] have been demonstrated to reduce capillary leakage by an unknown mechanism. Potentially, they may therefore reduce fibrin or white cell leakage into the pericapillary tissues. Paroven® 500mg twice-daily (Zyma UK) was prescribed in a prospective randomized double-blind placebo controlled trial. In addition all patients received class II compression stockings. Of 138 patients who were followed up for 18 months, no benefit was found at the end of this time in 23% randomized to Paroven® recurring at 12 months increasing to 34% at 18 months compared with 22% and 32% for placebo.[17]

Surgery

The principle behind venous surgery to reduce recurrence is simply to remove the venous hypertension, which has been the cause of all the skin changes. However, achieving this simple aim, is far from simple. Whereas in the past it was thought that all venous ulcers were the result a 'post-phlebitic' limb, we know that in the majority of patients with venous ulcers there has never been any deep vein thrombosis (Fig. 2). In this study of 117 limbs, 87% had superficial disease and 38% had deep venous disease.

The mixture of disease raises several questions. If there is both superficial incompetence and perforator incompetence do the perforators become competent once the superficial veins have been operated on? If there is superficial and deep

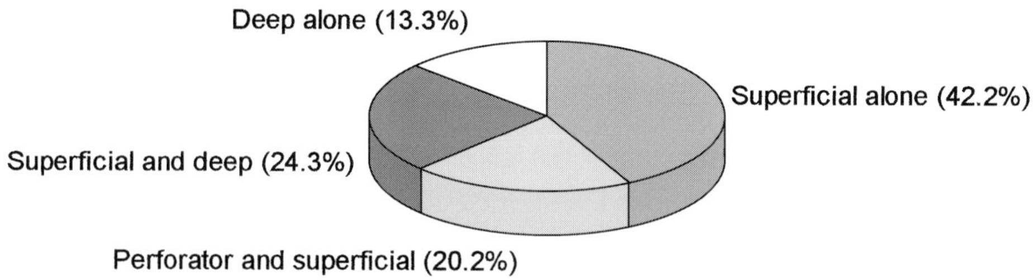

Fig. 2. Site of venous incompetence in 117 limbs with healed venous ulcers.

disease is there any point in only operating on the superficial veins? Can we predict which operations will be successful using functional tests such as photoplethysmography with and without tourniquets or using foot volumetry? Does successful venous surgery offer any benefit over good compression hosiery? What is the place of deep vein surgery? This chapter will not discuss the place of perforator surgery as it is covered in the next chapter by Meyer and Burnand (p. 275).

Preoperative assessment

If the aim is to abolish venous hypertension then a full venous assessment needs to be made before embarking on surgery. The main tool now in use is colour duplex ultrasonography. As with all methods of investigating veins it is heavily user-dependent. However, a skilled technologist will be able to demonstrate not only sites of major incompetence but also perforators. A full examination of deep veins will demonstrate if there has been previous thrombus leading to incompetence of deep veins, continued obstruction or recanalization. It is also possible to see isolated sections of deep venous incompetence which may be very difficult to demonstrate with ascending and descending venography due to competent valves either side of the affected segment. Functional assessment with plethysmography or measurement of ambulatory venous pressures can give additional information particularly with mixed venous disease. If tests are repeated with and without occlusion of superficial veins it is possible to predict which patients will benefit most from surgery. In addition Bradbury and Ruckley showed that if foot volumetry was used to assess venous function pre- and postoperatively it is possible to predict which patient's ulcers will recur on the basis of a failure to maintain improvement in the test.[21]

Surgery to the long and short saphenous systems

As indicated in Table 3, 43–69% of patients have superficial venous incompetence alone. For these patients superficial surgery with appropriate ligation of the incompetent saphenous junctions, removal of incompetent long saphenous vein in the thigh and removal of superficial incompetent veins with multiple avulsions should abolish the venous hypertension and reduce recurrence of the ulcer. Nash reported 42 such patients and there was only one minor recurrence within 3 years.[22] In our series on the Wirral reported above, one of 17 patients experienced recurrence

Table 3. Site of major venous incompetence in patients with venous ulcers

No of limbs	*Superficial*	*Superficial and deep*	*Deep*	*Ref*
235	43	35	22	23
117	62	24	13	24
95	44	39	7	25
120	69	31	?	26
82	59	41	50	27

over a mean of 30 months. However, superficial surgery is not always successful. Akesson looked at 30 limbs with a median 3½ year follow-up: 24% recurred but if the ambulatory venous pressure (AVP) was reduced to below 60 mmHg then only 11% recurred compared with 30% recurrence in those with higher AVPs postoperatively.[28] This serves to underline the benefit of functional testing to assess prognosis. Sethia and Darke showed that with careful superficial surgery the dorsal foot vein pressure is normalized even without carrying out perforator surgery.[29] They put this into practice with 54 patients and only six (11%) reulcerated within 3½ years. In these, missed short saphenous or popliteal incompetence accounted for persistence of venous hypertension.[23]

Most would therefore agree that patients with superficial venous incompetence and ulceration should be offered surgery. However, this is not straightforward, as the patients are often elderly and otherwise infirm. The mean age of our ulcer patients on the Wirral is 73 years and 19% died during the 2- to 3-year follow-up. Other reports do not mention the mortality rate in their patients. While carrying out the randomized trial of Paroven® in healed ulcers we assessed all 138 patients and only 48 were recommended for superficial surgery. The remaining 65% of patients were either not fit for surgery, did not want to consider surgery or also had deep disease.[17]

Perforator surgery

Open surgery is covered in the next chapter by Meyer and Burnand (p. 275) and endoscopic surgery in an earlier chapter by Stansby and Lintott (p. 241).

Deep venous disease causing ulceration

It is only in the last 15 years that it has been recognized that the classical appearances of the 'post-phlebitic' limb with lipodermatosclerosis, haemosiderin deposition, atrophy blanche and eczema may exist in the absence of any deep vein thrombosis. However, without doubt some people who have deep vein thrombosis progress to having the skin changes described above (Fig. 2). The majority of people who develop a truly post-phlebitic limb with ulceration have never been given adequate instructions on elevation and wearing of compression hosiery. About 6% of these patients subsequently develop ulceration, but even if they have not worn compression hosiery soon after their deep venous thrombosis, there is demonstrable benefit from starting compression later.[30] In a recent prospective study of 86 limbs for 1–11 years, only 12 limbs showed clinical deterioration and 3% developed new ulcers over that period. These data suggest that the prognosis is not nearly as bad as was reported in the 1950s.[31,32]

Following deep venous thrombosis two patterns emerge. First there is the obstructed limb which presents with swelling, 'venous claudication', skin changes and ulceration. Second there is the limb where the thrombosis recanalizes leading to destruction of deep venous valves and subsequent incompetent deep veins which is frequently associated with superficial and perforator incompetence as the blood seeks the easiest route to return to the heart.

Surgery for relief of venous obstruction

Saphenous vein cross-over bypass graft (Palma's operation)

There is a small group of patients that benefit from operation who have a unilateral iliac or iliofemoral occlusion. Ideally one should wait for about 4 years after the thrombosis so that maximum venous collaterals have had time to build up. Prerequisites are that there should be a healthy normal leg on the other side with a good long saphenous vein and iliac vein. On the diseased side there needs to be a clear section of femoral vein. This simple operation was devised by Palma to reroute the venous drainage from the femoral vein on the diseased side to the contralateral side. It is performed by swinging the contralateral long saphenous vein across the pubis and anastamosing it to a section of patent femoral vein on the diseased side. Some have added a temporary arteriovenous fistula distally to enhance flow initially. This is probably the only deep venous operation carried out in many centres in the UK which is a tribute to the success of the procedure although we could not find any recently published significantly large series.

Surgery for incompetent deep vein valves

Superficial venous surgery for segmental deep venous incompetence

If there is deep venous incompetence of, for example, the superficial femoral vein but there is competence of the popliteal vein below it, this can be considered to be segmental incompetence. In a mixed series Sottiurai found that, based on venography, in the presence of above-knee segmental incompetence, 14 of 33 (44%) ulcers healed.[33] In a separate study which included pre- and postoperative duplex scanning of 325 limbs 15% were found to have segmental deep venous incompetence; 42 limbs had superficial venous surgery alone and this resulted in abolition of reflux in 52% of these limbs. Where the segment of preoperative reflux was above the knee, 75% resolved with superficial surgery alone. In those with ulcers in this group, 83% healed their ulcer compared with 64% of those that had segmental reflux below the knee.[34] Therefore in this selected group of patients surgery is very rewarding.

Brachial valve transplant

This procedure consists of excision of a section of brachial vein containing one or two valves and then interposing this in the femoral or popliteal vein. However, the pressures exerted on arm vein valves are considerably lower than in the leg and the results have been poor. Cheatle reported a series of 21 patients; ten thrombosed soon after the operation and the transplanted valve continued to function in only two.[35] Sottiurai has reported that 39% of brachial venous valves were incompetent from the start.[33] Currently research is in progress to assess the possible use of a section of saphenous vein containing a valve which then has a metal stent attached at either end before placement in the popliteal vein as an endovascular procedure.[35]

Transposition

The incompetent vein, usually the superficial femoral vein is divided and re-inserted end-to-side, incorporating a competent valve in the adjacent vein, e.g. deep femoral vein or long saphenous. This has also not been very successful but series are small. Cheatle performed eight operations in combination with superficial surgery; two thrombosed, one developed recurrent reflux and two developed recurrent ulceration.[35]

Valve repair

Various approaches to an incompetent major valve have been described. Although most series say this is their preferred option in terms of functional results, clearly many patients who have had previous thrombosis do not have residual valves, as they have been destroyed in the thrombotic process. Where incompetent valves are found in the superficial femoral, popliteal or occasionally common femoral vein, competence is restored by direct suturing of the valve cusps to tighten them at their attachments to the vein wall. Alternatively external banding has been reported. When combined with superficial venous surgery ulcers have recurred in about one-third of patients.[33,36,37] A complete analysis of this procedure can be read in a previous chapter by Kroese (pp. 249–262).

Conclusion

While some centres have given hope for patients with intractable symptoms due to deep venous incompetence, many of these procedures are not carried out for venous ulceration. At a recent meeting of the Venous Forum of the Royal Society of Medicine held in Edinburgh, no-one in an audience of 250 people from all over the UK admitted to currently carrying out any of these procedures.

Skin grafting

Skin grafting has been shown to increase the healing rate of large venous ulcers.[38] However, there is very little information on the recurrence rates. As large ulcers are more commonly grafted and also large ulcers more commonly recur it is difficult to interpret the long-term results.[10] However, with new skin culture techniques being developed this is being actively studied. There are two types of cultured graft being pioneered. The first involves taking an 8mm punch biopsy from the patient; this can be transformed into 30cm^2 of keratinocyte culture in 3 weeks. The second type is a 'true' skin with both a dermis and epidermis and is a non-immunogenic culture of neonatal skin. It remains to be seen if either of these techniques will reduce recurrence. Theoretically the lack of scarred skin contracture with normal skin may be an advantage over keratinocyte culture.

CONCLUSION

Venous ulceration by its very nature is a chronic recurring condition. Although the mean age of patients is old, the age of presentation with a first ulcer is often many years earlier. Active intervention after first presentation significantly reduces episodes of recurrence and when recurrence does occur, early treatment with multilayer compression bandaging has been shown to achieve healing much more rapidly than if there is delay in recommencing full therapy. For the healed ulcer, good quality compression hosiery is essential and this needs to be renewed 6 monthly as the hosiery loses its elasticity. This strategy leads to demonstrable improvements in the affected leg. Pharmacological agents have not shown any significant benefit.

Full venous assessment will identify those patients in whom surgery is most likely to be of benefit. Where there is only superficial and perforator disease the superficial defects should be corrected first. On reassessment after this, if perforator disease persists there may be a place for perforator surgery but if there has been a previous deep venous thrombosis, this is not very successful. Isolated perforator disease is very rare. If there is segmental deep venous disease, superficial surgery may be of great benefit. However if there is deep venous incompetence, the results of surgery are mixed and deep vein surgery is not practised in the UK.

REFERENCES

1. Moffatt CJ, Franks PJ, Greenhalgh RM, McCollum CN *et al.*: Community clinics for leg ulcers and impact on healing. *Br Med J* **305**: 1389–1392, 1992
2. Moffatt CJ: Recurrence of leg ulcers within a community ulcer service. *J Wound Care* **4**: 57–61, 1995
3. Blair SD, Backhouse CM, McCollum CN: Sustained compression and healing of chronic venous ulcers. *Br Med J* **297**: 1159–1161, 1988
4. Simon DA, Freak L, McCollum CN *et al.*: Community leg ulcer clinics : a comparative study of two health authorities. *Br Med J* 312: 1648–1651: 1996
5. Moffatt CJ, Franks PJ, Greenhalgh RM: Community leg ulcer clinics: a four year review. *Proceedings 3rd European Conference on Advances in Wound Management, Oct 19–22 1993.* London: MacMillan Magazines, 1994
6. Nelzen O, Bergqvist D, Lindhagen A: Venous and non-venous leg ulcers: clinical history and appearance in a population study. *Br J Surg* **81**: 182–187, 1994
7. Callam MJ, Harper DR, Dale JJ, Ruckley CV: Chronic ulcer of the leg: clinical history. *Br Med J Clin Res* **294**: 1389–1391, 1987
8. Hansson C, Adersson E, Swanbeck G: A follow-up study of leg and foot ulcer patients *Acta Derm Venerol Stockh* **7**: 496–500, 1987
9. Cornwall J. Update on leg ulcer survey. *J Dist Nurse* **8**: 9–10, 1990
10. Franks PJ, Sharp EJ, Moffatt CJ: Risk factors for leg ulcer recurrence: A randomised trial of two types of compression stocking. *Age and Ageing* **24**: 490–494, 1995
11. Monk BE, Sarkany I: Outcome of treatment of venous stasis ulcers. *Clin Exp Dermatol* **7**: 397–400, 1982
12. Falanga V, Bucalo B: Use of a durometer to assess skin hardness. *J Am Acad Dermatol* **29**: 47–51, 1993
13. Mayberry JC, Moneta GL, DeFrang RD, Porter JM: The influence of elastic compression stockings on deep venous hemodynamics. *J Vasc Surg* **13** : 91–99, 1991

14. Abu-Own A, Shami SK, Chittenden SJ *et al.*: Microangiopathy of the skin and the effect of leg compression in patients with chronic venous insufficiency. *J Vasc Surg* **19**: 1074–1083, 1994
15. Partsch H: Compression therapy of the legs. *Dermatol Surg Oncol* **17**: 799–805, 1991
16. Samson RH, Showater DP: Stockings and the prevention of recurrent venous ulcers. *Dermatol Surg* **22**: 373–376, 1996
17. Wright DDI, Blair SD, McCollum CN: Oxerutins in the prevention of recurrence in chronic venous ulceration: randomized controlled trial. *Br J Surg* **78**: 1269–1270, 1991
18. Harper D, Nelson E, Gibson B *et al.*: A prospective randomised trial of class 2 and 3 compression in the prevention of venous ulceration. *Phlebology* **10**(Suppl 1): 872–873, 1995
19. McMullin G, Watkin G, Coleridge-Smith P et al.: The efficacy of fibrinolytic enhancement with stanozolol in the treatment of venous insufficiency. *Phlebology* **6**: 233–238, 1991
20. Stacey MC, Burnand KG, Layer GT, Pattison M: Transcutaneous oxygentensions in assessing the treatment of healed venous ulcers. *Br J Surg* **77**: 1050–1054, 1990
21. Bradbury AW, Ruckley CV: Foot volumetry can predict recurrent ulceration after subfascial ligation of perforators and saphenous ligation. *J Vasc Surg* **18**: 789–795, 1993
22. Nash TP: Venous ulceration: factors influencing recurrence after standard surgical proceedures. *Med J Austral* **154**: 48–50, 1991
23. Darke SG, Penfold C: Venous ulceration and saphenous ligation. *Eur J Vasc Surg* **6**: 4–9, 1992
24. Blair SD: Imaging to select patients with venous ulceration suitable for venous surgery.In: Greenhalgh RM (Ed) *Vascular Imaging for Surgeons* pp. 503–515. London: WB Saunders Co, 1995
25. Hanrahan LM, Araki CT, Rodriguez AA *et al.*: Distribution of valvular incompetence in patients with venous stasis ulceration. *J Vasc Surg* **13**: 805–812, 1991
26. Van Ridj AM, Solomon C, Christie R: Anatomic and physiologic characteristics of venous ulceration. *J Vasc Surg* **20**: 759–764, 1994
27. Scriven JM, Hartshorne T, London NJM *et al.*: Single visit venous ulcer assessment clinic : the first year. *Br J Surg* **84**: 334–336, 1997
28. Akesson H: Long-term clinical results following correction of incompetent superficial and perforating veins in patients with deep venous incompetence and ulcers. *Phlebology* **8**: 120–124, 1993
29. Sethia KK, Darke SG: Long saphenous incompetence as a cause of venous ulceration. *Br J Surg* **71**: 754–755. 1984
30. McCollum CN: Avoiding the consequences of deep vein thrombosis. *Br Med J* **317**: 696, 1998
31. Milne AA, Ruckley CV: The clinical course of patients following extensive deep venous thrombosis. *Eur J Vasc Surg* **8**: 56–59, 1994
32. Palma EG, Esperon R: Vein transplants and grafts in the surgical treatment of the post-phlebitic syndrome. *J Cardiovasc Surg* **1**: 94, 1960
33. Sottiurai VS: Surgical correction of recurrent venous ulcer. *J Cardiovasc Surg* **32**: 104–109, 1991
34. Bello AM, Scriven JM, London NJM *et al.*: The effect of superficial venous surgery on segmental deep venous reflux. *Proceedings Venous Forum* Edinburgh, 1998
35. Cheatle TR, Perrin M: Surgical Options in Post-thrombotic Syndrome. *Phlebology* **8**: 50–57, 1993
36. Scriven JM, Bello AM, London NJM *et al.*: The laboratory development of an endovenous valve transplantation device for the correction of popliteal vein reflux. *Proceedings Venous Forum* Edinburgh, 1998
37. Schanzer H, Skladany M, Peirce II EC: The role of external banding valvuloplasty in the surgical management of chronic deep venous disease. *Phlebology* **9**: 8–12, 1994
38. Poskitt KR, James AH, McCollum CN *et al.*: Pinch skin grafting or porcine dermis in venous ulcers: a randomised clinical trial. *Br Med J* **294**: 674–676, 1987

Commentary

There is no doubt that many patients in the community can expect more favourable outcomes as a result of the improvements in bandaging and nurse training documented by Blair and Hamsho. This improvement has to a considerable extent masked the fundamental problem of chronic leg represented by the hard core of intractable and recurrent ulcers. Data reviewed in this chapter show that even the most favourable series report around 30% of ulcerated legs failing to heal at 6 months, some never. Furthermore a substantial proportion, also around 30%, suffer recurrence of ulceration within 3 years, even with close attention to follow-up compression therapy.

Most chronic leg ulcers are of mixed aetiology so that it is usually more germane to talk of chronic leg ulcer than chronic venous ulcer. Experience suggests that the delays in management which a conservative approach incurs tend to reduce the prospects of success when the underlying vascular disorders are eventually tackled. The case for early diagnosis and early intervention is therefore cogently made by these authors. The problem of course, as these and other authors in this book point out, is that the deployment of surgical interventions is not evidence-based and often therefore not resourced. The case for better quality clinical research could not be more starkly apparent. *CVR*

The durability of perforating vein surgery for venous ulceration

FJ Meyer and Kevin G Burnand

INTRODUCTION

A venous ulcer is a solution of the continuity of the skin of the lower limb caused by an abnormality of the veins draining the limb.[1] There is no single venous abnormality that is always associated with ulceration and most of the changes in the skin and the ulcer base are non-specific.[2] The exact incidence of venous ulceration is thus difficult to ascertain. Epidemiological studies have estimated the prevalence of active leg ulceration in the United Kingdom at between 0.1 and 0.3%, with approximately 1% of the population being affected at some time in their lives.[3,4] About 70% of leg ulcers are associated with venous disease[3,4] and compression bandaging has been the mainstay of their treatment for centuries.[5] Randomized, controlled trials have shown that although 67–95% of venous leg ulcers will heal with compression bandaging within a year,[6,7] large numbers recur despite good medical treatment.[8] The greatest challenge in venous ulceration is to maintain skin integrity once an ulcer has healed and so prevent recurrence.

The deep and superficial venous systems of the lower limb are joined by communicating veins with valves that direct the blood from the superficial to the deep system. The two venous systems are separated by the deep fascia which is pierced by the communicating veins, hence the alternative label, perforating veins. They were first described by Verneuil in 1855[9] and more than 150 perforating veins have since been documented[10,11] although many of these are considered unimportant.[1] It has been suggested that medial calf perforating vein incompetence has an important aetiological role in the development of venous ulcers and that perforating vein ligation is important in healing and preventing recurrence.[12] To prove that this is the case, it must be shown that incompetent perforating veins are present in patients with venous ulceration, that perforating vein surgery improves venous function and that such surgery prevents ulcer recurrence.

PREVALENCE OF PERFORATING VEIN INCOMPETENCE IN VENOUS ULCERATION

Several groups have attempted to determine the prevalence of perforating vein incompetence in patients with leg ulcers. The results of these studies are summarized in Table 1. Although the methods used to determine perforating vein incompetence in these studies are somewhat inaccurate,[1] Haegar has stated that the calf perforating veins are always incompetent in patients with venous ulceration.[13] This echoes papers published as early as 1938 by Linton,[12,14] Cockett[15–17] and Turner-Warwick[18] suggesting that perforator incompetence is a prerequisite for ulcer development. Several studies have shown, however, that isolated perforator reflux occurs in only around 1–2% of ulcer patients.[19,20] It seems likely that while most venous ulcers are associated with perforator incompetence, this often co-exists with superficial or deep venous abnormalities and these may be responsible for most of the calf pump dysfunction observed.

Table 1. Incidence of perforating vein incompetence in limbs with venous ulcers

Authors	*Investigation techniques*	*Limbs*	*Incompetent perforating veins*	
			No	*%*
Dodd and Cockett (1956)[21]	Operative exploration	135	96	71
Haeger (1966)[13]	Operative exploration	54	54	100
Arnoldi and Haeger (1967)[22]	Operative exploration	509	509	100
Hoare *et al.* (1982)[23]	Ultrasound	80	71	88
Sethia and Darke (1984)[24]	Operative exploration	60	59	99
Negus (1985)[25]	Operative exploration	109	108	99
Thomas *et al.* (1986)[26]	Operative exploration	44	43	99
Pierik *et al.* (1997)[27]	Subfascial endoscopy	40	43 (+ 5 not identified by duplex)	100
	Duplex	40	46	100

Modified from Ref. 1

EFFECTS OF PERFORATING VEIN LIGATION ON VENOUS FUNCTION

In 1868, John Gay was the first to recognize that calf perforating veins might be involved in the genesis of venous ulceration. His theories were based on cadaveric dissections and later confirmed by animal experiments. He observed that ligating the femoral vein in dogs caused 'repletion of the intercommunicating veins and cutaneous capillary injection'.[28] Then John Homans, apparently unaware of Gay's work, reiterated and expanded the same ideas in 1917. Homans subdivided communicating vein incompetence into those associated with and presumably caused by the varicose process and those secondary to thrombosis.[29] He believed that the latter 'develop as an overflow or safety vent from the deep veins'. This hypothesis has never been disproved.

In the 1970s, Bjordal performed a series of elegant pressure-flow measurements which showed that ankle communicating vein reflux has a much smaller effect on calf pump function than saphenous incompetence.[30–34] This was not confirmed in similar studies by the St Mary's group, however.[35] Then in 1977, the Department of Surgery at St Thomas' compared foot vein pressure profiles before and after surgery in patients with a variety of phlebographically confirmed venous abnormalities.[36] It was found that although superficial venous surgery greatly improved pressure profiles, ligation of incompetent perforators in those patients with isolated perforator or combined deep venous and perforator incompetence did not restore calf pump function to normal. As the pressure profiles were similar in both the latter groups, it was suggested that those patients with isolated perforator incompetence probably had changes in their deep venous system which were not detected. These studies provide circumstantial support for Homans' views and also suggest that perforator surgery does not improve calf pump function.

Åkesson and colleagues[37] have examined the effect of staged surgical procedures on limb haemodynamics evaluated by occlusion plethysmography, foot volumetry and ambulatory venous pressure. This comprised superficial surgery followed by incompetent perforator eradication at least 6 months later. They found that perforator surgery conferred no measurable haemodynamic improvement after superficial surgery. Bradbury and Ruckley have investigated the ejection fraction and half refilling time in patients before and after perforator surgery (combined with superficial surgery where appropriate) and at the time of ulcer recurrence.[38] They found that limbs with both non-recurrence and recurrence showed significant haemodynamic improvements in the immediate postoperative period but that this was not maintained in patients whose ulcer recurred. This suggests that these individuals have previously undiagnosed deep venous pathology.

Other groups have examined the effects of saphenous surgery alone on perforator status. Campbell and West performed duplex ultrasonography in 185 limbs before and after superficial varicose vein surgery without perforator ligation.[39] They found that 80% of incompetent perforating veins regained competence postoperatively. Another study from Edinburgh also investigated the effects of saphenous surgery on perforator reflux.[40] In limbs with a normal deep venous system, they found that many incompetent perforators became competent following superficial surgery. A small minority, however, had residual communicating vein incompetence despite no duplex reflux being demonstrated. In those patients with deep venous reflux, a substantial number of perforators remained incompetent. This suggests that a small number of patients might benefit additionally from perforator ligation. Alternatively, it is possible that at least some of them have undetected deep venous damage. These papers discuss the effects of saphenous and perforator surgery on venous physiology, but they do not address the question of whether perforator ligation prevents ulcer recurrence.

RESULTS OF PERFORATING VEIN LIGATION

Calf perforating vein ligation was first described by Robert Linton in 1938[12] (Fig. 1). Alternative techniques have been proposed by Cockett,[15–17] De Palma,[41] Albanese[42] and others. De Palma and Albanese in particular were exploring methods of minimizing the skin trauma incurred during conventional perforator ligation. This has been dramatically reduced recently by the inception of subfascial endoscopic perforator ligation (SEPS) by Hauer in 1985[43] (Fig. 2). This innovation has rekindled interest in perforating vein surgery but there are few adequate data concerning its efficacy.

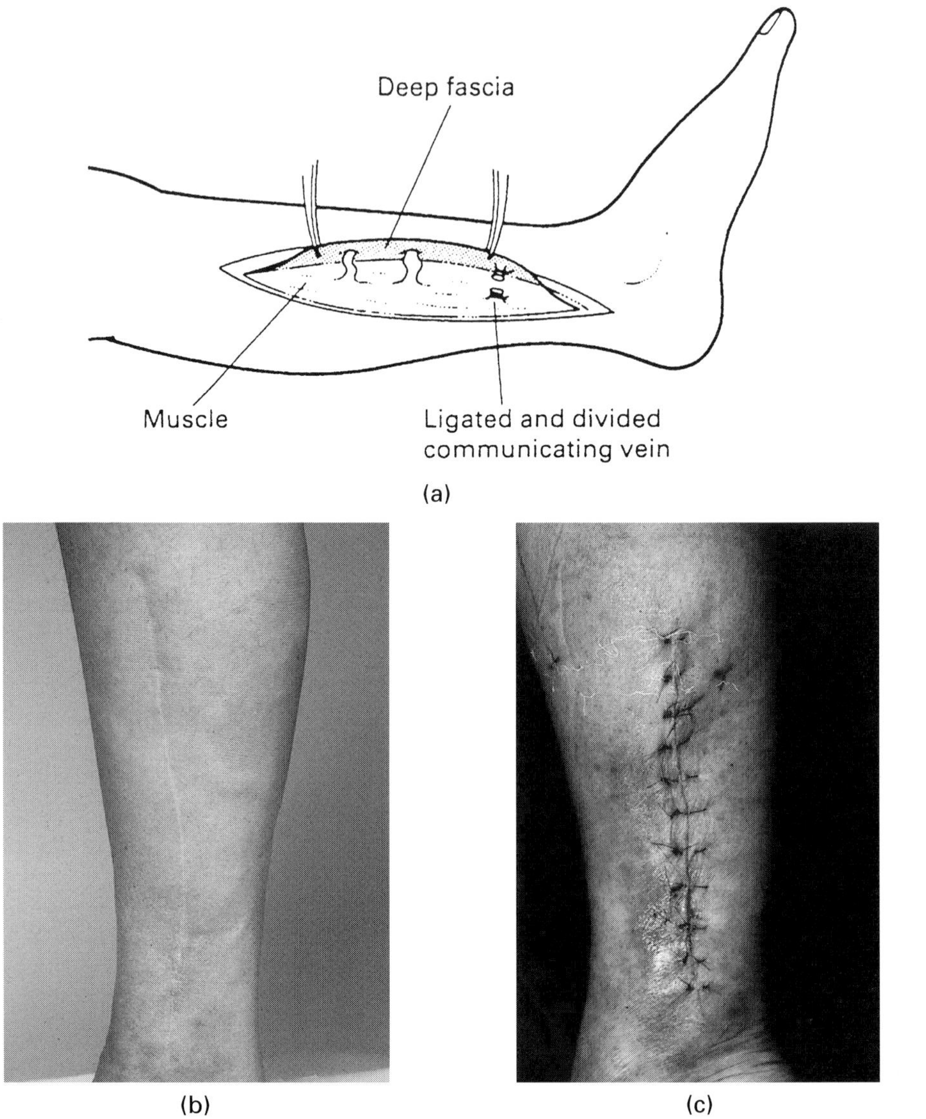

Fig. 1. Open subfascial ligation of medial calf perforating veins. (a) Operative approach. (b) Good wound healing 20 years after a Cockett's procedure. (c) Posterior skin flap necrosis following a Cockett's procedure.

There are no published prospective, randomized, controlled trials of perforator surgery for venous ulceration and most papers describe personal series of heterogenous patient groups. Reported ulcer recurrence rates vary between 0 and 51% depending on the nature of venous disease, concomitant venous surgery, use of postoperative compression hosiery and the length and adequacy of follow-up. A summary of studies identified from the literature is shown in Table 2.

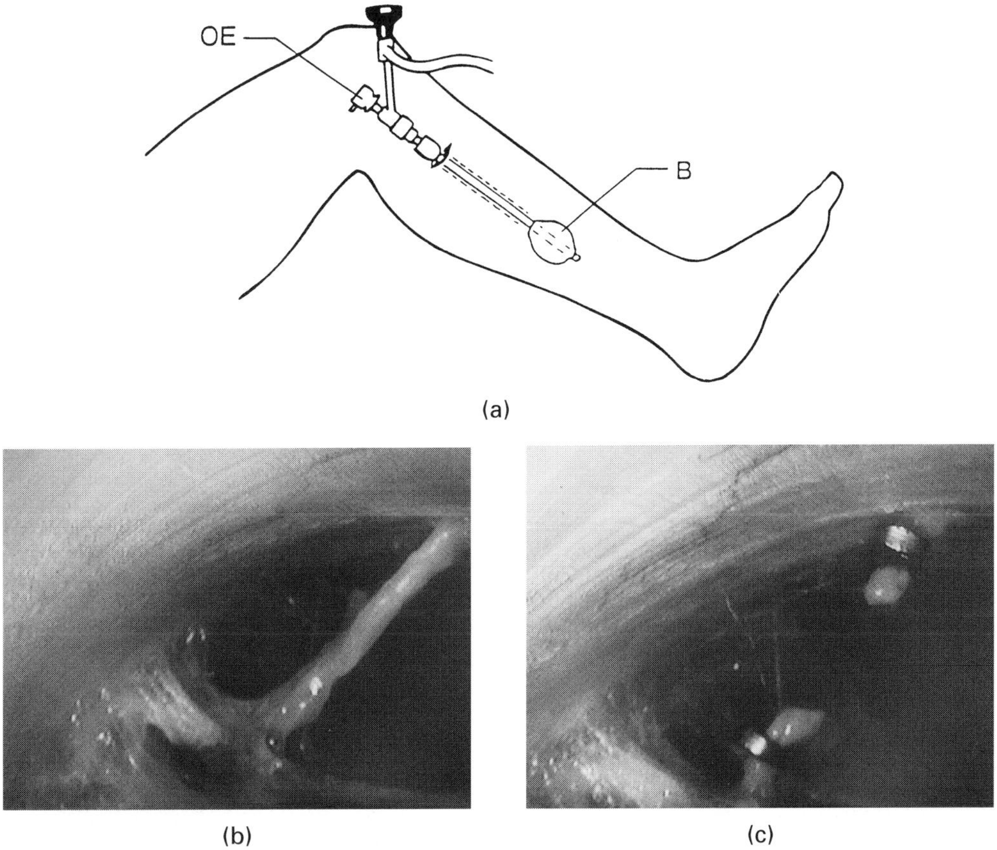

Fig. 2. Subfascial endoscopic ligation of medial calf perforating veins. (a) Operative approach: the operating endoscope (OE) inserted through a small incision, tissue dissection by balloon dilatation (B). (b) A perforating vein viewed through the operating endoscope. (c) The same perforator clipped and divided.

In 1976, the Department of Surgery at St Thomas' Hospital retrospectively examined the 5-year ulcer recurrence rate following combined superficial and perforator surgery in 41 patients.[44] None of the patients had been prescribed elastic stockings postoperatively. Phlebograms were performed on all subjects and reported as normal or post-phlebitic by an observer who was blinded to the clinical status of the patients. It was found that 23/24 patients with post-phlebitic limbs had ulcer recurrences at 5 years, whereas only 1/17 ulcers recurred in patients with normal phlebograms. More recently, Bradbury and co-workers also found that all their patients whose ulcers recurred had popliteal segment reflux.[45]

These results have not been reproduced by all other workers. Negus and Friedgood reported an overall recurrence rate of only around 15%, although there are some problems with this series.[46] The patient group was a mixture of those with normal and post-thrombotic deep veins. The extent of follow-up of the post-thrombotic patients is unclear and all subjects wore compression stockings postoperatively. Boggon's group also describe a recurrence rate of approximately 15% but there were few post-thrombotic patients included.[26] More recently, Pierik's group randomized patients to conventional or endoscopic perforator surgery.[47] They reported no recurrences in either group during a mean follow-up of 21 months but the deep venous status of these patients was not clear. Gloviczki and colleagues also published promising early results from SEPS.[48] They presented a later follow-up of these patients this year, however, which yielded a recurrence rate of 30% at 3 years.[49] Echoing the St Thomas's work of over 20 years ago, they showed that deep venous obstruction was a strong predictor of ulcer recurrence ($p < 0.0001$). None of this work compares surgery with medical treatment.

Table 2. The results of perforating vein surgery

Author	*Operation*	*Patients*	*Recurrence rate (%)*	*Follow-up*
Field and van Boxel (1971)[50]	Open	51	2	1–8 years
Silver *et al.* (1971)[51]	Open	28	10	64% >5 years
Thurston and Williams (1973)[52]	Open	89	13	3–84 months
Bowen (1975)[53]	Open	55	34	6 months–15 years
Burnand *et al.* (1976)[44]	Open	41	Postphlebitic 100% Others 6% (1/17)	up to 5 years
Blumenburg and Gelfland (1978)[54]	Open	16	4	6 months–6 years
de Palma (1979)[55]	Open	53	6	6 months–12 years
Hyde *et al.* (1981)[56]	Open	83	33	mean of 10 years
Almgren *et al.* (1982)[57]	Open	41	22	?
Negus and Friedgood (1982)[46]	Open	77	13	6 months–6 years
Cheung *et al.* (1985)[58]	Open	32	34	5 months–4 years
Johnson *et al.* (1985)[59]	Open	37	22	1 year
			41	3 years
			51	5 years
Wilkinson and Maclaren (1986)[60]	Open	108	2	6 months–9 years
Thomas *et al.* (1986)[26]	Open			
Szostek *et al.* (1988)[61]	Open	148	14.5	6 months–10 years
Cickrit *et al.* (1988)[62]	Open	32	22	6 months–10 years
Nash (1991)[63]	Open	90	18	3 years
Robison *et al.* (1992)[64]	Open	17	37	42 months
Bradbury *et al.* (1993)[45]	Open	53	26	3–144 months
Pierik *et al.* (1997)[47]	Open/SEPS	39	0	16–29 months
Gloviczki *et al.* (1998)[49]	SEPS	48	30	3 years

In view of the paucity of adequate data, we have conducted a randomized, controlled trial comparing the ulcer recurrence rate in 105 patients treated with either stanozolol (which has been shown to enhance fibrinolysis[65]) or surgery. Patients with healed venous ulcers were randomized to receive either 6 months oral stanozolol 5mg twice-daily or undergo superficial and perforator venous surgery and avulsions of minor varicosities as appropriate. All patients wore standard Sigvaris graduated compression stockings. In a separate study, a further 161 patients were treated conservatively and randomized to receive either Venosan 2002 or Scholl duofine (available on FP10) compression hosiery. The exclusion criteria used for both trials are listed in Table 3. All patients were followed up for 5 years or until their ulcer recurred, whichever was sooner. All affected limbs were assessed with foot volumetry and ascending and descending phlebograms. The results of both studies are summarized in Tables 4 and 5.

Table 3. Surgery versus stanozolol trial: exclusion criteria

Factors relating to ulcer aetiology	*Factors relating to stanozolol*
Ankle-brachial index <0.9	Prostatic carcinoma
Diabetes mellitus	Impaired hepatic function
Rheumatoid arthritis	Impaired renal function
SLE	Women under 40 years
Positive sickle cell test	Men under 18 years
Half refilling time >15s	Uncontrolled congestive cardiac failure
Clinically non-venous ulcers	Anticoagulant therapy
	Known stanozolol sensitivity

SLE: Systemic lupus erythematosus

Table 4. Results of surgery versus stanozolol

	Surgery	*Stanozolol*	*Statistical significance*
No of patients randomized	55	50	NS*
Number of patients completing treatment	42	41	NS*
Mean age (range)	58 (23–80)	59 (29–84)	NS*
No of patients with post-phlebitic change on phlebography	11	23	p <0.01*
Recurrence rate	10/42 (24%)	13/41 (32%)	NS*

* = $\chi 2$ test. NS: Not significant

Table 5. Results of Venosan versus Scholl stockings

	Venosan	*Scholl*	*Statistical significance*
No of patients randomized	84	77	NS*
Non-compliance with stockings	10/84 (11.9%)	18/77 (23.3%)	p <0.05*
No of patients with post-phlebitic change on phlebography	25/74 (34%)	23/45 (51%)	p <0.1*
Stockings only recurrence rate	37/74 (50%)	19/45 (42%)	NS*

* = $\chi 2$ test. NS: Not significant

This trial shows no significant benefit of surgery over stanozolol and stockings, despite the higher incidence of post-thrombotic damage in the pharmacological group. Both groups show an improvement compared with stockings alone. This concurs with earlier uncontrolled series which have suggested that superficial surgery decreases ulcer recurrence rates in those patients with normal deep veins.[66] In the stockings only study, the cheaper Scholl duofine FP10 hosiery was found to be as effective as the more expensive Venosan equivalent in compliant patients. The Venosan stockings were better tolerated, however, and a significant number of patients stopped wearing the Scholl stockings altogether.

CONCLUSIONS

The durability of perforating vein surgery for venous ulceration, particularly in the prevention of recurrence, remains unproven. Haemodynamic studies support Homans' ideas that perforator incompetence is caused by 'overflow' from refluxing superficial or deep venous systems. Many incompetent communicating veins become competent following long saphenous surgery provided the deep venous system is normal. There may be a small number of patients with isolated perforator incompetence who would benefit from perforator ligation. Endoscopic perforator surgery has reduced the complication rate following this type of procedure[47] but the increased incidence of peripheral nerve injury[67] in particular with this technique suggests that it should not be used indiscriminately. A multicentre, prospective, randomized, controlled trial of conservative management, SEPS alone, saphenous surgery alone and combined saphenous and perforator procedures in patients without post-phlebitic change on phlebography or popliteal vein incompetence on duplex has been proposed[68] and is vital to determine the role of perforator ligation in ulcer prevention.

REFERENCES

1. Browse NL, Burnand KG, Thomas ML: *Diseases of the Veins*. London: Edward Arnold, 1988
2. Rutter AG: Chronic ulcer of the leg in young subjects. *Surg Gyn Obstet* **98:** 291, 1954
3. Cornwall JV, Lewis JD: Leg ulcer revisited. *Br J Surg* **70:** 681, 1983
4. Callam MJ, Ruckley CV, Dale JJ, Harper DR: Chronic ulceration of the leg: extent of the problem and provision of care. *Br Med J* **290:** 1855, 1985
5. Marmasse J: La methode compressive a travers les ages. *Phlébologie* **32:** 119, 1979
6. Blair SD, Wright DDI, Backhouse CM *et al.*: Sustained compression and healing of chronic venous ulcers. *Br Med J* **297:**1159–1161, 1988
7. Burnand KG, Meyer FJ, Lagattolla NRF, Eastham D: unpublished data.
8. Browse NL: Venous ulceration. *Br Med J* **286:** 1920–1922, 1983
9. Verneuil A: Du siège réel et primitif des varices des membres inferieurs. *Gaz Méd Paris* **10:** 524, 1855
10. Raivió E: Untersuchungen über die Venen der unteren extremitaten mit besonderer berucksichtigung der gegenseit igen verbindugen zwischen den oberflachigen und tiefen Venen. *Ann Med Exp Finn* **26:** 1, 1948
11. van Limborgh J: L'anatomie du système veineux de l'extrémité inférieux en relation avec la pathologie variquese. *Fola Angiol* **8:** 3, 1961
12. Linton RR: The communicating veins of the lower leg and the operating technics for their ligation. *Ann Surg* **107:** 582, 1938
13. Haeger K: Three to six year results with standardized surgical therapy to venous ulcers. *Vasc Dis* **3:** 106, 1966
14. Linton RR, Hardy IB: Post-thrombotic syndrome of the lower extremity. Treatment by interruption of the superficial femoral vein and ligation and stripping of the long and short saphenous veins. *Surgery* **24:** 452, 1948
15. Cockett FB, Jones DE: The ankle blow-out syndrome. A new approach to the varicose ulcer problem. *Lancet* **i:** 17, 1953
16. Cockett FB: Diagnosis and surgery of high pressure venous leaks in the leg: a new overall concept of surgery of varicose veins and venous ulcers. *Br Med J* **2:** 1399, 1956
17. Cockett FB: The pathology and treatment of venous ulcers of the leg. *Br J Surg* **43:** 260, 1955

18. Turner-Warwick W: *The Rational Treatment of Varicose Veins and Varicocele (with notes on the obliterative method of treatment to other conditions)*. London: Faber and Faber, 1931
19. Hanrahan LM, Araki CT, Rodriguez AA *et al.*: Distribution of valvular incompetence in patients with venous stasis ulceration. *J Vasc Surg* **13:** 805–812, 1993
20. Labropoulous N, Delis K, Nicolaides AN *et al.*: The role of the distribution and anatomic extent of reflux in the development of signs and symptoms of chronic venous insufficiency. *J Vasc Surg* **23:** 504–510, 1996
21. Dodd H, Cockett FB. *The Pathology and Surgery of the Veins of the Lower Limb*. Edinburgh: Livingstone, 1956
22. Arnoldi CC, Haeger K: Ulcus Cruris Venosum – Crux medicorum. *Läkartidningen* **64:** 2149, 1967
23. Hoare MC, Nicolaides AN, Miles CR *et al.*: The role of primary varicose veins in venous ulceration. *Surgery* **92:** 450, 1982
24. Sethia KK, Darke SG: Long saphenous incompetence as a cause if venous ulceration. *Br J Surg* **71:** 754, 1984
25. Negus D: Prevention and treatment of venous ulceration. *Ann Roy Coll Surg Engl* **67:** 144, 1985
26. Thomas AMC, Tomlinson PJ, Boggon RP: Incompetent perforating vein ligation in the treatment of venous ulceration. *Ann Roy Coll Surg Engl* **68:** 214, 1986
27. Pierik EG, van Urk H, Wittens CH: Efficacy of subfascial endoscopy in eradicating perforating veins of the lower leg and its relation with venous ulcer. *J Vasc Surg* **26:** 255–259, 1997
28. Gay J: *Varicose Disease of the Lower Extremities and its Allied Disorders: Skin Discolouration, Induration and Ulcer*. London: Churchill, 1968
29. Homans J: The etiology and treatment of varicose ulcer of the leg. *Surg Gyn Obstet* **24:** 300, 1917
30. Bjordal RI: Simultaneous pressure and flow readings in varicose veins of the lower extremity. *Acta Chir Scand* **136:** 309, 1970
31. Bjordal RI: Pressure patterns in the saphenous system in patients with venous leg ulcers. *Acta Chir Scand* **137:** 495–501, 1971
32. Bjordal RI: Circulation patterns in incompetent perforating veins in the calf and in the saphenous system in primary varicose veins. *Acta Chir Scand* **138:** 251–261, 1972
33. Bjordal RI: Blood circulation in varicose veins of the lower extremities. *Angiology* **23:** 163–73, 1972
34. Bjordal RI: Circulation patterns in the saphenous system and the perforating veins in the calf of patients with previous deep vein thrombosis. *VASA* **3** (Supp): 1–41, 1974
35. Zukowski AJ, Nicolaides AN, Szendro G *et al.*: Haemodynamic significance of incompetent calf perforating veins. *Br J Surg* **78:** 625–629, 1991
36. Burnand KG, O'Donnell TF Jr, Lea Thomas M, Browse NL: The relative importance of incompetent communicating veins in the production of varicose veins and venous ulcers. *Surgery* **82:** 9–14, 1977
37. Åkesson H, Brudin L, Cwikiel W *et al.*: Does the correction of insufficient superficial and perforating veins improve venous function in patients with deep venous insufficiency? *Phlebology* **5:** 113–123, 1991
38. Bradbury AW, Ruckley CV: Foot volumetry can predict recurrent ulceration after subfascial ligation of perforators and saphenous ligation. *J Vasc Surg* **18:** 789–795, 1993
39. Campbell WA, West A: Duplex ultrasound audit of operative treatment of primary varicose veins. *Phlebology* **1** (Suppl): 407–409, 1995
40. Stuart WP: Perforator Surgery: What is its role? In: Ruckley CV, Fowkes FGR, Bradbury AW (Eds) *Venous Disease: Epidemiology, Management and Delivery of Care* pp. 132–138. London: Springer-Verlag, 1999
41. de Palma RG: Surgical therapy for venous stasis. *Surgery* **76:** 910, 1974
42. Albanese AR: New instruments of varicose vein surgery. *J Cardiovasc Surg* **6:** 65, 1965
43. Hauer G: Die endoscopische subfasciale Diszision der Perforansvenen: vorlaufige Hitteilung. *VASA* **14:** 59–61, 1985
44. Burnand KG, Thomas ML, O'Donnell T, Browse NL: Relation between postphlebitic

change in the deep veins and the results of surgical treatment of venous ulcers. *Lancet* **i:** 936–938, 1976

45. Bradbury AW, Stonebridge PA, Callam MJ *et al.*: Foot volumetry and duplex ultrasonography in patients with recurrent venous ulceration after saphenous and perforating vein ligation. *Br J Surg* **80:** 845–848, 1993
46. Negus D, Friedgood A: The effective management of venous ulceration. *Br J Surg* **70:** 623–627, 1983
47. Pierik EG, van Urk H, Hop WC, Wittens CH: Endoscopic versus open subfascial division of incompetent perforating veins in the treatment of venous leg ulceration: a randomized trial. *J Vasc Surg* **26:** 1049–1054, 1997
48. Gloviczki P, Cambria RA, Rhee RY *et al.*: Surgical technique and preliminary results of endoscopic subfascial division of perforating veins. *J Vasc Surg* **23:** 517–523, 1996
49. Gloviczki P, Rhodes JM, Canton LG, Rooke T: The management of incompetent perforating veins. *XIII World Congress of Phlebology* Abstract 55: 53, 1998
50. Field P, van Boxel P: The role of the Linton flap procedure in the management of stasis dermatitis and ulceration in the lower limb. *Surgery* **70:** 920–926, 1971
51. Silver D, Gleysteen JJ, Rhodes GR et al: Surgical treatment of the refractory post-phlebitic ulcer. *Arch Surg* **103:** 554–560, 1971
52. Thurston OG, Williams HTG: Chronic venous insufficiency in the lower extremity: pathogenesis and surgical treatment. *Arch Surg* **106:** 537–539, 1973
53. Bowen FH: Subfascial ligation (Linton operation) of the perforating leg veins to treat post-thrombophlebitic syndrome. *Am Surg* **41:** 148–151, 1975
54. Blumenburg RM, Gelfland ML: The posterior stocking seam approach to radical subfascial clipping of perforating veins. *Am J Surg* **136:** 202–205, 1978
55. de Palma RG: Surgical treatment for venous stasis: results of a modified Linton operation. *Am J Surg* **137:** 810–813, 1979
56. Hyde GL, Litton TC, Hull DA: Long-term results of subfascial vein ligation for venous stasis disease. *Surg Gyn Obstet* **153:** 683–686, 1981
57. Almgren B, Bowald S Eriksson I, Forsberg O: The posterior approach for the subfascial ligation of perforating veins. *Acta Chir Scand* **148:** 243–245, 1982
58. Cheung PS, Lim ST, Ng A: Evaluation of the posterior approach for subfascial ligation of perforator veins. *Aust NZ J Surg* **55:** 369–372, 1985
59. Johnson WC, O'Hara ET, Corey C *et al.*: Venous stasis ulceration: effectiveness of subfascial ligation. *Arch Surg* **120:** 797–800, 1985
60. Wilkinson JE, Maclaren IF: Long term review of procedures for venous perforator insufficiency. *Surg Gyn Obstet* **163:** 117–120, 1986
61. Szostek M, Skorski M, Zajac S *et al.*: Recurrences after surgical treatment of patients with post-thrombotic syndrome of the lower extremities. *Eur J Vasc Surg* **2:** 191–192, 1988
62. Cickrit DF, Nichols WK, Silver D: Surgical management of refractory venous stasis ulceration. *J Vasc Surg* **7:** 473–478, 1988
63. Nash TP: Venous ulceration: Factors influencing recurrence after standard surgical procedures. *Med J Aust* **154:** 48–50, 1991
64. Robison JG, Elliot BM, Kaplan AJ: Limitations of subfascial ligation for refractory chronic venous stasis ulceration. *Ann Vasc Surg* **6:** 9–14, 1992
65. Davidson JF, Lockhead M, McDonald GA, McNichol GP: Fibrinolytic enhancement by stanozolol: a double blind trial. *Br J Haematol* **22:** 543, 1972
66. Darke SG, Penfold C: Venous ulceration and saphenous ligation. *Eur J Vasc Surg* **6:** 4–9, 1992
67. Whiteley MS, Galland RB, Smith JJ: Subfascial endoscopic perforator vein surgery (SEPS): current practice among British surgeons. *Ann Roy Coll Surg Engl* **80:** 104–107, 1998
68. Ruckley CV, Makhdoomi KR: The venous perforator. *Br J Surg* **83:** 1492–1493, 1996

Commentary

'Perforator surgery' as a descriptive term for a surgical procedure is rather like 'vagotomy', that former happy hunting ground for gastric surgeons. Many different techniques have been described. Technical prowess is related to the number of serves (veins) located. There is uncertainty as to the physiological functions of the target structures and 'incompleteness' may be associated with recurrence.

The analogy falls short, however, as judged by the studies reviewed by Meyer and Burnand, in that physiological (haemodynamic) tests, unlike the insulin secretion test, cannot be used to measure the success or otherwise of perforator interruption. Anatomically the task falls to duplex scanning. Therapeutically, clinical trials are awaited. Qualitative reports contribute little.

The whole field of perforator surgery lacks precision and objectivity. Until perforator surgery is prefaced by analysis of valvular incompetence, not merely of perforators but also of their connecting deep and superficial systems, and until it is followed by measurement of the completeness of the perforator interruption, together with objective analysis of short- and long-term clinical outcome in precisely defined diseases, the indications will remain obscure and we will continue to flounder in our current intellectual quagmire. *CVR*

PERIPHERAL VASCULAR DURABILITY CONTROVERSIES

Methodological problems related to follow-up and patency assessment

Leif Panduro Jensen and Torben Veith Schroeder

INTRODUCTION

A number of studies are concerned with outcome in terms of patency or survival of special groups of patients – for example those having a distal bypass and suffering from diabetes. Vascular surgeons today know the basics of how to assess these parameters using life-table methods. However, a large number of methodological factors, starting with the design of the study are important too.[1–4]

STUDY DESIGN AND DATA COLLECTION

The optimal design is a prospective protocol which includes a consecutive quite large number of patients within a short period of time. Patients can then be expected to be treated relatively equally. However, many published series are retrospective, or more recently, data may be collected prospectively in a registry, but the questions are asked retrospectively. In such instances, the handling of patients may not necessarily have followed a well-defined protocol, especially so if data have been collected over a 5- or 10-year period.

In a controlled prospective trial the course and handling of data are clearly defined. This need not be the case in less controlled settings, as may be the case with a registry, in which a number of doctors complete the forms to the best of their ability. The data quality suffers under these circumstances. Efforts should be directed towards minimizing the effect of different sources of errors:

1. All data entry points should be accompanied by clearly stated definitions, preferably in accordance with international standards, to avoid interpersonal differences in the registration.
2. Also the outcome indicators (events) should be clearly defined. A classical problem is criteria for patency: only objective findings are acceptable whether based on pressure measurements or imaging modalities.
3. All entry points should be exclusive and exhaustive, thus achieving no overlapping of data and matching of any variable entries.
4. Minimize the number of data transformations, e.g. from datasheets to computer, to avoid random (typing) errors.

Equally important is the data validation, for errors and completeness.[5] Errors are unavoidable, and the validation process seeks to identify as many as possible. In many instances the errors can be corrected, but in others it is impossible. It is then important to get an impression of the magnitude of problem, which should be clearly stated when presenting the data. This goes for completeness as well; if some data are missing it will influence the results.

STATISTICAL ESTIMATION OF OUTCOME – SURVIVAL ANALYSIS: ANALYSIS OF DICHOTOMOUS OUTCOMES

In follow-up studies of, for example, patency or survival, the outcome variable of interest is the time until an event occurs. Patients are likely to have been observed for a varying length of time, some having had surgery a long time before, others having been operated on recently. Some grafts will have occluded or patients will have died, at times which can be ascertained relatively accurately; others may have been lost to follow-up for various reasons between one examination and the next or withdrawn from the study for medical reasons, perhaps by the intervention of some other disease or by an accidental death. In general, the methods used for analysis allow for the proper recognition of incomplete data from patient drop-out. Data may be affected by the following three factors:

1. Withdrawal before an event occurs.
2. An intervening event prohibits further observation.
3. Observation is terminated before an event occurs.

Withdrawals are assumed to be subject to the same probabilities of event as the non-withdrawals. This is a reasonable assumption for withdrawn patients who are still in the study and will be available for future follow-up. However, patients lost to follow-up may be lost for health reasons and that assumption could be wrong. Another assumption is that the probabilities remain reasonably constant over time. Finally no survival information is available for periods of follow-up longer than the maximum observed in the study and it is important to include the initial failure or deaths, a fact that has been forgotten in some older publications.

The graphical representation should also include information to allow the validity of the data to be checked. Underwood considered how to present the validity of life-table plots and suggested that the graphic presentation should include the number of patients at risk.[6] He also considered demanding presentation of the number of patients lost to follow-up, but concluded that the number at risk would be sufficient, as weak data would be revealed through this parameter alone. Alternatively, the standard error for each estimate can be displayed and when the 95% confidence interval of the event rate estimate exceeds ±10% the curve should either not be shown, or made dotted. As shown in Fig. 1 this recommendation is not always followed.[7]

Life-table methods of reporting were widely adopted during the 1970s and 1980s, both in the USA and Europe.[1,2,8] In 1986 an *Ad Hoc Committee on Reporting Standards* in USA stated that 'the life-table method is probably the best commonly used way of presenting patency data'. It was suggested, that reports with patency

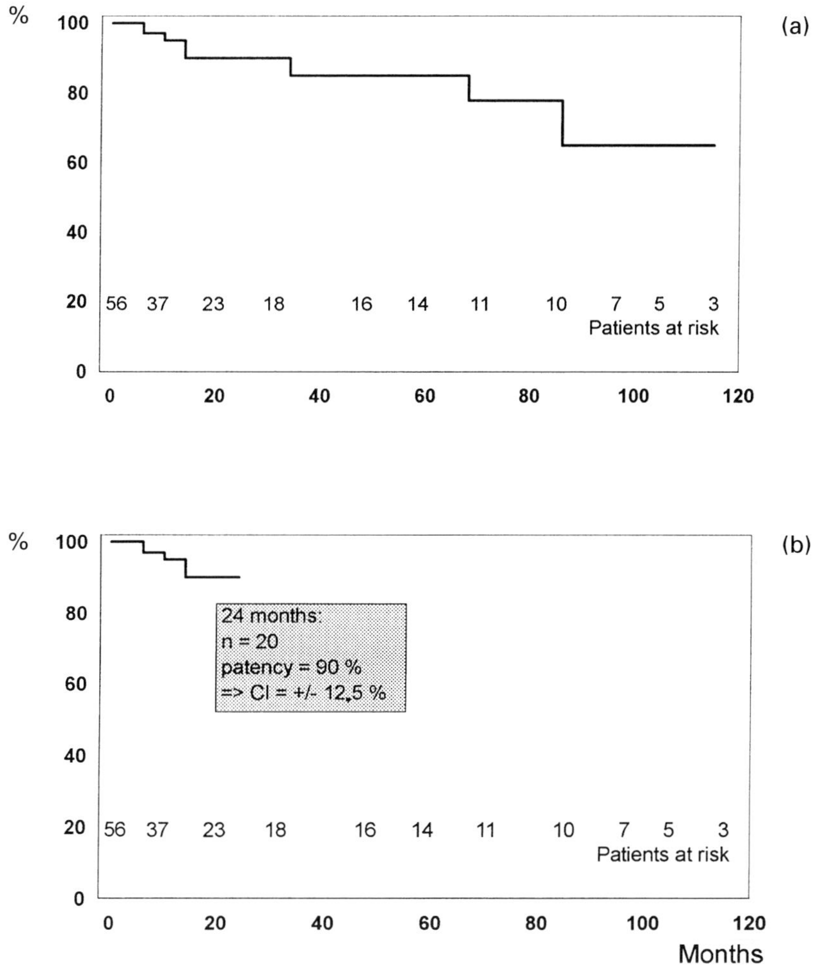

Fig. 1. (a) Long-term survival after carotid endarterectomy in 56 patients followed for up to 10 years, as reported in Ref. 7. (b) Same data as in (a), but patency curve is not shown when the 95% confidence interval of the event rate estimate exceeded ±10%

data for each time interval besides the cumulated patency should include tables on number of grafts at risk, number of occluded grafts and number of withdrawn patent grafts, subdivided into the withdrawal due to short duration, death or loss to follow-up. It is suitable when data are presented at intervals, but in recent years it has become common to present data in Kaplan–Meier plots with a continuous time axis, which would result in an extensive table corresponding to the graphical presentation.[9]

SURVEY OF CLINICAL FOLLOW-UP PAPERS PUBLISHED 1997/98

Suspecting that the reporting of survival data may be variable, we analysed papers published in *European Journal of Vascular and Endovascular Surgery*, 1997/98. Of 135 original articles, 41 (30%) were clinical with some element of follow-up. These 41 publications were examined for completeness of follow-up and fate of patients lost to follow-up/withdrawals as well as the presentation of patency rates, specifically whether numbers were stated for the patients at risk at the start of each interval, when using life-table methods, or periodically, when using the Kaplan–Meier survival estimate.

Most articles were based on prospective studies (21; 51%) or prospectively collected data (5; 12%), while 15 (37%) were based on retrospectively collected data. Defining complete follow-up as 90% or more, 12 (29%) papers met this requirement, while in eight (20%) papers follow-up was less complete. Surprisingly, 21 (51%) articles did not contain sufficient information to permit assessment of the completeness of follow-up (Table 1). Moreover, the cause of withdrawal or the reason that some patients were lost to follow-up were not stated in 10 (24%) of the papers.

Follow-up results were presented graphically in 23 (56%) papers, but in seven (30%) without stating the numbers for the patients at risk at various time intervals.

Table 1. Result of a survey of 41 clinical follow-up papers published in *Eur J Vasc Endovasc Surg* 1997/98

	No of studies	*Completeness of follow-up uncertain*		*Fate of lost patients uncertain*	
		No	*(%)*	*No*	*(%)*
Prospective	21	9	(43)	6	(29)
Retrospective studies based on prospective registry data	5	2	(40)	1	(20)
Retrospective	15	10	(67)	3	(20)

VASCULAR REGISTRIES

In recent years vascular registries have multiplied as part of an imperitive to audit.[10–14] Life-table calculations on large groups of patients have been greatly simplified. However, routine registry-based data always increases the number of patients lost to follow-up compared with a prospective study. This is easily forgotten when large groups of patients are observed: at the time of follow-up, hundreds of patients may remain at risk and the Kaplan–Meier calculations produce narrow standard deviations, indicating a high degree of data validity. Still, some patients may be lost without invalidating the life-table calculations. At least this has been the general impression, because withdrawn patients were considered to have the same distribution of events as the patients with a complete follow-up.[3,4]

VALIDATION OF OUTCOME IN PATIENTS LOST TO FOLLOW-UP

Some years ago we questioned the assumption that patients lost to follow-up behaved like patients with complete follow-up, by comparing patency rates calculated on the basis of a standard vascular registry with those obtained as part of a prospective, randomized trial in which follow-up was complete. Since 1989 all patients undergoing infrainguinal bypass procedures have been offered a standard follow-up programme using 3 months intervals and all data have been recorded

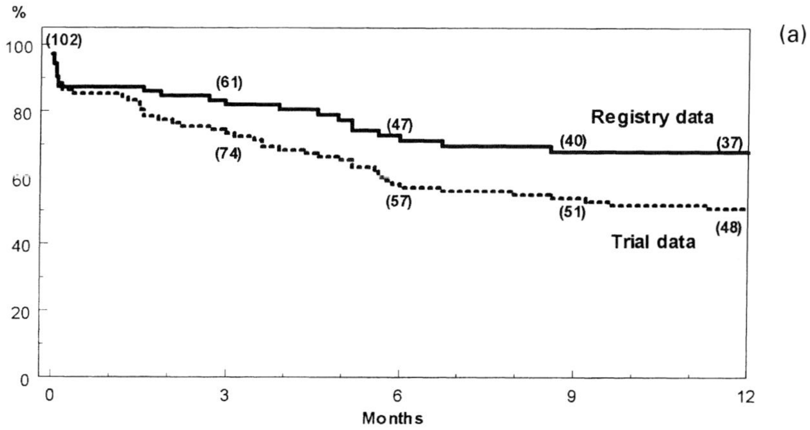

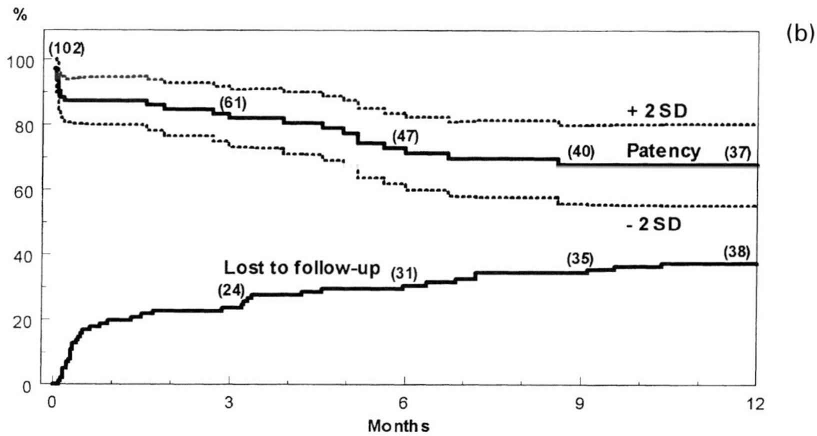

Fig. 2. (a) Comparison of the cumulated primary patency between the registry data (__) and the trial data (....).[15] (b) Primary patency as reported by the vascular registry (__), including 95% confidence intervals (...). In addition to the standard presentation of the number of patients at risk, data on number of patients lost to follow-up are presented as absolute numbers at given time, as well as a graphic

prospectively in a vascular registry.[15] As part of a randomized trial on adjuvant medication in femorocrural bypass surgery, 102 patients, operated on between 1990 and 1992 were independently and simultaneously monitored. This subgroup was examined 3 and 12 months postoperatively and 100% follow-up was obtained. After completion of the trial we calculated the patency and survival rates using life-table methods and compared the results based on the vascular registry with those achieved in the clinical trial.

A marked discrepancy appeared between the calculated figures: primary (68% in the registry and 52% in the trial) (Fig. 2) and secondary patency rates (90% vs 63%), limb survival (97% vs 77% as well as patients survival rates (95% vs 85%). The differences could be explained by a substantial number of patients being lost to follow-up according to the vascular registry database and the fact that these patients turned out to have a significantly increased rate of graft thrombosis, limb amputation and death, respectively (Table 2).

Table 2. Number of events for patients with complete 1-year follow-up and for the patients who were lost to follow-up in the vascular registry

	Complete follow-up			*Lost to follow-up*			*χ^2-test*
	No.	*Events*	*%*	*No.*	*Events*	*%*	*p*
Primary patency	64	26	41	38	23	61	0.05
Secondary patency	58	9	16	44	29	66	< 0.0005
Limb survival	52	2	4	50	20	40	< 0.0005
Patient survival	51	4	8	51	13	26	0.0005

Data from Ref. 15.

DISCUSSION

Since reporting standards for vascular surgery were widely adopted in the mid-1980s,[1,3,8,9] there is still a significant proportion of clinical papers, at least in the *European Journal of Vascular and Endovascular Surgery*, that do not report the results in accordance with these standards. This lack of standardized reporting leads to difficulty in the interpretation of data. One has to have confidence in the authors to have achieved complete follow-up, and not to have overstated their conclusions. Our survey of the papers with follow-up data in the *European Journal of Vascular and Endovascular Surgery* demonstrated that there is still a tendency not to report the number of patients in graphic survival presentations, and also to present survival data beyond the 95% confidence level of ±10%, where data become dubious. Not only does the presentation of data create problems, but also complete data, especially follow-up data, are often lacking. We made the unpleasant discovery that life-table statistics may inadvertently become unreliable if a larger proportion of patients is lost to follow-up, since failure to examine the patient for any reason may be related to the patient's health.

We believe that these observations may reflect a general problem in interpreting retrospective as well as prospectively collected data, including data from vascular registries and that reports tend to be too optimistic, if complete or near complete follow-up is not obtained. The lack of explicit information on the number of patients lost to follow-up in the reported survey indicates that this problem might be more frequent than realised. If any information exists it is usually in the form of total number withdrawn.

This raises the need for a fairly simple method of establishing the quality of follow-up data from the vascular registry. In addition to the number of patients at risk we suggest that any life-table calculations should include the number of patients lost to follow-up, presented as a number at a given time interval, or better, presented graphically as part of the Kaplan–Meier plot (Fig. 2b). In both instances, the validity of the follow-up can be estimated at a glance. Moreover, it is important to define when patients are considered lost to follow-up, i.e. the acceptable time interval between the last follow-up and the time of analysis or death. Increasing the acceptable time interval raises the risk that the event in question has occurred, but remain unregistered.

RECOMMENDATIONS

The increasing use of vascular registries and reporting of results from these, necessitates a simple way of stating the validity of follow-up. We recommend, that standards for analysing and reporting are used more carefully – in fact we suggest, that the basic rules put down in the guidelines to authors in the *European Journal of Vascular and Endovascular Surgery* are enforced. Explicitly, life-table data should always contain information on the number of patients lost to follow-up, the reason for premature termination of follow-up, in addition to the number of patients at risk. Moreover, it is suggested, that life-table plots could include visual information on the number of patients lost to follow-up. If follow-up is not complete, results tend to be too optimistic – an important observation to bear in mind when reading an article.

REFERENCES

1. Rutherford RB, Flanigan DP, Gupta SK *et al.*: Suggested standards for reports dealing with lower extremity ischemia. *J Vasc Surg* **4**: 80–94, 1986
2. Rutherford RB, Baker JD, Ernst C *et al.*: Recommended standards for reports dealing with lower extremity ischemia: revised version. *J Vasc Surg* **26**: 517–538, 1997
3. Armitage P: Survivorship tables. In: Armitage P. *Statistical Methods in Medical Research* pp. 408–415. Oxford: Blackwell Scientific Publications, 1980
4. McNeil D: *Epidemiological Research Methods* pp. 195–232. New York: John Wiley, 1996
5. Steering Committee of Swedvasc: Auditing Surgical Outcome. Ten years with the Swedish vascular registry – Swedvasc. *Eur J Surg* **164** (Suppl 581) 1–47, 1998
6. Underwood J, Faragher B, Charlesworth D: The uses and abuses of life-table methods in vascular surgery. *J Surg* **71**: 495–498, 1984
7. Eckstein HH, Schumacher H, Laubach H *et al.*: Early carotid endarterectomy after non-disabling ischaemic stroke: Adequate therapeutical option in selected patients. *Eur J Vasc Endovasc Surg* **15**: 423–428, 1998

8. Bonnevie O, Juhl E, Andersen B, Winkel P: Survival models in clinical research. *Ugeskr Læg* **133**: 1859–1864, 1971
9. Kaplan E, Meier P: Nonparametric estimation from incomplete observations. *J Am Stat Assoc* **53**: 457–481, 1958
10. Jensen LP, Schroeder TV, Lorentzen JE: *In situ* saphenous vein bypass surgery in diabetic patients. *Eur J Vasc Surg* **6**: 533–539, 1992
11. Bergqvist D, Troëng T, Einarsson E *et al.*: Vascular surgical audit during a 5-year period. *Eur J Vasc Surg* **8**: 472–477, 1994
12. Kuukasjärvi P, Salenius JP and the Finnvasc Study Group: Perioperative outcome of acute lower limb ischaemia on the basis of the National Vascular Registry. *Eur J Vasc Surg* **8**: 578–583, 1994
13. Van den Akker PJ, van Bockel JH, Brand R, van Schilfgaarde R: Computerised vascular data managment: a flexible modular registry suitable for the evaluation of long-term results in patients subjected to multiple interventions. *Eur J Vasc Surg* **5**: 459–465, 1991
14. Jensen LP, Schroeder T, Madsen PV, Lorentzen JE: Vascular registers in Denmark based on personal computers. *Ann Chir Gyn* **81**: 253–256, 1992
15. Jensen LP, Nielsen OM, Schroeder TV: The importance of complete follow-up for results after femoro-infrapopliteal vascular surgery. *Eur J Vasc Endovasc Surg* **12**: 282–286, 1996

Commentary

The authors have recognized that a wide ranging standard of reporting continues and have based their data on two volumes of the *European Journal of Vascular and Endovascular Surgery* until June 1998. They have made a number of points, but especially they have noted the difference in quality of data of prospective studies compared with registries. Often doctors filling in forms for registries have no sense of ownership of the data and such data must, inevitably, be of lower quality than the data from prospective studies where individuals have a much greater sense of ownership and responsibility for the data which will be published in their name. The authors indicate how easily life-table analyses can be performed on registries, but that there are always many more patients lost to follow-up in audit registries than in prospective studies. It would not matter if those lost to follow-up had similar outcomes as those remaining in consideration. However, the authors have shown that this is not always the case and that some data can easily be very misleading. The Kaplan–Meier method of reporting with a continuous time axis is recommended and at the same time a clear demonstration of numbers lost to follow-up at each point. The chapter is a sharp reminder for those who believe that the reporting standards of papers accepted in good journals are universally of high quality. The sentiments of the authors are echoed in a recent publication by Bland and Altman,[1] who make virtually exactly similar points and call for the Kaplan–Meier method of reporting and warn of some of the pitfalls particularly in patients failing to attend follow-up. *RMG*

Reference

1. Bland JM, Altman DG: Statistics notes: Survival probabilities (the Kaplan–Meier method). *Br Med J* **317**: 1572, 1998

Introduction of the Hemashield Vantage® graft for above-knee femoropopliteal bypass

K Balzer, D Raithel, H Scholz and S Horsch

INTRODUCTION

There are numerous choices of synthetic graft material available for performing peripheral arterial bypass procedures. No graft currently available has all the characteristics of the 'ideal' vascular graft. Newly developed products need to be carefully evaluated to see if their design intentions have been met and to determine their clinical performance. This multicentre study was undertaken to confirm the clinical utility of a uniquely designed vascular graft in infrainguinal procedures, and to provide an opportunity for surgeons to appraise its handling qualities in this application.

MATERIALS AND METHODS

A total of 100 patients with superficial femoral artery disease entered a study at four centres between May 1995 and June 1996. Patients with previous above-knee femoropopliteal bypass in the study limb were excluded. Reconstruction was performed with a new collagen-impregnated woven polyester vascular graft, the Hemashield Vantage® (Meadox BSC) which is designed specifically for peripheral vascular reconstruction. The graft has no crimps, and yet has longitudinal elasticity (i.e. both stretch and recoil). Graft diameters were 6 and 8 mm. Typically,[1] the patients, mean age 65 years, were made up of 73% males, 76% smokers, 40% diabetics; 55% were undergoing treatment for hypertension and 53% had raised lipid levels. The series included 80 claudicants, and 20 with rest pain (Fig. 1), excluding from calculation those patients with non-compressible vessels. Runoff was poor (no or one vessel) in 17% of patients and good (two or three vessels) in 83%.

Proximal anastomosis was to the common femoral artery in all but two patients, in whom the superficial femoral was used. Distal anastomoses was performed in all cases to the above-knee popliteal artery, with 87 to the suprageniculate and 13 to the popliteal segment between the superior and inferior geniculate arteries. Ankle brachial pressure index (ABPI) was monitored at 1, 3, 6, 12, 18 and 24 months and patency was determined by feeling pulses and noting ABPI change and by history. Primary and secondary patency rates were calculated by the life-table method.[2]

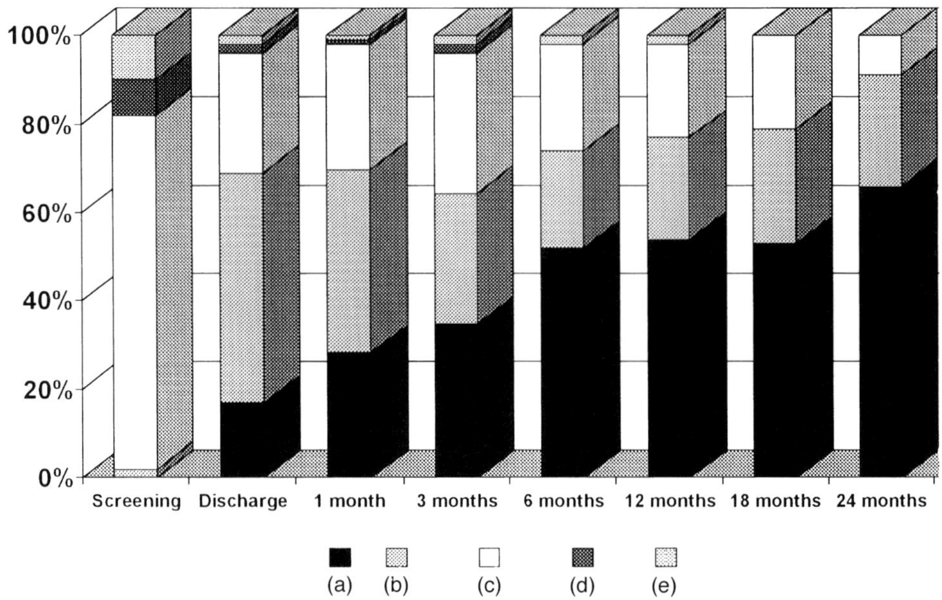

Fig. 1. Symptomatic outcome. (a): Asymptomatic; (b): mild intermittent claudication; (c): severe intermittent claudication; (d): ischaemic rest pain; (e): tissue loss – ulceration or gangrene.

RESULTS

The outcome in terms of symptoms is shown in Fig. 1, in which the effectiveness of bypass in these terms is plotted.

Primary and secondary patency are given in Fig. 2. The mean ABPI before operation was 0.47 and at discharge was 0.95%; these results remained stable through 24 months follow-up (mean 0.97).

At 24 months (n = 57 patients) no patient had rest pain or gangrene, 34% of patients had intermittent claudication and 66% of patients were asymptomatic.

During the study period, 24 grafts occluded and in 23 of these, thrombectomy was successful. In six patients with recurrent thromboses, one required a new bypass and two others had below-knee amputations. Local complications included lymphocoele (five) – of which three responded to conservative treatment and the other two required surgical intervention. There have been four late graft infections (30 days), two of which resulted in graft explantation. Otherwise there was one case of wound infection and six haematomas. During follow-up, four patients died – three of whom had myocardial infarct. The follow-up was up to 2 years but 14 patients did not attend follow-up clinics at all.

Status of the graft at discharge and follow-up
N=100

	PP Population (N=73)		ITT Population (N=100)		Cumulative		
	Primary patency	Secondary patency	Primary patency	Secondary patency	With-drawn	Lost to follow-up	Death
At discharge	95% (69/73)	95% (69/73)	95% (95/100)	95% (95/100)	5	0	
At follow-up 1 month	93% (68/73)	93% (68/73)	94% (94/100)	94% (94/100)	7	1	
At follow-up 3 months	92% (67/73)	92% (67/73)	92% (92/100)	92% (92/100)	8	6	
At follow-up 6 months	89% (65/73)	89% (65/73)	88% (88/100)	90% (90/100)	9	7	1
At follow-up 12 months	84% (61/73)	84% (61/73)	84% (84/100)	86% (86/100)	10	10	2
At follow-up 18 months	81% (59/73)	82% (60/73)	82% (82/100)	85% (85/100)	11	16	3
At follow-up 24 months	71% (52/73)	79% (58/73)	75% (75/100)	73% (73/100)	15	25	4

Four patients died due to reasons not related to graft implant. Two of them never came for follow-up and two died having a patent graft at their last visit. Cause of death was myocardial infarction in three patients and unknown in one patient.

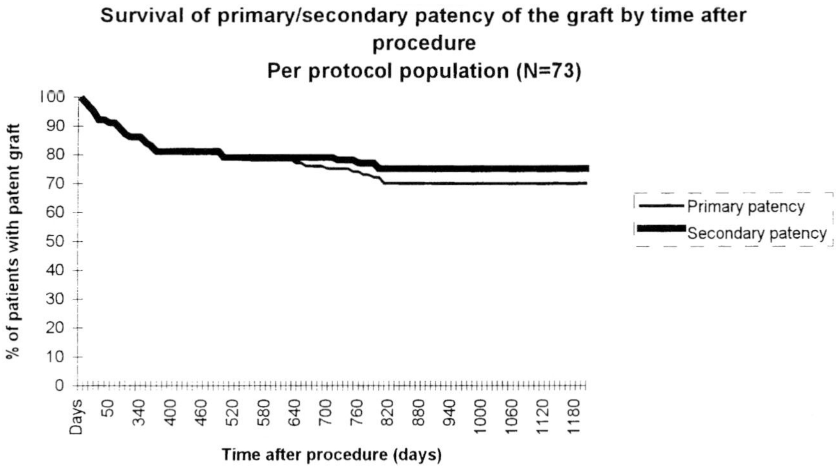

Fig. 2. Survival of patency per protocol population.

DISCUSSION

Currently, autologous saphenous vein grafts and expanded polytetrafluoroethylene (ePTFE) grafts are the most common choices for peripheral procedures. However, certain limitations apply to each of these choices. While vein grafts are known to have superior patency[3] over synthetics, vein harvest lengthens surgical time. An adequate vein may not be available in a particular patient, or there may be concomitant risk factors suggesting that the vein should be conserved for subsequent distal or coronary artery bypass.

Expanded PTFE grafts are known to be prone to prolonged suture hole bleeding and may exhibit poor transmural healing. Their minimal longitudinal stretching ability also poses problems; if cut too long, the graft may kink and occlude, if cut too short, excessive stress is placed on the anastomoses. Even the more recently available stretch version of ePTFE is not optimal since it has no recoil and once stretched is as difficult to manipulate as the original ePTFE.

Historically, polyester grafts were commonly used for infrainguinal procedures. A pivotal study comparing 100 polyester and 100 ePTFE grafts in claudicants found no difference in patency between the two graft types at 5 or 10 years.[4] A similar study in which 80% of the patients had rest pain, gangrene or ulcers showed polyester and ePTFE graft to have comparable patency at 2 years.[5] Pevec *et al.* showed that polyester grafts gave somewhat better clinical results than ePTFE,[6] utilizing a graft with no internal velour. This suggests that a smoother, non-velour luminal surface could be more beneficial for smaller diameter polyester grafts than the typical double velour construction.

Results of a 240-patient study have recently been published, demonstrating equivalent patency for a collagen-impregnated knitted polyester graft for above-knee femoropopliteal bypass.[7] The polyester graft used in that study has a double velour, crimped construction. The use of crimps is intended to impart longitudinal stretch and to maintain the graft's cylindrical shape. However, crimping can disturb laminar blood flow[8] and can make it less easy to fashion a 'hood'.

The Hemashield Vantage®, is a polyester woven graft which is different from any other textile product available (Fig. 3). It has a smooth inner surface for a thinner

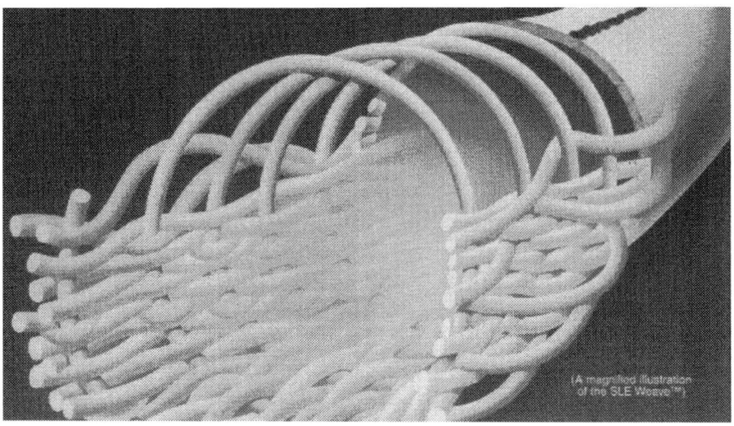

Fig. 3. Textile structure of the Hemashield Vantage® prosthesis.

fibrous capsule, an external velour to promote the adventitial healing needed for stabilization in surrounding tissue, a non-crimped wall for superior hemodynamics, a self-supporting wall without the need for a support coil to maintain graft shape, longitudinal elasticity, conformability for easy anastomosing, and minimization of suture line bleeding by virtue of collagen impregnation.

REFERENCES

1. McDaniel MD, Cronewett JL: Basic data related to natural history of intermittent claudication. *Ann Vasc Surg* **3**: 273–277, 1989
2. Ad Hoc Committee on Reporting Standards: Society for Vascular Surgery, International Society for Cardiovascular Surgery. Suggested standards for reports dealing with lower extremity ischemia. *J Vasc Surg* **4**: 80–94, 1986
3. Michaels JA: Choice of material for above-knee femoropopliteal bypass graft. *Br J Surg* **76**: 7–14, 1989
4. Rosenthal D, Evans RD, McKinsey J *et al.*: Prosthetic above-knee femoropopliteal bypass for intermittend claudication. *J Cardiovasc Surg* **31**: 462–468, 1990
5. Simone ST, Dubner B, Safi AR *et al.*: Comparative review of early and intermediate patency rates of polytetrafluoroethylene and autogenous saphenous vein grafts for lower extremity ischemia. *Surgery* 991–999, 1981
6. Pevec WC, Darling RC, L'Italien GJ, Abbott WM: Femoropopliteal reconstruction with knitted, nonvelour Dacron versus expanded polytetrafluoroethylene. *J Vasc Surg* **1**: 60–65, 1992
7. Abbott WM, Green RM, Matsumoto T *et al.*: Prosthetic above-knee femoropopliteal bypass grafting; Results of a multicenter randomized prospective trial. *J Vasc Surg* **25**: 19–28, 1997
8. Herring M, Dilley R, Gardner A, Glover J: The effects of crimping on the healing of prosthetic arterial grafts. *J Cardiovasc Surg* **21**: 596–603, 1980

Commentary

The author from Mulheim is joined by colleagues in Nuremberg, Berlin and Cologne to report 100 patients of above-knee femoropopliteal bypasses with a newly introduced Vantage® graft by Meadox. It is described as a polyester graft with external velour to encourage tissue ingrowth. It has a smooth internal lining and is not crimped. The word Dacron is not used, but it seems to be a type of Dacron without crimp and with external velour and it is of a woven type. The weave is presumably so loose as to require collagen impregnation to prevent bleeding. The authors have implanted 100 of these into patients into the femorosuprageniculate position and the operations are fairly standard; only two were anastomosed to the superficial femoral artery and the majority to the common femoral artery. All were anastomosed to the popliteal artery above the knee and most above the suprageniculate branch. The follow-up was up to 24 months and most of the criteria mentioned in the previous chapter by Jensen and Schroeder have not been applied. The patency has presumably been achieved by feeling pulses and looking at the ankle brachial pressure index and deciding on clinical grounds if a bypass is patent. The symptomatic outcome in Fig. 1 shows a growing number of patients becoming asymptomatic over 24 months, but it does not say how many patients were in each group at the time. The chapter does say that 14 failed to attend follow-up at all. We can assume nothing about these as the previous chapter explains. Equally in the cumulative patency rates for primary and secondary patency, numbers at the points on the curve are not given. No comparison of this newly introduced graft with any other graft material is made in this study. It is therefore essentially an early report to show that there is a new graft on the market which can be implanted in the femorosuprageniculate position. Experience is far too short to make any claims for durability, although early results and graft handling have pleased the investigators. *RMG*

Is the durability of the management of the diabetic foot affected by patient presentation?

Bruce Campbell

INTRODUCTION

This chapter is about the success and durability of local surgery for the infected and /or ischaemic diabetic foot, avoiding amputation at ankle level or above. The discussion is centred on the influence of patient presentation on outcome, but it presupposes three fundamental principles in management. First, good foot care; second, good general medical care; and third, the goal of a functional foot.

Good long-term foot care[1] involves a team approach, including an orthotist, and a podiatrist or chiropodist. The primary aim of the foot-care team is to prevent the feet of diabetics reaching a stage at which surgery is required, but after any operation their involvement is vital to reduce the chance of further problems. Education of the patient is an essential part of this process.

Good general medical care means expert control of diabetes, proper management of coexisting medical problems and appropriate early antibiotic treatment for infection.

A functional foot means one on which the patient can walk. Ideally this is a fully healed foot (the usual definition of 'success' for local amputation procedures), but an acceptable alternative may be an unhealed yet stable foot which allows walking. Preservation of a foot on which the patient cannot walk is usually less satisfactory than a well healed major amputation and a prosthesis.

WHY DO DIABETICS HAVE PROBLEMS WITH HEALING IN THE FEET?

Atherosclerosis is common in diabetics, occurring at a younger average age, and affecting particularly distal vessels (both tibial arteries and arteries in the foot). In addition, there are functional abnormalities in the microcirculation, with impaired vasomotor responses.[2] Sensory neuropathy disturbs pain and temperature sensation, while motor neuropathy affects the muscles of the foot causing deformities and pressure points. Reduced sweating leads to dry, cracked skin. Infection occurs more readily and tends to spread rapidly in the diabetic. All these factors may contribute in varying degree to the occurrence of foot ulcers, necrosis and infection in the diabetic foot, and then militate against healing.

Even when there are no special problems, the time taken to heal open wounds after amputation or debridement of the diabetic foot may be considerable: dressings are often needed for several months.

WHAT TYPES OF LOCAL PROCEDURE ARE COMMONLY DONE?

The aim of surgery is to evacuate pus and to remove necrotic tissue. Sometimes opening up of an abscess, sinus or fistula is sufficient, with local removal of infected tissue, without amputation of any digit (we define this as 'debridement') (Fig. 1). Amputations of individual toes or of a 'ray' of the foot are done in our practice by division of bone at the metatarsal neck or near the metatarsal base, respectively (Figs 2, 3). Transmetatarsal amputation (of all the toes) is usually through the metatarsal necks, and tarsal amputations are done at any level among the tarsal bones which allows adequate debridement while preserving enough vascularized plantar skin. Use of unconventional amputations at tarsal level has also been advocated by Chang *et al.*[3]

We usually leave the operative wound open for packing, while partially closing larger defects (especially after excision of the first or fifth ray) (Fig. 4). Transmetatarsal, tarsal and 'clean' toe amputations are generally closed with a single layer of interrupted sutures, but always with a drain.

Some accounts consider a Symes amputation to have 'preserved the extremity', but for the purposes of this review any amputation requiring a prosthesis is regarded as 'major'. Our own practice has not included Symes amputations.

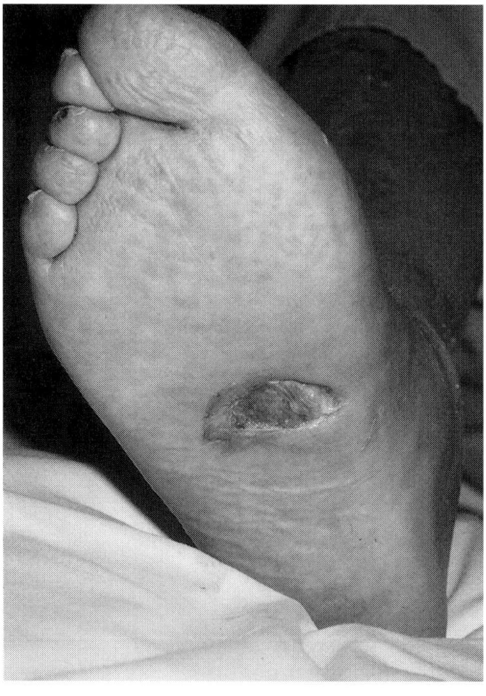

Fig. 1. A plantar sinus, which required debridement of necrotic plantar fascia, but which healed after femoropopliteal bypass grafting.

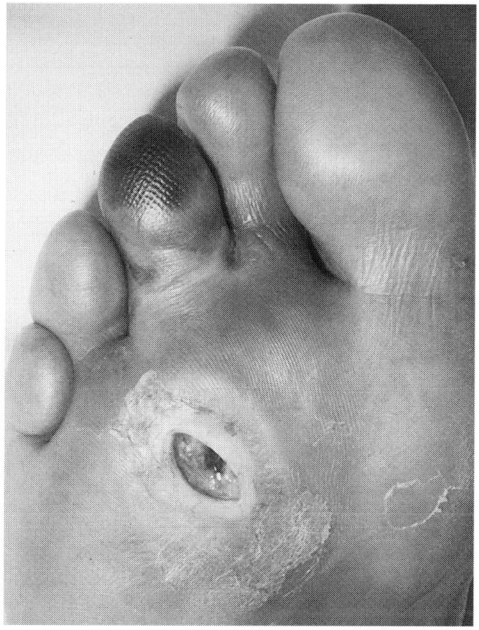

Fig. 2. Necrotic third toe, together with an infected sinus involving the third metatarsal. Ray amputation was required.

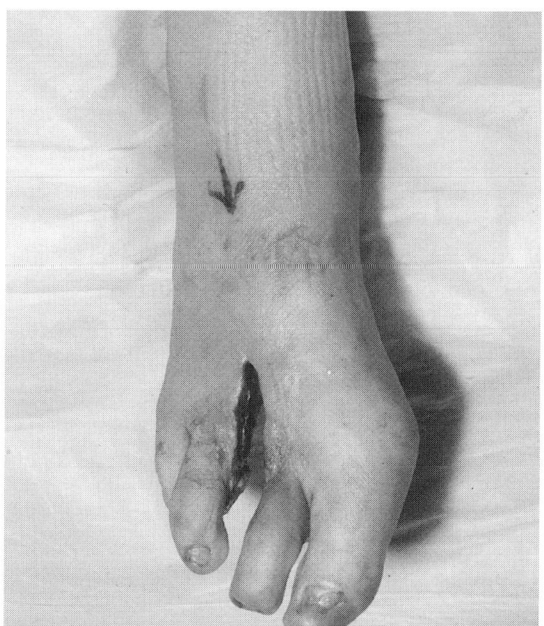

Fig. 3. Ray amputation of the third toe, through the base of the metatarsal. The extent of the original infection was similar to that shown in Fig. 2.

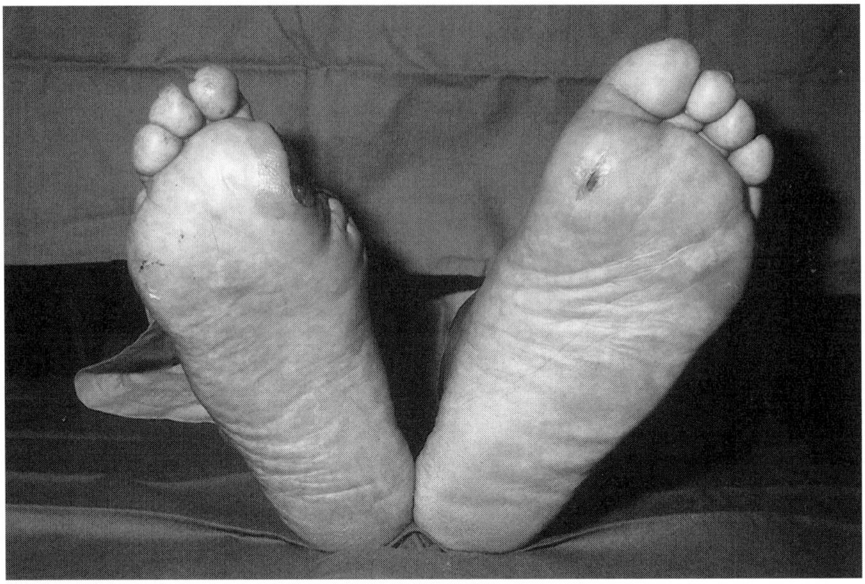

Fig. 4. Ray amputation of the right hallux through the metatarsal neck, with closure of the proximal part of the wound. Note the sinus beneath the first metatarsophalangeal joint of the left foot.

WHY DO REPORTED RESULTS VARY?

Types of series

The literature on local surgery for the diabetic foot is difficult to review and interpret in any scientific or comparative way.[4] This is an area in which randomized studies do not exist. Patient populations vary widely: they may include only patients who have had one type of local foot amputation,[5,6] or amputees of all kinds,[7] and may mix diabetics and non-diabetics:[8] others include only patients who have had revascularization.[9,10] Few present a comprehensive picture of all diabetics who have required foot surgery,[11] and even then case-mix comparisons with other series may be difficult.

Surgeon bias

Whatever the case-mix of a series, the bias of different surgeons will influence results. Surgeons who attempt local foot procedures even when there is a high risk of failure[7] will present different results from surgeons who advise primary major amputation in similar circumstances.

Definitions

Definitions vary.[4] In particular, the diagnostic criteria for arterial disease and for neuropathy differ between publications. In retrospective series data may be missing.[6]

Details of the severity of infection and necrosis are not always explicit: the most commonly used classification is that of Wagner (see below),[12] but this does not take into account the vascularity of the foot. By contrast, the modern concept of the ischaemic, neuropathic or neuroischaemic foot[1] simply describes the basic underlying problem, and not the state of the extremity in terms of the extent of infection or necrosis.

The terms used to describe foot problems differ between reports. For example, the terms ulcer ('superficial' or 'deep'), and mal perforans may have different meanings when used by different authors; and the terms 'necrosis' and 'gangrene' may be used with varying implications.

Finally, the definition of 'success' and the duration of follow-up differ between series. There is a difference between getting the foot healed and keeping it healed. Few series have reported the long-term outcome of unselected patients having local foot procedures, and one purpose of the present chapter is to describe our own experience in this regard.

HOW DOES PRESENTATION OF THE FOOT INFLUENCE PROGNOSIS?

The extent of necrosis and infection

The depth and extent of necrosis or infection are important.[4,12] Assuming adequate blood supply, superficial ulcers (Wagner Grade One foot) will often heal with good local care, including dressings and protection from pressure. These include ulcerated callosities and superficial ulcers over bunions. Larger superficial ulcers (<2cm) may benefit from surgical debridement, but often heal.

In a Grade Two foot ulceration is deeper, involving bone, joint capsule, ligament, or tendon but without established infection of those deeper structures. Sometimes healing can be achieved with good local care but surgical debridement is often required, and amputation of affected digits or rays may be neccessary.

A Grade Three foot means that deep structures have become infected, with osteomyelitis, pyoarthrosis, infection of tendon sheaths or abscess in the deep plantar space. Infection is frequently more widespread than clinical examination suggests and its real extent only becomes clear at the time of surgery. Once these deeper structures are involved, some kind of local surgery is required, often involving amputation of one or more digits or rays, but chances of healing are good, provided there is adequate blood supply.

A Grade Four foot has some gangrene of the toes or forefoot and surgery is almost always required. Prognosis depends on the extent of necrosis and the blood supply. Grade Five describes a foot with gangene so extensive that major amputation is inevitable.

Determining the extent of tissue damage

Determining the depth and extent of infection can be difficult, especially in the early stages when osteomyelitis or involvement of a joint may produce no obvious radiological changes. Bony destruction or gas in the tissues on radiographs are late signs. Gentle probing of a sinus may be helpful and some surgeons recommend sinograms.[4] Magnetic resonance imaging can be helpful in demonstrating the extent of deep necrosis and infection.[13] However, the amount of tissue which needs to be excised often becomes clear only at the time of operation.

Site of ulceration, oedema, and pain

In addition to the depth and local extent of necrosis, other features can affect prognosis. Larsson *et al.*[14] have documented heel ulcers, multiple ulcers, and ulcers causing intractable pain as associated with the need for major amputation. The group from Lund[15] have also described an association between the presence of peripheral oedema and failure to heal local foot procedures, neccessitating major amputation (primary healing after foot surgery in 26% with oedema compared with 63% overall). Oedema was also associated with increased mortality. Congestive cardiac failure was the most commonly identified cause, while neuropathy and deep vein thrombosis were responsible in some patients.

Urgency of referral

Related factors which may influence prognosis are the urgency of presentation (gross cellulitis or abscess, as opposed to chronic grumbling sepsis) and the speed of referral of such cases for surgery. The acutely infected foot needs aggressive antibiotic treatment, but this should not delay surgical referral if there is the possibility of contained pus, which must be drained (Fig. 5). Goodman *et al.*[16] noted that the

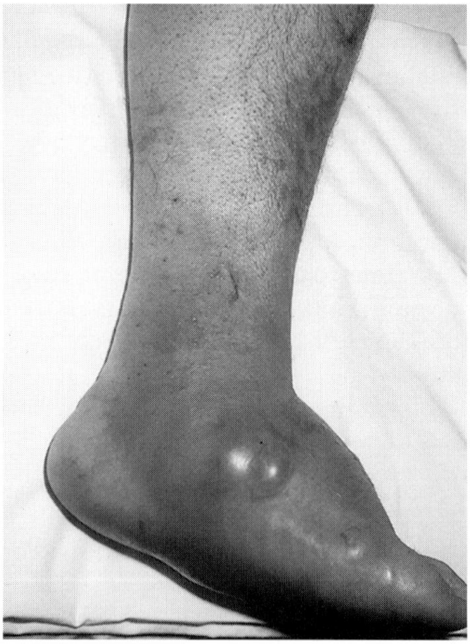

Fig. 5. Abscess in a diabetic foot, requiring urgent drainage. In this case sepsis was extensive.

severity of associated systemic infection (assessed by temperature and leucocytosis) influenced the prognosis for healing of a local foot procedure.

WHAT IS THE INFLUENCE OF ARTERIAL DISEASE ON HEALING?

Provided the extent of necrosis and infection allows a local procedure, the presence of peripheral arterial disease is then the most important determinant of healing.

Pulses and clinical examination

At one extreme, the foot with palpable pulses and normal ankle pressure indices (i.e. no significant arterial disease) usually heals,[8,12,17] although this is not invariable.[15] At the other extreme, the profoundly ischaemic foot with unrecordable ankle pressures will almost certainly not heal after local surgery. Between these extremes prediction of healing is not straightforward. In 1974 Williams[18] exemplified these categories by documenting three clinical groups of patients in a series of diabetics with foot necrosis of an extent which was amenable to local excision. Among 29 patients with 'necrosis in a hot foot' all healed after local surgery: among 23 with 'necrosis in a warm foot' 11 of 23 healed, while 12 required major amputation: among 31 with 'necrosis in a cold foot' all had major amputation.

Doppler ankle pressures

Determination of ankle systolic pressure (and ankle systolic pressure index – ASPI) is routine, and has some relationship with the likelihood of healing after local foot surgery,[19] but its predictive accuracy in controversial and unreliable. First, many diabetics have calcified tibial arteries, which are either incompressible or which give artefactually elevated pressure readings. The latter can cause confusion for the unwary: it is essential to listen to the signal quality. Another potential trap is occlusion or severe disease of the posterior tibial and dorsalis pedis arteries, with the best or only pressures in the peroneal: it is very important to examine the peroneal artery when assessing ankle Dopplers in the diabetic. These pitfalls should be borne in mind when interpreting the literature: for example, Schwartz *et al.*[20] concluded that there was 'no difference in mean ankle Doppler pressure between the healed and failed groups' (after toe and forefoot amputation), but noted that there was a significant difference 'if falsely elevated values were excluded'!

Differing thresholds have been described for ankle pressures likely to allow healing of the foot. Verta *et al.*[21] found ankle pressures of >40mmHg or ASPI >0.43 to be associated with healing both in diabetics and non-diabetics, while no feet healed with an ankle pressure <35mmHg. A similar ASPI threshold was described by Wagner[12] (in a series of 71 patients whose ankle pressure status was unknown to the surgeon) but absolute ankle pressure associated with healing in his series was 70mmHg, and other reports concur with this higher figure. In a small study from the same era Baker and Barnes[22] found a mean ankle pressure of 79mmHg in seven of 20 diabetics who failed to heal minor forefoot amputations, and no patient (including 30 non-diabetics) healed with a pressure <60mmHg. This finding was similar to that of Carter[23] who observed that healing of the foot was unlikely with ankle pressures <55mmHg in diabetics. Welch *et al.*[24] observed a mean ankle pressure of 89mmHg in a group of diabetics who failed to heal forefoot amputations – no different statistically from diabetics who did heal.

Toe pressures

In addition to the problem of arterial calcification, ankle pressures suffer the disadvantage that they take no account of arterial disease in the foot, which is common in diabetics. Toe pressure measurements overcome this difficulty. Both Lee *et al.*[25] and Schwartz *et al.*[20] found that toe pressures (measured by plethysmography) <20mmHg were associated with failure to heal forefoot procedures, while pressures of >40mmHg usually predicted success.

Skin blood flow measurements

Measurements of skin blood flow have been studied for prediction of healing in the diabetic foot. For example, Welch *et al.*[24] used clearance of ^{125}I-iodoantipyrine in 17 diabetics having forefoot amputation, and found a that a threshold value of 7–8ml/100g/min blood flow separated those who healed from those who did not heal. However, a substantial proportion of their patients had values very close to this threshold, and this kind of measurement has not become widely used in clinical practice.

In summary, the obviously cold, ischaemic foot, with an ankle systolic pressure less than about 70mmHg, or toe pressure <20mmHg is very unlikely to heal after a local operation.

WHAT OTHER PATIENT FACTORS MAY INFLUENCE HEALING?

In a consecutive series of 187 diabetics with foot ulceration requiring surgery in Lund (Sweden), Larsson *et al.*[11] found that older age (>74 years), a history of cerebrovascular disease, and lower haemoglobin level were associated with the need for amputation above the level of the ankle. These were all significant independent predictors, but none was reliable, and the authors emphasized that amputation level should be chosen on the basis of the whole clinical picture. In this series, congestive cardiac failure also had some association with amputation above the ankle, and it was suggested that both this and history of cerebrovascular disease were simply markers of advanced generalized atherosclerosis. In addition, long duration of diabetes was associated in this study with healing at below ankle level, but the series was dominated by Type I diabetics. There was no relationship between healing and the presence of retinopathy.

In a report of two cohorts of diabetics with various foot problems, Faglia *et al.*[19] also found an association between the need for major amputation and history of stroke, but no relationship with haemoglobin level. A reverse relationship with haemoglobin level – healing of the foot with low haemoglobin – has been reported in one other series.[26]

Faglia *et al.*[19] observed that prior major amputation of the contralateral limb was associated with progress to a major amputation. The frequency of bilateral major amputation in diabetics was observed many years ago,[27,28] and in our own practice diabetics predominate among bilateral amputees.[29]

DOES THE OPERATING SURGEON MAKE A DIFFERENCE?

Two studies have reported that the seniority of the surgeon influences the success of local foot procedures for diabetics. In a consecutive series of 68 patients reported by Turnbull and Chester[17] the initial foot operation was done by a consultant in 31% cases, and by a junior surgeon in 69%. Of those requiring revision, only 12% had originally been dealt with by a consultant, while 88% had been operated upon by a junior. In a retrospective series from Singapore, Wong *et al.*[30] also observed that operations done by senior surgeons were more likely to heal. However, their paper suggested that surgical decisions had been made by juniors without any senior input, and it may be that inexperience in making the decision to do a local foot procedure (and deciding its extent) is as important as technical operative skill in these cases.[31]

WHAT IS THE INFLUENCE OF ARTERIAL RECONSTRUCTION?

There can be no doubt that successful revascularization of the diabetic foot allows healing of local procedures in many limbs which would otherwise require major amputation, and impressive series have been published in recent years emphasizing the role of distal reconstruction.[9,32–34]

Eckstein *et al.*[35] pointed out that a significant proportion of patients requiring pedal bypasses have limited life expectancy, but in their series (71% diabetics) nearly two-thirds of patients who died did so without having suffered major amputation. In some diabetic patients, healing fails to occur despite technically successful bypass grafting[29] (Fig. 6).

WHAT IS THE LIFE EXPECTANCY OF PATIENTS WHO HAVE SURGERY FOR DIABETIC FOOT PROBLEMS?

In 1961 Wheelock reported a series of 428 diabetic patients who had transmetatarsal amputation during a 14-year period: their mortality was 23% at 2 years and 77% at 5 years. A series from Oxford by Finch *et al.* published in 1980[36] showed no diabetics surviving much longer than 3 years, following major, transmetatarsal, or Symes amputation. More recently Larsson *et al.*[37] described mortalities of 15%, 38% and 68% at 1, 3 and 5 years respectively among 189 diabetics having major or minor amputation: the mortality was higher after an initial major amputation. These series

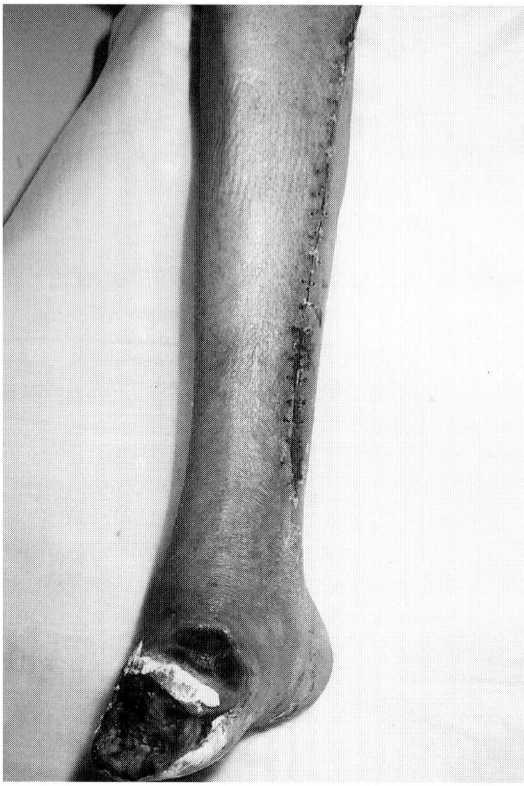

Fig. 6. Failure to heal despite a functioning distal bypass graft. The necrotic forefoot was amputated at the time of the femorotibial bypass, but the tissues of the foot show no sign of vascularity or healing.

give some insight into the poor survival of these patients, with over half of those having minor amputations of the foot being dead 5 years postoperatively.

The high subsequent mortality means that many foot salvage procedures are performed for diabetic patients whose life expectancy is short. The 'durability' of the salvage operation is then limited by the survival of the patient, rather than by failure of the procedure in the longer term. Provided a pain free and functional foot can be achieved for the patient's lifetime, then a local amputation (with or without associated arterial reconstruction) must be considered a success. By the same token, prolonged failure to heal after local amputation which results in disability may mar the whole remaining existence of a patient. Even those local procedures which heal often take a very long time to do so – median 29 weeks (range 3–191 weeks) in the comprehensive series by Larsson *et al.*[37] The latter study is one of the few to examine long-term prognosis for diabetics having local foot amputations. We have undertaken a similar exercise, reviewing the outcome for these patients some 6–10 years after surgery.

WHAT IS THE LONG-TERM OUTCOME FOR DIABETICS HAVING LOCAL FOOT PROCEDURES?

We have recently reviewed the outcome of 75 consecutive diabetic patients who had local surgery to the feet for sepsis or gangrene during the years 1987–1992, with a median follow-up interval of 92 months (range 69–120 months).[38] During the period under study, 17 (24%) had surgery to both feet and a total of 136 operations were done (Table 1); 59 (79%) patients were male and the median age was 68 years; 34 were taking insulin, 37 oral hypoglycaemic agents and four were on a prescribed diet only.

These patients were referred to the author, who at that time provided vascular surgical services single handed for a population of about 320 000. Most were inpatient referrals from a variety of physicians at a time when the present highly organized diabetic service in our hospital was still developing. Their initial treatment included antibiotics and general medical care, with a median period of 7 days inpatient treatment before first referral to the vascular surgical team. This delay was rather less (median 4–5 days) for patients already known to the vascular team.

Arterial disease had been diagnosed in 57% limbs, on the basis of ankle systolic pressure index <0.8, or incompressible arteries with impalpable pulses and damped Doppler signals (the status of six limbs was not recorded). Toe pressures were not measured. Neuropathy had been diagnosed only on the basis of gross clinical signs, and had been documented in 60% patients; but most of the remainder almost certainly had less obvious or unrecorded neuropathy. (Latterly, all patients seen by our diabetologists have had detailed sensory testing.)

Among the 92 operated limbs, 21 (23%) had bypass grafting or angioplasty either before (8), at the same operation (8) or after (6) the procedure on their foot (one patient had angioplasty before, and then synchronous bypass grafting).

Healing of the local procedure was achieved in 53% of feet (48% in patients having surgery for one foot only and 58% for those having operations on both feet). Long-term details were missing for four limbs, and some patients who did not heal died without requiring major amputation.

Thirty-three (37%) of 88 limbs went on to major amputation. These amputations were done up to 7 years after the initial foot procedure, but the median interval was

Table 1. Indications for surgery and types of operation (136 operations in 92 feet)

Indications	
Ulceration	17
Deep infection	40
Gangrene	17
Combination	62
Types of operation	
Debridement	18
Amputation of 1–4 toes	99
Transmetatarsal amputation	9

24 days. This concurs with the experience of Murdoch *et al.*,[6] who observed that nearly all major amputations required after removal of the hallux were done in the first year. Among the arteriopathic limbs, 52% went on to major amputation, compared with 18% of those without arterial disease.

At follow-up of 69–120 months (median 92 months) only 20 (25%) patients were still alive. Sixteen (80%) were male and their median age at the time of the initial procedure had been 59. Of their 23 operated feet 17 (74%) remained healed. Among these survivors only 25% were arteriopaths, and no patient who had undergone bypass grafting or angioplasty had survived. Two of only five (40%) arteriopaths who survived had required major amputation, compared with two of 14 (14%) of those without arterial disease.

This retrospective study provides evidence for the impression of many vascular surgeons and diabetologists that patients with arterial disease and foot problems fare comparatively badly. Following local foot surgery both healing and survival are lower in arteriopaths and based on our experience the need for arterial reconstruction is associated with particularly poor prognosis in this group of patients. By contrast, those with neuropathy often remain healed in the longer term with good foot care.

CONCLUSION

Our documented knowledge of the long-term outcome after diabetic foot surgery is sparse. The majority of reports concern prediction of healing, rather than long-term durability and the influence of patient presentation even on initial healing is fickle. The published data provide observations and guidelines, but no certainty for the individual patient. Healing often takes months and the limited survival of many diabetics means that a substantial proportion (perhaps all) of their remaining lifespan is spent with a need for dressings after 'successful' surgery to the foot. In our experience the presence of arterial disease is of the greatest importance as an adverse factor for healing, durability of a healed foot and long-term survival.

Good foot care, with education of the patient, is now recognized as fundamental for avoiding serious foot problems in diabetics:[1] this cannot be overemphasized. For the healed foot after local amputation or debridement, orthotic and general care should be continued assiduously in the hope of maintaining a durable result.

REFERENCES

1. Edmonds M, Bouton A, Buckenham A *et al.* Report of the Diabetic Foot and Amputation Group. *Diabet Med* **13**: S27–S42, 1996
2. Flynn MD, Tooke JE: Aetiology of diabetic foot ulceration: a role for the microcirculation? *Diabet Med* **8**: 320–329, 1992
3. Chang BB, Bock DEM, Jacobs RL *et al.*: Increased limb salvage by the use of unconventional foot amputations. *J Vasc Surg* **19**: 341–349, 1994
4. O'Neal LW: Debridement and amputation. In: Marvin EL (Ed) *The Diabetic Foot* pp. 237–248. St Louis: CV Mosby, 1988

5. Wheelock, Jr FC: Transmetatarsal amputations and arterial surgery in diabetic patients. *New Engl J Med* **264**: 316–320, 1961
6. Murdoch DP, Armstrong DG, Dacus JB *et al.*: The natural history of great toe amputations. *J Foot Ankle Surg* **36**: 204–208, 1997
7. Porter JM, Bauer GM, Taylor LM: Lower-extremity amputation for ischaemia. *Arch Surg* **116**: 89–92, 1981
8. Little JM, Stephen MS, Zylstra PL: Amputation of the toes for vascular disease: fate of the affected leg. *Lancet* **ii**: 1318–1319, 1976
9. Pomposelli FB, Marcaccio EJ, Gibbons GW *et al.*: Dorsalis pedis arterial bypass; Durable limb salvage for foot ischemia in patients with diabetes mellitus. *J Vasc Surg* **21**: 375–384, 1995
10. Chang BB, Darling RC, Paty PSK *et al.*: Expeditious management of ischemic invasive foot infections. *Cardiovasc Surg* **4**: 792–795, 1996
11. Larsson J, Agardh CD, Apelqvist J, Stenstrom A: Clinical characteristics in relation to final amputation level in diabetic patients with foot ulcers: A prospective study of healing below or above the ankle in 187 patients. *Foot Ankle Int* **16**: 69–74, 1995
12. Wagner FW: The dysvascular foot: a system for diagnosis and treatment. *Foot Ankle Int* **2**: 64–122, 1981
13. Croll SD, Nicholas GG, Osborne MA *et al.*: Role of magnetic resonance imaging in the diagonsis of osteomyelitis in diabetic foot infections. *J Vasc Surg* **24**: 266–270, 1996
14. Larsson J, Agardh CD, Apelqvist J, Stenstrom A: Local signs and symptoms in relation to final amputation level in diabetic patients. *Acta Orthop Scand* **65**: 387–393, 1994
15. Apelqvist J, Larsson J, Agardh CD: The importance of peripheral pulses, peripheral oedema and local pain for the outcome of diabetic foot ulcers. *Diabet Med* **7**: 590–594, 1990
16. Goodman J, Bessman AN, Teget B, Wagner W: Risk factors in local surgical procedures for diabetic gangrene. *Surg Gyn Obstet* **143**: 587–591, 1976
17. Turnbull AR, Chester JF: Partial amputation of the foot for diabetic gangrene. *Ann Roy Coll Surg Eng* **70**: 329–331, 1988
18. Williams HTG, Hutchinson KJ, Brown GD: Gangrene of the feet in diabetics. *Arch Surg* **108**: 609–612, 1974
19. Faglia E, Favales F, Aldeghi A *et al.*: Change in a major amputation rate in a center dedicated to diabetic foot care during the 1980s: Prognostic determinants for major amputation. *J Diab* **12**: 96–102, 1998
20. Schwartz JA, Schuler JJ, O'Connor RJA, Flanigan DP: Predictive value of distal perfusion pressure in the healing of amputation of the digits and the forefoot. *Surg Gyn Obstet* **154**: 865–869, 1982
21. Verta MJ, Gross WS, van Bellen B *et al.*: Foefoot perfusion pressure and minor amputation for gangrene. *Surgery* **80**: 729–734, 1976
22. Baker WH, Barnes RW: Minor forefoot amputation in patients with low ankle pressure. *Am J Surg* **133**: 331–332, 1997
23. Carter SA: The relationship of distal systolic pressures to healing of skin lesions in limbs with arterial occlusive disease, with special reference to diabetes mellitus. *Scand J Clin Lab Invest* **31**: 239–243, 1873
24. Welch GH, Leiberman DP, Pollock JG, Angerson W: Failure of Doppler ankle pressure to predict healing of conservative forefoot amputations. *Br J Surg* **72**: 888–891, 1985
25. Lee BY, Trainor FS, Kavner D *et al.*: Noninvasive hemodynamic evaluation in selection of amputation level. *Surg Gyn Obstet* **149**: 241–244, 1979
26. Bailey MJ, Johnston CLW, Yates CJP *et al.*: Preoperative haemoglobin as predictor of outcome of diabetic amputations. *Lancet* **ii**: 168–170, 1979
27. Goldner, MG: The fate of the second leg in the diabetic amputee. *Diabetes* **9**: 100–103, 1960
28. Ecker ML, Jacobs BS: Lower extremity amputation in diabetic patients. *Diabetes* **19**: 189–195, 1970
29. Campbell WB, Kernick VFM, St Johnston JA., Rutter EA: Lower limb amputation: striking the balance. *Ann Roy Coll Surg Engl* **76**: 205–209, 1994
30. Wong YS, Lee JCH, Yu CS, Low BY: Results of minor foot amputations in diabetic mellitus. *Singapore Med J* **37**: 604–606, 1996

31. Sizer JS, Wheelock FC: Digital amputations in diabetic patients. *Surgery* **72**: 980–989, 1972
32. Shah DM, Chang BB, Fitzgerald KM *et al.*: Durability of the tibial artery bypass in diabetic patients. *Am J Surg* **156**: 133–135, 1988
33. Andros G, Harris RW, Salles-Cunha SX *et al.*: Lateral plantar artery bypass grafting: defining the limits of foot revascularization. *J Vasc Surg* **10**: 511–521, 1989
34. Stonebridge PA, Murie JA: Infrainguinal revascularization in the diabetic patient. *Br J Surg* **80**: 1237–1241, 1993
35. Eckstein HH, Schumacher H, Maeder N *et al.*: Pedal bypass for limb-threatening ischaemia: an 11-year review. *Br J Surg* **83**: 1554–1557, 1996
36. Finch DRA, Macdougal M, Tibbs DJ, Morris PJ: Amputation for vascular disease: the experience of a peripheral vascular unit. *Br J Surg* **67**: 233–237, 1980
37. Larsson J, Agardh CD, Apelqvist J, Stenstrom A: Long term prognosis after healed amputation in patients with diabetes. *Clin Orth Rel Res* **350**: 149–158, 1998
38. Campbell WB, Ponette D, Sugiono M: Long-term results following operation for diabetic foot problems: arterial disease confers a poor prognosis. 1999 (submitted for publication).

Commentary

This is a chapter emphasizing the particular whimsical strengths of this author. The section 'Why do reported results vary?' portrays the author in his element. Probing to analyse the differences in reporting and whether they are real or apparent. 'The aim of surgery is to evacuate pus ...' makes the matter sound very simple and to the point and this must be absolutely correct. The major difficulty is to know when pus is there, when to rely on antibiotics and when to drain. From this chapter and one's own experience, early aspiration for us and drainage wherever possible would indeed seem to be absolutely vital. Delay to relieve pus under pressure and in a confined space often leads to extension of infection proximately with disastrous results. Three principles of good foot care, good general medical care and the goal of a functional foot are well described in this chapter which emphasizes the value of the multidisciplinary approach to diabetic foot care. *RMG*

Vein graft surveillance is worthwhile

Andrew F Lennox and John H N Wolfe

INTRODUCTION

Autogenous vein grafts remain the optimal conduits for lower limb bypass procedures being performed for both occlusive atherosclerotic and aneurysmal disease. Over the last decade, surgical intervention for lower extremity ischaemia has increased, particularly for critical ischaemia, and now constitutes a large proportion of the workload in a vascular department. Unfortunately, the long-term success of this procedure is limited by the development of vein graft stenoses secondary to myointimal hyperplasia. This process can occur in up to 35% of patients within the first 2 years and threaten the patency of the graft.[1–10] Mills investigated the cause of acute graft occlusion, and found that graft stenosis due to myointimal hyperplasia was responsible for this complication in 65% of cases.[11] Once an autogenous graft occludes, it is difficult to improve secondary patency rates beyond 20–30%,[12] as radiological and surgical salvage procedures are less effective than for prosthetic grafts and a new graft remains the only option in the presence of persistent limb ischaemia. Despite advances in technique and experience, graft failure in the first postoperative year remains disappointingly high and attempts to reduce this by means of graft surveillance techniques have been widely adopted. Both retrospective and prospective studies have been published reporting the utility of regular surveillance protocols in improving graft patency rates; however there remains some controversy regarding the value of this policy with regards to its benefit over clinical assessment in detection, improvement in overall results and cost-effectiveness in today's climate of economic restraint.

MAGNITUDE OF THE PROBLEM

The European Consensus Document on critical ischaemia has determined that graft patency following infrainguinal bypass varies from 85% for above-knee autogenous vein grafts down to 25% at 1 year for distal prosthetic grafts.[13] The generally accepted principle is that longer grafts and/or prosthetic grafts are associated with reduced patency. The incidence of vein graft stenoses following bypass as demonstrated in Table 1 varies from between 15 and 35 within the first 2 years, the majority occurring in the first 12 months. As it has been shown that the majority of grafts that thrombose are secondary to a significant stenosis, these are patients who may benefit from a graft surveillance programme. A review of the role of graft surveillance by Giannoukas provided evidence that stenoses imposed a 3- to 6-fold risk of graft occlusion if they were left untreated.[14]

Table 1. Incidence of vein graft stenosis following lower limb bypass (1- to 2-year surveillance follow-up)

Author (Year)	*No of grafts*	*% Stenosed*
Bandyk *et al.* (1988)[1]	197	28
Moody *et al.* (1989)[2]	141	28
Taylor *et al.* (1990)[3]	412	16
Chang *et al.* (1990)[4]	350	20
Buth *et al.* (1991)[5]	116	37
Mills *et al.* (1993)[6]	227	13
Idu *et al.* (1993)[7]	160	36.2
Caps *et al.* (1995)[8]	61	34.4
Wilson *et al.* (1996)[9]	275	21.5

PATHOGENESIS AND IDENTIFICATION OF VEIN GRAFT FAILURE

In 1973, Szilagyi published the results of long-term angiographic follow-up in a large series of lower limb autogenous vein bypasses, and demonstrated that almost one-third of grafts developed significant defects either along the course of the graft or at the anastamoses.[15] The aetiology of vein graft failure remains debatable; however, the natural history of this complication suggests that the time course can be divided into three categories:

Early graft-related complications

Early graft-related complications within the first month of surgery are related to technical considerations that may have been undetected. Poor quality, damaged or twisted vein, inadequate inflow or runoff, intimal flaps, competent valve cusps (*in situ* grafts) or anastamotic imperfections are all frustrating technical problems. For this group, prevention is preferable to surveillance in reducing rates of graft failure, and techniques of pre- and intraoperative assessment have been suggested. B-Mode ultrasound has the ability not only to assess the diameter and distensibility of the vein that is to be used as a conduit but can also detect the presence of thick-walled or post-phlebitic veins that would be unsuitable for use as a graft. Davies *et al.* also showed a correlation between vein wall compliance and intimal thickening and found this to be associated with a higher incidence of subsequent vein graft stenosis.[16] However, others have had difficulty with this correlation.[17] Veins must also be handled and prepared carefully prior to insertion in order to limit the endothelial damage that may predispose to developing a later graft stenosis.

Various methods have been studied to assess the graft following anastamosis in order to identify structural and haemodynamic defects that can be surgically corrected prior to leaving the operating room. Continuous wave Doppler is limited in its ability to identify subtle but potentially 'at risk' lesions and angiography may also miss minor luminal defects as it is usually performed in a single plane view. Angioscopy is an excellent modality for imaging the lumen and anastamosis, particularly in identifying small webs and strands that could be a focus for intimal hyperplasia, although the ability to detect these lesions is not necessarily specific in predicting which grafts will ultimately progress to stenosis.[18] Some believe that the angioscope itself may damage the vein graft and for this reason do not support its use. The 'bucket test' is also useful and gives a broad haemodynamic assessment of graft function. With a pulse rate of 60, six pulsations of flow are collected and measured. The volume is multiplied by 10 to calculate the flow/minute, a rate of 150ml/min is considered the minimal acceptable flow rate.[19] Measurement of peripheral resistance is a further method to predict grafts that may have a poor outflow and therefore a lower chance of success.[20] Intraoperative duplex scanning is the best method for assessing the haemodynamics of the graft and sites of turbulent and compromised blood flow. Bandyk was able to achieve very low graft failure and high long-term patency rates by using this technique and correcting all haemodynamic defects that were identified at the time of surgery.[21]

Stenotic lesions

Stenotic lesions that develop within the first 12–18 months of surgery are due to myointimal hyperplasia or occasionally fibrosis at the valve cusps. This group constitutes the largest proportion of potentially identifiable and treatable graft lesions. Although several prospective studies utilizing a regular protocol of duplex surveillance with varied criteria for intervention have demonstrated an improvement in graft patency as a result,[3,7,22–25] the published literature in this field is limited by the lack of randomized trials comparing surveillance techniques and overall outcome in terms of graft survival and limb loss. It has been difficult to determine which grafts are at a higher risk of developing stenoses during this period of time. Some centres have attempted to identify patients whose grafts are at a lower risk of developing stenoses in whom a less intense surveillance programme may be required. They argue that surveillance should focus only on grafts that stenose in the first 6 or 12 months. Others have attempted to identify serological factors associated with graft stenosis. Smoking, elevated plasma fibrinogen[26,27] and homocysteine[28] levels are associated with an increased risk of graft stenosis and they may provide further evidence in determining which patients should have closer monitoring of the grafts within the first 2 years. The smooth muscle cells that are resistant to *in vitro* growth inhibition by heparin are also associated with an increased risk of graft stenosis.[29]

Late onset graft failure

Late onset graft failure is due predominantly to progression of the atherosclerotic disease process, not only distal disease but also affecting the proximal inflow. The risk appears to be approximately 2–3% per annum. We believe that attempts to reduce the incidence of graft failure in this group should be aimed at identifying risk factors that may benefit from either pharmacological or lifestyle interventions. Disease progression at this stage is now understood not only to increase graft-related complications but also to increase the morbidity and mortality related to coronary and cerebrovascular disease.

Brewster found that approximately 15% of grafts fail within the first month, almost 80% during the first 2 years and the remainder fail after this time.[30] From these percentages, it would seem that the biggest impact on reducing graft failure would be in the identification and treatment of graft stenoses.

IDENTIFICATION OF VEIN GRAFT STENOSES – WHICH IS THE BEST METHOD?

The ideal stenosis detection programme should provide non-invasive, accurate information regarding the patency and haemodynamics of the entire graft and anastamoses. The method should be safe, painless, easy to perform and cost-effective, and as many patients remain asymptomatic until the graft occludes, should also be able to detect lesions of varying degrees of stenosis and reliably monitor their progress over time.

Clinical assessment

Clinical palpation of a pulse within a graft is unreliable in detecting significantly compromised grafts, as many grafts are not palpable despite being patent due to position or body habitus. Pulses may also be enhanced by reflected waves from a very high peripheral resistance, giving a false impression of haemodynamic stability. Clinical symptoms are also insensitive with 20–67% of patients reported to have no symptoms despite the presence of a significant stenosis on angiography or duplex.[14]

Ankle brachial pressure index (ABPI)

The addition of Doppler derived pressures over the last 25 years has improved the clinical sensitivity of identifying a failing graft. However, if an index drop of 0.15 alone is used as an indicator, then there is a large proportion of false positives.[31,32] Low ABPI measurements can reflect not only disturbed flow down the graft but also disease progression of the native inflow or runoff arteries, and can be difficult to interpret in the presence of calcified vessels in diabetic patients. An exercise treadmill test demonstrating a drop of > 0.2 may be more sensitive, but patients with significant lesions will also fail to be identified.

Duplex

The duplex scanner embodies both B-mode imaging and Doppler ultrasound, and can provide both anatomic and haemodynamic information. Flow within the graft can be calculated at any point as the product of the average velocity and the cross-sectional area. With the knowledge that flow at one point in a graft without branches equals flow at any other point, any reduction in luminal area will be associated with a proportional rise in velocity (see Fig. 1). Whereas it was initially postulated that failing grafts could be detected by low velocities, the concept of a velocity ratio is a much more reliable indicator of severe stenosis. Because the

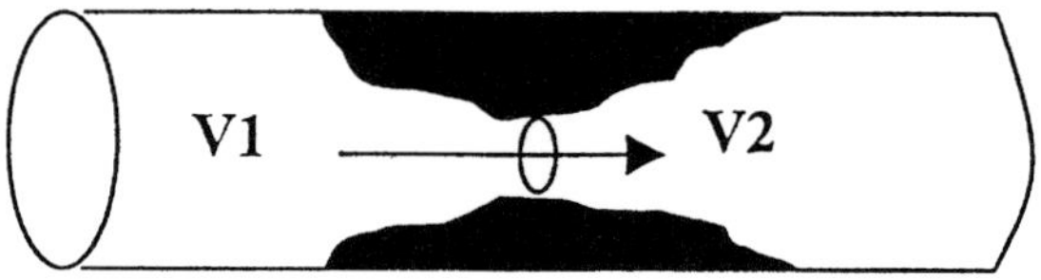

FLOW 1 = FLOW 2

Fig. 1. Velocity ratio V2/V1 is calculated at the stenosis (V2) and proximal to the lesion (V1) with flow equal at all points along the graft due to the absence of any branch points.

measurement is a ratio, changes in cardiac output and peripheral resistance do not alter the readings, and accurate comparisons over a period of follow-up can be made. The ratio also removes the single most important cause of error – the measurement of diameter. Small errors are compounded since the equation for measuring flow will take into account the squared value of the radius of the vessel at the site of the stenosis. Minor stenoses are defined as having a V2/V1 ratio < 2 and major stenoses have a ratio > 2. By using this technique in 75 patients, a close correlation with angiography has been demonstrated.[33] A V2/V1 ratio > 2 acts as screen and many of these patients with stenoses between 50% and 70% are managed conservatively. Others have therefore suggested a higher threshold of V2/V1 ratio of 2.5 or even 3.[34–36] This ratio is a reliable method for diagnosis in a graft stenosis, but a stenosis at the distal anastamosis, or just beyond, particularly in the popliteal fossa, may be difficult to evaluate. The absolute peak velocity < 45 cm/s is useful under these circumstances.[1] The peak velocity when used as the only criteria does, however, tend to miss localized lesions within the graft. We advocate using a combination of these two methods as shown in Fig. 2, where flow reduction due to a haemodynamically significant graft stenosis can be identified in all patients.[37] Figure 3 illustrates a long diffuse stenosis at the distal end of a graft where a discreet region of high velocity will not be found.

The addition of colour flow has made this technique quicker and more efficient, both in identifying the graft and locating sites of altered flow velocities as illustrated in Fig. 4 in comparison with angiography. However, there are still some limitations in assessing disease in the arteries of the calf. This method combined with clinical assessment and a fall in ABPI is generally accepted as the optimal combination in any surveillance programme. Any prospective study aimed at determining the worth of a surveillance programme will need to compare this combination with the benefits of clinical assessment alone, as performed in the only prosective randomized studies to date.[38,39] Duplex, which has the ability to accurately identify the exact site of the stenotic lesion within the graft, can be utilized to mark this location preoperatively to guide the surgical approach, particularly if the graft is tunnelled deeply and the segment of disease is short.

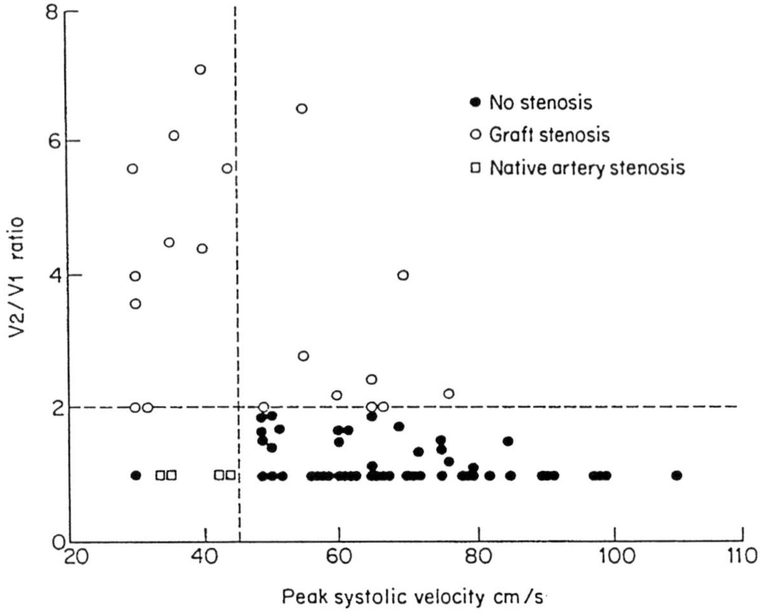

Fig. 2. V2 : V1 ratio findings compared with peak systolic velocity in grafts which are normal and stenosed on angiography. V2 : V1 ratio detects all stenoses within grafts but misses four patients with native vessel stenosis who were detected by a peak systolic velocity < 45 cm/s. (Reproduced with permission of *Eur J Vasc Surg*.)

Angiography

Multiplanar anigography remains the traditional 'gold standard' method against which other techniques are compared and will pick up twice as many lesions as clinical assessment.[40] Intravenous digital subtraction angiography (DSA) can be performed as an outpatient, but nevertheless is not an appropriate screening tool. It is costly, time-consuming and patients tolerance is low.

A prospective study conducted by Treiman has questioned the need for routine angiography following identification of a significant lesion prior to undergoing surgical revision.[41] Using the criteria of a V2/V1 ratio >2.5, a peak velocity > 250 cm/s or a distal velocity of < 45 cm/s, he was able to identify 31 grafts that required revision, only five of which were in patients with recurrent symptoms. Operation was performed with a 94% assisted primary patency rate at 3 years with minimal morbidity based only on the duplex scan identification and localization of the stenoses. Data reported by Caps *et al.* supports the belief that angiography is no longer the current 'gold standard' as the angiogram prior to surgery did not alter the management plan in any of their cases.[8]

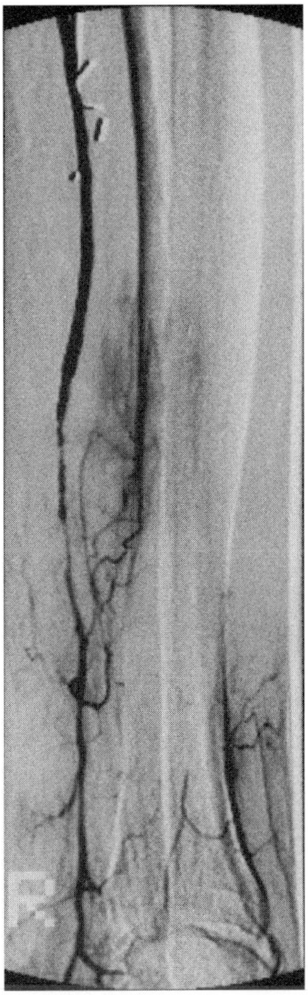

Fig. 3. Long diffuse stenosis at the distal end of an *in situ* graft possibly caused by the insertion of a valvulotome at the time of surgery. Diffuse lesions with poor runoff may not have a discreet site of elevated velocity.

DURATION AND FREQUENCY OF GRAFT SURVEILLANCE

Graft surveillance programmes are time consuming and expensive in a busy vascular service, and the length and frequency of scanning needs to be justified, based on the resources that are available. As most stenoses develop within the first 12–18 months, it is during this time that the value of surveillance will be most cost-effective. The current policy in our institution is to scan all vein grafts intensively for the first 6 months (at discharge, 6 weeks, 3 months and 6 months) and again at 9 and 12 months unless there are features of the graft or patient that warrants closer scrutiny on an individual basis such as the development of an early mild stenosis, poor quality vein used, runoff to an isolated popliteal segment or a prior graft that had stenosed or failed previously.[3] Some centres advocate a further scan at 18 months, although our experience suggests that the low number of extra grafts salvaged by adopting this policy does not justify the costs. We, of course, continue to scan all stenoses that have been identified and are being treated expectantly, but if there are no stenoses at 1 year the patient has no further surveillance.

Mills concluded that a normal early postoperative duplex scan exhibited a very low subsequent rate of stenosis and thus could be subject to a selective, less intense surveillance protocol.[11] Idu *et al.* recommend that these 'low risk' patients only require 6 months of surveillance in order to economize their protocol, despite the fact that a small proportion of patients with late onset stenosis would be missed.[42] This view was not supported by the Leicester group who found significant stenoses in 42% (11/26) grafts with a normal pre-discharge duplex scan.[43] Furthermore, they concluded that although the risk reduces after 1 year, there remains a 10% per year chance of developing a new stenosis, and thus graft surveillance should be life-long.[44] There is little evidence to support this as a cost-effective method and with cost

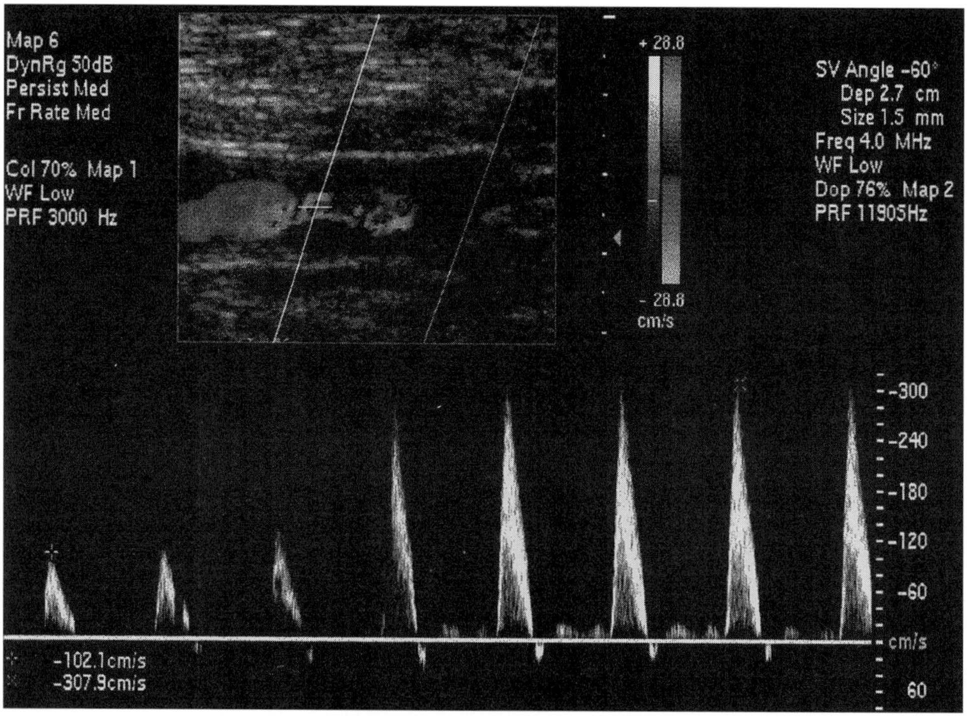

Fig. 4. Flow image demonstrating elevation of flow velocity at the site of a localized graft stenosis and a V2 : V1 ratio > 3.

restraints it will become necessary to determine which patients are at highest risk. It has been estimated that the cost of a failed femorodistal graft leading to a secondary amputation is four times the cost of a successful bypass[45] and a 5% reduction in amputation rates justifies a 1-year surveillance programme.[19] Currently, there is unlikely to be a definitive consensus on an appropriate policy, particularly as the only two randomized trials have resulted in conflicting conclusions regarding the benefits of graft surveillance over clinical assessment.[38,39]

DO PROSTHETIC GRAFTS REQUIRE SURVEILLANCE?

Prosthetic bypass grafts differ from autogenous vein in that they do not achieve full endothelial coverage except at the anastamosis. The current literature demonstrates only a limited benefit from a surveillance programme, as most of the prosthetic grafts that occlude do not have any predictive features on the preceding duplex scans.[46–48] Whilst patency rates for an above-knee femoropopliteal bypass are comparable with autogenous vein, more distal grafts are inferior to vein. Whereas great care is taken to preserve functioning autogenous vein grafts (to preserve valuable vein), prosthetic grafts are readily available and the prospect of intervening in an asymptomatic patient with a view to extending the graft to the infragenicular level is not appealing to most surgeons. The argument for asymptomatic intervention is weak and a new graft is probably the best option for an infrainguinal prosthetic graft thrombosis.

IS THE TREATMENT OF SURVEILLANCE-DETECTED GRAFT STENOSES SUCCESSFUL?

The significant incidence of stenoses, their association with graft failure and the current inability to prevent this complication are all powerful arguments for a postoperative surveillance programme. However, justification for embarking on detection programmes also depends on obtaining benefits for the patient. The identification of a haemodynamically significant graft stenosis can only alter the eventual outcome and be deemed a valuable addition to patient care if the subsequent management of the stenosis improves the patency rates and reduces costs, morbidity and rates of lower limb amputation.

The alternatives available to the surgeon after identifying a graft 'at risk' either clinically or with duplex/angiography are surgical correction, radiological intervention or continued monitoring. The repair of a stenosis essentially depends on the timing of intervention. If stenoses are repaired before they result in graft failure very satisfactory long-term patency rates > 80% at 5 years can be expected. In contrast, salvage patency rates following graft occlusions which require graft thrombectomy or thrombolysis followed by stenosis repair are considerably inferior (in the order of 20–37%).[12,49]

After early graft failure it has been proposed that the endothelial injury caused by the thrombectomy balloon catheter may accentuate the healing response involving platelet aggregation, smooth muscle cell proliferation and intimal thickening, thereby increasing the risk of further graft-related stenosis and reducing patency rate.[50] Robinson was also able to demonstrate the poor outcome following intervention for early graft failure, and although advocating a single attempt if the graft occludes, does not recommend further operation if the patient had occluded whilst being on anticoagulation or in those having revision bypass surgery.[51]

Surgery involves patch angioplasty usually with autogenous vein, interposition grafts or extension 'jump' grafts, particularly if the lesion is at the distal anastamosis. These methods are advocated by many authors and increase the primary assisted patency rates (as shown in Table 2), to levels that are comparable with primary patency rates of undiseased bypasses.[8,9,22,30,36,39,52–55] Surgical intervention often requires the use of short additional lengths of autogenous vein, but this is preferable to finding vein for an entirely new bypass graft, where sources such as the arm or short saphenous vein may be adequate for these purposes.

Radiological techniques include percutaneous transluminal angioplasty (PTA), directional atherectomy or endovascular stenting, but all have come under criticism when long-term success is compared with surgical methods. Some authors report poor patency in the order of 7–50% at 2–3 years, especially when treating long stenoses such as that shown in Fig. 3.[3,56,57] Other centres have had more success with patency rates of 65–90%.[58,59] Dunlop has also found that although many grafts could initially be treated successfully with PTA, restenosis rates were unacceptably high (42%), particularly in the distal one-third of the *in situ* graft where diameters are smaller.[60] Although many of these were salvaged with further PTA (a tempting, less invasive technique with low morbidity), there is little doubt now that PTA should only be used in grafts with short web stenoses as demonstrated in Fig. 5. Long (>2cm) and distal anastamotic stenoses (Fig. 6) are best treated by the surgical methods described above.

Directional atherectomy has also been recently reported to have benefit in improving the assisted primary patency rate to 79% at 3 years, approaching similar rates as surgical intervention.[61]

Table 2. Assisted primary patency rates following surgical correction of surveillance detected vein graft stenoses

Author (Year)	*Grafts*	*Primary patency*	*Assisted patency*
Berkowitz *et al.* (1981)[52]	134	67% 1 year	86% 1 year
Brewster *et al.* (1983)[30]	350	NA	31% 5 years
Bandyk *et al.* (1987)[53]	192	48% 3 years	89% 3 years
Grigg *et al.* (1988)[54]	80	79% 1 year	85% 1 year
Green *et al.* (1990)[36]	177	66% 5 years	80% 5 years
Mattos *et al.* (1993)[55]	170	NA	88% 2 years
Bergamini *et al.* (1995)[22]	615	56% 5 years	80% 5 years
Caps *et al.* (1995)[8]	61	44% 3 years	77% 3 years
Wilson *et al.* (1996)[9]	275	67% 1 year	77% 1 year
Ihlberg et al. (1998)[39]	185	56% 1year	65% 1 year

NA: Information not available.

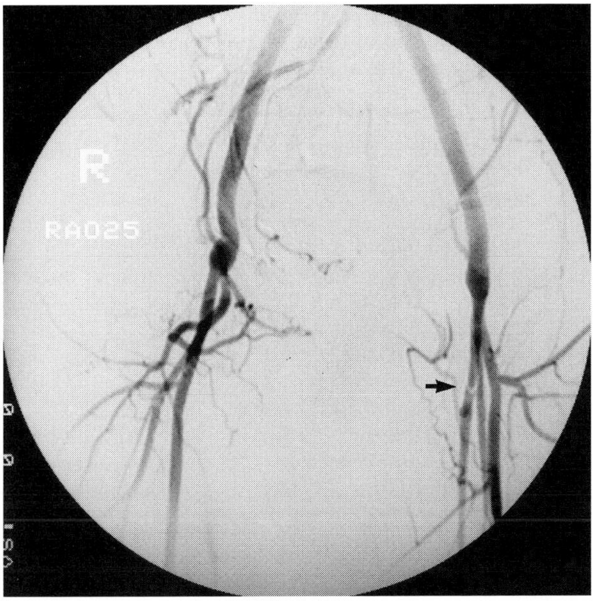

Fig. 5. Short web stenosis in the proximal segment of a femoropopliteal bypass graft suitable for treatment with balloon angioplasty.

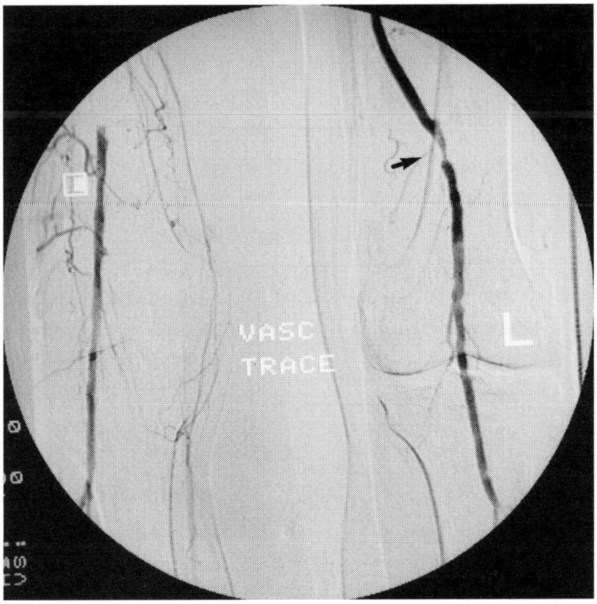

Fig. 6. Long (> 2 cm) stenosis at the distal anastamosis of the vein graft, more suitable for surgical correction.

Table 3. The potential advantages and disadvantages of the currently used radiological and surgical techniques of treating vein graft stenosis

Method	*Advantages*	*Disadvantages*
Percutaneous transluminal angioplasty (PTA) and Directional atherectomy (DA)	Quick/technically easy (PTA) Relatively inexpensive Low morbidity Short hospital stay Can be repeated Preserves native vein High patency rates (DA) Hyperplastic tissue can be removed (DA) Avoids redo surgical dissection	Limited success in long lesions (PTA) Restenosis in small grafts Hyperplastic tissue remains (PTA) Risk of dissection/ pseudoaneurysm
Surgical intervention	Established improvement in longer term patency Can remove fibrotic stricture	Morbidity of surgery Requires native vein to be used Difficulty of redo surgery

The potential benefits and disadvantages of interventional radiological techniques compared with surgical management are listed in Table 3. However, these factors have not been proven in a randomized trial.

CONCLUSIONS

Vein graft surveillance plays a valuable role in aiding clinical assessment in the maintenance of graft patency, thereby reducing the number of grafts that require replacement with the subsequent increased patient morbidity, extra workload and use of limited resources. The value of a regular protocol for at least 12 months and possibly even longer is now well established in a number of clinical studies. In particular, grafts that demonstrate some degree of haemodynamic or structural abnormality at the early postoperative surveillance scan pose a higher risk of subsequent failure and should be closely monitored for disease progression to allow intervention at an appropriate time. Although some would argue that that not all stenosed grafts proceed to occlusion, there is enough direct and indirect proof to warrant intervention in most cases.

REFERENCES

1. Bandyk D, Seabrook G, Moldenhauer R et al: Haemodynamics of vein graft stenosis. *J Vasc Surg* **8**: 688–695, 1988
2. Moody P, DeCossart LM, Douglas HM *et al.*: Asymptomatic strictures in femoropopliteal vein grafts. *Eur J Vasc Surg* **3**: 389–392, 1989
3. Taylor PR, Wolfe JHN, Tyrrell MR *et al.*: Graft stenosis: Justification for 1-year surveillance. *Br J Surg* **77**: 1125–1128, 1990

4. Chang BB, Leather RP, Kaufman JL *et al.*: Haemodynamic characteristics of failing infrainguinal *in situ* vein bypass. *J Vasc Surg* **12**: 596–600, 1990
5. Buth J, Disselhoff B, Sommeling C, Stam L: Colour-flow duplex criteria for grading stenosis in infrainguinal vein grafts. *J Vasc Surg* **14**: 716–728, 1991
6. Mills JL, Fujitani RM, Taylor SM: The characteristics and anatomic distribution of lesions that cause reversed vein graft failure: A five year prospective study. *J Vasc Surg* **17**: 195–206, 1993
7. Idu MM, Blankenstein JD, de Dier P *et al.*: Impact of a colour-flow duplex surveillance program on infrainguinal vein graft patency: A five-year experience. *J Vasc Surg* 17; 42–53, 1993
8. Caps MT, Cantwell-Gab K, Bergelin RO *et al.*: Vein graft lesions: Time of onset and rate of progression. *J Vasc Surg* 22; 466–75, 1995
9. Wilson YG, Davies AH, Curie IC *et al.*: Vein graft stenosis: Incidence and intervention. *Eur J Vasc Endovasc Surg* 11; 164–169, 1996
10. Harris PL: Vein graft surveillance-all part of the service. *Br J Surg* **79**: 97–987, 1992
11. Mills JL, Bandyk DF, Ghatan V *et al.*: The origin of infrainguinal vein graft stenosis: A prospective study based on duplex surveillance. *J Vasc Surg* **20**: 16–25, 1995
12. Whittemore AD, Clowes AW, Couch NP, Mannick JA: Secondary femoropopliteal reconstruction. *Ann Surg* **193**: 35–42, 1981
13. European Consensus Document on critical limb ischaemia: In Dormandy J, Stock G (Eds) *Critical Limb Ischaemia: Its Pathophysiology and Management*. Berlin: Springer-Verlag, 1990
14. Giannoukas AD, Androulakis AE, Labropoulos N *et al.*: The role of surveillance after infrainguinal bypass grafting. *Eur J Vasc Endovasc Surg* 11; 279–289, 1996
15. Szilagyi DE, Elliot JP, Hageman JH *et al.*: Biological fate of autologous vein implants as arterial substitutes: Observations in femoro-popliteal operations for atherosclerosis. *Ann Surg* **178**: 232–246, 1973
16. Davies AH, Magee TR, Baird RN: Vein compliance: a preoperative indicator of vein morphology and of veins at risk of vascular graft stenosis. *Br J Surg* **79**: 1019–1021, 1992
17. Varty K, Porter K, Bell PRF *et al.*: Vein morphology and bypass graft stenosis. *Br J Surg* **83**: 1375–1379, 1996
18. Miller A, Marcaccio EJ, Tannenbaum GA *et al.*: Comparison of angioscopy and angiography for monitoring infrainguinal bypass vein grafts: Results of a prospective randomized trial. *J Vasc Surg* **17**: 382–398, 1993
19. Grigg MJ, Nicolaides AN, Wolfe JHN: Can postoperative surveillance of femoro-distal vein grafts be justified? In: Greenhalgh RM (Ed) *Indications in Vascular Surgery* pp. 259–270. London: WB Saunders Co., 1998
20. Scott D, Vowden P, Beard J, Horrocks M: Non-invasive estimation of peripheral resistance using PGR before femoro-distal bypass. *Br J Surg* **77**: 391–395, 1990
21. Bandyk DF, Johnson BL, Gupta AK *et al.*: Nature and management of duplex abnormalities encountered during infrainguinal vein bypass grafting. *J Vasc Surg* **24**: 430–438, 1996
22. Bergamini TM, George Jr SM, Massey HT *et al.*: Intensive surveillance of femoropopliteal-tibial autogenous vein bypasses improves long-term graft patency and limb salvage. *Ann Surg* **22**: 507–516, 1995
23. Dunlop P, Hartshorne T, Bolia A *et al.*: The long-term outcome of infrainguinal vein graft surveillance. *Eur J Vasc Endovasc Surg* 10; 352–355, 1995
24. Golledge J, Beattie DK, Greenhalgh RM *et al.*: Have the results of infrainguinal bypass improved with the widespread utilisation of postoperative surveillance? *Eur J Vasc Endovasc Surg* 11; 388–392, 1996
25. Mills JL, Harris EJ, Taylor Jr LM *et al.*: The importance of routine surveillance of distal bypass grafts with duplex scanning: A study of 379 reversed vein grafts. *J Vasc Surg* 12; 379–389, 1990
26. Cheshire NJ, Wolfe JHN, Barradas M: Smoking and plasma fibrinogen, lipoprotein(a) and serotonin are markers for postoperative infrainguinal graft stenosis. *Eur J Vasc Endovasc Surg* **11**: 479–486, 1996
27. Hicks RC, Golledge J, Mir-Hasseine R, Powell JT: Vasoactive effects of fibrinogen on saphenous vein. *Nature* **379**: 818–820, 1996

28. Mireskandari M, Schachter M, Timms IGO *et al.*: Plasma homocysteine is an independent risk factor for vein graft stenosis. Abstract presented to Association of Surgeons Great Britain and Ireland Meeting 1998. *Br J Surg* **85** (Suppl): 27, 1998
29. Chan P, Patel M, Betteridge L *et al.*: Abnormal growth regulation of vascular smoth muscle cells in patients with restenosis. *Lancet* **341**: 341–342, 1993.
30. Brewster JC, LaSalle AJ, Robinson JG *et al.*: Femoropopliteal graft failures: Clinical consequeces and success of secondary reconstructions. *Arch Surg* **118**: 1043–1047, 1983
31. McShane MD, Gazzard VM, Clifford PC *et al.*: Duplex ultrasound monitoring of arterial grafts: Prospective evaluation in conjunction with ankle pressure indices after femorodistal bypass. *Eur J Vasc Endovasc Surg* **1**: 385–390, 1987
32. Dalsing MC, Cikrit DF, Lalka SG et al.: Femorodistal vein grafts: The utility of graft surveillance criteria. *J Vasc Surg* **21**: 127–134, 1995
33. Grigg MJ, Nicolaides AN, Wolfe JHN: Detection and grading of femorodistal vein graft stenoses: Duplex velocity measurements compared with angiography. *J Vasc Surg* **8**: 661–666, 1998
34. McShane MD, Gazzard VM, Clifford PC *et al.*: Duplex ultrasound assessment of femorodistal grafts: Correlation with angiography. *Eur J Vasc Endovasc Surg* **1**: 409–414, 1987
35. Olojugba DH, McCarthy MJ, Naylor AR *et al.*: At what peak velocity ratio value should duplex-detected infrainguinal vein graft stenoses be revised? *Eur J Vasc Endovasc Surg* **15**: 258–260, 1998
36. Green RM, McNamara J, Ouriel K, DeWese JA: Comparison of infrainguinal graft surveillance techniques. *J Vasc Surg* **11**: 207–215, 1990
37. Wolfe JHN, Taylor R, Cheshire NJ: Graft surveillance: A biased overview. In: Greenhalgh RM, Hollier LM (Eds) *The Maintenance of Arterial Reconstruction* pp. 119–128. London: WB Saunders Co., 1991
38. Lundell A, Lindblad B, Bergqvist D *et al.*: Femoropopliteal-crural graft patency is improved by an intensive surveillance program: A prospective randomized study. *J Vasc Surg* **21**: 26–34, 1995
39. Ihlberg L, Luther M, Tierala E, Lepantalo M: The utility of duplex scanning in infrainguinal vein graft surveillance: Results from a randomised controlled study. *Eur J Vasc Endovasc Surg* **16**: 19–27, 1998
40. Wolfe JHN, Lea Thomas M, Browse NL *et al.*: Early diagnosis of femorodistal graft stenosis. *Br J Surg* **74**: 268–270, 1987
41. Treiman GS, Lawrence PF, Galt SW *et al.*: Revision of reversed infrainguinal bypass grafts without preoperative arteriography. *J Vasc Surg* **26**: 1020–1028, 1997
42. Idu MM, Buth, J, Cuypers PH *et al.*: Economising vein-graft surveillance programs *Eur J Vasc Endovasc Surg* **15**: 432–438, 1998
43. Olojugba DH, Varty K, Hartshorne T *et al.*: Predischarge duplex imaging of infrainguinal vein grafts does not predict the development of stenoses. *Br J Surg* **85**: 1225–1227, 1998
44. McCarthy MJ, Olojugba D, Loftus IM *et al.*: Lower limb surveillance following autologous vein bypass should be life long. *Br J Surg* **85**: 1369–1372, 1998
45. Panayiotopoulos YP, Tyrell MR, Owen SE *et al.*: Outcome and cost analysis after femorocrural and femoropedal grafting for critical limb ischaemia. *Br J Surg* **84**: 207–212, 1997
46. Lalak NJ, Hanel KC, Hunt J *et al.*: Duplex scan surveillance of infrainguinal prosthetic bypass grafts. *J Vasc Surg* **20**: 637–641, 1994
47. Dunlop P, Sayers RD, Naylor AR *et al.*: The effect of a surveillance programme on the patency of synthetic infrainguinal bypass grafts. *Eur J Vasc Endovasc Surg* **11**: 441–445, 1996
48. Hoballah JJ, Nazzai MM, Ryan SM *et al.*: Is colour duplex surveillance of infrainguinal polytetrafluoroethylene grafts worthwhile? *Am J Surg* **174**: 131–135, 1997
49. Sladen JG, Gilmour JL: Vein graft stenosis: characteristics and effect of treatment. *Am J Surg* **141**: 549–553, 1981
50. Nielsen TG, Jensen LP, Schroeder TV: Early vein bypass thrombectomy is associated with an increased risk of graft related stenoses. *Eur J Vasc Endovasc Surg* **13**: 134–138, 1997
51. Robinson KD, Sato DT, Gregory RT *et al.*: Long-term outcome after early infrainguinal graft failure. *J Vasc Surg* **26**: 425–438, 1997

52. Berkowitz HD, Hobbs CL, Roberts B *et al.*: Value of routine vascular laboratory studies to identify vein graft stenosis. *Surgery* **90**: 971–979, 1981
53. Bandyk DF, Keabnick HW, Stewart GW, Towne JB: Durability of the *in situ* saphenous vein arterial bypass: a comparison of primary and secondary procedures. *J Vasc Surg* **5**: 256–268, 1987
54. Grigg MJ, Nicolaides AN, Wolfe JHN: Femorodistal vein bypass graft stenoses. *Br J Surg* **75**: 737–740, 1988
55. Mattos MA, van Bemmelen PS, Hodgson KJ *et al.*: Does detection of stenoses identified with colour duplex scanning improve infrainguinal graft patency? *J Vasc Surg* **17**: 54–66, 1993
56. Whittemore AD, Donaldson MC, Polak JF *et al.*: Limitations of balloon angioplasty for vein graft stenosis. *J Vasc Surg* **14**: 340–345, 1991
57. Thompson JF, McShaneMD, Gazzard V *et al.*: Limitations of percutaneous transluminal angioplasty in the treatment of femorodistal graft stenoses. *Eur J Vasc Surg* **3**: 209–211, 1989
58. Veith J, Weiser RK, Gupta SK: Diagnosis and management of failing lower extremity arterial reconstructions prior to graft occlusion. J Cardiovasc Surg **25**: 381–384, 1986
59. London NJM, Sayers RD, Thompson MM *et al.*: Interventional radiology in the maintenance of infrainguinal vein graft patency. *Br J Surg* **80**: 187–193, 1993
60. Dunlop P, Varty K, Hartshorne T *et al.*: Percutaneous transluminal angioplasty of infrainguinal vein graft stenosis: Long-term outcome *Br J Surg* **82**: 204–206, 1995
61. Porter DH, Rosen MP, Skillman J *et al.*: Mid-term and long-term results with directional atherectomy of vein graft stenoses. *J Vasc Surg* **23**: 554–563, 1996

Commentary

'Vein graft surveillance plays a valuable role in aiding clinical assessment in the maintenance and patency . . . The value of a regular protocol for at least 12 months and possibly even longer is now well established in a number of clinical studies.'

From this chapter one would conclude that there is nothing more to add, vein graft surveillance is mandatory. It is time to read on to the next chapter. *RMG*

Vein graft surveillance could be overrated

Paula Lee Kirby and Alun Huw Davies

INTRODUCTION

Vein graft surveillance has become an accepted part of follow-up for patients with vein bypass grafts.[1] It was known as early as 1973 that approximately 30% of vein grafts will developed a stenosis within the lumen of the graft;[2] a number of different modalities are routinely used to gain information on the performance of the graft postoperatively. The current available methods of surveillance are described below.

Clinical evaluation and ankle brachial pressure index (ABPI)

Alone, clinical investigations are only able to detect gross changes of graft performance, for example the loss of a palpable pulse in the graft or distal vessels. A decrease in resting ABPIs may be indicative of a problem within a graft but may miss up to 50% of stenoses.[3] It has been suggested that ABPIs may be useful as an initial screening test.[4,5]

Duplex

The ideal diagnostic tool? Duplex scanning combines a real-time B mode ultrasound image with Doppler blood flow waveform data. This technique has many advantages over angiography; it is non-invasive, repeatable, reproducible and has high detection rates. However, initial costs are high and require the skills of highly trained personnel to perform the test.

Angiography

Initially angiography was used to visualize the graft and distal vessels. However, this is by no means ideal for serial investigations, due to associated complications at the puncture site and exposure to contrast agents. One other disadvantage of angiography is the uniplanar image obtained which may miss irregular plaques within the lumen of the vessel. Oblique views would improve sensitivity but increase time and contrast usage. However, this technique is still adopted as the gold standard in imaging and is employed by many vascular surgeons before embarking on an intervention as indicated by a non-diagnostic method.

NATURAL HISTORY OF A VEIN GRAFT

It is difficult to predict which infrainguinal vein grafts will subsequently fail at the time of operation. Certain factors contribute to the success or failure of a graft, for example choice of vein, extent of trauma incurred whilst harvesting the vein or any pre-existing disease at the anastomotic sites. It is believed that there is a greater chance of long-term technical success if lesions are revised before the graft occludes. Although one prospective study indicated that *de novo* stenoses are uncommon in reversed and *in situ* vein bypasses, instead they result from an existing deficit or abnormality within the vein.[6]

Whittemore *et al.* defined three phases of graft failure; early (first month postoperatively), intermediate (1–12 months) and late (after 1 year).[7]

Early

The early failures are attributed to technical complications. In particular the vein may become damaged or ischaemic during mobilization. For the latter reason *in situ* grafts were originally favoured; however, subsequent results indicated no benefit in this technique over reversed vein bypass.[8,9] The balance in results may be due to the effects of passing a valulotome through the lumen of an *in situ* graft to strip the valve leaflets.

Intermediate

The majority of stenoses found within the body of a vein graft between 1 and 12 months are thought to be due to myointimal hyperplasia.[10,7] Less common events leading to the failure of a graft in this period are valve cusp fibrosis and aneurysmal dilatation of the vessel. Stenoses are commonly found at sites of turbulent flow through the vessel, such as anastomotic sites and areas of shear stress.[11] Other authors have suggested that it is dependent on the quality of the vein used.[12–14] The trigger for neointimal hyperplasia may be an injury to the endothelial lining of the vein leading to platelet aggregation and smooth muscle cell proliferation, causing a narrowing of the vessel lumen.[15] Such strictures may rapidly progress to occlusion of the graft.[2,16]

Late

Late failures are predominantly associated with progression of the underlying atherosclerotic disease of the native vessels. Particular poor prognosis is associated with patients who continue to smoke against medical advice and those with high plasma fibrinogen levels. It is difficult to say whether fibrinogen levels are causative or a reaction to the disease progression; however, it is significantly correlated with graft failure.[17]

The natural fate of a graft with a stenosis is difficult to evaluate, as most series report that once a haemodynamically significant stenosis is detected, intervention is planned. In one study of 80 grafts, all followed with duplex surveillance, 23% (5/22) with identified stenoses occluded and 7% (4/58) without a detected lesion occluded.[18] However, this was not considered to be statistically significant[19] and therefore could not be translated to an improved outcome. This was also true for 275 primary grafts followed in Bristol.[20] Eighty-five grafts developed a stenosis on surveillance. Twenty-four of these had no subsequent treatment to correct the lesion. A further 64 developed a *de novo* inflow or outflow problem due to disease progression, of which 28 were untreated. The cumulative 12-month patency rates in both the untreated (n=52) and treated groups (n=97) were not significantly different. Therefore it is quite possible that some stenoses will remain stable and not threaten graft viability.

INDICATION FOR SURGERY

Bypass operations are most commonly indicated for patients with critical limb ischaemia. However, a smaller proportion are performed for disabling claudication or popliteal aneurysms. Not all claudicants are considered suitable for bypass surgery; they may benefit best from percutaneous transluminal angioplasty and/or an established exercise regime, together with advice on smoking.

Unfortunately outcome measures of vein graft success can be difficult to interpret as the prognosis for operations performed for claudication is better than critical limb ischaemia (see definition of critical limb ischaemia in the European Consensus Document[21]). Outcome measures commonly quoted are patency rates (primary, primary assisted and secondary) and less frequently limb salvage. These are defined as: primary, uninterrupted patency with no procedures performed on the graft or anastomoses; primary assisted, intervention has been performed on a failing but still patent graft; secondary patency, flow is restored through most of the original graft including at least one of its original anastomoses.[22]

CRITERIA FOR IDENTIFYING THE AT-RISK GRAFT

The criteria for identifying an at-risk graft are dependent on the modality used for surveillance. A decrease of 0.2 in consecutive ABPI measurements will identify up to 50% of stenoses. A drop of 0.1 may identify up to 75% of stenoses, but this is close to the margin of error of the technique.[23] An area of >50% reduction in diameter of the vessel lumen, as determined by digital subtraction angiography, is also used.[24]

Criteria used in duplex scanning are: i) peak systolic flow velocity of < 45cm/s being indicative of poor flow through the length of the vessel[4] and ii) a local increase in velocity is associated with a narrowing of the vessel lumen.[25] The V2/V1 ratio at the site of a stenosis is often used to determine when to intervene but again the ratio at which the graft is considered to be at risk is centre, if not consultant, specific. The values of V2/V1 ratio quoted as being indicative of haemodynamically at risk grafts ranges from 1.5 to 3.0.[6,26,27]

UNNECESSARY INTERVENTION?

Early intervention may not always be advantageous; the techniques used to correct failing grafts, such as balloon angioplasty or further surgery (vein patch, interposition graft or jump graft surgery), may introduce extra risks to the graft. It has been suggested that if a radiological or surgical intervention procedure is performed to correct a stenosis, there is a greater chance of a recurrence of that stenosis or developing a second lesion.[10,2,25]

What is not known, though, is how many grafts with a small stenosis would remain stable if no intervention was performed.[26,28,29] There are few data available on the natural history of asymptomatic yet haemodynamically significant lesions. One small study showed that conservatively treated grafts with a non-haemodynamically significant stenosis had a 12-month patency rate of only 58%, although the majority of these patients avoided amputation of their limb despite having occluded grafts.[26] Mattos *et al.* also noted that most of the stenoses detected in their series of patients remained patent whether they were revised or not.[29]

DEVELOPMENT OF A SURVEILLANCE PROGRAMME AND COST

Duplex ultrasound scanning facilities are expensive to establish and maintain. The initial outlay for the machines, the cost of trained staff and any extra costs of interventions performed as a result of the duplex findings must all be considered. However, Grigg *et al.* estimated that if duplex surveillance of all vein grafts prevented 1–2% of patients needing an amputation then the saving would be great enough to justify the expense of establishing a surveillance programme.[30]

In addition to the financial cost to the budget holder, the benefit to the patient must also be considered. Whilst it is difficult to measure physical parameters and emotions, certain tools have been validated to compare patient populations, for example 'generic' quality of life questionnaires.[31] These are typically broken down into physical and psychological domains and can be compared between patient populations or with 'normal' populations. None of the studies reviewed in this chapter have addressed these issues in their patients.

IS DUPLEX REALLY NECESSARY?

To date only two small prospective studies have been performed comparing duplex surveillance with clinical follow-up in vein graft patients;[32,33] however, the use of duplex scanning has been recommended in the management of these patients. This has been concluded from a number of studies using series of patients receiving duplex scans at follow-up compared with historical controls.[18,34] Even if the groups are matched for age, indication for surgery and diabetes, certain factors cannot be accounted for in the analysis. Discrepancies between the two groups may include quality of the surgery performed and differences in the intensity of the follow-up regimes.[35]

A summation analysis of published series of vein grafts, up to 1995, comparing clinical follow-up and duplex surveillance showed that whilst patency rates appeared to be better in the duplex group, there was no significant difference in the amputation rates between the two groups.[35] However, there was inconsistent reporting of the amputation rates in these studies. It has been suggested that the amputation rates need to be improved to justify the cost of a surveillance programme.[30] However, without data to support the number of amputations in both groups it becomes difficult to observe any advantage in one regime over the other.

A survey, conducted by our vascular unit, of 112 vascular consultants in the UK, reported the absence of duplex surveillance in a significant number of both teaching hospitals (22%) and district general hospitals (44%).[36] The reasons for failure to use duplex were divided between lack of resources and non-belief in its efficacy. Therefore the use of duplex in the surveillance of vein bypass patients is not universal and before dedicating limited funds to machines and operators, surely it is best to have direct proof of the benefits of a technique?

The two prospective studies comparing duplex scanning and a clinical regime were both performed in single centres. Lundell *et al.* studied both vein and synthetic grafts and demonstrated an advantage to duplex scanning in the vein bypasses when comparing patency rates, but not amputation rate.[32] More recently, Ihlberg *et al.* could not demonstrate any statistical difference in primary patency (Fig. 1), assisted primary patency or limb salvage between duplex surveillance and clinical assessment in their randomized controlled trial.[33] In contrast to the previous trial, the patients in the clinical arm of Ihlberg's trial had significantly higher secondary patency rates than those followed with duplex; 84% ABPI vs 71% duplex, p=0.04 (Fig. 2). However

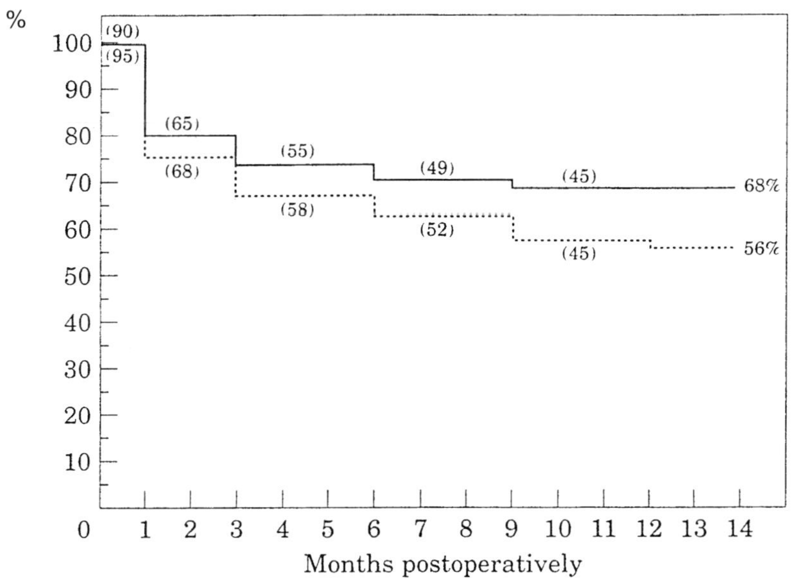

Fig. 1. There is no statistical difference in primary patency rate in the surveillance (68% at 14 months) compared with the non-duplex groups. (Reproduced from Ref. 33 with permission.)

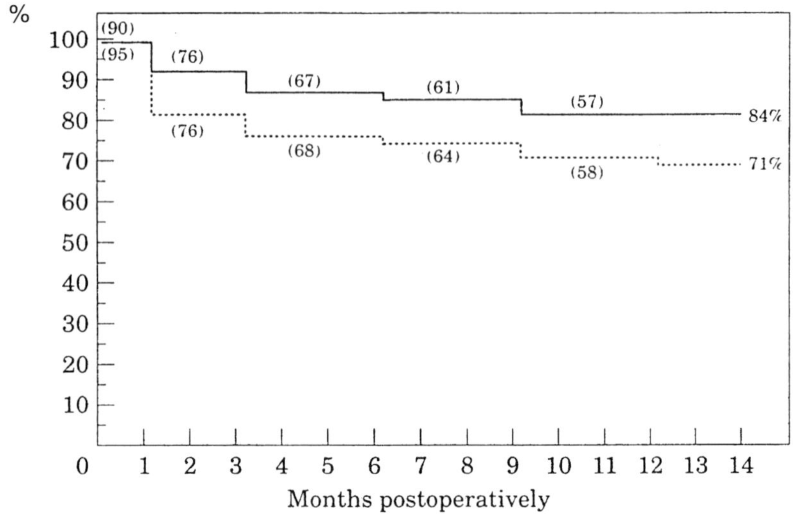

Fig. 2. Cumulative secondary patency was significantly higher in the non-surveillance arm at 14 months (84%) than in the surveillance arm of the study. (Reproduced from Ref. 33 with permission.)

Ihlberg *et al.* also reported difficulty in obtaining complete data on patients and had a small cohort of patients per group.

A summation analysis of these two sets of data at 1 year shows no difference in primary assisted patency; 70% ABPI (n=77), 71% duplex (n=88). The combined duplex group had a lower secondary patency than ABPI; 81% ABPI (n=86), 75% duplex (n=95). Further analysis of data was not possible as primary patency and limb salvage was only reported by Ihlberg and not Lundell. In summary, both papers concluded that there was a need for a large randomized controlled trial.

A LARGE MULTICENTRE RANDOMIZED CONTROLLED CLINICAL TRIAL

The Vein Graft Surveillance Trial (VGST) was established in 1997, and began recruiting patients in March 1998. It is a large multicentre randomized controlled trial to assess amputation rates, graft patency, quality of life and healthcare costs in 1200 vein bypass patients from 50 centres in the UK and Europe. The follow-up period for each patient is 18 months, with data collected at 6 weeks, then 3, 6, 9, 12 and 18 months. This is shown in Fig. 3.

Patients are randomized after 30 days of their operation, providing their graft is patent at that time, to either a clinical or duplex follow-up regime. Randomization is carried out by an independent computer system at the University of York and patient allocation is stratified by centre and indication for surgery (claudication or rest pain). Patients randomized to clinical follow-up have resting ABPIs measured and a clinical consultation, whereas the duplex group have the same plus a routine duplex scan at each appointment.

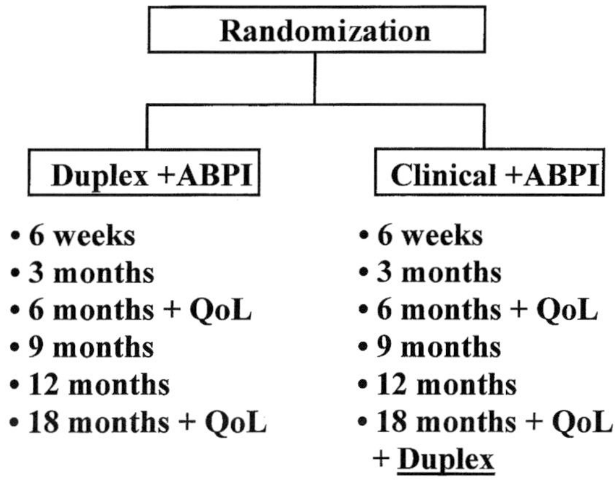

Fig. 3. Summary of the Vein Graft Surveillance Trial.

The main hypothesis to be tested in this trial is that there is no difference between duplex surveillance and clinical assessment following femorodistal vein bypass in with respect to limb salvage. However, graft patency, patient quality of life and cost analysis will also be measured. Quality of life data will be collected from the generic health questionnaires Medical Outcomes Survey Short Form 36 (MOS SF-36)[37] and EuroQol.[38,39] In the event that there is no difference between groups, a cost benefit analysis will be performed with respect to the budget holder and the patient.

CONCLUSION

More recently the emphasis has been placed on evidence-based medicine and the need for randomized controlled trials to influence a clinician's decision on how to provide the best medical care for their patients.[40] Randomized controlled trials are considered the least biased method of testing a new treatment, drug, investigation or device, provided that the randomization process is truly blind to the investigator.[41]

The use of duplex scanning has been adopted in the vascular unit as accepted practice without the results of a large prospective randomized controlled trial. The smaller prospective trials discussed within this chapter have not given a consistent answer and have concluded that such a large trial is required. We therefore propose that duplex surveillance may be overrated, until evidence is available to the contrary.

ACKNOWLEDGEMENTS

This study is funded by the British Heart Foundation Project Grant Number PG/97087.

REFERENCES

1. Harris PL: Vein graft surveillance – all part of the service. *Br J Surg* **79**: 97–98, 1992
2. Szilagyi DE, Elliott JP, Hageman JH *et al.*: Biologic fate of autogenous vein implants as arterial substitutes: clinical, angiographic and histopathologic observations in femoro-popliteal operations for atherosclerosis. *Ann Surg* **178**: 232–246, 1973
3. Wyatt MG, Muir RM, Tennant WG *et al.*: Impedance analysis to identify the at risk femorodistal graft. *J Vasc Surg* **13**: 284–291, 1991
4. Bandyk DF, Cato RF, Towne JB: A low flow velocity predicts failure of femoropopliteal and femorotibial bypass grafts. *Surgery* **98**: 799–809, 1985
5. Brennan JA, Walsh AK, Beard JD *et al.*: The role of simple non-invasive testing in infrainguinal vein graft surveillance. *Eur J Vasc Surg* **5**: 13–17, 1991
6. Mills JL, Bandyk DF, Gahtan V, Esses GE: The origin of infrainguinal vein graft stenosis: a prospective study based on duplex surveillance. *J Vasc Surg* **21**: 16–22, 1995
7. Whittemore AD, Clowes AW, Couch NP, Mannick JA: Secondary femoropopliteal reconstruction. *Ann Surg* **193**: 35–42, 1981
8. Sayers RD, Raptis S, Berce M, Miller JH: Long-term results of femorotibial bypass with vein or polyterafluoroethylene. *Br J Surg* **85**: 934–938, 1998
9. Harris PL, How TV, Jones DR: Prospectively randomized clinical trial to compare *in situ* and reversed saphenous vein grafts for femoropopliteal bypass. *Br J Surg* **74**: 252–255, 1987
10. Moody P, DeCossart LM, Douglas HM, Harris PL: Asymptomatic strictures in femoropopliteal vein grafts. *Eur J Vasc Surg* **75**: 737–740, 1989
11. Dobrin PB, Littooy FN, Endean ED: Mechanical factors predisposing to intimal hyperplasia and medial thickening in autogenous vein grafts. *Surgery* **105**: 393–400, 1989
12. Wilson YG: Vein quality in infrainguinal revascularisation: assessment by angioscopy and histology. *Ann Roy Coll Surg Engl* **80**: 3–15, 1998
13. Marin ML, Veith FJ, Panetta TF *et al.*: Saphenous vein biopsy: a predictor of vein graft failure. *J Vasc Surg* **18**: 407–414, 1993
14. Davies AH, Magee TR, Baird RN *et al.*: Vein compliance: a preoperative indicator of vein morphology and of veins at risk of vascular graft stenosis. *Br J Surg* **79**: 1019–1021, 1992
15. Davies MG, Hagen PO: Pathobiology of intimal hyperplasia. *Br J Surg* **81**: 1254–1269, 1994
16. Caps MT, Cantwell GK, Bergelin RO, Strandness-DE J: Vein graft lesions: time of onset and rate of progression. *J Vasc Surg* **22**: 466–474, 1995
17. Hicks RC, Ellis M, Mir HR *et al.*: The influence of fibrinogen concentration on the development of vein graft stenoses. *Eur J Vasc Endovasc Surg* **9**: 415–420, 1995
18. Moody P, Gould DA, Harris PL: Vein graft surveillance improves patency in femoropopliteal bypass. *Eur J Vasc Surg* **4**: 117–121, 1990
19. Beattie DK, Greenhalgh RM, Davies AH: Vein graft surveillance: is the case proven? *Ann Roy Coll Surg Engl* **79**: 1–2, 1997
20. Wilson YG, Davies AH, Currie IC *et al.*: Vein graft stenosis: incidence and intervention. *Eur J Vasc Endovasc Surg* **11**: 164–169, 1996
21. Second European Consensus Document on chronic critical leg ischaemia: *Eur J Vasc Endovasc Surg* **6** (Suppl A): 1–32, 1992
22. Rutherford RB: Standards for evaluating results of interventional therapy for peripheral vascular disease. *Circulation* **83** (Suppl 2): 6–11, 1991
23. Davies AH, Magee TR, Tennant SG *et al.*: Criteria for identification of the 'at-risk' infrainguinal bypass graft. *Eur J Vasc Surg* **8**: 315–319, 1994
24. Harris PL, Moody AP: The management of vein bypass strictures. In Greenhalgh RM, Hollier L (Eds) *The Maintenence of Arterial Reconstruction* pp. 169–178. London: WB Saunders Co, 1991
25. Grigg MJ, Nicolaides AN, Wolfe JH: Detection and grading of femorodistal vein graft stenoses: duplex velocity measurements compared with angiography *J Vasc Surg* **8**: 661–666, 1988
26. Nielsen TG: Natural history of infrainguinal vein bypass stenoses: early lesions increase the risk of thrombosis. *Eur J Vasc Endovasc Surg* **12**: 60–64, 1996

27. Sladen JG, Reid JD, Cooperberg PL *et al.*: Color flow duplex screening of infrainguinal grafts combining low- and high-velocity criteria. *Am J Surg* **158**: 107–112, 1989
28. Nehler MR, Moneta GL, Yeager RA *et al.*: Surgical treatment of threatened reversed infrainguinal vein grafts. *J Vasc Surg* **20**: 558–563, 1994
29. Mattos MA, Hodgson KJ, Ramsey DE *et al.*: Does correction of stenoses identified with color duplex scanning improve infrainguinal graft patency? *J Vasc Surg* **17**: 54–64, 1993
30. Grigg M, Nicolaides AN, Wolfe JH: Can postoperative surveillance of femoro-distal vein grafts be justified? In: Greenhalgh RM, Jamieson CW, Nicolaides AN (Eds) *Limb Salvage and Amputation in Vascular Disease* pp 259–270. London: W B Saunders Co, 1988
31. Sanders C, Egger M, Donovan J *et al.*: Reporting on quality of life in randomised controlled trials: bibliographic study. *Br Med J* **317**: 1191–1194, 1998
32. Lundell A, Lindblad B, Bergqvist D, Hansen F: Femoropopliteal-crural graft patency is improved by an intensive surveillance program: a prospective randomized study. *J Vasc Surg* **21**: 26–33, 1995
33. Ihlberg L, Luther M, Tierala E, Lepantalo M: The utility of duplex scanning in infainguinal vein graft surveillance: Results from a randomised controlled study. *Eur J Vasc Endovasc Surg* **16**: 19–27, 1998
34. Bandyk DF, Kaebnick HW, Stewart GW, Towne JB: Durability of the *in situ* saphenous vein arterial bypass: a comparison of primary and secondary patency. *J Vasc Surg* **5**: 256–268, 1987
35. Golledge J, Beattie DK, Greenhalgh RM, Davies AH: Have the results of infrainguinal bypass improved with the widespread utilisation of postoperative surveillance? *Eur J Vasc Endovasc Surg* **11**: 388–392, 1996
36. Gibbs RGJ, Beattie DK, Greenhalgh RM *et al.*: Vein graft surveillance: current trends. *Br J Surg* [abstract] **84**: 63, 1997
37. Garratt AM, Ruta DA, Abdalla MI *et al.*: The SF36 health survey questionnaire: an outcome measure suitable for routine use within the NHS? *Br Med J* **306**: 1440–1444, 1993
38. Brazier J, Jones N, Kind P: Testing the validity of the Euroqol and comparing it with the SF-36 health survey questionnaire. *Qual Life Res* **2**: 169–180, 1993
39. van Agt HM, Essink BM, Krabbe PF, Bonsel GJ: Test-retest reliability of health state valuations collected with the EuroQol questionnaire. *Soc Sci Med* **39**: 1537–1544, 1994
40. Kunz R, Oxman AD: The unpredictability paradox: review of empirical comparisons of randomised and non-randomised trials. *Br Med J* **317**: 1185–1190, 1998
41. Kerridge I, Lowe M, Henry D: Ethics and evidence based medicine. *Br Med J* **316**: 1151–1153, 1998

Commentary

This can hardly be described as an independent commentary as the commentator and authors work together and are joint applicants for the Vein Graft Surveillance Trial. Suffice it to say that there are those who have assumed that vein graft surveillance is worth the effort and that there is also a body of opinion that feels that this expensive practice should be justified. It could well be that it is justified. Some 10–15 years ago, the ankle brachial pressure index was certainly denigrated by those who had championed vein graft surveillance and it is rather remarkable that at this stage the vein graft surveillance is under scrutiny. Is any practice sacrosanct? Clearly it is not and we must have evidence these days for our practice. *RMG*

THE DURABILITY OF ENDOVASCULAR AORTIC ANEURYSM REPAIR

Do we learn anything from the Registry of Endovascular Treatment of Aneurysms (RETA) on the durability of stent grafts?

SM Thomas and JD Beard

INTRODUCTION

The Joint Working Party of the Vascular Surgical Society of Great Britain and Ireland and the British Society of Interventional Radiologists agreed the principles for the introduction of endovascular grafting of abdominal aortic aneurysms (AAA) in 1995.[1] Part of these principles included the establishment of a central registry to be maintained by the Joint Working Party. The Registry of Endovascular Treatment of Aneurysms (RETA) was therefore established and data collection began on 1 January 1996.

In an attempt to maximize submission to the registry and to ensure a high rate of follow-up, requested data have been kept to a minimum. Submission of data to the RETA registry is on a succinct case registration form which records: details of patient demographics, indications for repair, suitability for conventional repair, patient fitness, aneurysm morphology, type of device used, details of the procedure and immediate and 30-day outcomes. Single-sheet follow-up data forms are returned to the submitting centre annually.

Despite the problems with a registry it will usually provide a large amount of data and hopefully be a representative means to assess a new technology during its introduction into practice and prior to the preferred method of assessment; the randomized controlled trial. Although registration of all AAAs treated endovascularly is an important element of the RETA registry, giving useful information on the likely 30-day outcomes of patients treated in the UK, follow-up data are of equal or probably more importance. Such data are often lacking for the small numbers of patients in many of the reports of endovascular grafting of AAA,[2,3] though this is improving.[4] This chapter concentrates on the follow-up data collected on the RETA registry since its inception, in an attempt to address the question of durability of stent grafts in the treatment of AAA.

DEMOGRAPHICS AND EARLY OUTCOMES

To date, 473 patients have been submitted to the RETA registry from 28 centres (median 10.5 cases per centre, range 1–101). Most of the patients on the registry have had elective repair of asymptomatic aneurysms: 82.2% (n=388) had elective repair of an asymptomatic AAA, 14.2% (n=67) had elective repair for symptoms, nine (1.9%)

acute repair for a non-ruptured AAA, and eight (1.7%) acute repair for ruptures. A total of 88% (n=409) were American Society of Anesthesiology (ASA) grade I–III and 12% (n=56) ASA grade IV–V (missing data n=9) at the time of the procedure. In all, 20 (4.2%) had an aortic tube graft, 273 (57.7%) had an aorto-bi-iliac graft and 180 (38.1%) had an aorto-uni-iliac graft and a femerofemoral cross-over. Mean age was 71.8 years (range 44–91).

For the purposes of analysis the patients can be divided into those with an aortic tube graft or aorto-bi-iliac graft (the more endovascular technique) and those with an aorto-uni-iliac graft and a surgical cross-over (the more surgical technique). Those in the aorto-uni-iliac and cross-over group were slightly older (mean age 72.4 vs 71.4 ($p>0.05$, t-test)) but significantly more were unfit for conventional repair (Fig. 1).

In 358 (75.7%) cases (data missing n=2) the aneurysm was excluded at the end of the procedure with no procedural complications. In all, 26 (5.5%) patients required conversion to an open repair with 25 of these being immediate conversions; one being performed the day after the attempted stent graft procedure because the device was too small. Primary endoleaks* for which no treatment was deemed necessary immediately occurred in 11% (n=52).

At 30 days or discharge the aneurysm exclusion rate was 85.6% overall. Persistent primary endoleaks remained in 6.6%. There were three cases of macroembolization which lead to lower limb amputation. The mortality rate was 6.3% (n=30) overall, with those who had an aorto-bi-iliac or tube graft having a lower mortality (2.7% vs 12.2%). Even after adjusting for confounders of age and case mix using logistic regression this difference remained significant ($p<0.05$). Those unfit for conventional repair had a higher mortality at 23.2% and conversion carried a high mortality of 30.8% (Table 1).

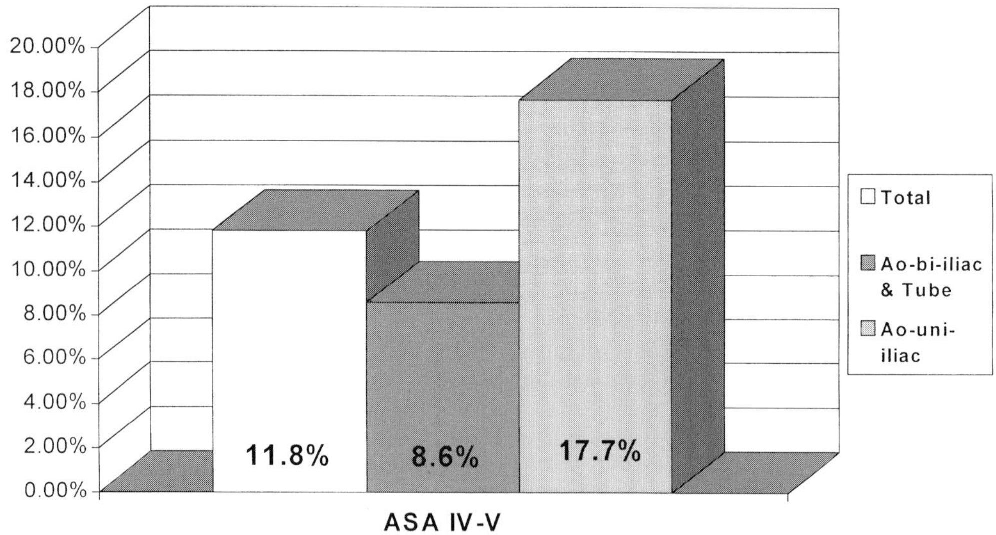

Fig. 1. Those considered unfit for conventional repair, total and by graft type. Chi-square: $p<0.005$.

* The description of endoleaks has not been standardized; the method used in this chapter follows that described by White *et al.*[9]

Table 1. The 30-day/discharge outcome

	n	*(%)*
Aneurysm excluded/repaired		
Aorto-bi-iliac and tube grafts	258/293	(88.1)
Aorto-uni-iliac + cross-over	147/180	(81.7)
	405/473	(85.6)
Persistent leak		
Aorto-bi-iliac and tube grafts	21/293	(7.2)
Aorto-uni-iliac + cross-over	10/180	(5.6)
	31/473	(6.6)
Major amputation	3	(0.6)
Deaths		
Aorto-bi-iliac and tube grafts	8/293	(2.7)
Aorto-uni-iliac graft + cross-over	22/180	(12.2)
ASA I–III	17/409	(4.2)
ASA IV–V	13/56	(23.2)
Conversions to open repair	8/26	(30.8)
Non-conversions	22/447	(4.9)
	30/473	(6.3)

1-YEAR FOLLOW-UP DATA

Requests for 1-year follow-up data were made to submitting centres for 230 of the 473 cases on the registry. Follow-up data were returned on 173, giving a follow-up rate of 75.2% at 1 year. This 173 1-year follow-up cohort form the bulk of available follow-up data for analysis. Monitoring of the aneurysm and stent graft was by computed tomography (CT) in 74.4% (n=128/172), Ultrasound/duplex in 33.1% (n=57/172), Angiography in 14% (n=24/172) and magnetic resonance imaging (MRI) in 1.2% (n=2/172) (missing data n=1).

Most of the patients on the registry have had elective repair of asymptomatic aneurysms. This is similarly reflected in the follow-up data: 84.4% (n=146) having had elective repair of an asymptomatic AAA, 13.3% (n=23) having elective repair for symptoms, one (0.6%) acutely for a non-ruptured AAA, and three (1.7%) acutely for contained ruptures. A total of 90.5% (n=152) were ASA grade I–III and 9.5% (n=16) ASA grade IV–V at the time of the procedure (missing data n=5);11 (6.4%) had an aortic tube graft, 97 (56.1%) had an aorto-bi-iliac graft and 65 (37.6%) had an aorto-uni-iliac graft and a femoral-femoral cross-over. The different devices for which 1-year follow-up is available are shown in Fig. 2.

The early outcome data showed that dividing the patients into those treated with an aortic tube graft or aorto-bi-iliac graft and those with an aorto-uni-iliac graft and a surgical cross-over is illuminating and the follow-up data have been similarly analysed. Once again those in the aorto-uni-iliac and cross-over group were older

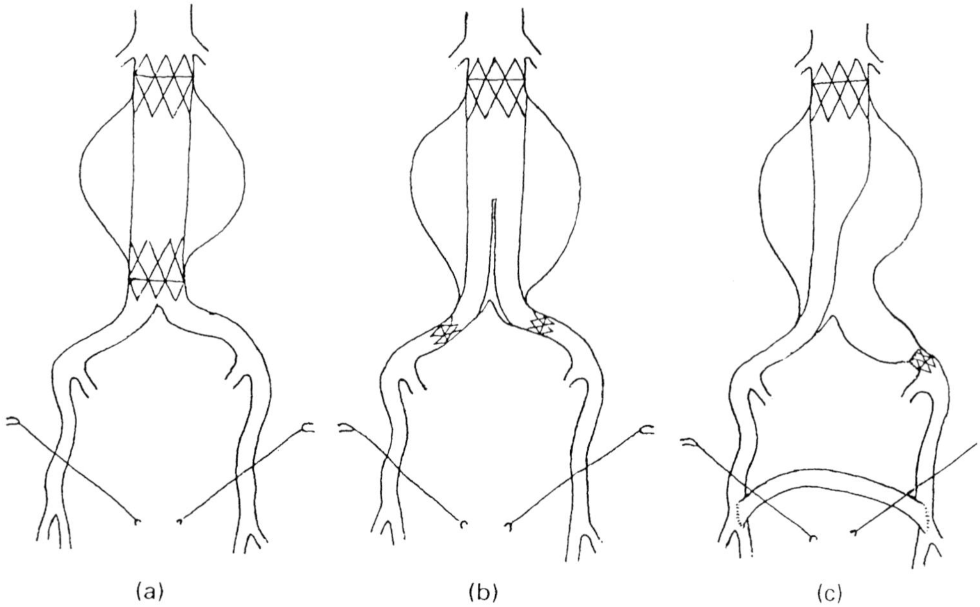

Aortic tube Grafts n=11 (6.4%)	Aorto-bi-iliac Grafts n=97 (56.1%)	Aorto-uni-iliac Grafts n=65 (37.6%)
Bard n=4 (36.4%)	EVT n=11 (11.3%)	EVT n=1 (1.5%)
Gianturco-Dacron n=1 (9.1%)	Perth n=3 (3.1%)	Gianturco-Dacron n=33 (50.8%)
Vanguard n=6 (54.5%)	Talent n=5 (5.2%)	Palmaz/PTFE n=30 (46.2%)
Vanguard n=78 (80.4%)	Talent n=1 (1.5%)	

Fig. 2. Different devices for which 1-year follow-up data are available.

(mean age 73 vs 70 ($p<0.05$, t-test)) and more unfit, though this was not statistically significant (Fig. 3).

Between discharge/30 days and 1 year there were 18 (10.4%) deaths. The majority of these were not directly related to the endovascular repair procedure or the AAA and were most commonly related to co-morbid conditions such as cardiovascular disease (Table 2). There were, however, two deaths due to rupture of the treated AAA (1.1% rupture rate). One patient's aneurysm was excluded at the primary procedure, but he re-presented at just over 1 year with a ruptured AAA and aortoenteric fistula. The second patient had a persisting primary proximal perigraft endoleak despite treatment with a Palmaz stent; in this case rupture occurred at 4 months post-procedure. Both ruptures occurred following repair using the Vanguard device. In all the other cases the AAA was excluded at death. The mortality rate in patients treated with aorto-bi-iliac or tube devices was 9.3% (n=10/108) compared with 12.3% (n=8/65) in those patients treated with aorto-uni-iliac devices, a difference which was not statistically significant. As expected, the

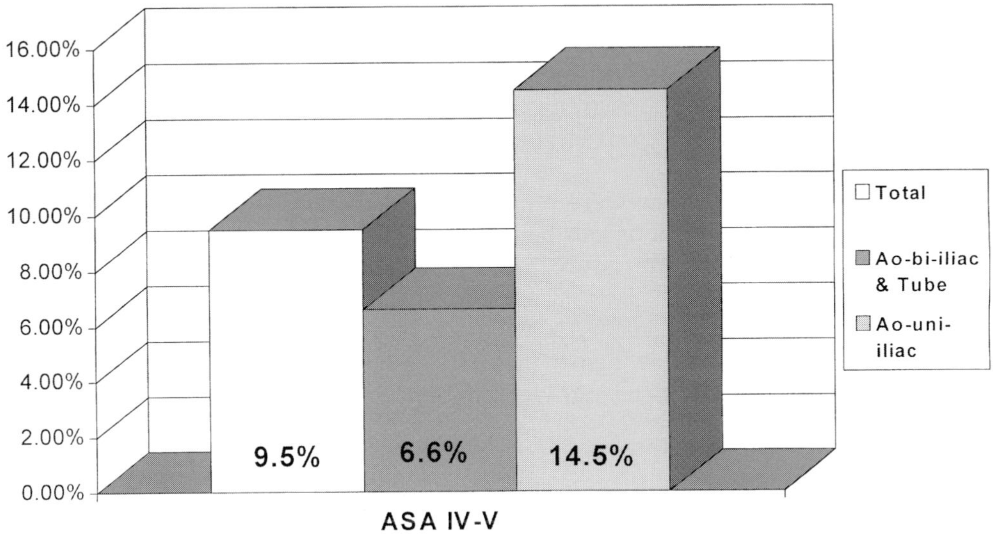

Fig. 3. Data for 1-year follow-up. Those considered unfit for conventional repair, total and by graft type. Chi-square: p=0.09.

Table 2. Cause of death in patients during the first year of follow-up

All causes	*n*	*(%)*
AAA rupture	2	(1.1)
Myocardial infarction	5	(2.7)
IHD/CCF	3	(1.7)
Thyrotoxic crisis	1	(0.7)
Renal failure	2	(1.1)
Pancreatic carcinoma	1	(0.7)
Sepsis/chest infection	3	(1.7)
Rupture of thoracic AA	1	(0.7)
	18	(10.4)

IHD: Ischaemic heart disease. CCF: congestive cardiac failure. AAA: Abdominal aortic aneurysm. AA: Aortic aneurysm.

mortality in the first year after the procedure was significantly higher in unfit patients being 8.6% (n=13/152) in those ASA class I–III and 31.3% (n=5/16) in ASA class IV–V ($p<0.005$, chi-squared test) (missing data n=5). The 1-year follow-up mortality rate was lowest for those treated electively for asymptomatic AAA at 8.9% (n=13/146), it was 17.4% (n=4/23) for elective symptomatic AAA, 0% (n=0/1) for acute non-ruptured and 33.3% (n=1/3) for acute ruptured AAA.

The 1-year follow-up data were available on six persisting primary endoleaks. The only persisting primary proximal perigraft endoleak has already been mentioned

(AAA ruptured 4 months post-procedure). In one case of bilateral persisting primary distal perigraft endoleaks, following bifurcating stent graft repair, extraperitoneal surgical banding of both common iliac arteries was required. Three endoleaks (two distal perigraft and one retrograde lumbar) sealed spontaneously. The final endoleak, a small distal perigraft endoleak, was being observed and the AAA had not increased in size.

A total of 36 complications were reported in 19.7% (n=34) of patients at 1-year follow-up. These complications can be divided into those related to the device or AAA, those related to the procedure, and other complications, which include new medical problems (Table 3).

There were 23 complications in 12.7% (n=22) of patients related to the device or AAA, the majority of these being primary or secondary endoleaks requiring treatment. Two secondary retrograde lumbar endoleaks, five distal perigraft

Table 3. Complications reported at 1-year follow-up

Device- or AAA-related complications	
Graft occlusion	
Surgical bypass performed	3
Endoleaks/stump dislocation	
Endovascular stent graft treatment	
± embolization of IIA	
successful exclusion	4
persisting endoleaks	2
limb thrombosis requiring surgery	1
Embolization alone	3
Surgical banding for persisting endoleaks at both distal anastomoses	1
Treatment awaited	1
Observing endoleak	1
Limb kink/stenosis – asymptomatic, observing	2
Limb occlusion – thrombolysis and stent insertion	1
Tube graft too short- extended	1
Limb kink – stented	1
Graft shrinkage- Intermittent claudication, no treatment	1
AAA increasing in size, no leak- observing	1
Procedure related complications	
Persisting groin lymph leak	2
CFA occlusion at cut-down – bypassed	1
Iliac artery dissection – stented	1
Incisional hernia	1
Groin infection MRSA	1
Other/Medical complications	
Myocardial infarction	2
General malaise and weight loss at 3–6 months	2
Progressive PVD	2
Iron deficiency anaemia- Warfarin post PE	1

IIA: Internal iliac artery; MRSA: methicillin resistant *Staphylococcus aureus*; PVD: peripheral vascular disease; PE: pulmonary embolism; CFA: common femoral artery; AAA: abdominal aortic aneurysm.

endoleaks (two persisting primary, three secondary), four stump dislocations with associated secondary perigraft endoleaks and one persisting primary proximal perigraft endoleak were reported to have been observed or treated in the 1-year follow-up period. These device or AAA complications occurred in 13.9% (n=15/108) of patients treated with aorto-bi-iliac or tube devices against 10.8% (n=7/65) of those treated with aorto-uni-iliac grafts and a cross-over, a difference which was not statistically significant. Of the individual devices the Vanguard had the highest rate of device- or AAA-related problems during the first year of follow-up at 17.9% (n=15/84), the PTFE/Palmaz aorto-uni-iliac device next at 13.3% (n=4/30) and then the Gianturco/Dacron aorto-uni-iliac device at 8.8% (n=3/34); differences which were not statistically significant. The other devices (Bard device, EVT, Perth and Talent) had no reported device or AAA problems in the first year but the numbers were small.

The rate of procedure-related complications and other complications were similar for both main types of device. Procedure-related complications occurred in 2.8% (n=3/108) of patients treated with aorto-bi-iliac or tube devices against 4.5% (n=3/65) of those treated with aorto-uni-iliac grafts and a cross-over. Other or medical complications occurred in 3.7% (n=4/108) of patients treated with aorto-bi-iliac or tube devices compared with 4.5% (n=3/65) of those treated with aorto-uni-iliac grafts and a cross-over. Two patients in this group experienced malaise and weight loss at approximately 3–6 months post-procedure. Both had been treated with the Vanguard device but had not experienced post-procedure pyrexia, which has been reported as part of the 'post-implantation syndrome' commonly seen with this device.[5,6] In both cases no cause was found and the symptoms settled spontaneously.

2-YEAR FOLLOW-UP DATA

Collection of 2-year follow-up data has been less successful than for the 1-year follow-up period and 91 requests for 2-year follow-up data were sent to submitting centres. Only 20 completed 2-year follow-up forms were returned, giving a rate of return of 21.9%.

One (5%) of the patients was treated with an aortic tube graft, 11 (55%) with an aorto-bi-iliac stent graft and eight (40%) with an aorto-uni-iliac graft and a cross-over. Twelve (60%) Vanguard devices, five (25%) Gianturco/Dacron and three (15%) PTFE/Palmaz devices were used.

The mortality rate in this group was 5% (n=1/20); the cause of death was a probable myocardial infarction, but whether the AAA was excluded was unknown.

In two cases, follow-up was available on complications noted at 1-year follow-up. An aneurysm which was enlarging but without leak identified at 1-year remained excluded. A Vanguard stump dislocation repaired during the first year of follow-up using another stent graft remained effectively sealed at 2 years.

Two (10%) secondary endoleaks developed in the second year of follow-up, both in Vanguard devices. One was a distal perigraft endoleak and the other a graft wall endoleak. Both were successfully excluded with the Passager stent graft. Treatment was necessary at 2 years post-insertion in both cases.

DISCUSSION

It is important to bear in mind the limitations of a registry when considering the results obtained from it. A registry is an observational data set and therefore comparing outcomes in different patient groups is problematic because of confounding. As submission of data is voluntary, there is a risk of bias in the data submitted to the registry. It is not usually possible to ascertain the amount and characteristics of data that were not submitted. This problem of validity has been recognized and is being addressed by the Joint Working Party. Principles have been agreed whereby centres submitting data to the registry will be selected at random for audit. This will involve verifying data submitted on the registration and follow-up forms and ensuring the number of cases entered from that centre are correct, from theatre and radiology records. The co-operation of companies supplying devices is also being sought with a view to cross-checking the total number of devices supplied in the UK since the registry began.

Obtaining follow-up data is another challenge. The coordinators of RETA ask submitting centres to provide appropriate follow-up data at yearly intervals. There has been a reasonable return rate for 1-year follow-up data. Supply of the second year follow-up data has, however, been problematic with such small numbers that few meaningful inferences can be made from this data at present. Despite these problems, the RETA registry has collected data on a large number of patients. The patients, treatments and outcomes are markedly heterogeneous and are probably representative for the UK population, making inferences reasonably generalizable.

The 30-day/discharge mortality of patients entered on to RETA is 6.3% overall, though there is a difference in mortality between those having aorto-bi-iliac and tube devices (mortality 2.7%) and those treated with an aorto-uni-iliac graft and a cross-over (mortality 12.2%). The patients in the aorto-uni-iliac group are more unfit but even allowing for confounders this difference remained statistically significant ($p<0.05$). This difference may be due to the more surgical approach required for the aorto-uni-iliac procedure.

Patients who survived to 30 days had a mortality rate of 10.5% in the first year following repair so that 89.5% survived to 1 year. At 2-year follow-up a further 5% of patients had died. The difference in mortality between the main device types, i.e. aorto-bi-iliac and tubes (9.3%) vs aorto-uni-iliac grafts with a cross-over (12.2%) was not statistically significant at 1 year. So it would appear that any excess mortality in the aorto-uni-iliac graft and cross-over group seen at 30 days is not carried over into the follow-up period. Mortality was lower in those fit for conventional repair with 91.4% survival at 1 year compared with 68.7% for those deemed unfit for conventional surgery (ASA IV), as one would expect because of the presence of severe co-morbidity. Most deaths during follow-up are attributable to co-morbid conditions such as cardiac disease. However, AAA rupture occurred in two patients (1.1%) from the 1 year follow-up group. In one of these cases the AAA had been excluded at the primary procedure and no leak had been identified at follow-up. The other patient had a persisting primary proximal endoleak despite attempted endovascular treatment with a Palmaz stent. This is the only persisting primary proximal endoleak which was not effectively sealed either endovascularly or surgically. The other persisting primary endoleaks had a much more benign course either being successfully treated or sealing spontaneously, though one small persisting primary distal endoleak is being observed.

The complication rate at follow-up has been relatively high with 12.7% of patients in the first year and 10% in the second year having a problem with the device or AAA for which treatment or close observation was deemed necessary. The majority of these complications were secondary endoleaks often due to stump dislocations. Whether these stump dislocations were related to changes in the morphology of the aneurysm post-thrombosis leading to kinking, was not clear as such data are not specifically collected on the registry. Such a problem has been previously reported[7,8] and may be a cause of late stent graft failure, though treatment with additional stent grafts is often successful. These dislocations and secondary endoleaks were most common with the Vanguard device, though it should be remembered that this is the device with which there is the largest and longest experience and whether these problems are specific to this device, only time will tell.

Complications related to the procedure such as wound infections, access artery occlusions and iliac artery dissections occurred in a small proportion of cases. Of interest was the reporting of two cases of general malaise and weight loss, in one case with a raised C-reactive protein. This occurred at 3–6 months post-procedure in both cases and no cause was found. The symptoms settled spontaneously and may be a late manifestation of the so called 'post-implantation syndrome' seen particularly with the Vanguard device.[5,6]

CONCLUSION

This chapter has concentrated on trying to use the data from the RETA registry to assess the likely long-term outcomes following stent-graft repair of AAA. Ruptures have occurred during follow-up and device-related complications occur in about 10% of cases per year.

We remain in the early phase of assessment of endovascular treatment of AAA and the RETA registry is as yet ill equipped to provide insight beyond the first year of follow-up. Also, stent grafting techniques and equipment are constantly evolving and new untested devices are becoming available for use in the UK. To learn more about these new devices and to assess the long-term effects of this treatment it is imperative that data submission to RETA continues and that follow up of this valuable cohort is maintained.

REFERENCES

1. Harris PL: Endovascular grafting for abdominal aortic aneurysms. *Ann Roy Coll Surg Engl* **78**: 23–24, 1996
2. Brewster DC, Geller SC, Kaufman JA *et al.*: Initial experience with endovascular aneurysm repair: comparison of early results with outcome of conventional open repair. *J Vasc Surg* **27**: 992–1003, 1998
3. Kato N, Dake MD, Semba CP *et al.*: Treatment of aortoiliac aneurysms with use of single-piece tapered stent-grafts. *J Vasc Intervent Radiol* **9**: 41–49, 1998

4. May J, White GH, Yu W *et al.*: Concurrent comparison of endoluminal versus open repair in the treatment of abdominal aortic aneurysms: analysis of 303 patients by life table method. *J Vasc Surg* **27**: 213–220, 1998
5. Blum U, Voshage G, Lammer J *et al.*: Endoluminal stent-grafts for infrarenal abdominal aortic aneurysms. *New Engl J Med* **336**: 13–20, 1997
6. Norgren L, Swartbol P: Biological responses to endovascular treatment of abdominal aortic aneurysms. *J Endovasc Surg* **4**: 169–173, 1997
7. Gould D, Edwards R, Harris P *et al.*: Mid-term results of endovascular repair of abdominal aortic aneurysm: sac length reduction and graft tortuosity (abstract). *Br J Radiol* **71**: 26, 1998
8. May J, White GH, Yu W, Sieunarine K: Importance of plain x-ray in endoluminal aortic graft surveillance. *Eur J Vasc Endovasc Surg* **13**: 202–206, 1997
9. White GH, Yu W, May J, Chaufour X, Stephen MS: Endoleak as a complication of endoluminal grafting of abdominal aortic aneurysms: classification, incidence, diagnosis, and management. *J Endovasc Surg* **4**: 152–168, 1997

Commentary

The RETA Registry has been of very considerable value. It has set the scene for the endovascular aneurysm repair (EVAR) trials for the future. The registry cannot be absolutely complete, although of recent months and in 1998, it must be assumed that almost all, if not all of the EVAR procedures are recorded in Sheffield because centres know that the RETA register is plotting the learning curves of the centres. The RETA data will provide the springboard for centres to become part of the EVAR trials 1 and 2 which will be in progress at the time of publication of this book. There have been a number of problems. The RETA registry underscores some of the strengths of EVAR in the UK in 1999. There is now a clear intention of collaboration of radiologists and vascular surgeons in the performance of these procedures. Without such co-operation, the stent graft systems will simply not be purchased under the NHS. Each centre must demonstrate that they have achieved a satisfactory learning curve and this learning experience will be plotted in Sheffield. The RETA data has been achieved through excellent collaboration of the joint working party of the two British societies for interventional radiology and vascular surgery and so it is highly appropriate that these data should pass from this registry to the trial management committee of the EVAR trials to establish participation in EVAR trials 1 and 2. The RETA data has established which patients are fit for an open repair and which are unfit. In simple terms, approximately two-thirds of EVAR procedures performed in Britain were performed as an alternative to open repair. Therefore, a choice has been made during this learning curve. In the future, patients will need to know whether EVAR or open repair is more satisfactory and which is more durable. Therefore a random controlled trial (EVAR 1) between EVAR and open repair is appropriate. Since the findings of the UK Small Aneurysm trial[1,2] have been known it is to be expected that patients with asymptomatic and non-tender aneurysms of greater than 5.5 cm diameter will be enrolled. There is currently no proof that EVAR is superior to open repair and therefore it is assumed that EVAR should be delayed until an aneurysm reaches 5.5 cm or becomes tender or grows more than 1 cm per year. The NHS will also recognize that as open repair was shown to be more expensive than surveillance for smaller aneurysms, EVAR repair for aneurysms smaller than 5.5 cm can scarcely be justified at the present time. Should a subsequent trial show the superiority of EVAR over open repair, then this issue could be reopened.

For patients unfit for open repair, the EVAR 2 trial will be performed and the RETA data indicate that a number of patients are having EVAR in the UK in this category in these 2 years reported. In EVAR 2, best medical treatment and EVAR is compared with best medical treatment alone, again in a random controlled trial. These are exciting times with respect to best medical treatment, as it has just been shown how matrix metalloproteinases can be interrupted by tetracycline derivatives[3] and how aneurysm expansion is slower in patients on indomethacin.[4] *RMG*

References

1. UK Small Aneurysm Trial Participants: Mortality results for randomised controlled trial of early elective surgery of ultrasonographic surveillance for small abdominal aortic aneurysms. *Lancet* **352**: 1649–1655, 1998.
2. UK Small Aneurysm Trial Participants: Health service costs and quality of life for early elective surgery or ultrasonographic surveillance for small abdominal aortic aneurysms. *Lancet* **352**: 1656–1660, 1998.
3. Thompson RW, Parks WC: Role of metalloproteinases in abdominal aortic aneurysms. *Ann N Y Acad Sci* **800**: 157–174, 1996.
4. Franklin IJ, Walton LJ, Greenhalgh RM, Powell JT: Targetting prostaglandin E_2 for the medical treatment of aortic aneurysms. *Br J Surg* **85**: 1557, 1998.

Failure of endovascular repair of abdominal aortic aneurysms: endoleak, adverse events and grading of technical difficulty

Geoffrey H White and James May

INTRODUCTION

This chapter examines modes of device or procedure failure that detract from the durability of endovascular graft repair operations for abdominal aortic aneurysms (AAA). In assessing device durability, it would be desirable to be able to stratify results according to patient selection groups. We propose the use of a grading system to predict the degree of difficulty of endovascular repair cases, so that the relative importance of device characteristics and patient anatomy can be recognized.

Endoluminal aneurysm repair is a procedure under trial. The feasibility and relative safety of the procedure has been demonstrated for a range of devices, but no reliable long-term data are yet available regarding device durability or patient outcome beyond the initial few years. The technology commenced with improvised or home-made stent-graft devices, and has now progressed to second-generation devices that are being produced by commercial companies. The process of testing and trialing these has been carried out within a wide range of ethical standards and scientific parameters, making it quite difficult to make a valid comparison. Gradual improvements have been made to increase user-friendliness, particularly with respect to achieving safer access to the vascular system and improved reliability in graft deployment. It is likely that the technology will advance rapidly, so that the current devices may become obsolete with surprising rapidity.

To date, this allows expression of personal preferences in graft choice, but we do not yet have sufficient evidence to judge which graft is best. As with the field of artificial cardiac valves, serious defects may become evident with any of the grafts currently under trial, either as short-term or late events. These may be due to graft material failure or metal fatigue, or to the relentless mechanical effects of the haemodynamics within the aorta. Recent evidence shows that the ability of endovascular grafts to cause shrinkage and regression of aortic aneurysms may have a paradoxical effect of distorting the endograft itself, thus causing geometric changes within the metallic framework and, ultimately, device failure.[1] Thus, the desired positive effect of the device may ironically lead eventually to its failure. In this field, long-term results will dictate which device is regarded as the best.

Within our vascular unit, we have had the oppportunity to study a range of endovascular graft devices, of both the improvised and the commercial varieties. The devices trialed and the incidence of one of the main early failure modes, endoleak, are presented in Table 1. We continue to trial each of the commercial devices currently available to us; each has individual advantages and disadvantages, and in

Table 1. The incidence of primary endoleak (CT scan at discharge), RPA Hospital, University of Sydney; Australia, May 1992–August 1998

Endograft type and incidence of primary endoleak						
Device	*No of cases*	*Graft-related type I endoleak*		*Retrograde II type II endoleak*	*Total*	
		n	*(%)*		*n*	*(%)*
Balloon-deployed						
Parodi	10	3	(30)	0	3	
White/Yu	110	5	(4.5)	1 (IMA)	6	(5.5)
Self-expanding						
EVT	19	2	(10.5)	1	3	(15)
Chuter	1	0		0	0	
Mintec	16	2	(12.5)	0	2	(12.5)
Vanguard	51	7	(14)	4 (IMA)	11	(22)
Talent	17	1	(12.5)	2	2	(18)
Bard	5	1		0	1	
AneuRx	32	10	(29)	1 (lumb.)	10	(34)
TOTAL	261	31	(12)	9 (3.5%)	40	(15.3)

our opinion none deserves a rating higher than 'adequate' at this stage of assessment. Many improvements will be made in the near future.

HOW TO JUDGE ENDOVASCULAR GRAFT DEVICES? METHODS OF OUTCOME ASSESSMENT

Conventional measures of surgical procedure outcome have had only limited applicability to the assessment of endovascular graft technology, particularly with respect to treatment of aortic aneurysms. It is clear that a successful implantation of the device does not guarantee successful patient outcome. A *technical success* may not necessarily lead to a *clinical success*. The published standards for reporting have proven of little benefit in comparing devices, particularly since there is no clear-cut definition of what constitutes procedure success. We believe that other factors should be taken into consideration, including the incidence of device technical complications (DTCs), analagous to critical incidents, the number of adverse events associated with the operation, the incidence of endoleak and of graft failure. These factors are considered in more detail later in this chapter.

ENDOLEAK

Endoleak is a condition associated with endoluminal vascular grafts defined by the persistence of blood flow outside the lumen of the endoluminal graft but within an aneurysm sac or adjacent vascular segment being treated by the graft.[2,3] Endoleak is usually due to incomplete sealing or exclusion of the aneurysm sac or vessel segment, as evidenced by imaging studies such as contrast-enhanced computed tomography (CT) scan, ultrasound or angiography. Endoleak may also occur when the blood flow into the aneurysm sac is due to retrograde flow from patent collateral vessels, particularly the lumbar arteries or inferior mesenteric artery, even when a complete seal has been obtained around the endoluminal graft.[3,4]

Classification of endoleak

A classification of endoleak is presented in Table 2. A distinction is made between endoleak related to incomplete seal around the graft device (type I endoleak), and endoleak associated with retrograde flow from collateral arterial branches (type II endoleak).[5]

We have also proposed that two further subgroups of this graft-related endoleak be recognized, both describing persistent flow related to the wall or mid-graft region of the endovascular graft or device.[6] Thus, endoleak due to fabric tears, graft disconnection or disintegration is called type III endoleak, and flow through the graft presumed to be associated with graft wall porosity is type IV endoleak.[6]

All subgroups may be further defined as primary (early) or secondary (late), or by site.[3]

Type I endoleak (perigraft endoleak or graft-related endoleak)

This occurs when a persistent perigraft channel of blood flow develops due to inadequate or ineffective seal at the graft ends (at the proximal, or distal graft aspects) or attachment zones.

Type II endoleak (retrograde endoleak or non-graft-related endoleak)

This type occurs when there is persistent collateral blood flow into the aneurysm sac flowing retrogradely from patent lumbar arteries, the inferior mesenteric artery, or other collateral vessels. In this case, there is a complete seal around the graft attachment zones so that the complication is not related directly to the graft itself.

Type III endoleak (fabric tear or modular disconnection)

Endoleak at the midgraft region may be due to leakage through a defect in the graft fabric, or between the segments of a modular, multisegment graft. This subgroup of endoleak is essentially due to mechanical failure of the graft, secondary to early component defect or late material fatigue. Some cases may be associated with the effects of haemodynamic forces or changes in aneurysm morphology with shrinkage.

Type IV endoleak (graft porosity)

This is any minor blush of contrast on completion angiogram or subsequent contrast studies, which is presumed to be emanating from blood diffusion across the pores of a highly porous graft fabric, or perhaps through the small holes in the graft fabric caused by sutures or stent struts, etc. This is usually an intentional design feature, rather than a form of device failure. In practice, differentiation of type IV endoleak

Table 2. A classification of endoleak

Classification	*Alternative terms*	*Forms*	*Rx alternatives*
Type I endoleak	Perigraft leak Perigraft channel Graft-related endoleak	Proximal graft attachment zone Distal attachment zone	Proximal or distal extension or cuff Embolization Secondary endograft Open repair
Type II endoleak	Retrograde endoleak Collateral flow Retroleak Non-grade-related endoleak	Patent lumbar artery Patent IMA Patent intercostal artery Others (accessory renal artery, internal iliac, subclavian, etc)	Conservative Coil embolization Laparoscopic clip application
Type III endoleak	Fabric tear Modular disconnection or poor seal	Midgraft fabric tear Contralateral stump disconnection	Secondary endograft
Type IV endoleak	Porosity	Graft wall fabric porosity; suture holes	Conservative
Endoleak of undefined origin			
Non-endoleak aneurysm sac pressurization	Endopressure Endotension Pressure-leak Pseudo-endoleak	High pressure in sac, but no endoleak shown Thrombotic seal	Secondary endograft Open repair ?Others

from type III will often prove very difficult, and may require postoperative, directed angiography. As yet, the long-term effects of type IV endoleak are unknown.

Endoleak: undefined origin

In many cases, the precise source of endoleak will not be clear from routine follow-up imaging studies and further investigation may be required. In this situation, it may be appropriate to classify the condition as 'endoleak, undefined origin' until the type of endoleak is defined by further studies.

Non-endoleak aneurysm sac pressurization (endopressure or endotension)

In these cases, no endoleak is demonstrated on imaging studies, but pressure within the aneurysm sac is elevated, and may be very close to systemic pressure.[6] The seal is formed by semi-liquid thrombus, and the pressure in the sac is similar to pressures measured in endoleak. The aneurysm will often be clinically pulsatile and wall-pulsatility may also be detected and monitored by specialized ultrasound techniques.[7]

In clinical practice, we have learnt that high pressure may be maintained within the AAA sac with no evidence of leak or bloodflow outside the graft, in cases where a rim of thrombus is interposed between the sac contents and the aortic lumen. We observed this in two patients where the proximal stent slipped distally within the proximal aneurysm neck; the aneurysm became pulsatile once more and was enlarging on progress CT scans, but no contrast media was detected outside of the graft (unpublished data). This condition, which some have referred to as 'endopressure' or 'pressure-leak' (Juan Parodi, personal communication), or as 'endotension' (Geoff Gilling-Smith, personal communication) does not fit conveniently into the definition of endoleak, but is obviously closely associated and probably represents an intermediate state. We believe, therefore, that this condition should be recognized as a related group ('non-endoleak aneurysm sac pressurization').

Precise classification of these various types of endoleak allows more meaningful communication and comparison of results from different investigators and different devices. In addition, treatment recommendations can be made according to the type of endoleak, as well as its site. For example, type III endoleak (fabric tear or modular separation) can be effectively treated in many cases by insertion of a further endograft to line and reinforce the graft wall or connection zone where the defect is detected,[8] whereas type II endoleak may be managed quite differently by transluminal coil embolization.[9,10] There is good case for conservative management of type II endoleak when there is no aneurysm enlargement; recent evidence demonstrated that there was no significant increase in AAA size over 18 months in a series of patients who had primary type II endoleak.[11] A further advantage of the proposed classification of endoleak is that it will permit similar follow-up studies to present differential information for each type of endoleak, so that their prognosis and best treatment can ultimately be determined.

As we have previously recommended,[5] further specificity can be gained by adding the qualifiers A or B, where A refers to endoleaks in which only an inflow channel can be imaged, and B refers to endoleak with demonstrated inflow and outflow channels. Secondary or late endoleak continues to be the major long-term complication of the endoluminal grafting technique.[3,12] Late endoleak of type I or type III classification is equivalent to aneurysm recurrence, and may be complicated by aortic rupture.[13–17] With respect to late endoleak, and in the absence of contradictory information, we continue to recommend that active intervention (percutaneous embolization of feeding vessels, secondary endoluminal graft procedures, conversion to open repair, or other interventions) be carried out in all patients who develope late endoleak (types I-IV), to prevent AAA rupture.

Timing of occurence of endoleak

Primary endoleak

Primary endoleak is considered to exist when it is detected during the perioperative (30-day) period. Since flow into the aneurysm sac may also become re-established as a late complication after apparent initial complete seal, a separate entity should be recognized as secondary endoleak.

Secondary or late endoleak (delayed or late endoleak)

Secondary or late endoleak is developing into the major long-term complication of the endoluminal grafting technique.[3,12,18] Late endoleak of type 1 classification is equivalent to aneurysm recurrence, and may be complicated by aortic rupture.[13,14,19] We recommend that active intervention (percutaneous embolization of feeding vessels, or secondary endoluminal graft procedures) be carried out in all patients who develope late endoleak, to prevent AAA rupture. Type II endoleak seems empirically far less likely to lead to aneurysm rupture (there have been no published reports of aneurysm rupture associated with late type II endoleak, to date). Nevertheless, it is instructive to consider that rupture has been reported due to backflow from collateral vessels of an AAA treated by surgical ligation and extra-anatomic bypass.[20] Thus, even though the current management of primary endoleak of type II origin is often conservative, late development of type II endoleak is treated by percutaneous embolization techniques.

Graft porosity and difficulties in differentiating source of endoleak

It is recognized that, with new thin-walled graft materials, endoleak in the early few days after endograft procedures may be due to graft porosity or to small holes in the graft wall caused by suture attachment of the metallic stent to the graft and that these pores may close spontaneously within a short period. In current experience with the AneuRx graft, for example, a blush of contrast is seen within the aneurysm sac on completion angiography in the large majority of cases undertaken, and contrast is demonstrated outside the graft on CT scan performed 2–5 days postoperatively in approximately one-quarter to one-third of cases. Many of these resolve within the first month.[21] This suggests that sealing of pores or flow channels has occurred.

Some have taken the viewpoint that such bloodflow through the graft wall is insignificant, that it is not a form of endoleak, and that sealing of these holes equates to a successful procedure.[21] The corollary of this attitude, which some investigators seem to have adopted, is that all early flow in the sac should therefore be regarded as harmless until it is proven not to be. There are several telling arguments against this attitude: (i) It can be extremely difficult to determine accurately if blush flow outside of the graft on completion angiography or on early postoperative CT scan is actually endoleak around the ends, or through a modular connection site, or simple flow through graft pores; (ii) it has been shown that endoleak through a hole of any size, even a very small one, results in identical high pressure within the AAA sac,[22] (iii) pressure in the aneurysm sac remains high after endoluminal repair with a porous graft, in benchtop model studies;[23] and (iv) the long-term outcome of this phenomenon is unknown, and it is feasible that graft porosity may be found to be associated with late complications such as continued enlargement of the aneurysm sac, recurrent endoleak, etc. A simple solution is to continue to include porosity within the definition of endoleak, but to recognize its different aetiology from other types of endoleak by defining it as type IV.

One aspect which should be investigated thoroughly is whether pressure reduction within the aneurysm sac is achieved as effectively when the seal of small channels in the graft wall is thrombotic rather than structural; thrombus (or fibrin plug) sealing a flow channel may possibly transmit higher pressures to the interior of the aneurysm sac leading to different pressure effects on the aortic wall in both the early and late stages. In fact, it has been demonstrated in experimental studies that coil embolization of endoleak channels associated with holes in the graft fabric does not effectively reduce sac pressure, even though no endoleak can be demonstrated after the thrombosis has been induced.[24] It is feasible, therefore, that there may be differences in pressure transmission through holes or pores of various sizes, which have been sealed by thrombus of varying composition, and that these differences may lead to a differential tendency for the thrombosed aneurysm sac to shrink or perhaps to enlarge.

It is likely that other subgroups of endoleak will be recognized as the design of endovascular grafts evolves, and as imaging techniques become more precise.

Incidence of endoleak

There has been wide variation in the incidence of endoleak reported in series to date. Moore and Rutherford reported a primary endoleak rate of 44% for the multicentre trial of the EVT device,[25] with more than half of these cases being short-term, self-sealing endoleak, leaving a persistent primary endoleak rate of 21%. Marin and Veith reported primary endoleak in 27% of cases,[26] including some which progressed to spontaneous thrombosis. Blum *et al.* (4%),[27] May *et al.* (9%)[28] and Parodi[29] have all reported incidence of 10% or less.

The incidence of primary endoleak probably depends on the device being used and the experience of the operative team in patient selection and implantation techniques. The incidence of endoleak with various devices in our own practice is presented in Table 2. Since some of these devices have been in use for less than a year, the relative incidence of late endoleak is not yet known.

Severity of endoleak

The severity of endoleak probably depends on the size of the perigraft channel and the flow within it, so that small endoleaks may have less tendency to cause major complications. It has been shown that endoleak may seal in the early postoperative stage or at a later time, presumably by a process of thrombosis. The long-term outcome of sealed endoleak is unknown. With further experience, it may become possible to further define degrees of endoleak as being minor (i.e. likely to seal safely by thrombotic process) or major (unlikely to seal, or sealed by unstable thrombus with maintained high pressure within the aneurysm sac or high potential for recurrence). Aneurysm rupture has been reported in patients with persistent major endoleak.[13,14,19] Pressure monitoring may be shown to have a valuable role in determining the severity and long-term behaviour of different degrees and types of endoleak.

Some have taken the viewpoint that a large calibre patent inferior mesenteric artery or large lumbars (particularly the fourth lumbar arteries) should be embolized preoperatively, or intraoperatively and if this proves to be true, then the presence of retrograde endoeak may come to constitute operator error in selected cases. Although the prognosis of this type II endoleak appears to be relatively favorable during the first 12 to 18 months,[11] it is also possible that longer term persistent retrograde perfusion of the aneurysm sac may go on to cause secondary changes to the biological reactions within the aneurysm thrombus, to the geometry of the aneurysm sac, or to the graft wall, any of which could result in late deleterious alterations in graft geometry or integrity. Certainly, rupture of surgically thrombosed aneurysm[30] and of excluded aneurysms[20] has been reported, so there is reason for some caution with regard to the outcome of uncorrected type II endoleak.

Until long-term data are available from closely monitored prospective studies, we believe that it is preferable to continue to include all forms of endoleak within the umbrella of the one diagnosis, but to recognize various subgroups of endoleak as an indication of their various aetiologies and patterns of behaviour.

Management of endoleak

Management of endoleak may be considered under five broad categories:

(i) *Conservative* (observation, with monitoring by repeat imaging).
(ii) *Embolization.* Percutaneous embolization and other endovascular interventions.
(iii) *Endograft.* Correction by further endoluminal graft procedure.
(iv) *Surgical* band-ligature of the aortic neck.
(v) *Conversion* to open repair of aneurysm.

Our previous report has emphasized the possibility of aneurysm rupture in patients with late endoleak where conservative management had been preferred to active intervention.[14] All three patients who suffered this complication survived emergency open repair of the ruptured aneurysm. In our experience, no patient with primary endoleak has yet suffered aneurysm rupture, although only small numbers of patients have not undergone active intervention to correct the endoleak.

The appropriate management depends on the severity of endoleak, the timing of detection and the medical status of the patient. Endoleak detected during the implant procedure on completion arteriogram can often be corrected by balloon dilatation of unexpanded graft segments, or by further endograft.

Correction of endoleak by further endoluminal graft implantation

It may be possible to close endoleak by placement of a further endoluminal graft or coated stent. The concept of having available a 'tool-box' containing a variety of such devices to enable immediate correction of endoleak or graft misplacement is attractive. In our experience, this has been more successful in the management of late endoleak, rather than primary endoleak.

Conversion to open repair

Open repair of the aneurysm may be required in some cases where the morphology of the aorta or the graft problem causing endoleak cannot be safely managed by endovascular techniques, or when attempts at secondary endovascular repair are unsuccessful.[31] If a patient is in an extremely high risk group, then it may be determined that it is safer to manage the case conservatively rather than to resort to open repair.

The incidence of secondary endoleak appears likely to increase gradually with follow-up, and may be associated with degenerative changes in the graft structure or fabric integrity over time, particularly beyond the initial 2–3 years. Closely monitored prospective studies of long-term outcome will be required before the durability, the ultimate role of endoluminal repair and best choice of devices can be defined.

GRAFT DEPLOYMENT SUCCESS

We believe that the concept of 'technical success' is not particularly valid as a means of comparing endovascular devices. Incidence of technical success probably is only useful as an index of the efficacy of the delivery system of the device, in addition to aspects of patient selection and operator experience.[32] The strictest definition of clinical success could be regarded to be 'the establishment of a patent, haemostatic endovascular graft, which: (i) does not have signs of endoleak at any stage; and (ii) which leads to decrease in AAA size; and (iii) which acts as a permanent protection from aneurysm rupture.'

DEVICE TECHNICAL COMPLICATIONS

Current reporting standards for surgical procedures emphasize patient outcome parameters and complications, but do not usually consider technical difficulties or device problems. In a prospective study, we evaluated the incidence of technical problems and deployment-related complications during a series of consecutive patients undergoing endoluminal grafting of AAA with a range of devices, in an analysis similar to critical incident reporting.[33]

Data regarding the occurrence of intraoperative technical difficulties and device complications were recorded prospectively for 55 consecutive AAA cases performed over a 12-month interval with balloon-expanded (n = 5) or self-expanding endovascular graft devices (Vanguard bifurcated graft; n = 38, Talent bifurcated endoluminal graft; n = 5, Bard endoluminal tube graft ; n = 4, Aneurx bifurcated graft; n = 3), in addition to the usual records of patient outcome and procedure complications. Secondary aortic procedures and thoracic or iliac cases were excluded. The critical incidents were classified as being related to: (i) ipsilateral sheath or delivery catheter, (ii) contralateral sheath, or (iii) general incidents (any intraoperative problem with guidewires, balloons, or endoluminal graft deployment). We also determined the effect of patient selection factors or surgeon error on the occurence of critical incidents.

Device technical complications occured in 41 of the 50 cases undertaken with self-expanding devices (82%), and four of five (80%) cases with balloon-expanded devices. A total of 103 problems were documented (range 0–10 per patient). The most common problem was graft foreshortening during deployment, which resulted in requirement for extension grafts in eight patients. Despite these problems, grafts were able to be implanted in all patients, and no patient required conversion to open repair. Primary endoleak occured in nine patients with self-expanding devices (perigraft endoleak n=6, retrograde flow from patent inferior mesenteric artery n=3). There were two deaths (3.6%) in the perioperative period. Other outcome parameters (graft deployment, conversion to open repair, technical and clinical success rates) were similar in an extended series of 83 self-expanding cases compared with 88 balloon expanded device cases.[33]

This study demonstrated a very high incidence of device technical complication or critical incidents with the current designs of endoluminal grafts. In this small sample, there were no significant differences in the rate of such events between the various devices. In addition to prospective studies of surgical outcome, careful recording and analysis of DTCs may have a valuable role in the assessment of new technologies, similar to the use of critical incident reporting in anaesthesia practice.

ADVERSE EVENTS FOLLOWING ENDOVASCULAR REPAIR OF ABDOMINAL AORTIC ANEURYSMS

Another method of assessing endovascular grafts is to document prospectively all adverse events that occur in the perioperative 30-day period, and in subsequent follow-up. An adverse event may be defined as any of the following: death, conversion to open repair, requirement for further interventions (percutaneous or surgical), renal failure, respiratory failure, wound complications, endoleak and AAA rupture. In a recent study, we compared two groups of patients who underwent endovascular repair of AAA in different time periods:[34] Group I (n=75) had their procedure during the initial 3-year period of our experience, whereas Group II (n=115) had their operations in the subsequent 2½ year period (Table 3).

A total of 110 adverse events occured in 88 of the patients. There was no significant difference in the total number of adverse events for Group I (37/75) versus Group II (51/115). It is surprising that despite improvements in technology and experience,

Table 3. Clinical characteristics of two groups of patients undergoing endoluminal abdominal aortic aneurysm repair during two successive periods of time

Age (mean in years)	*Group I* *n* = 75	*Group II* *n* = 115	*p Value*
	71	72	NS
Female/Male	6/69	9/106	NS
AAA diameter (mean cm)	5.5	5.4	NS
Co-morbidities	44%	30%	NS
Common iliac tortuosity >90°/90° or less	0/75	20/95	0.0002
Proportion first generation prostheses	75/0	45/70	<0.000001
Configuration tube/ Non-tube	39/36	17/98	<0.00001

NS: not significant.

adverse events continue to occur in a relatively high proportion (45%) of patients undergoing endoluminal repair.

No significant differences were found between individual categories of adverse events in the two time periods, with the exception of primary conversion from endoluminal to open repair which occurred more frequently in the early period (Table 4).

There are some possible explanations for this paradoxical situation where improvements in technology and increasing experience have failed to reduce the incidence of adverse events. New equipment may simply replace an old problem with a new problem. Endoleak, for instance, was an uncommon occurrence with endografts of aortoiliac/femoral configuration in the early period of time. In some cases, this resulted from the practice of hand suturing the distal end of the endograft which guaranteed freedom from distal endoleak. With the advent of endografts with

Table 4. Incidence of adverse events occurring in two groups of patients undergoing endoluminal abdominal aortic aneurysm repair during two successive periods of time.

	Group I *n*	*(%)*	*Group II* *n*	*(%)*	*p Value*
	75		115		
Perioperative (30-day) deaths	4	(5.3)	4	(3.5)	NS
Conversion: primary	12	(16.0)	5	(4.3)	0.007
secondary	6	(8.0)	4	(3.5)	NS
Supplementary endoluminal repair	7	(9.3)	5	(4.3)	NS
Lower limb ischaemia	7	(9.3)	17	(14.7)	NS
Haemodialysis required	3	(4.0)	4	(3.5)	NS
Failure to cure the AAA	5	(6.6)	17	(14.8)	NS
Wound complications	4	(5.3)	8	(7)	NS
Total adverse events	48	(64)	62	(54)	NS
Total patients with adverse events	37	(49)	51	(45)	NS

NS: not significant.

self-expanding metallic frames running throughout their length, hand suturing was no longer necessary. This had the advantage of being less invasive but the disadvantage of increasing the potential for distal endoleak.

Similarly, modular bifurcated endografts eliminated the problem of twisting in one piece bifurcated grafts, thus reducing the incidence of immediate conversion from endoluminal to open repair. Coinciding with this reduction in need for conversion, however, was a corresponding increase in the incidence of endoleak due to dislocation of component parts of modular prostheses.[34]

A disproportionately larger number of tube endografts were performed in the early time period and a disproportionately larger number of bifurcated endografts in the later period. While this change had the desirable effect of reducing the incidence of distal endoleak in patients with distal aneurysm necks of marginal or inadequate length who would previously have had a tube endograft, the bifurcated endograft brought its own complications. In particular, kinking and twisting of the limbs of bifurcated endografts resulted in distal ischaemia and the need for further intervention.

A further factor mitigating against a reduction in adverse events is the increasing willingness to attempt endoluminal repair in more technically challenging patients, that accompanies increasing experience. This factor is largely unrecognized and difficult to quantify. The most notable example of this is the comparison of Groups I and II regarding degree of tortuosity of the common iliac arteries. In Group I this did not exceed 90° whereas Group II patients frequently had common iliac arteries with degrees of tortuosity exceeding 90° and ranging up to 150°.

Reporting the incidence of adverse events provides a more accurate and descriptive picture of the morbidity of the endoluminal method than simply reporting cases as success or failure, and can be used to compare graft types. The similarity in the incidence of adverse events over the two time frames in this study suggests that there are inherent risks in the endoluminal method, and that the high incidence is not just an expression of the initial learning curve.

ENDOGRAFT STRUCTURAL DEFECTS AND DEVICE FAILURE

The endoluminal method of AAA repair has drawn attention to the changes in morphology of the aorta and iliac arteries that accompany increasing size of the aneurysm. Aneurysms increase in size longitudinally in addition to transverse expansion. This increase in longitudinal expansion is accommodated by a corresponding increase in tortuosity of the aorta and iliac arteries. It has long been recognized that iliac tortuosity has important implications for gaining access to the aorta for an endograft. Tortuosity in the proximal neck of the aneurysm may lead to migration and endoleak if the neck is short as well as tortuous.

The changes in morphology that accompany successful endoluminal repair have also been recognized since 1995 and reported by a number of groups.[35–39] These include a reduction in the maximum transverse diameter of the aneurysm and an increase in diameter of the proximal neck of the order of 10%. In addition to contrast-enhanced, CT demonstrating exclusion of the aneurysm sac from the general circulation, one of the important criteria of successful endoluminal repair is a reduction in maximum transverse diameter of the aneurysm.

A phenomenon which has been recognized only in the last 2 years is distortion in prostheses following endoluminal AAA repair. This may involve changes in shape and position and occurs most commonly in the form of kinking in the limbs of bifurcated prostheses at their junction with the trunk, but may also occur in tube endografts. These structural changes may lead to thrombosis of graft limbs, or result in either dislocation of component parts of a modular prosthesis or dislocation of the limbs of an endograft from the native common iliac arteries. Both forms of dislocation, of course, result inevitably in endoleak.

The possible causes of kinking distortion are:

1. increase in length of the prosthesis following deployment;
2. reduction in the length of the aneurysm sac; and
3. migration of the prosthesis from the proximal or distal anchoring sites in the native arteries.

In a recent study, we demonstrated that two commonly used self-expanding prostheses frequently lose up to 15% of their length during deployment.[40] This may be an inherent property of the self-expanding stent framework of the devices, exacerbated by longitudinal pushing forces applied to the graft during deployment, resulting in an accordion effect. Harris and his colleagues[1] from Liverpool noted a similar shortening from the listed length in 15 of 16 patients (21.5 mm mean). Such foreshortening of prostheses during deployment raises the question of subsequent re-expansion to the original length, resulting in graft kinking. Direct evidence for this, however, is lacking, but three explants with severe deformity reported by Stelter and his colleagues[41] from Frankfurt were found to be the same length as the packaged specifications. Stelter concluded from this that increase in length of the prostheses could not, therefore, be responsible for kinking. It could be argued, however, that since many prostheses deploy in a foreshortened state, the observations of Stelter may have represented re-expansion back to the original length with resulting distortion.

Harris *et al.* present convincing data on the relationship between longitudinal shortening of AAA and kinking.[1] Migration of the prosthesis from the proximal or distal anchoring sites in the native arteries is the third possibility in explaining the aetiology of kinking distortion. Such dislocation, however, might be the result of kinking rather than the cause of it. At this stage of our knowledge concerning the late effects of endografting, it would appear that all three possible causes of kinking may contribute to this problem, but that longitudinal foreshortening of the aneurysm sac is probably the major factor.

In addition to distortion, endoluminal prostheses are at risk of structural deterioration. This may involve fatigue fracture in the metal frame, disintegration of sutures holding the metal frame together or attaching the stents to the fabric, and fabric deterioration ranging from small defects to disintegration of the graft. These forms of structural deterioration may lead to graft distortion and failure. It seems very likely that the incidence of such material fatigue increases with time.

A GRADING SCALE FOR DEGREE OF DIFFICULTY FOR ENDOLUMINAL ABDOMINAL AORTIC ANEURYSM REPAIR PROCEDURES

Deployment of endovascular grafts is more difficult in patients who have unfavourable anatomic features such as tortuous, calcified or stenotic iliac arteries and/or short or angulated neck of the aneurysm. The early and long-term outcome of endovascular repair of AAAs may correlate with the degree of difficulty of implanting the graft. We have therefore proposed that a grading scale be applied to these features in an attempt to predict the degree of difficulty of obtaining a successful result.[42] This could potentially be used to differentiate the relative contribution of anatomical and patient selection factors versus device factors in determining procedure outcome and long-term durability.

It is clear that an endograft procedure performed in a patient with a long, straight proximal aortic neck, in association with relatively straight non-atherosclerotic iliac arteries, now has a very high prospect of resulting in a successful procedure. However, a patient with a short, or angulated, proximal neck with tortuous, stenosed iliac arteries, or iliac aneurysmal disease, will be far more difficult to treat successfully. Even if an initial good result is achieved, later complications due to these anatomic features may eventuate.

This grading scale has be structured similar to the methods used in the Glasgow Coma Scale. Weighted values are given to various anatomic factors, with the higher degree of difficulty correlating with a higher grading score.

An initial proposal for a Grading Scale For Degree of Difficulty of Endovascular Repair, using a number of relative value scores for various anatomic features is

Table 5. A grading scale to predict degree of difficulty of endovascular graft procedures for abdominal aortic aneurysms (SYDNEY Aneurysm Scale)

Relative value point scores for AAA difficulty	
Proximal neck	
length less than 15 mm	3 points
angulation greater than 45 degrees	3 points
thrombus layer thicker than 2 mm	3 points
Aortic sac	
angulation greater than 60 degrees	3 points
Iliac artery	
tortuosity greater than 90 degrees	3 points
stenosis (or requires dilatation to pass sheath)	3 points
severe circumferential calcification	3 points
Other features, such as patency of the inferior mesenteric artery, presence of eccentric thrombus in the lumen, etc, could be allocated relative values of 1–2 points, or more to produce a more complete system.	
Grade I	0–2 points
Grade II	3–5 points
Grade III	>5 points

presented in the accompanying table (Table 5). Since we are still in the early phases of knowledge regarding endovascular graft procedures, this table should be regarded as an preliminary attempt at forming a useful grading system and it is likely that this system will evolve with further discussion and input from other investigators. Clinical studies to test the validity of such a grading scale are in progress.

REFERENCES

1. Harris P, Brennan J, Martin J *et al.*: Longitudinal aneurysm shrinkage following endovascular aortic aneurysm repair is a source of intermediate and late complications. *J Endovasc Surg* **6**: 11–16, 1999
2. White GH, Yu W, May J: Endoleak – A proposed new terminology to describe incomplete aneurysm exclusion by an endoluminal graft. (letter) *J Endovasc Surg* **3**: 124–125, 1996
3 White GH, Yu W, May J *et al.*: Endoleak as a complication of endoluminal grafting of abdominal aortic aneurysms: Classification, incidence, diagnosis and management. *J Endovasc Surg* **4**: 152–168, 1997
4. Malina M, Ivancev K, Chuter TAM *et al.*: Changing aneurysmal morphology after endovascular grafting: Relation to leakage or persistent perfusion. *J Endovasc Surg* **4**: 23–30, 1997
5. White GH, May J, Waugh RC, Yu W: Type I and type II endoleaks: A more useful classification for reporting results of endoluminal AAA repair. *J Endovasc Surg* **5**: 189–191, 1998
6. White GH, May J, Waugh RC, Yu W: Type III and type IV endoleak: Toward a complete definition of blood flow in the sac after endoluminal repair of AAA. *J Endovasc Surg* **5**: 305–309, 1998
7. Malina M, Lanne T, Ivancev K *et al.*: Reduced pulsatile wall motion of abdominal aortic aneurysms after endovascular repair. *J Vasc Surg* **27**: 624–631, 1998
8. Maleux G, Rousseau H, Otal P *et al.*: Modular component separation and reperfusion of abdominal aortic aneurysm sac after endovascular repair of the abdominal aortic aneurysm. *J Vasc Surg* **28**: 349–352, 1998
9. Kato N, Semba CP, Dake MD: Embolization of perigraft leaks after endovascular stent-graft treatment of aortic aneurysms. *J Vasc Intervent Radiol* **7**: 805–811, 1996
10. Van Schie G, Sieunarine K, Holt M *et al.*: Successful embolization of persistent endoleak from a patent inferior mesenteric artery. *J Endovasc Surg* **4**: 312–315, 1997
11. Resch T, Ivancev K, Lindh M *et al.*: Persistent collateral perfusion of abdominal aortic aneurysm after endovascular repair does not lead to progressive change in aneurysm diameter. *J Vasc Surg* **28**: 242–249, 1998
12. Raithel D, Heilberger P, Ritter W, Schunn C: Secondary endoleaks after endovascular aortic reconstruction. *J Endovasc Surg* **5**: I-26–I-27, 1998
13. Lumsden AB, Allen RC, Chaikof EL *et al.*: Delayed rupture of aortic aneurysms following endovascular stent grafting. *Am J Surg* **170**: 174–178, 1995
14. White GH, Yu W, May J *et al.*: Three-year experience with the White-Yu endovascular GAD graft for transluminal repair of aortic and iliac aneurysms. *J Endovasc Surg* **4**: 124–136, 1997
15. Parodi JC: Endovascular repair of abdominal aortic aneurysms and other arterial lesions. *J Vasc Surg* **21**: 549–557, 1995
16. Torsello GB, Klenk E, Kasprzak B, Umsheid T: Rupture of abdominal aortic aneurysm previously treated by endovascular stentgraft. *J Vasc Surg* **28**: 184–187, 1998
17. Alimi YS, Chakfe N, Rivoal E *et al.*: Rupture of an abdominal aortic aneurysm after endovascular graft placement and aneurysm size reduction. *J Vasc Surg* **28**: 178–183, 1998
18. May J, White GH, Yu W *et al.*: Importance of graft configuration in outcome of endovascular repair. *Eur J Vasc Endovasc Surg* **15**: 406–411, 1999

19. Parodi JC: Endovascular repair of abdominal aortic aneurysms and other arterial lesions. *J Vasc Surg* **21**: 549–557, 1995
20. Resnikoff M, Darling C, Chang BB *et al.*: Fate of the excluded abdominal aortic aneurysm sac: Long-term follow-up of 831 patients. *J Vasc Surg* **24**: 851–855, 1996
21. Zarins CK *et al.*: AneuRx stent graft vs open repair of abdominal aortic aneurysms: multicenter prospective clinical trial. (Presentation at Society for Vascular Surgery, San Diego 6/98) *J Vasc Surg* **29**: 292–300, 1999
22. Schurink GWH, Aarts NJM, Wilde J *et al.*: Endoleakage after stent-graft treatment of abdominal aortic aneurysm: Implications on pressure and imaging – an *in-vitro* study. *J Vasc Surg* **28**: 234–241, 1998
23. Sanchez LA, Faries PL, Marin ML *et al.*: Chronic intraaneurysmal pressure measurement: an experimental method for evaluating the effectiveness of endovascular aneurysm exclusion. *J Vasc Surg* **26**: 222–230, 1997
24. Marty B, Sanchez LA, Ohki T *et al.*: Endoleak after endovascular graft repair of experimental aortic aneurysms: does coil embolization with angiographic "seal" lower intraaneurysmal pressure? *J Vasc Surg* **27**: 454–462, 1998
25. Moore WS, Rutherford R: Transfemoral endovascular repair of abdominal aortic aneurysm: Results of the North Americain EVT phase 1 trial. *J Vasc Surg* **23**: 543–553, 1996
26. Marin ML, Veith F, Cynamon J *et al.*: Initial experience with transluminally placed endovascular grafts for the treatment of complex vascular lesions. *Ann Surg* **22**: 449–465, 1995
27. Blum U, Langer M, Spillner G *et al.*: Abdominal aortic aneurysms: Preliminary technical and clinical results with transfemoral placement of endovascular self-expanding stent-grafts. *Radiology* **198**: 25–31, 1996
28. May J, White GH, Yu W *et al.*: Surgical management of complications following endoluminal grafting of abdominal aotic aneuryms. *Eur J Vasc Endovasc Surg* **10**: 51–59, 1995
29. Parodi JC: Endovascular repair of abdominal aortic aneuryms. In: *Advances in Vascular Surgery* pp. 85–106. St Louis: Mosby-Year Book, 1993
30. Schanzer H, Papa MC, Miller CM: Rupture of surgically thrombosed abdominal aortic aneurysm. *J Vasc Surg* **2**: 278–280, 1985
31. May J, White GH, Yu W *et al.*: Endoluminal grafting of abdominal aortic aneurysms: Causes of failure and their prevention. *J Endovasc Surg* **1**: 44–52, 1994
32. Ahn SS, Rutherford RB, Johnston KW *et al.*: Reporting standards for infrarenal endovascular abdominal aortic aneurysm repair. *J Vasc Surg* **25**: 405–410, 1997
33. White GH, May J *et al.*: High incidence of intraoperative technical difficulties and device complications with self-expanding stent-grafts used for endovascular repair of abdominal aortic aneurysms. *J Vasc Surg* 1999 (in press)
34. May J, White GH, Waugh RC *et al.*: Adverse events following endoluminal repair of abdominal aortic aneurysms: A comparison during two successive periods of time. *J Vasc Surg* **29**: 32–39, 1999
35. May J, White GH, Yu W *et al.*: A prospective study of changes in morphology and dimensions of abdominal aortic aneurysms following endoluminal repair: a preliminary report. *J Endovasc Surg* **2**: 343–347, 1995
36. May J, White GH, Yu W *et al.*: A prospective study of anatomico-pathological changes in abdominal aortic aneurysms following endoluminal repair: Is the aneurysmal process reversed? *Eur J Vasc Endovasc Surg* **12**: 11–17, 1996
37. Matsumara JS, Pearce WH, McCarthy WJ, Yao J: ST for the EVT Investigators. Reduction in aortic aneurysm size: early results after endovascular graft placement. *J Vasc Surg* **25**: 113–123, 1997
38. Malina M, Ivancev K, Chuter TAM *et al.*: Changing aneurysmal morphology after endovascular grafting: relation to leakage or persistent perfusion. *J Endovasc Surg* **4**: 23–30, 1997
39. Broeders IAMJ, Blankensteijn JD, Gvakharia A *et al.*: The efficacy of transfemoral endovascular aneurysm management: A study on size changes of the abdominal aorta during mid-term follow-up. *Eur J Vasc Endovasc Surg* **14**: 84–90, 1997

40. White GH, May J, Waugh R *et al.*: Shortening of endografts during the deployment phase in endovascular repair of AAA. *J Endovasc Surg* **6**: 4–10, 1999
41. Umscheid T, Stelter WJ: Time related alterations of shape, position and structure in selfexpanding modular stent grafts for treatment of AAA. *J Endovasc Surg* **6**: 17–32, 1999

Commentary

This is a very important contribution from the Sydney centre where Geoffrey White and James May have had such a wide experience from early on with endovascular aneurysm repair. Their classification of endoleaks is very helpful and the significance of endoleaks is currently a matter of the highest priority which will have an enormous impact upon the ultimate durability of this novel technique for aortic aneurysm repair. At present it is very beneficial to understand which endoleaks are important to the extent that further intervention is required. The interesting increase in pressure within the aneurysm sack after this novel technique is not always demonstrated by contrast and CT scan and has been noted by a number of groups as mentioned in this chapter. The significance of this is important to determine. At the time of writing, quite how important this phenomenon is, is somewhat unclear. It could be very important in which case it will be necessary to monitor the pressure of all endovascular repairs after implantation, or less important, in which case selective pressure measurements will be required. *RMG*

How is durability related to patient selection and graft design with endoluminal grafting for abdominal aortic aneurysm?

Michael MD Lawrence-Brown, James B Semmens, David E Hartley, Robert P Mun, Greg van Schie, Marcel A Goodman, Frank J Prendergast and Kishore Sieunarine

INTRODUCTION

The aim of intervention for abdominal aortic aneurysm (AAA) is to prevent death from rupture, because 75% of males and 90% of females with ruptured AAA will die.[1] Since rupture is related to the size of the aneurysm – size, currently measured by diameter, is the indication for intervention. Intervention is indicated when the risk of rupture exceeds the risk of the procedure – the long-term result depends on the durability of the repair. The introduction of endoluminal grafts requires evaluation of this new technology, re-evaluation of the old and the establishment of guidelines.

PATIENT SELECTION

For open surgery, the size at which intervention is recommended varies from unit to unit, and country to country from 45mm to 60mm, with 50mm being probably the least controversial size. Smaller aneurysms are probably associated with lower risk because of ease of operation due to longer healthier proximal necks, less involved iliac vessels and younger, generally fitter patients. The reported 30-day mortality for open repair varies from 2 to 10%: for experienced units this figure is expected to be ≤ 5% for open operation.[2–6] In Western Australia, 30-day mortality for open repair is 4.7%.[1] The survival thereafter is very good – with 93.9% relative survival to their peer group at 5 years.[7] The absolute survival at 5 years being 71.4% and 46% at 10 years. However, many patients offered open surgery are pre-selected for survival.

The introduction of endoluminal grafts during the 1990s has provided an alternative to open repair.[8–12] Endoluminal grafts are less stressful and invasive and this is reflected in the 30-day mortality (1.4% for 144 bifurcated endografts inserted in Western Australia between June 1994 and November 1998). As for open repair, smaller aneurysms present more suitable morphology for endoluminal repair. Most endografts can be inserted with minimal stress under general anaesthetic, epidural or even local anaesthetic. In most cases blood loss is minimal, Intensive Care Unit admission unnecessary and postoperative care similar to hernia repair. With endoluminal grafts, the morphology of the AAA is more important, relatively, than fitness for operation because success is dependent on total exclusion of the aneurysm, which is directly related to morphology. Successfully excluded aneurysms will diminish in size and cease to pose a risk of rupture. Conversely, non-successful exclusions may increase the rate of expansion and thereby, rupture. Most early non-successful exclusions (apart from retroleaks) are the result of patient selection factors. The long-term results are dependent on suitable morphology of the AAA, understanding the forces that might cause an endograft to fail, using durable materials and combining these factors to develop guidelines for patient selection and indications for the procedure.[13,14]

ANEURYSM SELECTION FOR ENDOLUMINAL GRAFTING

The crucial factors in patient selection for endoluminal grafting are the proximal neck and the morphology of the iliac vessels.

The proximal neck

1. Length from renal artery to chamber of aneurysm.
2. The changes in angle.
3. Diameter.
4. Contour and shape.
5. Quality of the wall and presence of thrombus, atheroma and calcification.

The importance of these factors is in the prevention of proximal endoleaks and secure fixation (see Fig. 1).

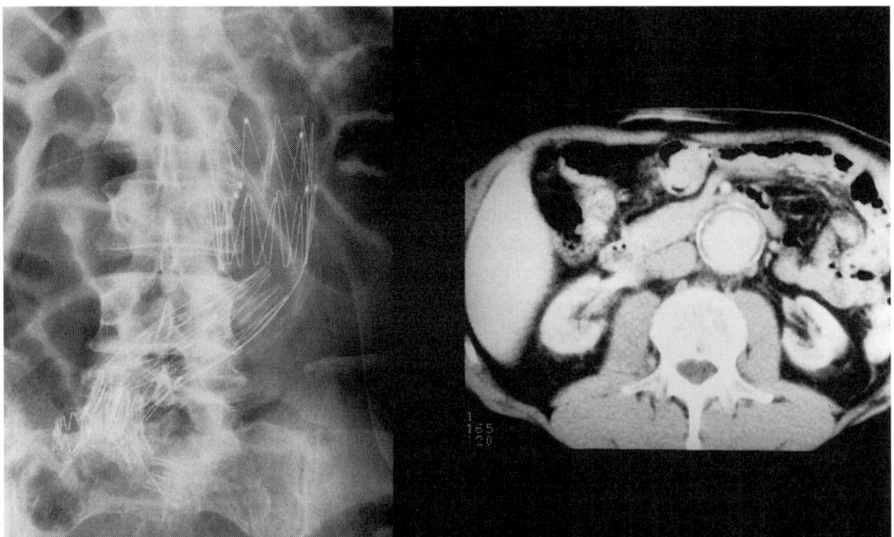

Fig. 1. Distal migration of the proximal end of an endoluminal graft from a large diameter neck containing thrombus.

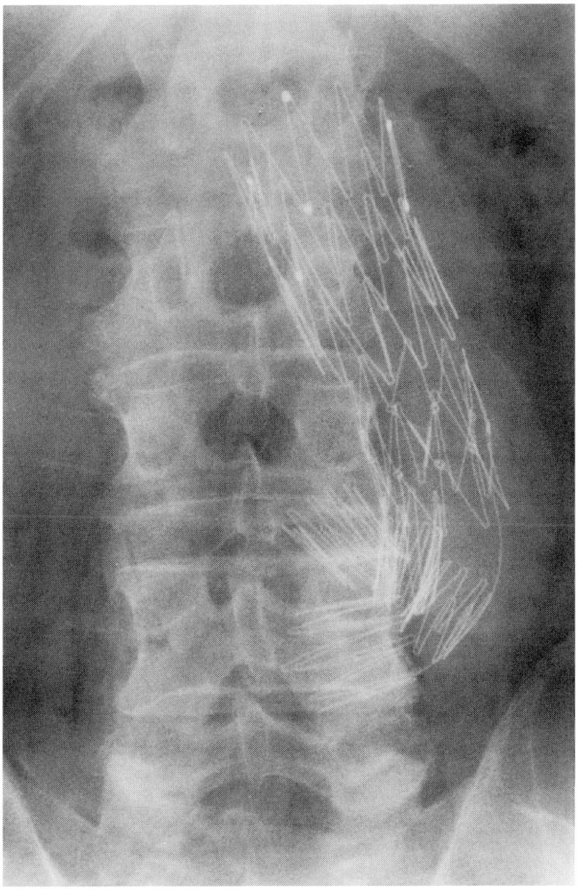

Fig. 2. Proximal migration of distal end out of the iliac vessels with kinking of the limbs of the endoluminal graft.

Iliac vessels morphology

1. Ease of access.
2. Ability to rotate a three-dimensional device and position accurately.
3. Distal fixation.

These factors relate to the preservation of outflow as well as prevention of endoleaks (see Fig. 2).

SECURITY OF ATTACHMENT

The security and durability of open grafting are the result of hand-sewing, demonstrable security of haemostasis (seal) at the time of operation, and the collapse and healing of tissue closely applied to the graft which becomes encased with tissue support.

The endoluminal graft must hang like a chandelier into the chamber of the aneurysm for a number of years – until the aneurysm shrinks to encase the graft within the chamber and provide the full length body support enjoyed by the open repair. Constant pounding and erosion forces work to disrupt and dislodge the graft within the chamber.

GRAFT DESIGN

The 8 years experience with endoluminal grafting has brought most workers in the field to a similar position with design. The features are as follows.

1. *A bifurcated graft* – restores normal anatomy perfusing both iliacs directly;
2. *A self-expanding graft* – accommodates for errors in diameter assessment and variation, a radial force (friction) at all contact points and resistance to compression;
3. *A modular system* – allows for endoluminal building of the bifurcated system via two ports; the ability to adjust for, and address, length assessment problems which result from variations in the final curved positions of graft lie, and optimize the landing zone in the iliac vessel;
4. *Full length metallic skeleton* – provides for maintenance of length and some pillar (column) strength; visibility for alignment and insertion and protection against kinking and twisting.

There are some controversial factors in graft design. One of these is the use of hooks, or staples, for proximal attachment vs reliance on friction forces and pillar strength. Another is the use of modules and assemblies with joints vs one-piece devices.

PROXIMAL ATTACHMENT

The long-term success of the procedure depends on continuing exclusion of the aneurysm chamber. Proximal security is important to prevent migration of the device and exposure of the aneurysm chamber to blood flow and pressure. In many cases friction alone or friction and pillar strength may be sufficient. However, in some cases these forces have been overcome and migration has occurred.

Pull out experiments have been performed using harvested pig aortas to examine the stability and durability of stents after deployment (Fig. 1). The method employed a simple spring force measuring device to pull on the deployed stent until it started to move and become detached. It was used to compare covered stents with stents on the outside and no hooks, covered stents with stents on the inside and no hooks, and covered stents attached by an anchor stent with hooks. The force required to pull out and displace a non-hooked stent was 5–6 Newton (600Gml) compared with 40–50 Newton for the hooked stents. This meant that up to 10-times the force is required to dislodge a graft by straightening the hooks. A sutured anastomosis has a rupture force around 125 Newton and this may involve arterial tear. Stapled anastomoses have been proposed and are expected to have the pull down strength of a sutured

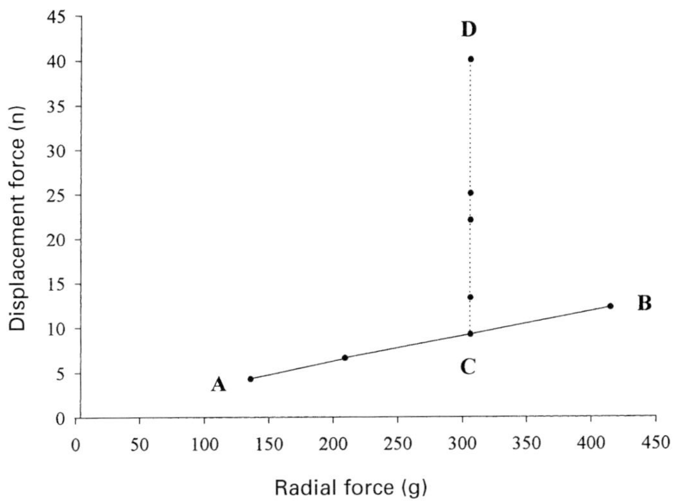

Fig. 3. Increasing pull out force with increasing radial force along A to B. Increasing pull out force required with increasing strength of hook attachment (C – D). The relationship of C – D is independent of the position along A – B.

anastomosis. Some workers object to penetration of the arterial wall, but this has to be balanced against the danger of migration, and has not been a problem for the authors to date.

MODULAR JOINTS AND THE FLOW OF BLOOD THROUGH A STENT GRAFT IN AN ANEURYSM

There are two main forces acting upon an endoluminal graft.[15–17] In the first instance, the simplest visualization of the force is to consider an unsupported flexible tube in a cavity. If the tube has a constant diameter and the flow is constant, the force on the wall of the tube is perpendicular to the wall at that point and proportional to the square of the change in velocity of the fluid at that point (Fig. 4). Thus, if the flow is constant, the tube will assume an even curvature, and the force will be equal at all points along the wall.

In reaction to the force on the wall of the tube, there must be a balancing force where it enters and exits the cavity (Fig. 5). This force must resist the pull of the force on the curve in the tube. With the even curvature of the tube, this force will be equal at the proximal and distal positions. Consider, however, if the diameter of the tube reduces in the direction of the flow, then the velocity of the blood will increase and the change in the velocity vector applied to the wall will be greater still. Consequently the force on the wall will be greater, with the force being inversely proportional to the fourth power of the diameter. The effect of this will be to shift the centre of the force further down stream, onto the lower half of the tube, and will

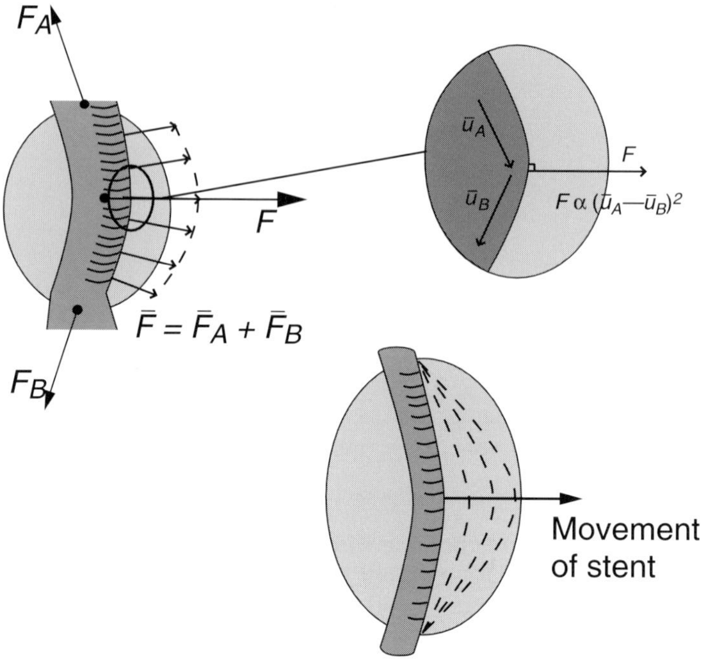

Fig. 4. On a constant diameter artery, the force will be constant along all points of the wall. Force F is the resultant force of all the velocity changes, i.e. the curvature and narrowing of the tube. The magnitude of the force (*F*) will increase as the curvature increases. *Fa* and *Fb* are the reaction forces that are required to balance force *F*. Over time, the cyclic action of the stresses on the stent will tend to move it until the wall of the aneurysm supports it. This will stress the joint at the proximal and distal points. The place of least resistance will be displaced. The maximum point of movement and stress per unit force, is in the centre of the tube or centre of the force.

result in non-even curvature of the tube. The curvature in the lower half of the tube will be greater than in the upper half. This increase in curvature will result in a higher rate of change in the velocity vector, which will further increase the force on the lower half of the tube until a balance is achieved.

The other effect of this movement of the centre of force is to increase the force on the distal end relative to the proximal end. This implies that if an endoluminal graft is curved in deployment in the cavity, it is more likely to be pulled from the distal entrance to the aneurysm than the proximal entrance with this force, but this is not the only force being applied.

The other force that acts on an endoluminal graft is that arising from the change in flow direction where the graft bifurcates (Fig. 6). At this point, the graft narrows, accelerating the flow and the flow also changes direction. The force in this case will act in the distal direction, and tend to pull the graft from the proximal entrance. The magnitude of this force is independent of the location of the bifurcation in the cavity. However, if the endoluminal graft is curved, and the bifurcation is above the centre

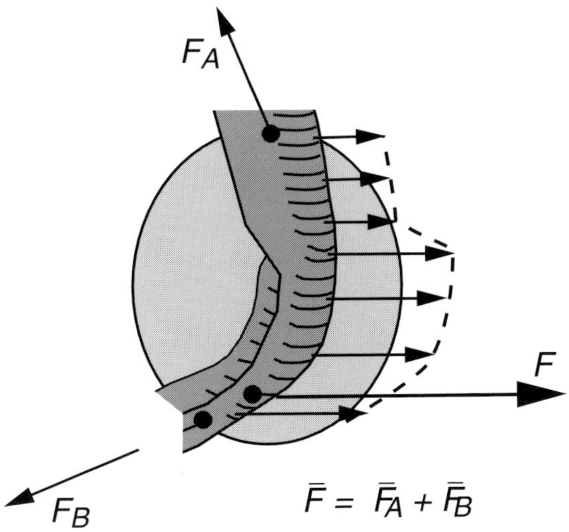

Fig. 5. As a tube (artery) narrows, the velocity increases, which increases the force applied to the narrow section of the tube, which in turn increases the degree of curvature. The force is proportional to the velocity squared. If there has to be a decrease in diameter, this should be as low as possible in the chamber to minimize the deforming force. (The forces are defined in Fig. 4.)

of the curvature it will tend to further increase the rate of curvature. The force vectors from the curvature of the graft, and the bifurcation, indicate that there must be a critical degree of curvature. If the graft is less curved than this, the net force will be to pull the graft from the proximal entrance. If it is greater than this, then the net force will tend to pull the graft from the distal entrance.

When the normal pulsating flow is considered, then the force at any point will oscillate between an upper and lower value. The difference between the maximum and minimum force will increase as the graft narrows or increases in rate of curvature. This force will place mechanical strain on the graft and any join in it, and the cyclic nature of this strain will tend to separate any joint or slide it open (see Fig. 7).

Furthermore, uneven flow in the legs after bifurcation will result in the direction of the downward force on the bifurcation being off-centre. The pulsating flow will cause this force to oscillate in direction and this will have the effect of working or rotating the overlapping joint and the proximal and distal landing zones from side to side. This could considerably enhance the effect of any direct force on moving the graft.

The above summarizes the effect of force on the graft, but it has not considered the actual displacement. The graft is fixed at two points, at the proximal and distal entrances to the cavity: it may be pinned at the proximal entrance. As the force

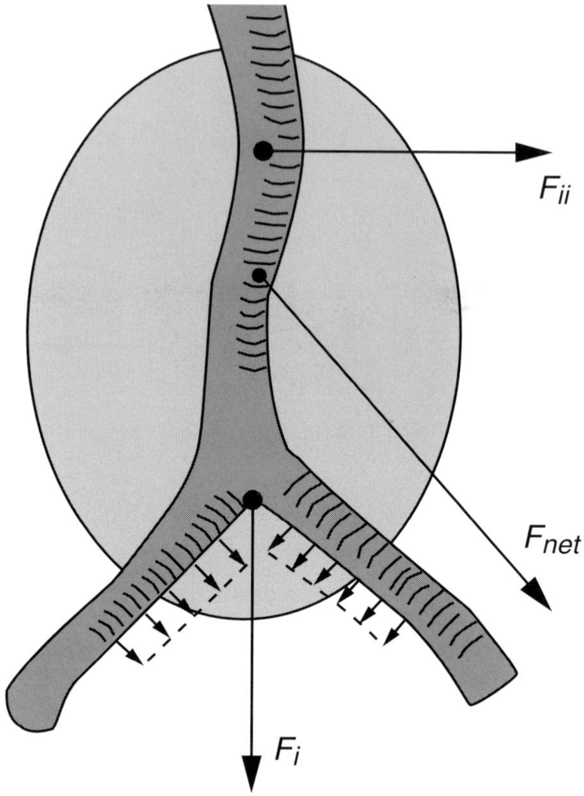

Fig. 6. The force acting on the bifurcation is a result of the change of velocity of the fluid at that point. The net force (F_{net}) acting on the stent is the sum of the forces acting on the bifurcation (F_i) and the force acting on the curvature (F_{ii}) of the stent.

applied to the graft oscillates, the displacement in the cavity will also oscillate. The degree of movement will be a function of the distance from the entrance to the cavity and the force applied. This displacement will attempt to pull the graft into the cavity to provide the extra length required. The possible points of movement are the:

proximal entrance;
distal entrance; and
overlapping joint.

In each case, the movement can only be inward, to increase the curvature within the cavity. This movement will continue until the graft becomes supported by the cavity wall or the force is insufficient to cause movement. The graft can reach the cavity wall in two ways. The cavity can shrink, or the joint can separate sufficiently to allow it to reach the wall. If the overlap in the join is insufficient to allow this latter result, then there is a risk of separation at the join.

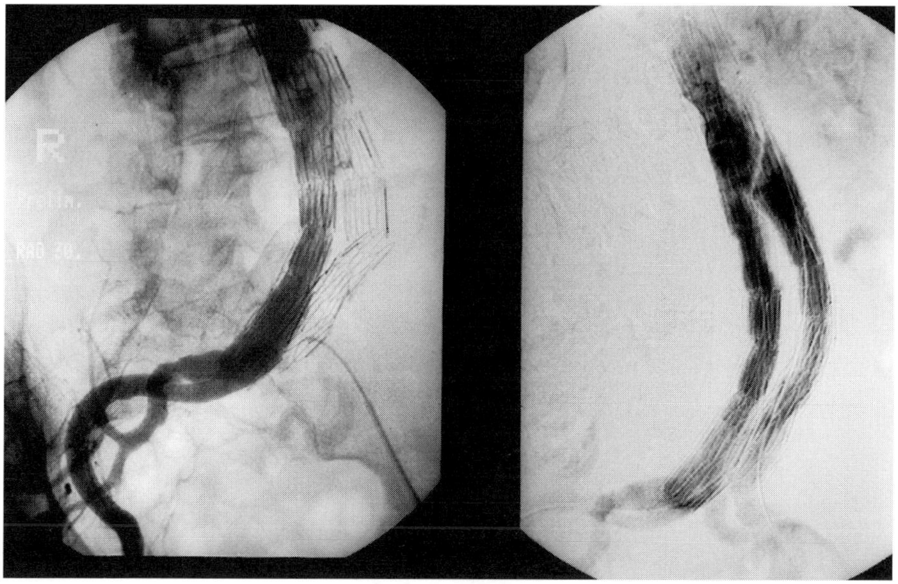

Fig. 7. Dislocation of the joint within an enlarged aneurysm chamber at 1 year due to inadequate joint overlap at the time of deployment – and correction with a bridging stent.

The movement of the graft and tendency to separate is greatest at the centre of the cavity, and least at the top or bottom. Consequently, to minimize the risk of joint separation, the joint must be located at a position of relatively low stress and movement. This is likely to be found at the top or bottom of the cavity, rather than in the centre (Fig. 8). Further, it is desirous to minimize the actual and potential curvature of the graft, to minimize the risk of joint separation, and to ensure that the overlap in the join is sufficient to allow the graft to reach the wall of the cavity without separating.

None of the above has yet considered the effect of the elastic nature of the wall, nor has consideration been made on the nature of the rheological properties of blood, such as the momentum of the particulate matter. These will further complicate the solution of the problem, though they are unlikely to affect the nature of the results.

DURABILITY OF THE ENDOLUMINAL GRAFT

The required durability of an endoluminal graft is related to the life expectancy of patient, the security of attachment and assembly, and the durability of the materials. If the risk of the procedure is lowered, and is more appealing to the patient, then the size of the aneurysm determining intervention is reduced. In which case the morphology of the aneursym is much kinder to the security of attachment and assembly of the endoluminal graft: the shrinking required to encase the graft is much

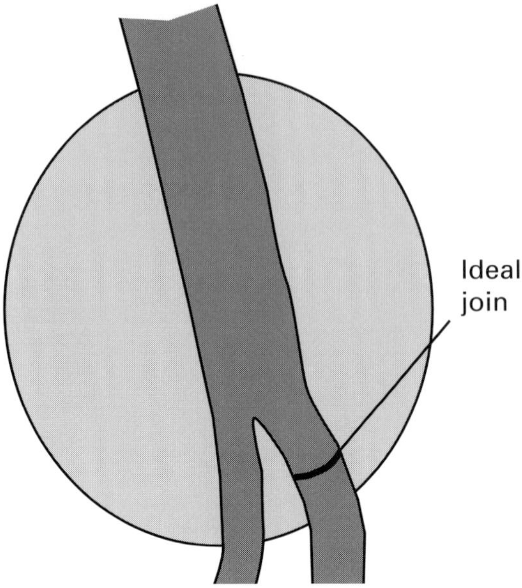

Fig. 8. The location of the centre of force, and the action of each reaction force then becomes important in determining where the join in the stent should be located in the aneurysm. The current work suggests that the best placement for the join may be as close to the proximal or distal entrance to the aneurysm as possible.

less and once encased the graft is secure. If the above is true and intervention is performed earlier, then the repair will have to last longer and the emphasis shifts towards the materials.

The conclusion of this argument is that the indications for endoluminal grafting and patient selection will take on a different perspective to open graft repair of AAA because the risk benefit analysis is different. We predict that endoluminal grafting for AAA will reduce the size indication for prophylactic repair to approximately 40mm. Endoluminal grafting is feasible with a larger aneurysm but the demands on the devices are greater.

REFERENCES

1. Semmens JB, Lawrence-Brown MMD, Norman PE *et al.*: The quality of surgical care project: benchmark standards for open repair of abdominal aortic aneurysm in Western Australia. *Aust NZ J Surg* **68**: 404–410, 1998
2. Ingoldby CJ, Wujanto R, Mitchell JE: Impact of vascular surgery on community mortality from ruptured aortic aneurysms. *Br J Surg* **73**: 551–553, 1986
3. Soreide O, Lillestol J, Christensen O *et al.*: Abdominal aortic aneurysms: survival analysis of four hundred and thirty-four patients. *Surgery* **91**: 188–193, 1982

4. Mutirangura P, Stonebridge PA, Clason AE *et al.*: Ten-year review of non-ruptured aortic aneurysms. *Br J Surg* **76**: 1251–1254, 1989
5. Johnston KW: Influence of sex on the results of abdominal aortic aneurysm repair. *J Vasc Surg* **20**: 914–923, 1994
6. Rutledge R, Oller D, Meyer A, Johnson G: A statewide, population-based, time-series analysis of the outcome of ruptured abdominal aortic aneurysm. *Ann Surg* **223**: 492–505, 1996
7. Norman PE, Semmens JB, Lawrence-Brown MMD, Holman CDJ: Long-term relative survival following surgery for abdominal aortic aneurysm in Western Australia. *Br Med J* **317**: 852–856, 1998
8. Parodi JC, Palmaz JC, Barone HD: Transfemoral infraluminal graft implantation for abdominal aortic aneurysms. *Ann Vasc Surg* **5**: 491–499, 1991
9. Chuter TA, Green RM, Ouriel K: Transfemoral endovascular graft placement. *J Vasc Surg* **18**: 185–197, 1993
10. Yusuf SW, Baker DM, Hind RE *et al.*: Endoluminal transfemoral abdominal aortic aneurysm repair with aorto-uni-iliac graft and femorofemoral bypass. *Br J Surg* **82**: 916, 1995
11. Lawrence-Brown M.M.D., Hartley D, MacSweeny S *et al.*: The Perth endoluminal bifurcated graft system – development and early experience. *J Cardiovasc Surg* **4**: 706–712, 1996
12. Gordon M, Lawrence-Brown MMD, Hartley D *et al.*: A self-expanding endoluminal graft for treatment of aneurysms: results through the development phase. *Aust NZ J Surg* **66**: 621–625, 1996
13. van Schie G, Sieunarine K, Lawrence-Brown MMD, Hartley D: The Perth bifurcated endovascular graft for infrarenal aortic aneurysms. *Semin Intervent Radiol* **15**: 63–69, 1998
14. Lawrence-Brown MMD, Sieunarine K, Hartley D *et al.*: The Perth HL-B bifurcated endoluminal graft: A review of the experience and intermediate results *J Cardiovasc Surg* **6**: 220–225, 1997
15. Ziegler F: *Mechanics of Solids and Fluids* 2nd edn. New York: Springer-Verlag, 1995
16. Anenis M, Stancampiano AP, Wakhloo AK, Lieber BB: Modelling of flow in a straight stented and non-stented side wall aneurysm model. *J Biomed Eng* **119**: 206–203, 1997
17. Perktold K, Hofer M, Rappitsch G *et al.*: Validated computational of physiologic flow in a realistic coronary artery branch. *J Biomechanics* **31**: 217–218, 1998

Commentary

This experience in Perth is greatly admired and the thinking, which has led to the evolution of the Perth System, emerges clearly in this chapter. So much depends upon the forces exerted on the implanted device and this has led to design changes. The analysis of these co-workers is such that they have now recommended the use of suprarenal anchoring of all endografts for aneurysm repairs and the whole of the graft systems are supported down the length of the fabric with stands. The explanation for this is clearly to be found within this chapter. *RMG*

The durability of the AneuRx stent graft system

Frans L Moll, Rudolf P Tutein Nolthenius and Jos C van den Berg

INTRODUCTION

With the development of a modular system for endovascular stent graft repair of infrarenal abdominal aortic aneurysms (AAA) a breakthrough was reached in the application of this endovascular technique. In the early days of stent grafts only tubes were available and fewer than 10% of patients had aneurysm morphology suitable for endovascular tube grafts.[1]

The development of bifurcated stent grafts opened up a larger group of patients, but each graft had to be customized and ordered in advance for the individual patient's needs. The specially designed stent graft had to fit in one session and last minute adaptations are intraoperative corrections were not possible. The introduction of systems with modular components not only widens the clinical applications, but also allows timing of the procedure at any moment preferred.

MODULAR STENT GRAFT SYSTEM

A modular system which comes up to these expectations is the Medtronic AneuRx stent graft (Figs 1, 2). The graft is made of woven polyester with its proven compability to the arterial system. It is fully externally supported by a nitinol mesh (memory metal) to stent the graft both longitudinally as well as radially. This 'coat of mail' allows good flexibility whilst maintaining column strength and radial force. The system consists of several segments in different length and diameter: a bifurcated body with one short 'pant-leg' and one long iliac limb, solitary iliac 'legs' to be connected with the short pant-leg and extender cuffs for the proximal aortic side and for the distal iliac areas. With a 10–20% oversizing of the diameter of the stent graft compared with the diameter of the aorta and iliaca arteries, the risk for migration is low because of adequate friction and hoop strength of the stent. Meanwhile, the chances are low that the stent graft incites aneurysm degeneration at the attachment sites. The stent is made of nitinol and therefore the graft is self-expandable. Balloon dilatation may be reserved to stenotic iliac areas or irregular vessel sections.

STENT GRAFT IMPLANTATION

After animal studies[2] the AneuRx stent graft implantation started in patients in June 1996 in the USA in an FDA sanctioned clinical trial. It was first introduced in Europe in December 1996 in the St Antonius Hospital, Nieuwegein, The Netherlands.

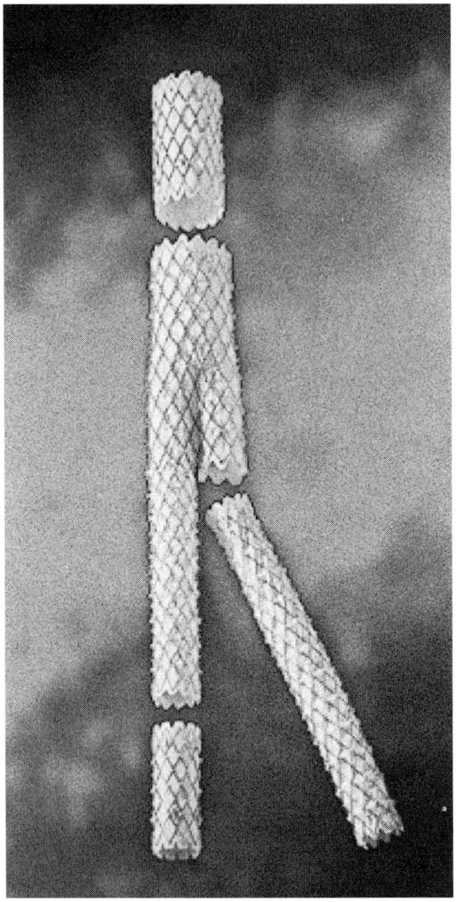

Fig. 1. AneuRx modular stent graft system.

The aneurysm-related inclusion criteria are:

- proximal infrarenal aortic neck length > 10 mm;
- a proximal neck diameter of 16–26 cm;
- the minimal iliac diameter to allow the introduction system is 6 mm, with a maximum diameter of 18 mm.

Patients with excessive iliac tortuosity and severely calcified stenosed segments are excluded. Preoperative evaluation is done with angiography and spiral computed tomographic (CT)-scanning.

Device selection is based on these investigations. Intravascular ultrasound is recommended at the time of intervention to determine definitive aortic and iliac diameters and length in order to confirm graft size selection. Length measurements are made using the catheter pull-back method, measuring distance between renal

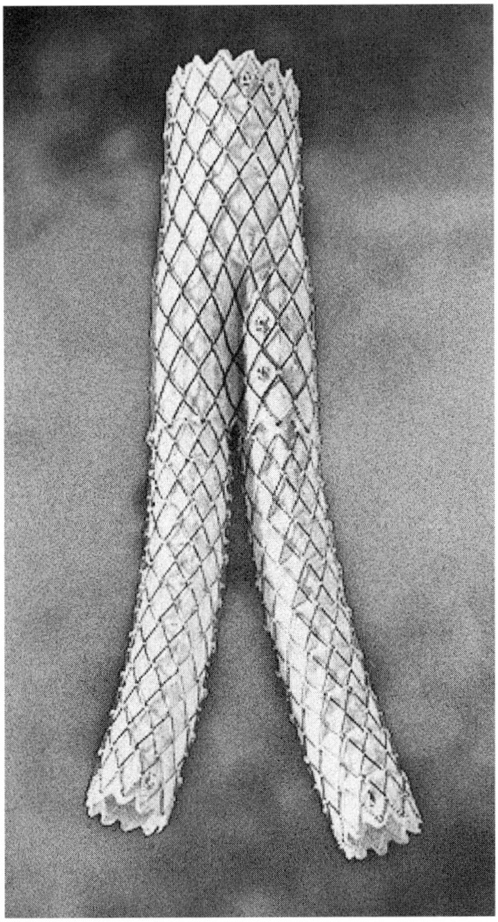

Fig. 2. AneuRx modular bifurcated stent graft.

arteries, aortic bifurcation and hypogastric arteries. Postoperatively all patients undergo spiral CT-scanning or duplex evaluation 2–3 days after the procedure to check the stent graft position and to detect possible endoleaks. An often-used postoperative follow-up schedule is spiral CT-scanning with contrast at 3, 6 and 12 months, and annually thereafter.

CLINCAL EXPERIENCE

Until October 1998, 474 patients were treated with the AneuRx stent graft in 12 clinics in the USA. The first pilot study ended in September 1996 and the phase II study ended in April 1997. Outside the USA more than 800 patients have been treated and the inclusion is still going on. There is no obligatory registration for follow-up, but the majority of patients are included in some kind of national or multinational registration by professional organizations. Data compiled from the Eurostar registration including the Dutch contribution (n = 106, December 1996–October 1998), the Italian registration (RITA, n = 177, January 1998–October 1998), the British Users Group (n = 137, October 1997–October 1998) make a total of 420 patients suitable for analysis, most of them with short-term follow-up.

Technical success was achieved in 96% and of course this is mainly determined by following the inclusion criteria. By exploring the limits of the device, the introduction system becomes stranded in small heavily calcified and tortuous iliac arteries or blocks the possibility of hooking up the contralateral iliac stent graft into the short pant leg of the stent bifurcation. Correction of malpositioning of the proximal attachement side infrarenally can be corrected by extender cuffs. The same applies to the iliac location. Misplacement of the stent graft has nothing to do with the durability of the procedure, but with technical error and experience of the operating team.

The short-term advantages of stent graft procedures are short hospital stay and recovery, less blood loss and a short procedure time compared with the traditional surgical procedure. The mean hospital stay in the stent graft group is 4½ days and 98% of patients operated under general anaesthesia are extubated the same day. In general, intensive care unit-care is not necessary. In the Italian experience 32% are even treated under epidural anaesthesia. The average blood loss per procedure is 450 cc, but this is clearly the subject of the team's learning curve and dependent on introduction sheaths with well functioning haemostatic valves. Procedure time varies from 3.1 hours in the USA to 2.5 hours in Europe.

EARLY FOLLOW-UP

Endoleaks are to be divided into the time of onset – acute, persistent and late – and the anatomical location – attachment or anastomotic side, graft leakage and continuous blood flow to the AAA by lumbar and visceral arteries.

When spiral CT-scanning is performed before discharge, backbleeding from the lumbar and visceral vessels is often seen (acute endoleaks 16% US and 11% Europe). Attachment leaks are noted in 5% and 4% respectively.

Initial oozing through the woven graft at the time of implantation in the heparinized patient seen intraoperatively at the post-deployment angiography usually disappears at pre-discharge spiral CT-scans.

1-YEAR FOLLOW-UP

In 44 patients with a documented 1-year follow-up, 8% had a persistent endoleak from backbleeding lumbar and visceral arteries. These are followed conservatively, because the aneurysm volume is not growing. When the aneurysms with persistent endoleaks are groing, most physicians treat these patients either by selective embolization of the lumbar and visceral arteries, or by injection of a siccative agent, such as tissue col into the aneurysm sac. So far, it is unknown how many patients are treated this way, but the numbers are to be collected in order to anticipate the problem at the time of operation and advise for future protocols.

Migration of the stent graft during follow-up is not reported, either in the USA nor in Europe. Occlusion of stent graft limbs due to kinking is less than 3%. Shrinking of the AAA, not only transversally, but also longitudinally does curve the stent graft. Up until now the uninterrupted 'exoskeleton' of the AneuRx stent graft prevents kinking and therefore occlusion of the graft limb. In our own experience, we saw one limb occlusion in a not fully deployed graft limb with a pre-existing and untreated common iliac artery stenosis. It is recommended to balloon dilate such areas at the time of stent graft implantation.

DURABILITY

Stent graft construction

Integrity of the stent graft is a prerequisite for the durability. Woven polyester has a proven compability with arterial blood flow, but is known for a poor ingrow into the

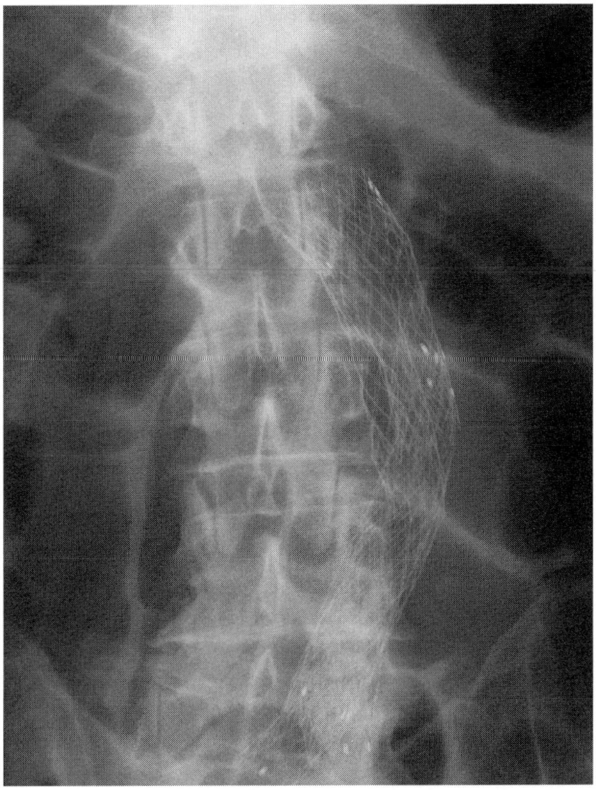

Fig. 3. A 73-year-old man with AneuRx bifurcated stent graft implantation.

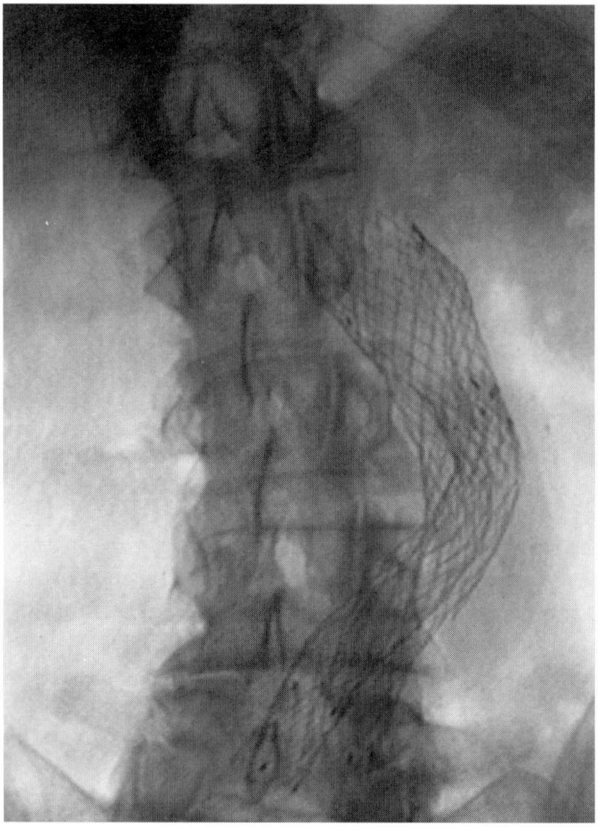

Fig. 4. (Same patient as in Fig. 3) AneuRx bifurcated stent graft curving after 1 year follow-up and aneurysm shrinkage.

arterial wall. Stents with a correct balance between hoop strength and friction do ingrow and do not migrate. However, when aneurysms shrink, especially longitudinally, the forces to migrate from attachment sides are strong. This is accentuated when the graft is stented longitudinally, giving column strength. To relieve the forces at the attachment sides, the stent coat of mail should allow curving, meanwhile preventing kinking and occlusion of graft limbs (Figs 3, 4). In stent grafts with interruptions of the exoskeleton, occlusions may occur due to kinking of these interrupted areas when aneurysms are shrinking. Theoretically, the shape of the stents must be smooth and not perforating or eroding the polyester fibre of the graft when bending and stretching occurs in the postoperative period. Long-term and close control of these types of stent grafts is mandatory to answer those questions because mechanical graft perforation could be lethal.[3]

Stent graft anatomical position

Correct anatomical positioning is a second condition for durable results. A minimum of at least 1 cm of a non-aneurysmatic infrarenal aorta is necessary for good sealing.

Irregular calcified circumferences of the aortic neck increase the risk of late endoleaks, because the hoop strength of the stents might be insufficient to reform the calcified neck into a suitable circular area. The same is true for thrombus in the neck. The lack of stent friction against the arterial wall increases the risk of migration and thrombus may dissolve under pressure in interrupted areas, causing endoleaks. For

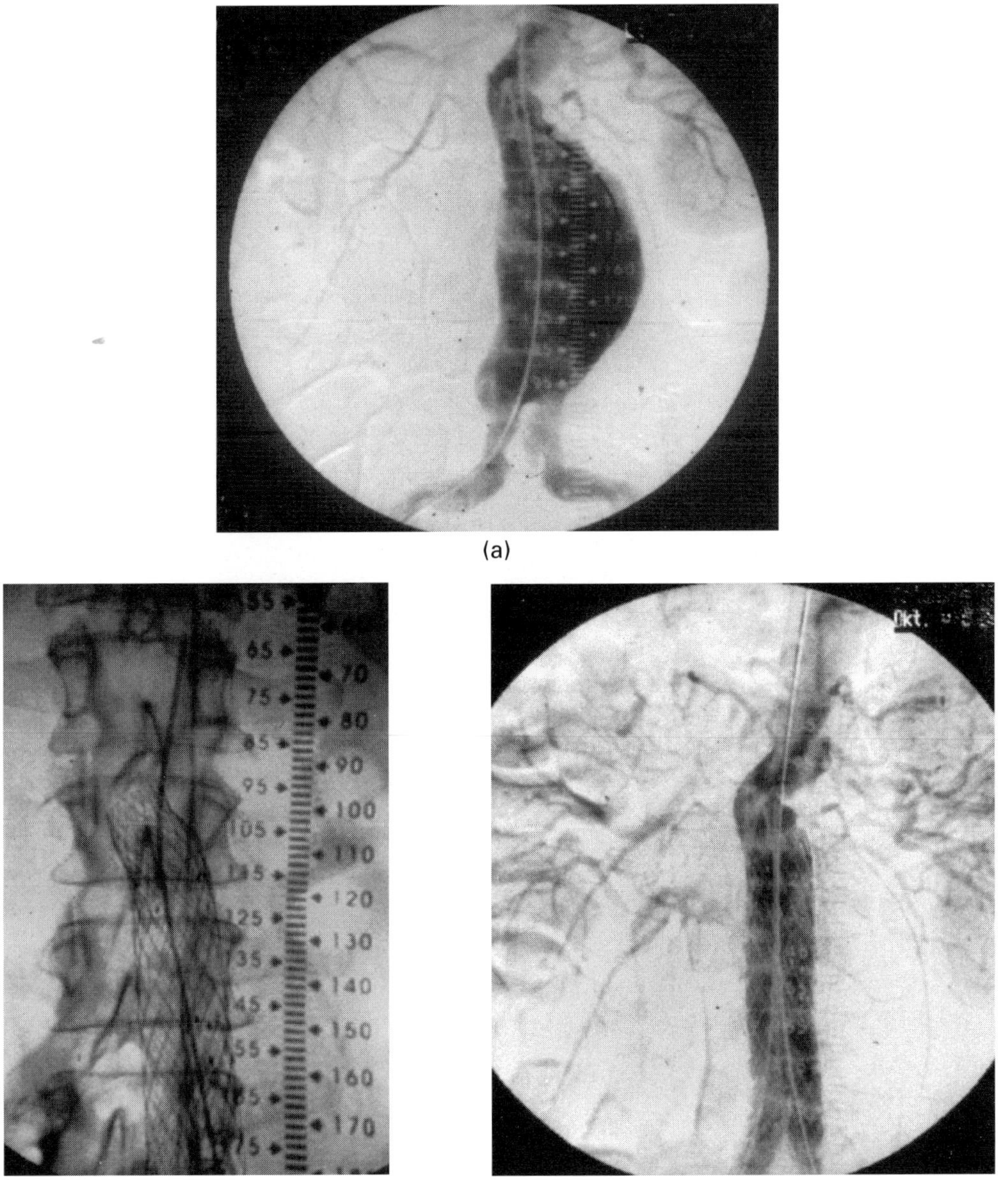

Fig. 5. Angulated infrarenal aortic neck and an AneuRx bifurcated stent graft with adequate sealing and tapering of the stent graft at the site of angulation.

angulated necks, specific attention must be made to overlap the angulation generously and to attach immediately below the origin of the renal arteries. In our experience, two patients developed late endoleaks after 1 year of adequate sealing at the angulated area and were discovered before aneurysms volume expansion. AneuRx aortic extender cuffs were placed between the area of angulation and the renal arteries. No additional endoleaks are present thus far (Figs 5, 6).

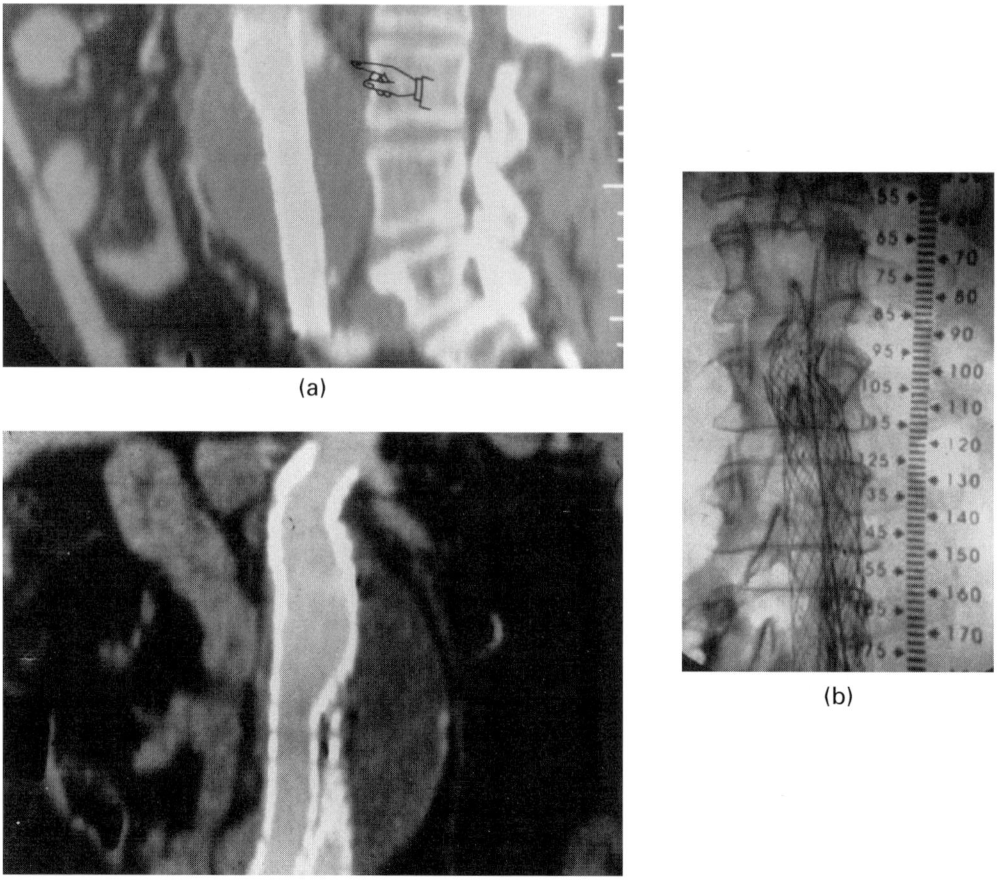

(a) (b) (c)

Fig. 6. Late proximal endoleak after more than 1 year and sealing with an aortic extender cuff, indicating the necessity to overlap the angulation for durable results.

CONCLUSION

The results of this modular AneuRx stent graft system with an uninterrupted memory shaped alloy (nitinol) exoskeleton and adequate hoop and column strength of the stent are encouraging. Based on this short-term follow-up, these endovascular stent grafts can be selected as first option in elderly and high-risk patients, and application in other patients is advised to be done in a trial setting It is too early to think in terms of satisfactory long-term results yet and so our views on durability must be reserved and careful postoperative monitoring of this system continued.

REFERENCES

1. Allen RC, White RA, Zarins ChK *et al.*: What are the characteristics of the ideal endovascular graft for abdominal aortic aneurysm exclusion? *J Endovasc Surg* **4**: 195–202, 1997
2. White RA, Fogarty TJ, Kopchok GE *et al.*: Evaluation of a modular endovascular bifurcation prosthesis in a canine aortic aneurysm model. *J Vasc Surg* **24**: 1034–1942, 1996
3. Buth J *et al.*: Personal communication Eurostar experience.

Commentary

These authors from Nieuwegein have had considerable experience using the AneuRx device since June 1996. They feel that this modular device satisfies many of the criteria that they were seeking. They have used intravascular ultrasound to determine definitive aortic and iliac diameters at the time of implantation and recommend this. The authors have described experience with AneuRx in the USA and Europe and how postoperative complications have been managed. On durability, the authors comment that the fabric used is woven Dacron and they note that this material has poor ingrowth into the arterial wall. The importance of this expected lack of ingrowth cannot be estimated at this stage. It has not been an important matter in patency comparing woven and knitted Dacron for bypass, but tissue growth could be an important factor for stent graft technique for aortic aneurysm in terms of durability. Time will tell. We simply do not know how important it is for this novel technique for the Dacron material to generate an adherence of its own. The AneuRx device is certainly very user friendly in the experience of these authors and in my own experience. The memory-shaped alloy and the oversizing should ensure a powerful fit. The complete 'coat of mail' throughout the modular system should discourage late kinking. In terms of long-term durability, it will be interesting to know how this device responds to changes in artery wall shape which will inevitably happen. It seems set to do well in terms of avoidance of kinking, but whether it will remain equally as adherent by using woven Dacron and a memory-shaped alloy whose diameter is determined by the temperature of the blood at the time of implantation, is to be seen in due course. At present, users are extremely happy with AneuRx. The authors have been very fair in their analysis of this system and are calling for careful monitoring during follow-up.
RMG

The durability of the Vanguard® system

Peter L Harris

INTRODUCTION

Stentor (MinTec) which was the precursor of the Vanguard® system (Boston Scientific Corp) was the first device for endovascular aneurysm repair to be marketed commercially. Designed by Claude Mialhe[1] it was also the first modular system – in which the endograft is constructed *in situ* from separate components, and the first to combine the endograft and its introducer as a complete package. Being the first available it was also the device with which many clinicians gained their first experience of endovascular grafting for aneurysms, especially those practising in Europe.

There are advantages and disadvantages from being first in the market place. The obvious advantage, from a commercial view-point, is the absence of competition. However, despite patent laws, this benefit is likely to be short-lived if the product is successful. The main disadvantage of being first, with a technique that is clinically unproven, is that you are most vulnerable to unforeseen pitfalls in what is essentially uncharted territory.

The Stentor system was marketed in Europe in 1994, and was replaced by the Vanguard system in 1996 after the Boston Scientific Corporation acquired the MinTec Company. Approximately 1500 Stentor devices were implanted, mostly in Europe, and at least twice this number of Vanguard devices have been implanted, world-wide, subsequently. The combined total number of implants of these devices far exceeds that of any other type of system. Therefore, there is more information about their performance in clinical practice than there is about any other device.

STRUCTURE OF THE VANGUARD SYSTEM

Both the Stentor and Vanguard devices are constructed from a nitinol wire stent with a thin Dacron covering on the outer side. The physical properties of the nitinol wire are temperature-dependent. At body temperature the stent exerts maximal radial force, while at lower temperatures it is relatively compliant. Cooling the system, by irrigating it with iced saline, facilitates its passage through the introducer sheath during deployment.

The stent, itself, is constructed from separate rows of nitinol wire that are loosely connected by polypropylene sutures. Similar sutures attach the fabric to the stent at regular intervals. At the proximal end of the device there is a row of the stent that is uncovered by fabric. A number of barbs to prevent distal migration of the device are deployed at intervals around the circumference at this junction. The Dacron fabric in the Vanguard device is of considerably better quality than that employed originally in the Stentor system and a longitudinal seam that was a point of weakness in the Stentor device was eliminated. Both the Stentor and Vanguard bifurcated endografts are composed of two modular parts. There is a body and limb together that are deployed first and a second limb that is deployed separately from the opposite groin. The second limb forms a seal with the body by overlapping into a short, slightly tapered stump. All modular systems, introduced subsequently by other manufacturers, have copied this basic arrangement.

The system depends upon contiguity of the rows of the stent for column strength and articulation between the rows for flexibility. The first of these properties is considered necessary for its stability *in situ* and the second is a requirement for successful navigation of the vascular system during deployment. Appreciation of the structure of Stentor and Vanguard endografts is of importance when considering the relevance of changes that have been observed in some of them following implantation (see below).

THE EUROSTAR PROJECT

The most comprehensive source of information on the durability of the Vanguard system is the Eurostar Registry. This is a multicentred, international, European project that was established in 1996 to assess the clinical effectiveness of the endovascular approach for aortic aneurysm repair. Data is gathered on all types of endograft, including Stentor and Vanguard. Currently, 38 centres of vascular surgery in 11 European countries contribute and in excess of 1500 patients had been registered by the end of 1998.

By coincidence, the Eurostar Registry was initiated at the time that the Stentor system was being replaced by Vanguard. No other commercial systems were available at this time. Data on the Vanguard endograft has been collected prospectively with employment of the 'Intention to treat principle'. However, retrospective data on the Stentor system was also accepted so that comparisons between these, first- and second-generation, devices are possible. At the time of analysis the total number of Stentor devices registered with Eurostar was 316 and there were 335 patients, who had received the Vanguard system.

EARLY RESULTS

The Eurostar Registry shows that endovascular repair of abdominal aortic aneurysms using Stentor and Vanguard devices is associated with a very low risk of operative complications. Over 97% of devices were deployed successfully and the combined 30-day mortality rate was 3.7%. Technical complications were encountered during the course of the procedure in 156 patients (24%), but in most cases these were resolved successfully and in only seven patients was conversion to open repair necessary – three Stentor and four Vanguard. These excellent early results are compatible with other reports.[2]

The most important finding at this stage was an unexpectedly high incidence of early endoleaks. In all, 14% of patients were reported to have unresolved endoleaks on discharge from hospital.

LATER RESULTS (DURABILITY)

The Eurostar Protocol specifies objective follow-up assessment of aortic endografts within 1 month and at 3, 6, 9, and 12 months following operation and then yearly thereafter.

The intention is for all patients to be followed for at least 5 years after operation. The standard method of examination employed to examine the patients under consideration, to date, has been contrast-enhanced computed tomography (CT) scanning. Most have also been assessed by plain abdominal X-ray in four planes, and all had angiography at 1 year. Additional examinations have been carried out by whatever method was deemed appropriate by the clinician in charge according to clinical indications.

Late endoleaks

New endoleaks have been observed at all intervals after operation. The cumulative endoleak-free rate at 12 and 24 months for the Stentor endograft was 82% and 76% respectively (Fig. 1), while for the Vanguard endograft the endoleak free rate at 12 months was 72% (Fig. 2). It is likely that the higher rate of endoleaks associated with the Vanguard system is a reflection of more liberal patient selection rather than being related to the device itself. Unfortunately, there is no sign, so far, to indicate that the incidence of new endoleaks will diminish with time.

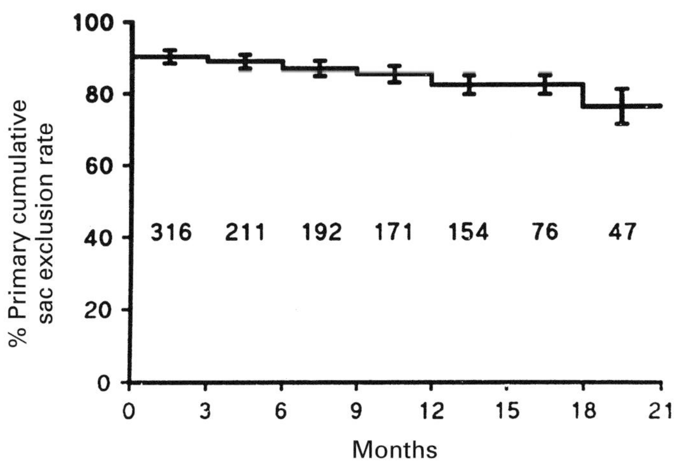

Fig. 1. Cumulative rate of freedom from endoleak following treatment of infrarenal abdominal aortic aneurysms using the Stentor endograft (n = 316).

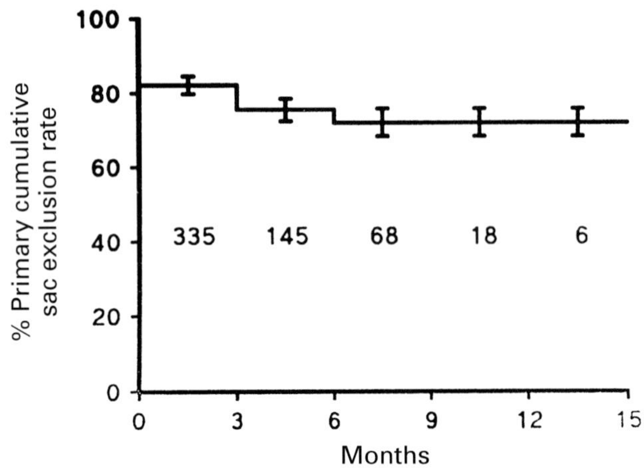

Fig. 2. Cumulative rate of freedom from endoleak following treatment of infrarenal abdominal aortic aneurysms using the Vanguard endograft (n = 335).

In contrast to early endoleaks, which included roughly equal numbers of proximal and distal graft-related endoleaks, and reperfusion endoleaks from aortic side-branches, late endoleaks arose predominantly from the distal anastomoses or from the main body of the graft. Late proximal endoleaks have been exceptionally rare, only one being reported to date. This would suggest that fears of problems due to continuing expansion of the neck of the aneurysm were probably unfounded.

The causes of late endoleaks identified to date include proximal dislocation of the limbs from the iliac arteries, dislocation of the second limb from the stump on the body of the graft and fabric tears. While distal stent migration and second limb dislocation may occur in isolation, often they appear to be associated with structural deformation of the stent graft itself. Similarly, late tears in the fabric may be secondary to structural changes in the stent.

Although 37% of early endoleaks reported to the Eurostar Registry sealed spontaneously, this development must be regarded with caution since there is no guarantee that the aneurysm sac does not remain pressurized through thrombus under these circumstances. The majority of late endoleaks were resolved by secondary endovascular interventions.

Correlation between changing diameter of the aneurysm sac postoperatively and the presence or absence of an endoleak confirms that this complication is likely to have an important influence upon the durability of the intervention. In patients in whom no endoleak has been observed following operation, the mean maximum transverse diameter of their aneurysm sacs reduces significantly. In those in whom an endoleak has been identified and successfully treated, the mean transverse diameter of their aneurysm sacs also reduces. However, in patients with a persistent endoleak, the mean maximum transverse diameter increases. Therefore, it can be concluded that the presence of a persistent endoleak indicates that the patient remains at risk from rupture of his aneurysm and it is important to draw a distinction between these and transient endoleaks. This is likely to apply equally to Vanguard and all other types of endograft for aneurysm repair. Analysis of aggregated data on a total of 865 endografts included in the Eurostar Registry shows that, whereas the rate of freedom from all endoleaks at 18 months after operation was 74%, the rate of freedom from persistent endoleaks was 90%.[3]

It is important to note that there are patients within the Eurostar database in whom the aneurysm sac is expanding without any endoleak having been identified, and conversely there are patients with endoleaks in whom the aneurysm sac is decreasing in size. Therefore, the visualization of endoleak alone is not a completely reliable indicator of failure of treatment, and this is likely to be true not only of the Vanguard system, but also all other devices for endovascular aneurysm repair. Prediction of failure or durability of endovascular repair is therefore more complex than may at first seem to be the case.

The definitive indicator of success or failure of treatment is the number of deaths from ruptured aortic aneurysm prevented. To date, there are insufficient data from any source to draw conclusions on this point. Rupture of the aneurysm following endovascular repair has been reported to the Eurostar Registry in six patients, three of whom died as a consequence. The cumulative survival rate for patients with Stentor endografts was 95% and 89% at 12 and 18 months (Fig. 3), and for those with Vanguard endografts it was 62% at 12 months (Fig. 4). But these calculations take into account deaths from all causes. Once again, the less favourable results with Vanguard are likely to reflect the tendency of clinicians to broaden the indications to include less favourable patients as they gain experience with the technique. There are no data to indicate that Vanguard endografts are associated with a higher incidence of potentially fatal device-related complications.

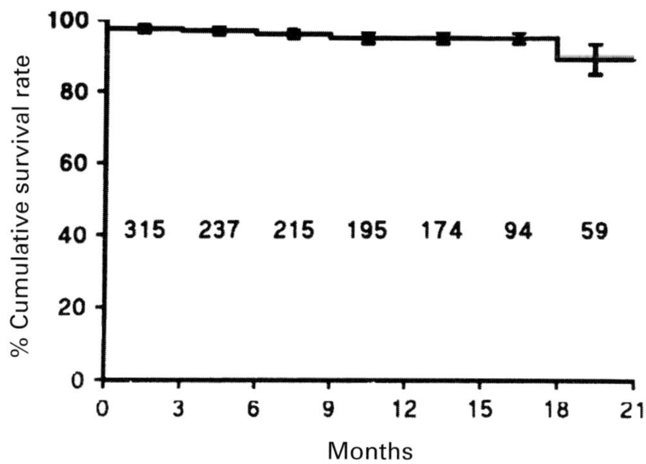

Fig. 3. Cumulative rate of survival of patients following treatment of infrarenal abdominal aortic aneurysms with the Stentor endograft (n = 315).

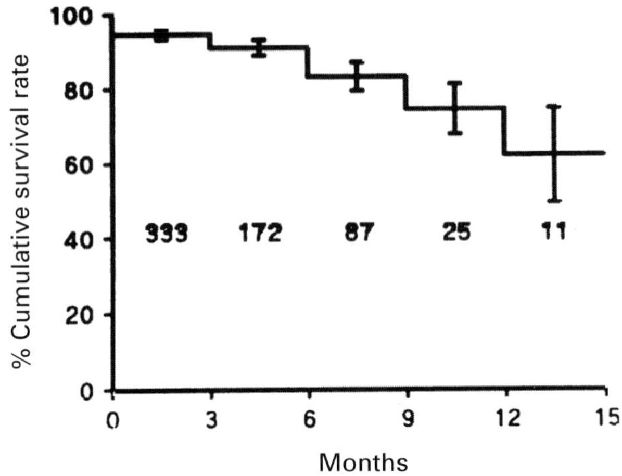

Fig. 4. Cumulative rate of survival of patients following treatment of infrarenal abdominal aortic aneurysms with the Vanguard endograft (n = 333).

Postoperative structural changes in the Vanguard system

During 1997 the Boston Scientific Corporation temporarily withdrew Vanguard endografts from the market after first reports of suture break involving the polypropylene sutures connecting the rows of the stent, and the fabric to the stent. It had been observed on straight abdominal X-rays that in some patients separation had occurred between rows of the stent.[4] Following disclosure of this problem the Eurostar organization was commissioned by the Boston Scientific Corporation to conduct a survey on the incidence of suture break and to ascertain what, if any, were the clinical implications. A total of 93 patients were examined by straight X-rays at their next scheduled attendance for follow-up examination. The time interval after operation varied from 1 to 18 months. The X-rays were taken in four planes, anteroposterior, lateral and left and right oblique. Evidence of suture break (Fig. 5) was found in 50% of these patients. Although a number of clinical complications had been reported within this population of patients including endoleak, graft limb thrombosis and stent migration, there was no statistical correlation between these complications and the presence or absence of suture break. Although the phenomenon of suture break does not appear to have had any significant impact upon the clinical performance of the Vanguard system to date, most surgeons are likely to regard it, with unease, as evidence of structural fatigue in the Vanguard device.

At the same time that the issue of suture break came to light, Eurostar collaborators began to report progressive distortion of many Vanguard and Stentor devices as time passed after implantation. The endografts were becoming buckled and, in some cases, acutely angulated or kinked (Fig. 5). In Liverpool, review of 28 patients with Vanguard devices that had been implanted for more than 1 year showed that 17 (61%) had become kinked, defined as an increase in angulation of more than 30

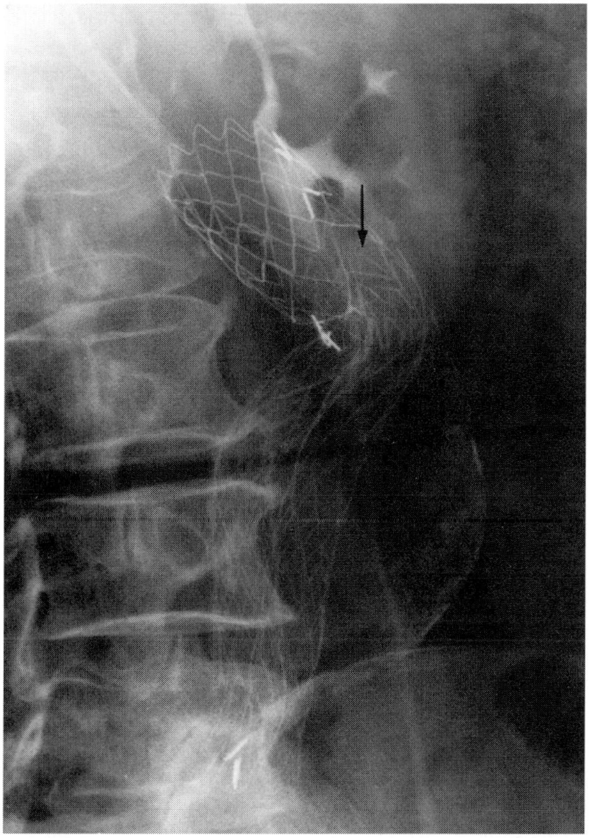

Fig. 5. Straight X-ray showing distortion of a Stentor endograft 12 months after implantation. The arrow indicates separation of rows of the stent associated with suture break.

degrees, and another five (18%) showed similar but lesser degrees of distortion. Of the 17 patients with kinked grafts, four had developed dislocation of the second limb from the body of the device resulting in a mid-graft endoleak, three had developed occlusion of one limb of the graft and another two had developed distal endoleaks. Therefore, it seems probable that late deformity of Stentor and Vanguard devices is an important cause of late complications particularly endoleaks and graft limb occlusion. Structural deformation of the device could also be the cause of late mid-graft and distal endoleaks.

Possible causes of buckling of endografts include: 1) elongation of the device after implantation; 2) migration of either proximal or distal ends of the stent; and 3) shortening of the aneurysm sac. In a study undertaken in Liverpool, detailed measurements taken from spiral CT scans with three-dimensional reconstruction of the aneurysm and endograft indicate that, of these, shortening of the aneurysm sac is by far the most important. An aneurysm, which is effectively excluded from the circulation by an endograft contracts not only in its transverse diameter, but also in length. A reduction in the length of the sac after 12 months of 15–20% is usual. The contiguous articulated stent of the Vanguard device seems to be unable to accommodate shortening of this degree without becoming buckled or kinked, and in some cases this may lead to clinical complications.

Further information about postoperative structural changes in the Stentor device has been obtained by a study of explants retrieved either at late conversion to open repair or at post-mortem examination. The Eurostar organization has been collaborating with Professor Robert Guidoin of the Biomaterials Institute in Quebec City in a study of these explants. Suture break has been a universal finding, and this has been associated not only with separation of the rows of the stent, but also overlapping of the stent creating an irregular surface. This, in turn, could be a cause of frictional damage to the overlying fabric in some individuals.

The studies undertaken in Quebec City have further raised concerns regarding the biostability of the nitinol wire from which the stent is constructed. Although all of the devices have been removed within 1 year after implantation, evidence of early corrosion has been observed in some cases. The significance of this finding is supported by first reports, to the Eurostar Registry, of nitinol wire fractures observed on postoperative radiographs.

CONCLUSION

Experience with Stentor and Vanguard endografts, to date, has provided considerable insight into long-term problems associated with endovascular aneurysm repair in general. In contrast to the treatment of occlusive arterial disease where stents are supported by the vessels into which they are introduced, the durability of endovascular aneurysm repair depends entirely upon the integrity of the device itself. On average, these devices are subjected to 37 million pressure pulses every year in an environment that exposes them to a high risk of biodegradation and corrosion. Furthermore, the geometry and anatomical disposition of the vessels changes as a direct consequence of deployment of the device and the natural forces involved are likely to be extremely powerful. Future evolution of the Vanguard system and all other similar endografts will need to take these factors into account if this approach to the treatment of abdominal aortic aneurysms is to yield durable results.

REFERENCES

1. Mialhe C, Amicabile C, Becquemin J-P: Endovascular treatment of infrarenal abdominal aneurysms by the Stentor system: Preliminary results of 79 cases. *J Vasc Surg* **26**: 199–209, 1997
2. Blum U, Voshage G, Lammer J *et al.*: Endoluminal stent-grafts for infra-renal abdominal aortic aneurysms. *New Engl J Med* **336**: 13–20, 1997
3. Cuypers P, Buth J, Harris PL *et al.*: Realistic expectations for patients with stent-graft treatment of abdominal aortic aneurysms: Results of a European multicentre registry. *Eur J Vasc Endovasc Surg* 1999 (in press)

4. Stelter W, Umscheid T, Zeigler P: Three-year experience with modular stent-graft devices for endovascular AAA treatment. *J Endovasc Surg* **4**: 362–369, 1997

Commentary

The experience of the Vanguard device in Europe is clearly described in this chapter and the problem of endoleak is brought out extremely well. The endoleak rate of discharge of 14% must have worried the operators, but the figure of 90% freedom from persistent endoleaks in due course is more reassuring. The vital importance of change of size of aorta after implantation is evidently very important and where aortas have not diminished in size and endoleaks have persisted, the concern level is understandably very high. This chapter describes six aortic ruptures after Vanguard implantation, three of which were fatal. The rupture of aortic aneurysms following endovascular graft deployment must have come as a great surprise, but I have to confirm that I have also had experience of this in a Zenith graft. In our patient, the aneurysm sac discharged into the psoas region and the patient had absolutely no symptoms whatsoever; he was lucky. This chapter raises the massive question of how best to monitor endoleaks and at the time of publishing this book, it is a major issue. *RMG*

Late risks of endograft for aortic aneurysm: observations from the United States Vanguard® trial

Hugh G Beebe

INTRODUCTION

This chapter summarizes the relatively early results of the United States Vanguard® aortic endograft and serves as an introduction to aspects of endograft design and clinical application that may have lessons for all types of endografts used to treat abdominal aortic aneurysm. While technical details of endograft design fall within the province of the engineer, it is essential that clinicians treating patients be familiar with design features of these devices that are still appropriately regarded as investigational. Since these design features may be relevant to ultimate clinical outcomes, a working knowledge of endograft design considerations allows doctors to best inform patients about risks and benefits. Also, during a time when endovascular techniques are evolving, device developers need a meaningful dialogue with those physicians and surgeons who use endografts.

DEVELOPMENT OF THE VANGUARD AORTIC ENDOGRAFT

The Vanguard aortic endograft has a historical lineage that sets the stage for understanding its results and for making broader generalizations about endografts. The original Vanguard design concept was derived from the Stentor endograft developed by Claude Mialhe and others made widely available in Europe by the MinTec Corporation during 1992. It was available in straight or bifurcated configurations in which the latter was modular, requiring assembly of components *in situ* within the aortoiliac segment. The potential advantages over single-piece aortoiliac bifurcation grafts were a smaller diameter delivery system and simpler operation of it. In addition, further advantages or potential advantages included capability for placing full-length stenting throughout the endoprosthesis that could be available in a modular system and a greater range of diameter and length dimensions to accommodate requirements for variable iliac artery morphology.

In April 1996, Meadox/Boston Scientific Corporation acquired the Stentor endograft technology and changes were instituted in response to the experience previously gained. Among these were the following:

1. A completely new woven polyester graft fabric to reduce water porosity to 200 cc per minute.

2. Elimination of a hand-sewn seam along the length of the prosthesis to achieve one-piece construction of the main fabric tube.
3. Replacement of the nitinol wire with a smoother surface, slightly thicker diameter section.
4. Refinement of the delivery system for simplicity and elimination of torque-induced realignment of components during delivery system passage.
5. Improvement in radiovisibility to enable fluoroscopic guidance.

This resulted in an adapted and significantly modified endograft, now called the Vanguard Endovascular Aortic Graft by Boston Scientific Vascular (Wayne, New Jersey, USA). Summaries of partial observations of the Stentor endograft experience have been published previously.[1–3]

It is important to recognize that the fundamental therapeutic concept common to all endografts *and* conventional vascular prostheses is replacement of the aneurysmal segment by a fabric tube. The methods of insertion of the fabric prosthesis differ greatly. Construction of endografts is highly variable from one design to another in three main areas: 1) attachment methods to secure the endograft in place; 2) adjunctive components that influence endograft physical properties such as circumfirential stents or longitudinal stiffeners; and 3) unibody/one piece versus modular design. Within each of these areas there are many details, but these basic features allow comparisons among different devices and serial observations of one device type.

Attachment of the Vanguard device within the zones of normal or undilated arterial anatomy adjacent to the aneurysmal portion is accomplished primarily by radial force of the segmental stents resulting in frictional contact with the aortic or iliac arterial walls. At the proximal end, there is an additional feature consisting of three wires shaped to form six barbs that can engage the surface of the aortic wall.

The Vanguard device is supported by nitinol zig-zag stents placed inside a single-piece, polyester, woven fabric tube. The stents are constructed of thermal-memory nitinol wire and arranged in a series of segments of variable diameter throughout the full length of the endograft. Within each of four sections of the endograft (upper, middle, transition and iliac limbs) a single length of wire is used to form successive segmental rings resulting in unitary spiral construction of each section. The entire assembly is joined with polypropylene ties (size 60) between stents at zig-zag apices. These ties do not traverse the fabric except at the endograft ends proximally and distally. A total of 320 polypropylene ties are used in the bifurcation Vanguard device. Twenty-one additional polyester sutures attach the fabric to stent components at the proximal end of the endograft and by some of the polypropylene ties at the distalmost end (Figs 1a,b).

These polypropylene ties are intended primarily as a deployment aid to keep components aligned as the delivery system is operated. The flexible and segmental nature of the supporting stent structure allows movement of the zigs relative to each other such that they may not remain in the original alignment relative to one another. This allows relief of structural stress or changes in geometry and adaptation to accommodate change in morphology of the excluded aneurysm.

The bifurcated endograft has two components – an aortic trunk, which is integral with a unilateral iliac segment, and a contralateral iliac limb that is added to the

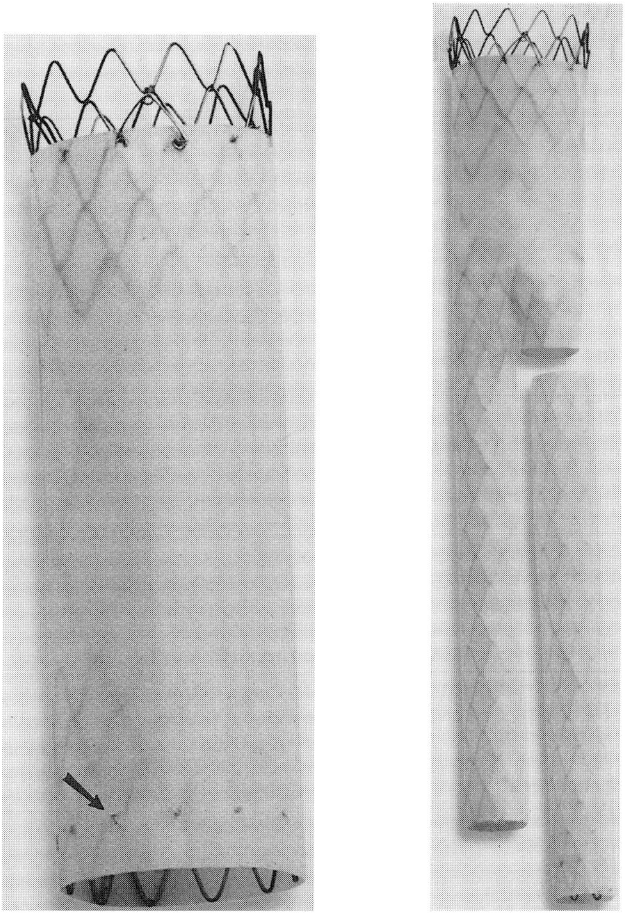

(a) (b)

Fig. 1. (a) The Vanguard endograft in straight configuration. Ties at the ends of the prosthesis that traverse the fabric can be seen (arrow). (b) The bifurcation modular prosthesis showing the main aortic trunk that is integral with the ipsilateral iliac limb and the separate contralateral iliac limb alongside.

primary component by contralateral vascular access using a separate delivery system. This is a so-called modular endovascular graft that is assembled *in situ* within the aortoiliac anatomy. The component containing the aortic trunk and ipsilateral iliac limb is delivered using a 21 French catheter while the contralateral limb utilizes a 12 French delivery system. Iliac artery extensions, the 'Passager' prosthesis, can be added as needed. Appropriately sized choices of diameter and length of endoprostheses are available to accommodate most patients who have suitable attachment zones, although aortoiliac morphology must be precisely and accurately measured to ensure the highest chance of technical success.

The delivery system of concentric sheaths containing the endoprosthesis is advanced over a guidewire into the segment to be treated. The endograft is deployed by retracting the outer sheath while holding the supporting inner catheter stationary. Upon exposure to body temperature, the nitinol wire frame self-expands to its pre-set diameter and excludes the aneurysm. A balloon on the end of the delivery catheter is used to model the stent frame and fabric from within. The endoprosthesis is radiopaque but is not known to cause magnetic resonance imaging artifacts.

Thus, features of the Vanguard design utilized in the US trial include:

1. Utilization of stent support throughout the full length of the endoprosthesis.
2. Placement of the supporting stents inside the fabric tube.
3. Numerous ties used to connect component stents.
4. Absence of suture fixation between the supporting stents and the fabric except at the ends of the device.
5. Self-expanding stents at the arterial attachment zones as contrasted with balloon-expanded stents.
6. A relatively flexible structure that can conform to changes in aortoiliac morphology.
7. A relatively non-porous fabric that aids performing and interpreting completion arteriography at the time of insertion.

Each of these features may have an influence on both early and late results. At present, data for the Vanguard device and all other endografts are still being acquired. It is too early in the world-wide endograft experience to draw firm conclusions about which of these details of endograft construction are important or to know whether others may prove to be so later on. Certainly it is not possible to make a definitive analysis from data available in the US Vanguard trial since that study began in mid 1997. However, results of preliminary evaluation reveal some important observations that will be discussed in detail as they are of interest for late outcomes and durability of endografts.

PRELIMINARY RESULTS OF THE UNITED STATES VANGUARD TRIAL

Use of the Vanguard aortic endograft in the USA as a Food and Drug Administration (FDA)-approved study of the safety and efficacy of the device, for treatment of standard risk patients, began on 6 August 1997. Evaluation is underway at 17 investigational sites and the protocol requires joint participation of vascular surgeons and interventional radiologists at each site. The following is a brief summary of the US Vanguard trial status at November 1998.

Methods

The primary objectives of this protocol are to evaluate the effectiveness of the Vanguard device in excluding infrarenal aortic aneurysms or aortoiliac aneurysms in patients who would otherwise require conventional surgical repair, and to assess the safety of the endovascular technique in comparison with conventional surgical repair. A secondary objective of the trial is to evaluate the clinical utility of the endovascular procedure when compared with conventional surgical repair.

The study was designed as a comparative clinical trial of two methods for electively treating infrarenal aortic aneurysms or aortoiliac aneurysms in patients who are surgical candidates of average risk. Patients were allocated to treatment by one of three approaches: conventional open surgical repair; a straight configuration endograft for exclusion of aortic aneurysm; or a bifurcated endograft for exclusion of aortic or aortoiliac aneurysm. Patients were enrolled with an infrarenal abdominal aortic aneurysm with or without iliac aneurysms.

Selection criteria included acceptable surgical candidates with at least 4.0 cm aortic diameter measured by computed tomography (CT), > 200% of adjacent normal aortic diameter or with documented expansion > 5mm in the past year requiring surgery. Patients with aortoiliac aneurysms were also included, as long as both internal iliac arteries did not need to be occluded to exclude the aneurysms.

Patients were excluded from the trial if they had: a ruptured aneurysm with clinical instability; serum creatinine > 1.7 mg/dl; signs that inferior mesenteric artery blood flow was significant to prevent bowel ischaemia; required chronic anticoagulant therapy; findings suggesting mycotic aneurysm; presence of a horseshoe kidney; or factors that would preclude acquiring outcome data for the study.

All patients entered into any study cohort met identical risk criteria. Allocation to study group was determined primarily by anatomical criteria and was contemporaneous. Patients in the conventional open surgery group all received infrarenal prosthetic grafts.

Follow-up protocol was primarily based upon imaging data including completion arteriography for evaluation of device position and sealing and discharge CT scanning and ultrasound. At 1, 3, 6, 12, 18 and 24 months serial imaging studies are being obtained to assess aortoiliac morphology change, device position, presence of endoleak and prosthesis patency in addition to clinical evaluation.

Results

By 26 June 1998, 352 patients were enrolled in the trial: 86 surgical controls, 243 bifurcation endograft cohort and 23 straight endograft cohort. In addition, 36 patients were treated for emergency or compassionate use indications in patients at considerably higher risk than specified in the investigational protocol. These off-protocol patients are not included in this summary and will be the subject of a separate high risk analysis.

Primary technical success by intention-to-treat analysis defined as 30-day survival with endovascular aneurysm exclusion, free of direct endoleak, was achieved in 246 (95.3%) of all patients assigned to endograft treatment.

Thirty-day all-cause mortality occurred in two (0.8%) patients with bifurcation endograft, none with straight endograft and three (3.4%) open surgical patients ($p = 0.18$). The cause of death was cardiac in three and respiratory failure in one. One patient in the open surgical repair group died as a result of mesenteric infarction.

Conversion to laparotomy for open aneurysm repair occurred in five (1.8%) patients allocated to receive endograft treatment. In three cases the combination of iliac artery tortuosity and calcification prevented accomplishing the procedure and attempts to pass the delivery system resulted in significant iliac artery trauma in two. In one case, severe aortic angulation prevented satisfactory device deployment. In these four cases, patient selection for an endograft procedure was judged retrospectively to have been inappropriate or marginal. The fifth conversion was due to operator error resulting in malposition of a portion of the endograft in too proximal a position that could not be subsequently adjusted. There was no mortality among these five patients.

Primary endoleak occurred in 13/258 (5.0%) of endograft patients. Of these, five were closed with a secondary endovascular manoeuvre. The secondary endovascular procedures, all performed on the same day, were additional insertion of an endograft extension proximally or distally in three, balloon angioplasty and stenting at the iliac level in one and coil occlusion of a lumbar artery in another case. Eight endoleaks were classified as minor and thought to be due to aortic branch-flow from a patent lumbar or inferior mesenteric artery. These are being observed during follow-up and three have already been reclassified as cases of sealed endoleak when contrast was not observed on subsequent imaging.

Complications of any sort, including minor self-limiting ones, occurred at a rate of 41.3% in bifurcation endograft, 13% straight endograft and 64.4% of open surgery patients. The lesser rate of complications in endograft patients was significant ($p < 0.01$). Severe complications occurred in eight (3.3%) of bifurcation endograft, two (8.7%) straight endograft and five (5.8%) open surgery patients but were not significantly different among groups.

Arterial occlusion occurred in seven (2.7%) of endograft patients during 30 days. Four were technically related, occurred during the procedure and were repaired. Three were occlusions of an endograft limb and were resolved by secondary procedures without limb loss. Non-fatal cardiac events occurred in four (1.5%) endograft patients and 11 (12.2%) open surgical controls ($p < 0.001$).

By November 1998, adjudicated follow-up observations were: 286 1-month visits, 275 3-month visits, 188 6-month visits and 50 12-month visits.

BREAKAGE OF TIES BETWEEN VANGUARD STENTS

In Europe during 1997, an observer reviewing follow-up plain abdominal X-rays to assess device alignment or migration, fortuitously noted that there had been separation of two adjacent stent apices and reasoned that this could only have occurred if the polypropylene ties uniting them had broken. This resulted in a detailed and widespread review of many follow-up data throughout Europe including independent radiologist scrutiny of patient images. A careful prospective focus was organized in the USA anticipating similar occurrences. Detailed information was presented in November 1997 to the United States FDA, the government agency that provides regulatory oversight of investigational devices in sanctioned trials. This report included conclusions from investigation of 455 European patients that disclosed no explicit linkage between tie breaks and adverse clinical status.

In the US trial all images from each investigational site were submitted to an independent core laboratory for review. The primary data for evaluation of presence of stent tie breaks was from plain radiography images of four orthogonal abdominal views to assess device integrity and geometric relationship of adjacent stent zig-zag apices (Fig. 2). Results of the US prospective analysis of tie breaks in 123 patients from 14 participating institutions are shown in Table 1 below.

Slightly more than one in five sets of films was classified as unreadable because either the quality of the image was inadequate for this type of analysis, for example excessive motion, or the degree of overlap of stent images interfered with interpretation in the area of greatest interest. Correlation with clinical outcome used three primary endpoints: endoleak, patency and conversion to open surgical procedure. Any lesser adverse events were also recorded in relation to stent tie breakage.

If uninterpretable images are subtracted from the total cohort (denominator), the number of patients with at least one tie break is approximately 20%. The relationship between tie breaks and aneurysm shrinkage is not fully understood yet, but it appears that there is an association. When an endoprosthesis resides in a vascular segment that is shrinking in diameter and perhaps in length as well, it will be affected by physical forces generating tension along the resultant curvature. The attachments by polypropylene ties between stents will become focal points for stress. It is not surprising that adaptation to this changing physical environment occurs partly by breakage of ties where the combination of focal stress and slight relative motion (fretting) is occurring. If this occurs without malpositioning of the stents, embolism of prolypropylene, or other adverse occurrence, it is possible to conceive of this stress-relieving change within the endograft as adaptive.

In addition, the Boston Scientific Corporation conducted *in vitro* testing of the Vanguard device, with various numbers of stent ties removed, to gather data on whether there were structural implications that could be measured by simulation

Table 1. Preliminary prospective analysis of tie breaks from the US Vanguard trial

Site	*Patients (n)*	*Intact*	*Unreadable*	*Tie breaks*
1	16	9	4	3
2	18	12	1	3
3	5	5	0	0
4	3	2	1	0
5	6	3	3	0
6	10	8	1	1
7	7	6	1	0
8	17	3	13	0
9	10	8	0	2
10	2	2	0	0
11	9	4	4	1
12	15	8	0	6
13	3	1	0	1
14	2	2	0	0
TOTAL	123	73 (59.3%)	28 (22.8%)	17 (13.8%)

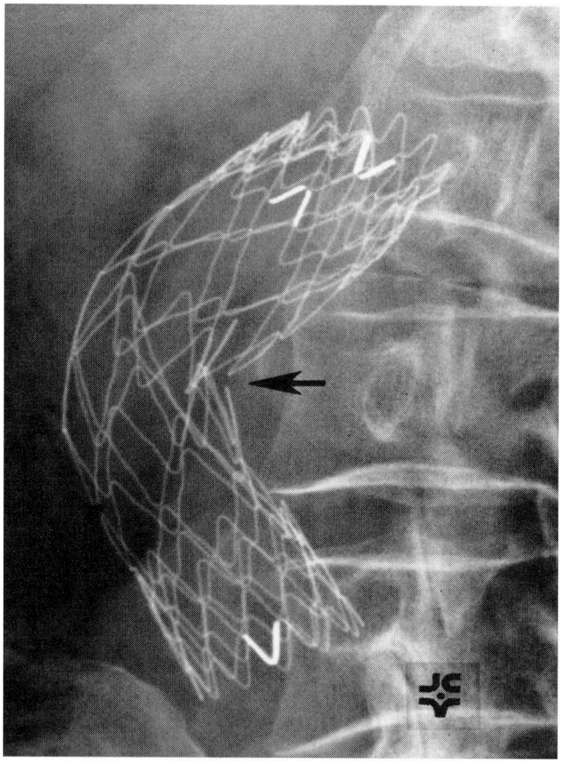

Fig. 2. This plain radiograph shows the stent of a straight endograft at 1 year after implantation. The aneurysm had decreased in size causing further angulation of the prosthesis. The distance between apices of two adjacent stents (arrow) is evidence of tie breakage that must have occurred to allow such separation.

testing methods. Two hypothetical causes of tie breaks were studied: 1) that tie breaks were induced by bending and twisting of the catheter delivery system during initial deployment manoeuvres; and 2) that changing vascular morphology induced tie breaks.

To test the first hypothesis, catheters loaded with stent grafts were subjected to different conditions that produced degrees of bending and twisting. An extreme simulation of high stress deployment was achieved by developing a passageway with a tight double curve bend radius that just allowed the catheter to be pushed through it without breaking. After the results of six different extreme stress models were obtained and analysed, additional iterations of testing with multiple Vanguard devices loaded into delivery systems was done using the worst case models. In summary, these tests resulted in either no tie breaks in many tests or one or two ties broken (out of a total of 320) in a minority of test cases.

To characterize the performance of the Vanguard device in a simulated clinical environment, an *in vitro* 'changing morphology' test fixture and method were developed. This apparatus provided for normothermic blood flow simulation with angulation and length change induced (Fig. 3) When the Vanguard device ties are intact, the mean radial force is 0.63 lb. When six to 18 randomly located ties are removed, radial force increases in the range of 0.83–0.92 lb.

Interpretation of the sum of all data from clinical observation and *in vitro* testing allows some interval conclusions to be formed and suggests the value of a heightened focus in some areas for ongoing future assessment of endograft durability.

Interval conclusions at the time of this writing are:

1. So far, it appears that the hypothesis that tie breaks are caused by bending and twisting forces during insertion of the Vanguard device has been disproved.
2. When up to 18 ties are removed in random pattern, radial force of the stents is increased.
3. Clinically, tie breakage is associated with shrinkage of the aneurysm, a process that results in stress on the endoprosthesis in a significant number of cases.
4. No adverse clinical event has been directly attributed to tie breaks *per se* in either the retrospective or prospective analysis.
5. It is possible that tie breaks represent adaptation of an endoluminal device to unmeasured forces of changing aortoiliac anatomy.
6. The frequency of tie breaks observed without adverse late outcome reinforces the concept of the primary function of the ties themselves as being an aid to insertion of the Vanguard device without dependence on them for continued satisfactory aneurysm exclusion function.

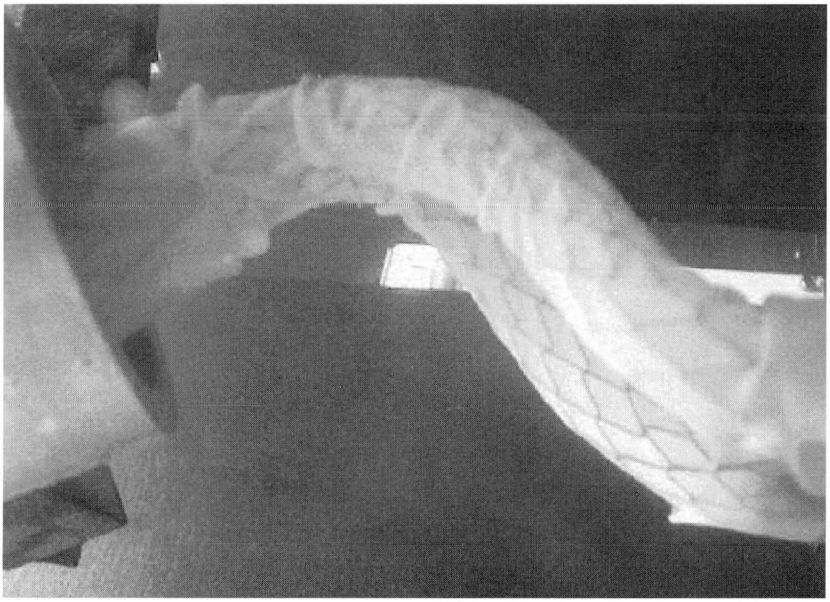

Fig. 3. Illustration showing the apparatus used to simulate pulsatile fluid flow through an endograft with curvature and angulation during bench testing.

Another aspect of the tie breaks issue reveals something about the interaction between physician users and medical device manufacturers of endovascular products being applied clinically in a stage of relatively early development. The observation of the Vanguard device tie breaks was not the first surprising revelation of evidence demonstrating structural change of an aortic endograft. In a trial of another endovascular device, an unexpected finding from routine follow-up X-rays showed that metal fatigue had caused late failure of hooks used to assist in proximal fixation of an aortic endograft manufactured by Endovascular Technologies, Inc. (EVT) (Menlo Park, CA) (Fig. 4).[4,5]

When that problem was identified, a thorough retrospective analysis was conducted to define the extent of structural changes in all available patients who had received the Endovascular Technologies straight endografts; the bifurcation model had yet to be released for use. In the case of the Endovascular Technologies endograft, an actual clinical adverse event characterized by a graft migration occurred and was linked with the radiological finding. The process of putting these observations into appropriate clinical perspective was different from the analysis of the Vanguard tie breaks in two respects: 1) association with real clinical events moves the analysis out of the theoretical realm to concrete estimates of clinical risk; and 2) the failure mode analysis of the Endovascular Technologies device was entirely negative in context. Hook fracture could only be conceived as completely adverse. The Vanguard tie break analysis was more complex since it appeared that a case

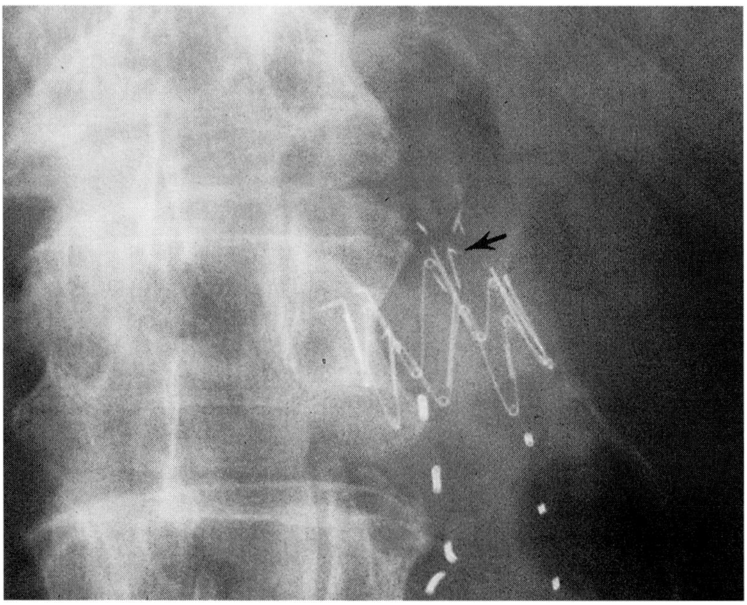

Fig. 4. An angled hook at the proximal stent of the Endovascular Technologies prosthesis can be seen to have separated from the zig-zag main portion of the stent (arrow). This resulted in revision of this aspect of the endograft which has resolved the problem in subsequent use (From Ref. 4, with permission.)

could be made for tie breaks reflecting conformity to changes in aortic morphology in a way that was relieving stress on the prosthesis.

This latter point had significant impact on the dialogue between company engineering and research and development staff and the physician users of the device whose advice was sought. Indeed physician interpretation of the evidence of tie breaks was heavily relied upon *because* there was an absence of observed clinical adverse events. The decision was made, with appropriate communication to physician participants in the US Vanguard trial and regulatory agencies, to continue the investigational study. This illustrates the great importance of physician users having a solid working familiarity with design details of medical devices in clinical investigation.

ENDOPROSTHESIS FABRIC EROSION

In July 1998, a patient previously treated in Europe with a Vanguard device presented with a ruptured aneurysm. The endograft had been implanted, without any recognized difficulty, 8 months prior to rupture for treatment of a 5-cm infrarenal aneurysm. A follow-up CT scan at 3 months showed no evidence of endoleak. A CT scan done at 7 months showed evidence of a small endoleak probably arising from the body of the endograft. Plain films were interpreted as normal in post-procedure appearance, showing stable position of the Vanguard device with only slight angulation. An arteriogram confirmed the presence of endoleak in the mid-graft. While considering therapeutic options, the patient developed symptoms of ruptured aneurysm and was treated by conventional surgery with a clinically successful outcome. Examination of the explanted Vanguard device disclosed a previously unreported finding – the presence of three holes in the endograft fabric component.

As of November 1998, there have been a total of six reported cases, one among the US Vanguard trial cohort, that have been analysed and are considered to represent a similar cause of late endoleak. These cases have been the subject of intensive study accompanied by *in vitro* simulation testing to assist in understanding aspects of the failure that cannot be evaluated from clinical data.

Although prospective data seeking such occurrences have not been previously acquired, these cases represent only six such events among over 3000 Vanguard devices implanted world-wide through October 1998. Some generalizations about these six cases can be made:

1. All patients presented with symptoms; four were thought to represent rupture or contained rupture.
2. Four presented within 1 year of implantation (an observation of possible importance in explaining cause; see below).
3. All patients converted to open repair survived except an 82-year-old woman with known cardiac and renal failure that had previously disqualified her as an elective surgical candidate.
4. Explanted devices were observed to contain multiple holes.
5. These holes are located primarily in the middle portion of the endograft.

6. The portion of the endograft with holes was located within the aneurysm sac.
7. There was no consistent relationship with presence or absence of tie breaks as judged by follow-up imaging and by examination of explants.

A representative case from the US trial is of interest. A 76-year-old female in poor general health with a history of hypertension, cirrhosis, anaemia, diabetes and multiple previous laparotomies presented with an asymptomatic 5.1 cm aneurysm. Treatment in April 1998 by a bifurcation Vanguard device proceeded uneventfully with a total operative time of 115 minutes. An early postoperative CT scan with contrast was consistent with a small branch endoleak (Fig. 5).

Retrospective reanalysis of the early postoperative CT scan shows a small endoleak that was probably due to lumbar branch blood flow. In October 1998, 6 months post-procedure, complaint of abdominal pain led to a CT scan showing evidence of aneurysm expansion to 6 cm, clear evidence of a massive endoleak and appearance of periaortic fluid consistent with rupture (Fig. 6). At operation no frank rupture of the aorta was found. The endograft was explanted and conventional open repair was accomplished with a satisfactory clinical result.

This explanted endograft was studied in detail as have the other specimens returned for evaluation. The findings reveal some definite and important evidence that leads to a partial understanding of the failure mode when combined with data

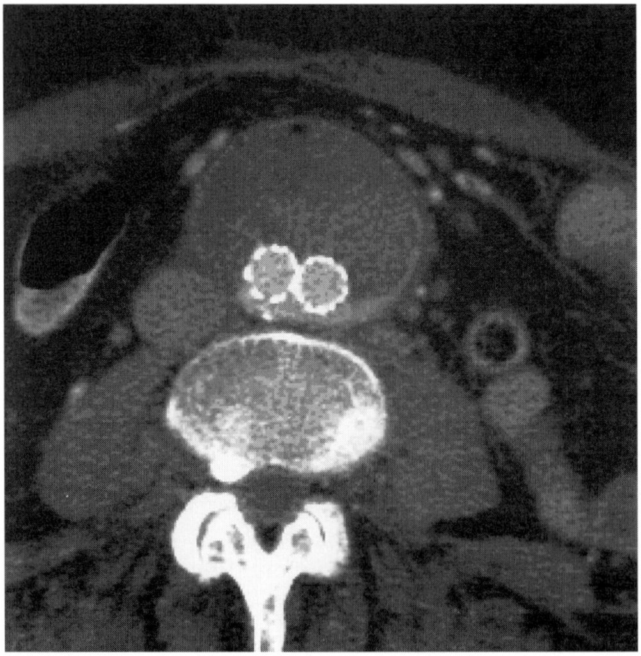

Fig. 5. This CT scan with contrast was obtained 2 days after endograft insertion and shows contrast along the posterior aspect of the aneurysm sac with a slender crescent extending around the left side toward the inferior mesenteric artery origin.

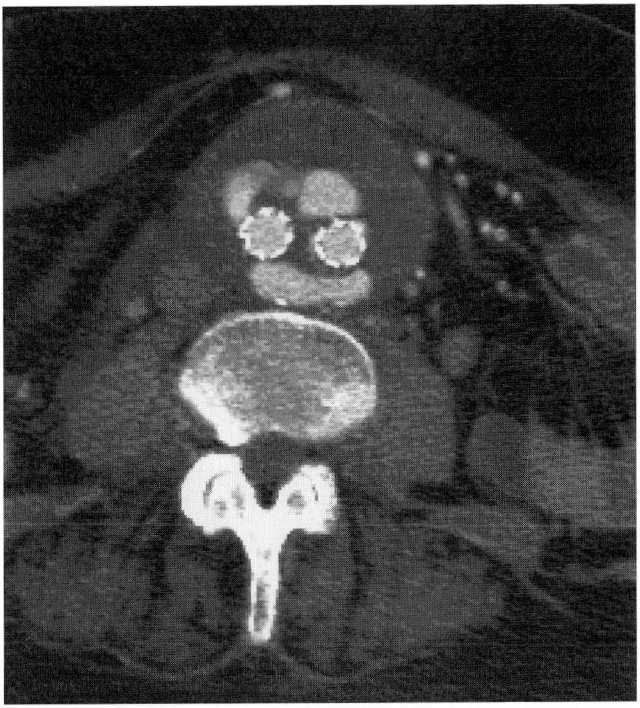

Fig. 6. An obvious major endoleak is readily seen on the CT scan obtained at 6 months follow-up. The appearance suggests the presence of multiple sites of origin but does not prove that this exists.

from *in vitro* testing in provocative models. Together, these data allow for informed but still theoretical consideration of a unifying hypothesis.

Structural changes observed in this case provide a graphic record of physical forces interacting within the endograft *in situ* (Fig. 7). These observations, both clinical and *in vitro*, are internally consistent and seem to provide compelling evidence to explain the observed fabric erosion. Impacting of the apex of a zig-zag stent on the adjacent fabric is an initiator of fabric wear. In the presence of enabling factors, these early changes can progress to extended tearing of the fabric beyond the initial point of the process. Such enabling factors may be conditions that permit or promote relative motion between the fabric and the adjacent stents. The presence of an endoleak might be such a factor because the fabric outside the underlying stents is not constrained by solid thrombus in the aneurysm sac.

However, this does not address two other questions that demand attention: why are the holes observed to be caused by fabric erosion located where they are clustered and why are these few patients different from the majority who are not known to have similar problems so far? Although the reporting of five cases among over 3000 implanted Vanguard devices implies a low prevalence of this problem, the data are not complete or of best quality. There is no prospective analysis to establish an

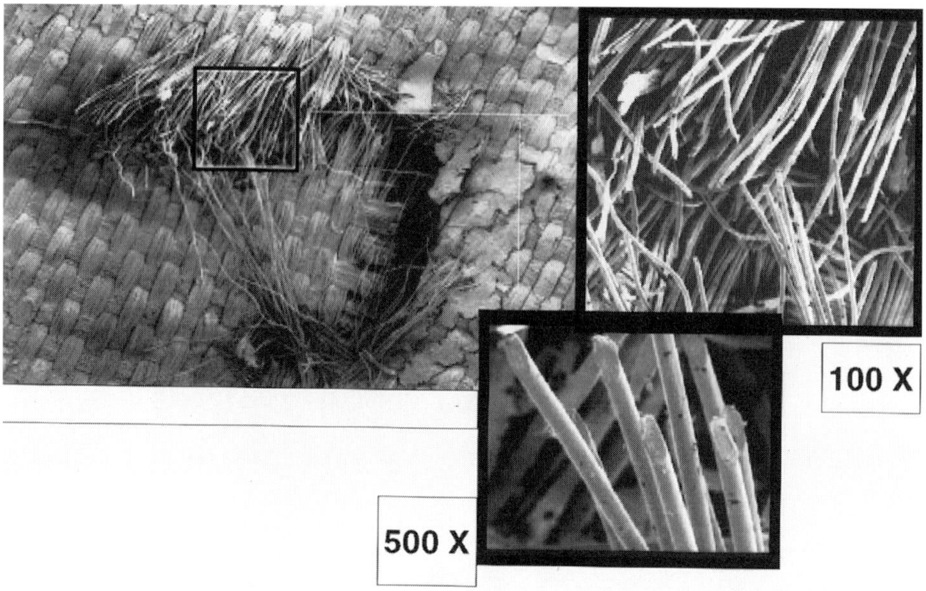

Fig. 7. Photographs at various magnifications of an area of graft fabric erosion. The pattern of the fabric tear follows the shape of the underlying stent.

incidence of fabric erosion that can be relied upon confidently as an estimate of risk. Data are accumulating from the Eurostar registry of endografts.[6] These are not audited data and the level of observation accuracy may vary among reporting centres, but it is clearly more valuable than what is known to date. Probably the best quality data bearing on this issue, though in a smaller patient cohort, will come from analysis of the US Vanguard trial. All follow-up imaging studies are subjected to double reading by an independent core laboratory and all clinical observations are audited and independently reviewed by an adjudication committee. When time allowed for follow-up permits a later assessment, prevalence of the fabric erosion problem should be better known. If this remains a very infrequent problem, it may be regarded as being another cause of late or secondary endoleak and managed as such.

There are a number of late or secondary endoleak causes that have been observed to occur with the use of every type of endograft presently in use. Among them are late fabric failure in the Stentor device associated with its full-length hand-sewn seam, detachment of the contralateral limb inserted into the main, aortic trunk of the prosthesis and migration of the distal iliac end of bifurcation endografts resulting in pulling out of the common iliac artery attachment zone. There may be others yet to be discovered. The point is that secondary endoleak happens because of a variety of causes and requires a variety of solutions to the problem. If graft fabric erosion such as described here proves to be a consistently rare occurrence, is it appropriate to regard this as simply another form of late secondary endoleak or ought it to be regarded similarly to the Endovascular Technologies device hook fracture problem which required a redesign of elements of the prosthesis? The answer to this question involves another consideration – what is the operative risk for the patient?

One of the most appealing features of endograft treatment of aortic aneurysm is the ability to provide treatment of a life-threatening condition for patients who have poor operative risk or who indicate prohibitive operative risk for conventional open repair. If a known late failure risk exists but occurs at a very low rate, it would seem ethically straightforward to construct an argument still favouring endovascular treatment for carefully selected patients. The same may not be true for patients who represent a good or average risk for conventional open surgical repair of aneurysm which has proved effective over the long term and increasingly safe in experienced vascular centres that report average elective mortality rates of less than 3%.

In summary, the early experience in aortic aneurysm exclusion with a modular, fully stent-supported prosthesis, the Vanguard aortic endograft, demonstrates satisfactory early, acute results. However, later observations reveal the need for close and continuing follow-up, prompt response to the occurrence of late endoleak, a thorough knowledge of prosthesis design and construction by clinical endograft users, and an active dialogue between device manufacturers and physicians involved in exploring this new method of treatment for aneurysm.

REFERENCES

1. Beebe HG, Blum U: Experience with the Meadox Vanguard endovascular graft. In: Yao JST, Pearce WH (Eds) *Techniques in Vascular and Endovascular Surgery* pp. 421–432. Stamford, CT: Appleton & Lange, 1998
2. Mialhe C, Amicabile C, Becquemin JP: Endovascular treatment of infrarenal abdominal aneurysms by the Stentor system: Preliminary results of 79 cases. *J Vasc Surg* **26**: 199–209, 1997
3. Blum U, Voshage G, Lammer J *et al.*: Endoluminal stent-grafts for infrarenal abdominal aortic aneurysms. *New Engl J Med* **336**: 13–20, 1997
4. Moore WS: The EVT tube and bifurcated endograft systems: Technical considerations and clinical summary. EVT Investigators. *J Endovasc Surg* **4**: 182–194, 1997
5. Moore WS, Rutherford RB: Transfemoral endovascular repair of abdominal aortic aneurysm: Results of the North American EVT phase 1 trial. EVT Investigators. *J Vasc Surg* **23**: 543–553,1996
6. Harris PL, Buth J, Mialhe C *et al.*: The need for clinical trials of endovascular abdominal aortic aneurysm stent-graft repair: The EUROSTAR Project. EUROpean collaborators on Stent-graft Techniques for abdominal aortic Aneurysm Repair. *J Endovasc Surg* **4**: 72–77, 1997

Commentary

The American experience with Vanguard augments the previous chapter very well. The authors speak of the US Clinical Trial in which patients are allocated to open repair, straight stent graft system or bifurcated system. The allocation is by anatomical criteria and certainly not by random allocation of patients suitable for all methods. Therefore the series are different from the start and any differences can be attributed to the differences between the series, not necessarily through the way in which the aneurysm was managed. Aortas are included with aneurysms greater than

4 cm diameter. The authors are able to report significant experience of stent graft single systems as well as bifurcated systems. Patients operated on for open repair may easily have had more extensive aneurysm not suitable for any form of stent graft repair. The US experience is, however, extremely valuable as an audit procedure and in this chapter, very many lessons are learnt. The authors in both this and the previous chapter speak of the difficulties of the broken ties and the significance of this. It is good that such careful audit in Europe and the USA is taking place. *RMG*

The durability of the EVT® (Endovascular Technologies) stent graft system

Jan D Blankensteijn, Ivo AMJ Broeders, Jan J Wever and Bert C Eikelboom

INTRODUCTION

Endovascular aneurysm repair can be performed effectively, as reported by many centres during the past few years.[1–8] In order to compete with transabdominal aneurysm surgery this new technique must also provide long-term exclusion of the abdominal aneurysm.

A number of systems have been developed to provide a durable fixation of the endograft to the aortic attachment areas. Three principles to keep the endograft in position are used: outward radial forces of the stents, columnar strength of fully stented endografts, and hooks penetrating the aortic wall.

The design principle of the Endovascular Technologies (EVT®) device (Endovascular Technologies, Guidant, Menlo Park) device is to mimic the conventional aortic graft as closely as possible. The EVT endograft consists of a standard woven polyester graft with crimped iliac limbs. Contrary to some other products, no new materials or graft designs have been used and therefore the durability of the EVT endovascular design can be considered exclusively dependent on the attachment systems. After endovascular abdominal aortic aneurysm repair, migration of the entire endoprothesis or one of its components may cause late complications of endovascular abdominal aortic aneurysm repair, such as secondary endoleaks.[9] This may be the consequence of insufficient fixation of the endoprosthesis to the aortic wall or by changing morphology of the abdominal aorta during follow-up. Dilation of the proximal and distal aneurysm necks has already been demonstrated, but a relation to graft migration remains to be proven.[2,8,10]

The attachment systems of the EVT endografts have been designed to create an anastomosis-like fixation using a Gianturco type stent, armed with hooks that penetrate the aortic wall.[11–14] The aim of this study is to investigate the efficacy of this system in preventing endograft migration after endovascular aneurysm repair, in the perspective of morphologic changes of the abdominal aorta during follow-up.

PATIENTS

All patients treated world-wide with a first- or second-generation EVT endograft were candidates for this study; those with a postoperative and at least a 12-month follow-up computed tomographic (CT) scan available for measurements were included (n=125). The median follow-up period was 24 months (range 12–48 months). In all, 61 patients had a follow-up period of 1–2 years; 42 patients a period of 2–3 years; and 22 patients a period of 3–4 years.

A total of 111 patients were male; the median age at the time of operation was 71 years (range 41–87 years). The median aneurysm diameter at the time of the operation was 53 mm (range 35–77 mm). All patients had been enrolled in prospective clinical studies; 101 patients in the phase 1 and 2 USA trials and 24 patients in an international trial. A first-generation EVT endograft had been inserted in 87 patients and a second-generation graft in 38.[13,14] Tube and bifurcated endografts were used in 106 and 19 cases respectively.

METHODS

The same investigator performed all measurements. The immediate postoperative contrast enhanced CT images were used as a reference and the last available follow-up images for comparison.

Investigation of endograft migration: definition of the reference levels and the position of the proximal and distal attachment systems

Registration of the position of the attachment systems was performed by measuring the distance between anatomic and prosthetic landmarks, using the vertical axis as a scale.

The ostium of the left renal artery was used as the reference level for defining the position of the proximal attachment system. When the ostium of the left renal artery was projected on more than one axial CT images, follow-up images were compared with the immediate postoperative CT images with the closest morphologic resemblance. In case the left renal artery could not be identified on the postoperative or the follow-up CT images, the right renal or superior mesenteric artery was used as a reference. The most cephalic CT image showing any parts of the attachment system frame or hooks was used to define the most cephalic position of the proximal attachment system.

The aortic bifurcation was utilized as the reference level for the distal attachment system of the tube endograft. The aortic bifurcation was defined as the first image demonstrating complete separation of the left and right common iliac arteries. The most caudal image showing parts of the frame or hooks was used to mark the most caudal position of the distal attachment system of a tube endograft. A similar method was applied to define the position of the distal attachment systems of a bifurcated endograft; the most cephalic images showing complete separation of the left and right external and hypogastric arteries were used as reference levels.

The distance between the reference levels and the levels of the proximal and distal attachment systems on the postoperative scans was compared with the corresponding measurements on the last follow-up scans.

Investigation of morphologic changes of the abdominal aorta: methodology and definition of the levels of measurement

Size changes of the abdominal aorta were investigated by measuring the aortic cross-sectional area in the axial plane at three levels on the immediate postoperative and last follow-up scans: the suprarenal aorta at 10 mm above the most cephalic renal artery, the proximal aneurysm neck at 10 mm below the most caudal renal artery and the distal aneurysm neck at 10 mm cephalic to the aortic bifurcation (tube endografts only). Assessment of the cross-sectional area was performed by outlining the outer aortic circumference of scanned CT images. Automated computer calibrated cross-sectional area measurements were subsequently obtained using UTHSCSA Image Tool (University of Texas Health Science Center; San Antonio USA).

Length changes of the infrarenal aorta were investigated comparing the distance between the level of the ostium of the left renal artery with the level of the aortic bifurcation, on the immediate postoperative and last follow-up CT images. Only those cases that had comparable images of the postoperative and follow-up CT scans available for measurement were included. Changes in the suprarenal aorta and proximal aneurysm neck were investigated in 80 and 111 patients respectively. Changes in the distal neck in tube graft cases were determined in 86 patients. Changes in length could be studied in all cases.

Definition of measurement accuracy

Each axial CT slice represents a volume of the scanned subject, projected in a two-dimensional plane perpendicular to the body axis. The anatomic and prosthetic landmarks may be positioned anywhere along this axis of this slice volume. Therefore, the inaccuracy of the investigation of both endograft migration and length changes is determined by the slice thickness of the postoperative and follow-up CT images. A maximum slice thickness of 2–3 mm was encountered in 35 patients; a maximum thickness of 4–5 mm in 37 and of 6–10 mm in 53. Migration was defined as a change between the level of anatomic landmark and the level of the attachment system, exceeding the maximal slice thickness.

A change in distance between the renal artery and the aortic bifurcation exceeding the maximal slice thickness of both the postoperative and the follow-up images was interpreted as lengthening or shortening; length changes within the maximum slice thickness were regarded as 'no change'. The intra-observer variability of cross-sectional area registration was based on randomly repeated measurements of 30 axial images, using the method described by Bland and Altman.[15] The 95% confidence interval for cross-sectional area assessment – defined as 1.96 SD and expressed in percentiles – was ± 9%. Changes between the postoperative and follow-up images smaller than 9% of the postoperative cross-sectional area were regarded as non-significant and defined as 'no change'. An increase of 9% or more was regarded as neck dilation, a decrease of 9% or more as shrinkage. Any tendency of size changes of the abdominal aorta based on the described length and cross-sectional area measurements were tested for statistical significance using the Wilcoxon rank test.

RESULTS

Endograft migration

Migration of the endograft attachment systems was found in four of 125 patients (3.2%; Table 1). Downward migration of the proximal attachment system was encountered in one of 125 cases (0.8%). The proximal attachment system of this first-generation endograft was deployed 20 mm caudal to the renal arteries, in a long proximal aneurysm neck. Multiple stent fractures were presumed to be the cause of migration and considered an indication to convert the patient to transabdominal aneurysm repair.

Upward migration of the distal attachment system of a tube endograft was found in three of 106 patients (2.8%). In two of these three cases, the distal attachment system was positioned at 8–10 mm proximal to the aortic bifurcation in a wide distal aneurysm neck (both 500 mm^2, maximal diameter 27 mm and 29 mm respectively). Inaccurate positioning during deployment of the distal stent appeared to be the cause of migration in these two cases. A third case was associated with a persistent distal endoleak.

The design of the EVT attachment systems was thoroughly revised after detection of hook breaks. Neither endograft migration nor attachment system breaks were encountered in patients with second-generation endografts (n=38).

Table 1. Description of cases demonstrating migration of the endograft

Case	*Diagnosis (months po)*	*Generation device*	*Attachment system*	*Migration (mm)*	*Probable cause*	*Outcome*
A	24	First	Distal	13	Incorrect deployment, late endoleak	Conversion 24 months po
B	24	First	Distal	16	Persistent endoleak	Conversion 24 months po
C	15	First	Distal	20	Incorrect deployment, late endoleak	Conversion 25 months po
D	15	First	Proximal	11	Multiple hook breaks	Conversion 17 months po

po: postoperatively.

Changes in aortic cross-sectional area

No significant changes in aortic cross-sectional area were found in the suprarenal aorta (z=0.32, p=0.8; Table 2).

A significant median yearly increase in cross-sectional area of 4.1% (–19 to 47%) was demonstrated in the proximal aneurysm neck (z=4.3, p<0.001; table 3). Aortic dilation at this level was found in 49 of 111 patients (44%, Table 3). Dilation of the proximal aneurysm neck was not demonstrated in the patient with migration of the proximal attachment system.

In patients with a tube endograft, a significant median yearly increase in cross-sectional area of 5.3% (–22 to 62%) was found in the distal aneurysm neck (z=4.2, p<0.001; Table 2). An increase in size was demonstrated in 41 of 86 cases (48%, Table 3). Significant distal neck dilation was also found in the patient with persistent distal endoleak.

Table 2. Changes in cross-sectional area (CA) during follow-up

Level of measurements	*Postoperative CA*	*Final CA*	*Change in absolute values*	*Change in % yearly*
Suprarenal aorta	458 (290–762)	462 (286–780)	0 (–187 to 157)	–0.7% (–18 to 36%)^{NS}
Proximal aneurysm neck	456 (200–689)	475 (242–677)	37 (–208 to 158)	4.1% (–19 to 47%)***
Distal aneurysm neck	394 (186–1428)	425 (235–1199)	27 (–502 to 334)	5.3% (–22 to 62%)***

(Cross-sectional areas are presented in mm^2 and expressed as a median value (range) (*** $p<0.001$; NS: not significant)

Table 3. Changes of cross-sectional areas during follow-up

Level of measurements	*Decrease*	*No change*	*Increase*
Suprarenal aorta (n=80)	17	46	17
Proximal aneurysm neck (n=111)	14	48	49
Distal aneurysm neck (n=86)	12	33	41

All follow-up measurements found within ± 9% of the postoperative measurements were defined as 'no change'

Length changes of the infrarenal aorta during follow-up

The median length of the infrarenal aorta – defined as the difference between the renal arteries and the aortic bifurcation – was 11.8 cm (8.9–15.9 cm) after operation and 11.8 cm (9.0–16.0 cm) at the last follow-up examination. The median change in length during follow-up was 0 cm (range –1.3 to 2.1 cm). Lengthening was seen in 17 of 125 patients (14%, median increase 0.8 cm (0.3–2.1 cm)). Shortening was found in 11 of 125 cases (9%; median decrease 0.9 cm (0.6–1.3 cm)). No significant changes in length were found in 97 of 125 cases (77%). Length changes of more than 1 cm were encountered in 8 of 125 patients (6%; lengthening four, shortening four). Migration of the endograft was not encountered in any of these patients.

DISCUSSION

Acceptable perioperative morbidity and low operative mortality after endovascular abdominal aortic aneurysm repair have been reported.[1–8,10,11,16,17] With growing experience, device- and technique-related complications are encountered necessitating reevaluation of patient selection and endograft design.[8,14,16,18] One critical issue is the prevention of endograft migration. The design of the endografts used in this study appeared effective in this respect. During follow-up, 97% of the endografts retained their initial position. Three of four cases of endograft migration concerned the distal attachment system in grafts of tubular design. No migration was demonstrated in endografts of bifurcated design. However, bifurcated grafts were not available during the first 2 years of EVT endograft trials. Currently, no more than 10% of all candidates for endovascular abdominal aortic aneurysm repair appear suitable for a tube endograft.

In case a suitable distal neck is present, accurate positioning of the distal stent is challenging because the endograft delivery system is hard to position in line with the aortic axis. This is caused by the marked angle between the common iliac artery and the aortic axis. Malalignment may result in endograft deployment at some distance from the aortic bifurcation, losing a few millimeters of indispensable distal attachment area. This technique-related problem was encountered in two of three cases of distal migration in this study. May *et al.*[19] reported on mid-term results using various types of endografts. In their experience, results of tube endografts were poor compared with endografts of bifurcated or monoiliac design. Treatment of suitable candidates with a large diameter or diseased distal aortic cuff should therefore preferably be performed by endograft extending into the iliac arteries.

All currently available systems use stents to hold the endograft in its desired position.[13,20–25] Circumferential arterial fixation relies on the friction forces between stent and wall. As the stents are usually oversized by a few millimeters compared with the aortic diameter, both self-expanding stents and balloon expandable stents generate an inward force of the radially stretched artery. In self-expanding stents the inward force is counteracted by the outward radial force of the stent and in balloon expandable stent by its so-called hoop strength. In both situations there is equilibrium of inward and outward forces. The potential harmful effects of outward forces are a matter of debate. Dilation of proximal and distal aneurysm necks in the years following endovascular repair has been reported.[2,8,10]

The average diameter of the infrarenal aorta increases by a few millimeters during a lifetime.[26] A much higher rate has been found after aneurysm repair by both endovascular and transabdominal methods.

Matsumura *et al.*[2] and Broeders *et al.*[8] independently reported on a non-significant dilation of the proximal aneurysm neck of 0.3–0.6 mm per year after endovascular aneurysm repair, while a significant increase in median diameter of the distal aneurysm neck of 0.9–1.2 mm was found. Malina *et al.*[10] found a median increase of 2 mm at the level of the proximal neck 12 months. These findings are confirmed by the results of this study.

Exact data on the impact of self-expanding stents on aortic neck dilatation are not yet available. Progression of aneurysmal disease might be another factor contributing to neck dilatation during follow-up. A dilated proximal or distal neck is generally considered an exclusion criterion for endovascular aneurysm repair. Nevertheless, pathologic changes of the arterial wall may be present before dilatation, as experienced in open aneurysm repair. Illig *et al.*[27] found a mean increase of the proximal aortic cuff of 0.6 mm per year in a group of 33 patients who underwent transabdominal aneurysm repair. Significant dilatation was found in 55% of these patients, with the amount of dilatation depending on the neck size at the time of operation. Neck dilatation experienced during follow-up may therefore be explained partly by progression of arterial disease in patients with aortic aneurysm.

The radial forces exerted to the arterial wall and thereby the friction forces between stent and wall will decrease when the inner arterial circumference approaches the nominal stent circumference. Theoretically, endografts not fixed by other means may be prone to dislodgment and migration in case of continuing aortic neck dilation. Long-term observation of attachment areas of endografts is required to evaluate the durability of endograft fixation.

Additional protection against graft migration is claimed by stenting the full length of the endograft trunk and limbs.[28] This provides columnar strength that will help the endograft to resist the downward forces of a pulsatile blood flow. This may indeed reinforce the vascular prosthesis. However, it limits the capacity of an endograft to adapt to changes in length of the aorta and iliac arteries during follow-up. Although upward migration of fully stented devices due to shortening of the aneurysm after exclusion is an uncommon problem, disintegration of fully stented modular systems has been associated with changing morphology of the excluded segment of the aorta and iliac arteries.[18]

A tendency towards shortening or lengthening of the infrarenal aorta after endovascular repair could not be demonstrated in this study. However, it should be noted that changes in length were measured along the vertical body axis, while changes in aortoiliac anatomy in aneurysmal disease occur in a multiplanar orientation. Investigation of endograft position in relation to morphologic changes of the excluded arterial segment should therefore preferably be performed by more sophisticated measurement techniques, such as analysis of central lumen lines and three-dimensional reconstructions.[29–31]

Length changes of more than 1 cm were found in eight patients (6.5%) included in this study. Graft migration was encountered in none of these cases, suggesting adequate adaptation of the non-stented endograft body. In conclusion, fixation of endografts by hooks embedded in the arterial wall provides a durable protection against migration at mid- to long-term follow-up. Although proximal and distal aneurysm necks dilate after endovascular aneurysm repair, this did not induce endograft migration in this study. Likewise, changes in the length of the infrarenal aorta were not related to displacement of the endograft.

REFERENCES

1. Blum U, Voshage G, Lammer J, Beyersdorf F, Tollner D, Kretschmer G *et al.*: Endoluminal stent-grafts for infrarenal abdominal aortic aneurysms. *New Engl J Med* **336**: 13–20, 1997
2. Matsumura JS, Pearce WH, McCarthy WJ, Yao JS: Reduction in aortic aneurysm size: early results after endovascular graft placement. EVT Investigators. *J Vasc Surg* **25**: 113–123, 1997
3. Blum U, Voshage G, Beyersdorf F *et al.*: Two-center German experience with aortic endografting. *J Endovasc Surg* **4**: 137–146, 1997
4. May J, White GH, Yu W *et al.*: Repair of abdominal aortic aneurysms by the endoluminal method: outcome in the first 100 patients. *Med J Aust* **165**: 549–551, 1996
5. Yusuf SW, Whitaker SC, Chuter *et al.*: Early results of endovascular aortic aneurysm surgery with aortouniiliac graft, contralateral iliac occlusion, and femorofemoral bypass. *J Vasc Surg* **25**: 165–172, 1997
6. Dyet JF: Pictorial review: endovascular repair of abdominal aortic aneurysms. *Br J Radiol* **69**: 1069–1074, 1996
7. Moore WS, Rutherford RB: Transfemoral endovascular repair of abdominal aortic

aneurysm: results of the North American EVT phase 1 trial. EVT Investigators. *J Vasc Surg* **23**: 543–553, 1996
8. Broeders IA, Blankensteijn JD, Gvakharia A *et al.*: The efficacy of transfemoral endovascular aneurysm management: a study on size changes of the abdominal aorta during mid-term follow-up. *Eur J Vasc Endovasc Surg* **14**: 84–90, 1997
9. White GH, Yu W, May J *et al.*: Endoleak as a complication of endoluminal grafting of abdominal aortic aneurysms: classification, incidence, diagnosis, and management. *J Endovasc Surg* **4**: 152–168, 1997
10. Malina M, Ivancev K, Chuter TA *et al.*: Changing aneurysmal morphology after endovascular grafting: relation to leakage or persistent perfusion. *J Endovasc Surg* **4**: 23–30, 1997
11. Colburn MD, Moore WS: Endovascular repair of abdominal aortic aneurysms using the EGS tube and bifurcated graft systems. *World J Surg* **20**: 664–672, 1996
12. May J, White GH, Yu W *et al.*: Early experience with the Sydney and EVT prostheses for endoluminal treatment of abdominal aortic aneurysms. *J Endovasc Surg* **2**: 240–247, 1995
13. Moore WS: The EVT tube and bifurcated endograft systems: technical considerations and clinical summary. EVT Investigators. *J Endovasc Surg* **4**: 182–194, 1997
14. Broeders IAMJ, Blankensteijn JD, Eikelboom BC: The EndoVascular Technologies System. In: Hopkinson B, Yusuf W, Whitaker S, Veith F (Eds) *Endovascular Surgery for Aortic Aneurysms* pp. 105–122. London: WB Saunders Co., 1997
15. Bland JM, Altman DG: Statistical methods for assessing agreement between two methods of clinical measurement. *Lancet* **i**: 307–310, 1986
16. Parodi JC, Barone A, Piraino R, Schonholz C: Endovascular treatment of abdominal aortic aneurysms: lessons learned. *J Endovasc Surg* **4**: 102–110, 1997
17. White GH, Yu W, May J *et al.*: Three-year experience with the White-Yu Endovascular GAD Graft for transluminal repair of aortic and iliac aneurysms. *J Endovasc Surg* **4**: 124–136, 1997
18. Stelter W, Umscheid T, Ziegler P: Three-year experience with modular stent-graft devices for endovascular AAA treatment. Abstract *Endovascular Symposium Sydney*; December 1997.
19. May J, White GH, Yu W *et al.*: Importance of graft configuration in outcome of endoluminal abdominal aortic aneurysm repair. *ESVS 11th Annual Meeting Abstract Book* Abstract, **11**: 62–63, 1997
20. Lawrence-Brown MM, Hartley D, MacSweeney ST *et al.*: The Perth endoluminal bifurcated graft system – development and early experience. *Cardiovasc Surg* **4**: 706–712, 1996
21. Chuter TA, Risberg B, Hopkinson BR *et al.*: Clinical experience with a bifurcated endovascular graft for abdominal aortic aneurysm repair. *J Vasc Surg* **24**: 655–666, 1996
22. May J, White GH, Yu W *et al.*: Endoluminal repair of abdominal aortic aneurysms: strengths and weaknesses of various prostheses observed in a 4.5-year experience. *J Endovasc Surg* **4**: 147–151, 1997
23. Ivancev K, Malina M, Lindblad B *et al.*: Abdominal aortic aneurysms: experience with the Ivancev–Malmo endovascular system for aortomonoiliac stent-grafts. *J Endovasc Surg* **4**: 242–251, 1997
24. Wilson GJ, Klement P, Kato YP *et al.*: A self-expanding bifurcated endovascular graft for abdominal aortic aneurysm repair. An initial study in a canine model. *ASAIO J* **42**: 386–393, 1996
25. Mialhe C, Amicabile C, Becquemin JP: Endovascular treatment of infrarenal abdominal aneurysms by the Stentor system: preliminary results of 79 cases. Stentor Retrospective Study Group. *J Vasc Surg* **26**: 199–209, 1997
26. Ouriel K, Green RM, Donayre C: An evaluation of new methods of expressing aortic aneurysm size: relation to rupture. *J Vasc Surg* **15**: 12, 1992
27. Illig KA, Green RM, Ouriel K *et al.*: Fate of the proximal aortic cuff: implications for endovascular aneurysm repair. *J Vasc Surg* **26**: 492–499, 1997
28. Allen RC, White RA, Zarins CK, Fogarty TJ: What are the characteristics of the ideal endovascular graft for abdominal aortic aneurysm exclusion? *J Endovasc Surg* **4**: 195–202, 1997
29. Broeders IA, Blankensteijn JD, Olree M *et al.*: Preoperative sizing of grafts for transfemoral

endovascular aneurysm management: a prospective comparative study of spiral CT angiography, arteriography, and conventional CT imaging. *J Endovasc Surg* **4**: 252–261, 1997
30. Balm R, Stokking R, Kaatee R *et al.*: Computed tomographic angiographic imaging of abdominal aortic aneurysms: implications for transfemoral endovascular aneurysm management. *J Vasc Surg* **26**: 231–237, 1997
31. Balm R, Kaatee R, Blankensteijn JD *et al.*: CT-angiography of abdominal aortic aneurysms after transfemoral endovascular aneurysm management. *Eur J Vasc Endovasc Surg* **12**: 182–188, 1996

Commentary

This chapter comments that the Endovascular Technologies (EVT) device durability depends 'exclusively on the attachment system'. The authors comment on the migration of the endograft in four of 125 cases. They describe migration upwards and comment on the change of the aortic shape after implantation. Because of this phenomenon, the endovascular device has to stand buckling and considerable changes of shape and only time will tell how the device will cope with these changes.
RMG

The Talent® abdominal aortic aneurysm stent graft: technical approaches and results of aneurysm exclusion

Frank J Criado, Omran Abul-Khoudoud, Eric Wellons, Timothy Mims and Marcos Sanchez

INTRODUCTION

The Talent® stent graft (World Medical Manufacturing Corporation, Sunrise, Florida) is a modular design, self-expandable endoprosthesis that was developed for endoluminal treatment of aortic aneurysms (Fig. 1). It is made of a series of serpentine nitinol stents, spaced discontinuously along a full-length spine that provides longitudinal stability (Fig. 2); the metal stents are completely embedded into the woven

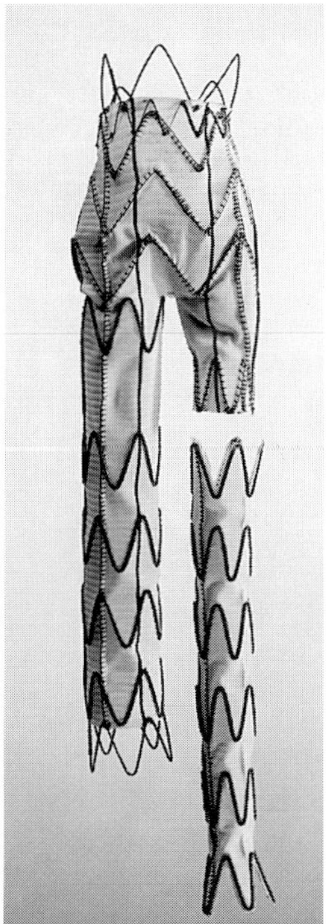

Fig. 1. Talent abdominal aortic aneurysm stent graft system.

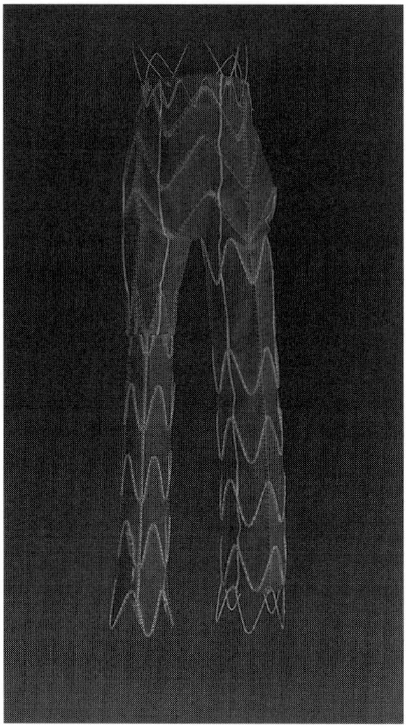

Fig. 2. Photonegative of device. Note serpentine stents spaced discontinuously, and longitudinal nitinol spine.

Table 1. Talent abdominal aortic aneurysm stent graft system

Aortic graft size	*Delivery system size*
20 mm	22F
22-30 mm	24F
32-36 mm	25F
> 36 mm (thoracic)	27F

Dacron fabric. The delivery system is a coaxial sheath with push rod and a compliant built-in polyurethane balloon that is used to optimize attachment to the inner surface of the aortic wall and to ensure complete expansion of the Dacron fabric throughout the length of the stent-graft system. The size profile of the delivery system containing the main section of the device ranges from 22F to 27F outer diameter (OD) (Table 1). A more recent technological development has been the creation of a thinner Dacron fabric (Talent Low-Profile System, LPS) that has resulted in a very significant reduction of delivery sheath OD by 2–4F sizes (Table 2).

Table 2. Talent low-profile system

Graft size	*Delivery system size*
Abdominal aortic aneurysm	
18–20 mm	20F
22–30 mm	22F
32–36 mm	24F
Thoracic	
28–36 mm	22F
38–46 mm	24F

Unique features of the Talent abdominal aortic aneurysm system include the proximal 15 mm-tall bare spring (Fig. 3), and manufacturer's customization to fit a wide range of sizes and morphologic configurations as determined preoperatively by computed tomography (CT) imaging and angiography.

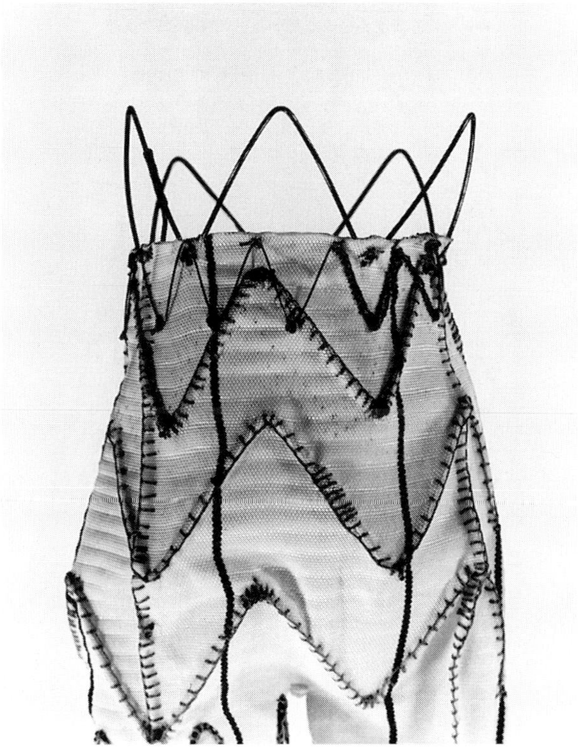

Fig. 3. Uncovered bare nitinol spring designed for aortic wall fixation across renal artery origins.

IMPLANT PLANNING AND DEVICE CUSTOMIZATION

The importance of precise preoperative measurements and morphologic characterization cannot be overemphasized. We continue to prefer the use of both spiral CT imaging and contrast angiography in most patients. On occasion, particularly with patients who have significant renal dysfunction, CT imaging (with three-dimensional reconstruction) is used as the sole modality of anatomical evaluation and sizing. Figure 4 describes the basic diagram used by World Medical engineers to plan the implant strategy and device customization for a given case. The lead implant surgeon (or interventionist) has an opportunity to participate in this process and to suggest modifications or special features that may be of importance in certain situations. The wide range of available diameters and configurations (Table 3) is of great practical use when fitting the patient's individual anatomy and special requirements. Aortic cuffs (proximal) and iliac (distal) extensions are always

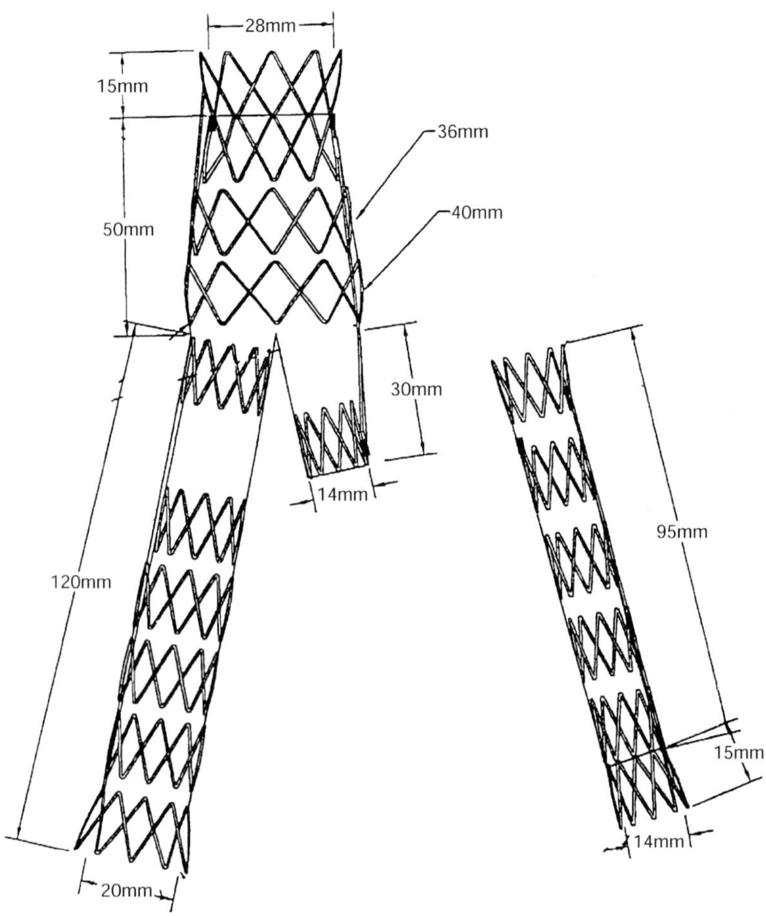

Fig. 4. Basic diagram for device planning and customization.

Table 3. Talent abdominal aortic aneurysm stent graft system

Size availability for customization	
Main section (usable on 14–34 mm aortas)	
Proximal neck diameter	16–36 mm
Length	5–12 cm
Iliac extensions (usable on 8–20 mm vessels)	
Diameter	8–22 mm
Length	7–13 cm

available in order to seal potential endoleaks and optimize the endoluminal exclusion procedure at the time of initial intervention. One additional option involves the use of a non-standard design whereby the aortic section and ipsilateral limb are made very short in order to have the flexibility to adjust distal length as needed (Fig. 5); this

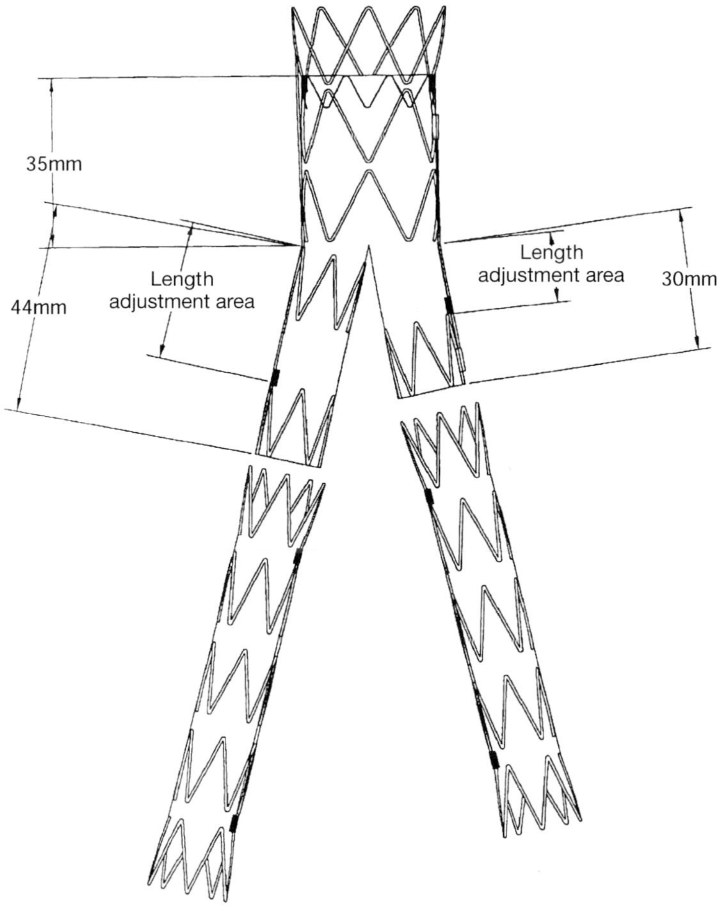

Fig. 5. Talent double short leg system. Modified design for greater flexibility to adjust length of iliac limbs.

has been found to be a practically useful option in situations precluding complete preoperative evaluation – i.e. ruptured aneurysms. Proximal neck assessment (length and diameter) only is required; distal landing and sealing can always be adjusted by adding iliac extension grafts as determined by retrograde reflux angiographic imaging (following deployment of the aortic section).

The implant procedure is of course guided by fluoroscopy and contrast angiography. We have used intravascular ultrasound imaging and found it useful, but do not view it as an obligatory adjunct in every case.

BRIEF TECHNICAL DESCRIPTION

A complete description of the implantation techniques and all available options would be well beyond the scope of this chapter. However, it is appropriate to include a brief account of commonly used technical approaches in order to enhance understanding of the capabilities of the Talent stent graft system to achieve success with exclusion of aortic aneurysms. These techniques have evolved over the past 1½ years in the authors' personal experience with over 65 abdominal aortic aneurysms implants. Naturally, the opinion and advice of many investigators worldwide (2500 plus implants) and of World Medical's engineering/technical team have also had significant influence.

1. The intervention commences (in our practice) with percutaneous catheterization of the left brachial artery and placement of a 5F introducer sheath. The brachial artery catheter has been found to be exceedingly safe and very helpful in several steps of the procedure including pre-deployment aortography, simple antegrade antegrade wire crossing of the short contralateral leg, and brachial–femoral 'body-flossing' to overcome tortuous iliac arteries. It also allows quick 'puff' angio injections during precise juxtarenal placement when the neck is very short, and completion angiography for final control.
2. The bilateral common femoral arteries are exposed surgically (by vertical groin incisions) from the inguinal ligament to the femoral bifurcation.
3. Systemic anticoagulation is induced with intravenous heparin to achieve an activated clotting time (ACT) of 300 seconds or higher. It is maintained at this level throughout the implant procedure by monitoring ACT every 15 minutes, with additional amounts of heparin being given as necessary.
4. A superstiff Amplatz 0.035 guidewire, 260 cm in length, is inserted transfemorally utilizing exchange technique. It is advanced to the top of the aortic arch, where it is maintained until deployment has been completed. It is useful to have visual control of the wire position at all times by relating it to an external reference point on the table (Fig. 6). This latter manoeuvre is extremely useful as control of the leading point of the wire is not practically achievable during the aortic implant procedure, leading potentially to inadvertent advancement into one of the branches of the aortic arch or heart chambers causing potentially serious complications.
5. The delivery sheath, containing the main section of the device, is advanced retrograde over the wire to the level of the renal arteries. A transverse femoral arteriotomy is used for endovascular introduction of the sheath.

6. Transluminal iliac access difficulties are a common source of complications or technical failure in a number of cases. One technique that we have found extremely useful for challenging iliac-anatomy situations, or even to negotiate angulated aortas, involves use of a goose-neck nitinol snare device (Microvena) that is introduced through a 6F left brachial artery sheath to capture and hold the transfemoral wire in the lumen of the thoracic aorta (Fig. 7). As the wire is held from the top, continuous downward pull will create a very firm and stable 'railroad' that enables introduction of the delivery sheath through tortuous and

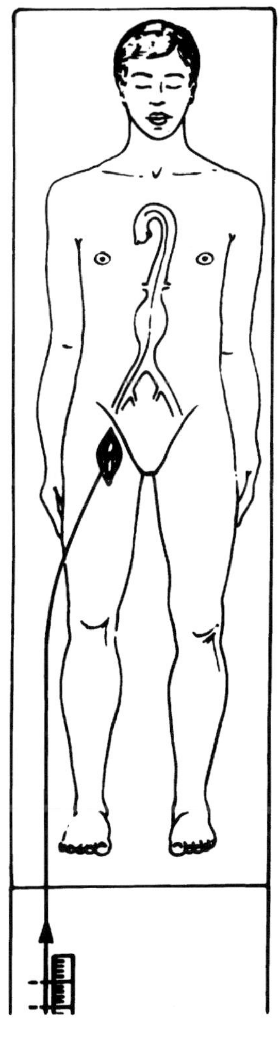

Fig. 6. Femoral guidewire is maintained at desired location by external control using a reference point as illustrated. This is particularly useful during difficult advancement of delivery sheath to the aorta.

kinked arteries. As with the 'body flossing technique' with a through-and-through brachial femoral guidewire (Fig. 7), these manoeuvres risk injury to the subclavian artery and aortic arch from a 'cheese-cutting' effect; a 5 or 6F catheter over the wire – as with the snare device where the 6F catheter is part of the kit – must be used to prevent such potentially catastrophic complications.

7. Contrast angiography of the abdominal aorta is now obtained with the aid of a power injector, utilizing the 5F pigtail catheter introduced from the left brachial sheath. The image intensifier of the X-ray machine is centred on L1-L2 in order to minimize parallax by having the juxtarenal aortic segment and renal arteries in the centre of the fluoroscopic field.
8. Deployment of the device is effected by gradually withdrawing the outer sheath as the pusher rod is held frozen in place. We recommend strongly that deployment begins above the level of the renal arteries, with expansion of the first two stents. The entire device is then brought down as a unit, and repositioned to the desired level, having the uppermost border of the Dacron fabric positioned immediately below the origin of the lowermost renal artery (Fig. 8). 'Ideal placement' consists of transrenal fixation of the bare spring, that often reaches near the origin of the superior mesenteric artery. When in doubt about possible coverage of one or both renal arteries by the Dacron fabric, a 'puff aortogram' can easily and quickly provide clues as to whether the device should be pulled down further to a lower level. Transrenal fixation may not be strictly necessary when a long proximal neck is present; even in these situations, however, we insist on juxtarenal placement of the Dacron fabric, and transrenal fixation and attachment of the proximal bare spring.
9. Deployment of the aortic segment/ipsilateral limb is completed by withdrawing the sheath all the way down.
10. The polyurethane balloon is used, meticulously and sequentially, to expand the stent graft throughout its length.
11. Assessment of adequacy of sealing and level of landing of the iliac limb can be quickly achieved by limited reflux retrograde angiogram performed through a 7F introducer sheath that is placed from the ipsilateral femoral artery over the wire (Fig. 9). Inadequacies in iliac limb landing may be addressed immediately by further balloon dilatation, or the addition of an iliac extension graft.
12. Guidewire access across the short contralateral leg is easily and quickly achieved from the top by passing a 260 cm long 0.035 Wholey (or similar) steerable guidewire through the left brachial catheter. The wire is advanced antegrade into the aneurysm and then out the iliac artery, and down to the exposed femoral artery where it is extracted through a transverse arteriotomy. Alternative techniques for gaining wire access to the contralateral leg exist (retrograde, cross-over) but none is as simple or fast as the top-down antegrade approach.
13. Following appropriate exchange for a superstiff Amplatz guidewire, the contralateral limb is deployed in standard manner, ensuring proper overlap in order to achieve a good haemostatic seal at the junction (Fig. 10).
14. A final contrast aortogram is obtained to document proper positioning of the entire device, and the absence of a significant endoleak. If an endoleak is identified, it can be addressed by further balloon expansion of the implanted endograft, and/or the addition of a proximal aortic cuff or distal iliac extension.

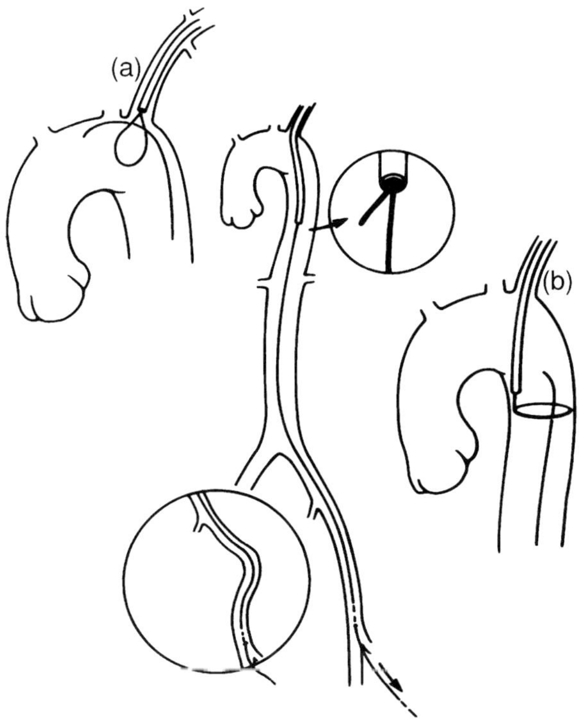

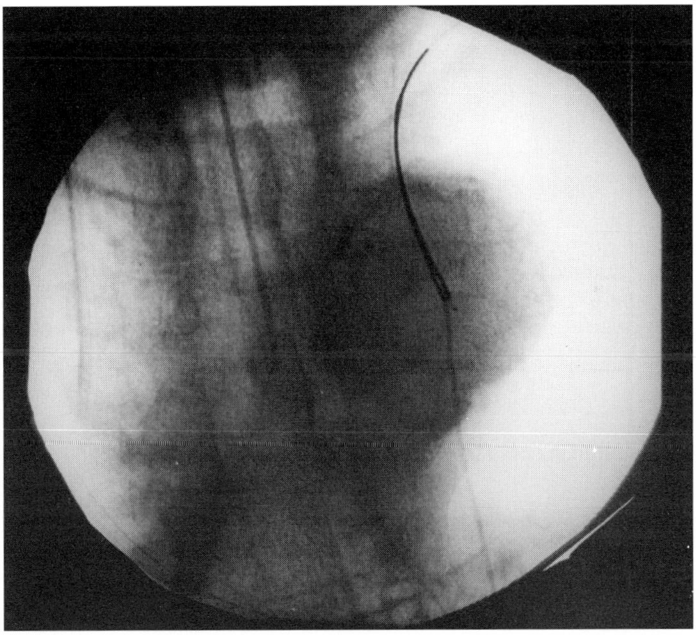

(c)

Fig. 7. Description of brachial snare technique to stabilize and tense transfemoral wire. This can be achieved in one of two ways: (a) advancing the wire through the snare loop formed in the lumen of the distal portion of the arch, right off the origin of the subclavian artery; or (b) with a larger snare loop (35 mm) positioned in the upper descending thoracic aorta. Recent clinical example of brachial snare technique (c).

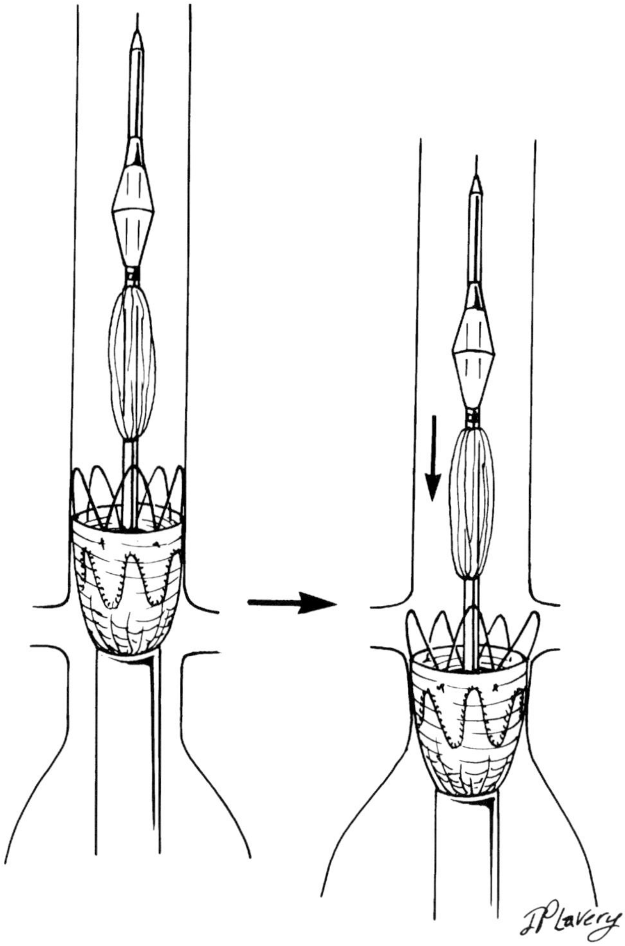

Fig. 8. Deployment of Talent device begins above the renal arteries by expansion of first two stent segments. Reposition down to desired location enables precise juxtarenal placement.

ADDITIONAL TECHNIQUES AND TROUBLESHOOTING

The two most common challenges are related to morphology and length of the proximal aortic neck; and iliac artery access difficulties related to anatomy and/or disease.

Morphology and length of the proximal aortic neck

Minimum requirement of a 1 cm length of the proximal neck is generally regarded as sound and realistic for most Talent implants. However, we have personally achieved

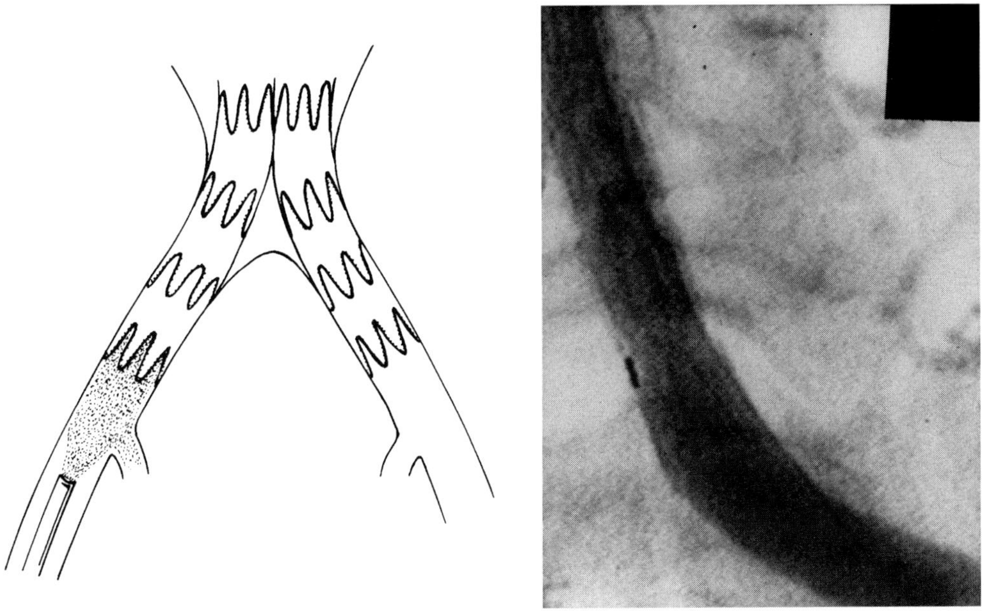

(a) (b)

Fig. 9. Reflux iliac angiogram confirms adequacy of distal limb placement and seal (a,b).

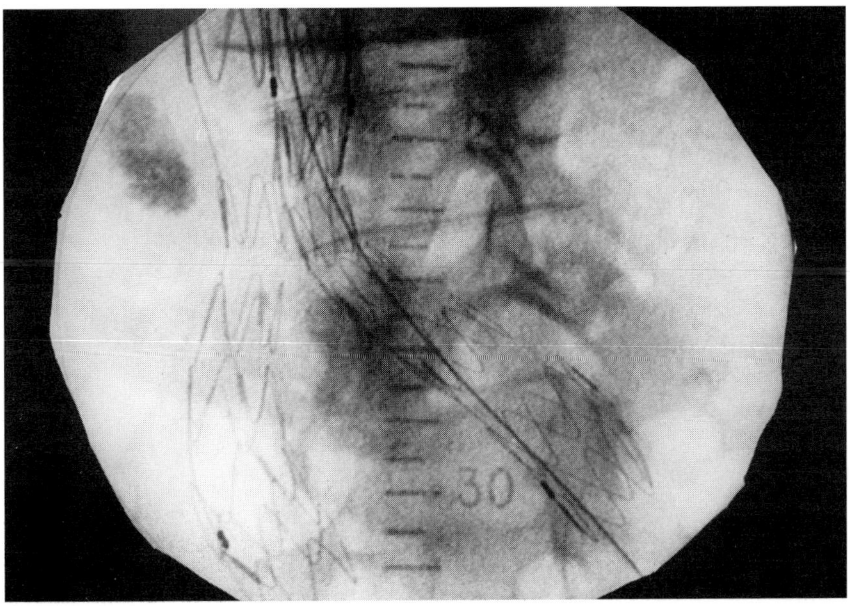

Fig. 10. Completed bifurcated stent graft. Note design customization to accommodate large iliac limbs through a narrow aortic bifurcation.

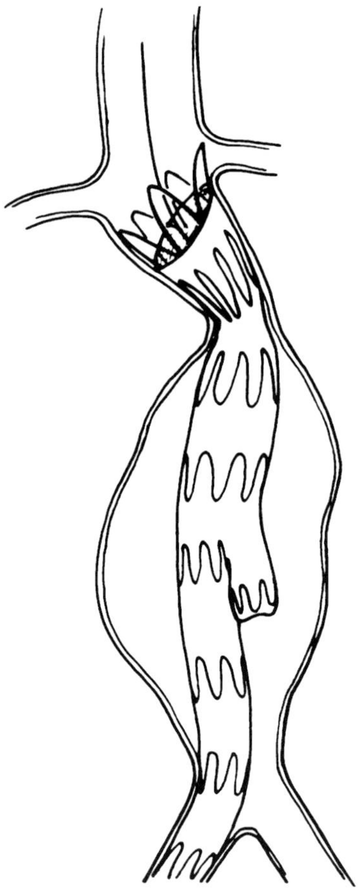

Fig. 11. Proximal end of the device may tilt significantly in the face of marked angulation, especially when the neck is short. The potential for endoleak is obvious.

success with abdominal aortic aneurysms exclusion on patients with upper necks of 0.5–0.8 cm in length. Complex morphology, especially when involving significant angulation, may constitute insurmountable impediments to successful endovascular exclusion (Fig. 11). As with other endograft devices, heavy circumferential calcification, and a thick layer of laminated thrombus at the neck on CT imaging constitute former contraindications to the procedure.

Iliac artery access difficulties

Troubleshooting for iliac artery access difficulties has been described (at least in part) with use of the transbrachial snare-device technique. Focal stenoses require preliminary balloon dilatation prior to passage of the delivery sheath. It is also important to know that small, non-diseased iliac arteries, can be dilated significantly with graduated dilators (Coon dilators) or even by means of balloon angioplasty techniques, permitting the passage of a delivery sheath with an outer diameter that may be larger than the preoperatively measured internal diameter of the artery. Extreme caution must be exercised, however, in order to avoid extensive dissection of the iliac arteries and prevent catastrophic rupture during forced introduction and delivery of the endograft: *do NOT forcibly dilate diseased, calcified arteries.*

Diameter oversizing by 10–15% is important, and used routinely to maximize sealing at the proximal attachment site. In most cases, the Talent system is designed to be 4 mm larger than the target juxtarenal aorta; and, occasionally, 6 mm. *The more challenging the neck, the greater the need for oversizing.* 'Aggressive' ballooning is felt to be a critical component of the procedure, especially when using graft oversize of more than 10%.

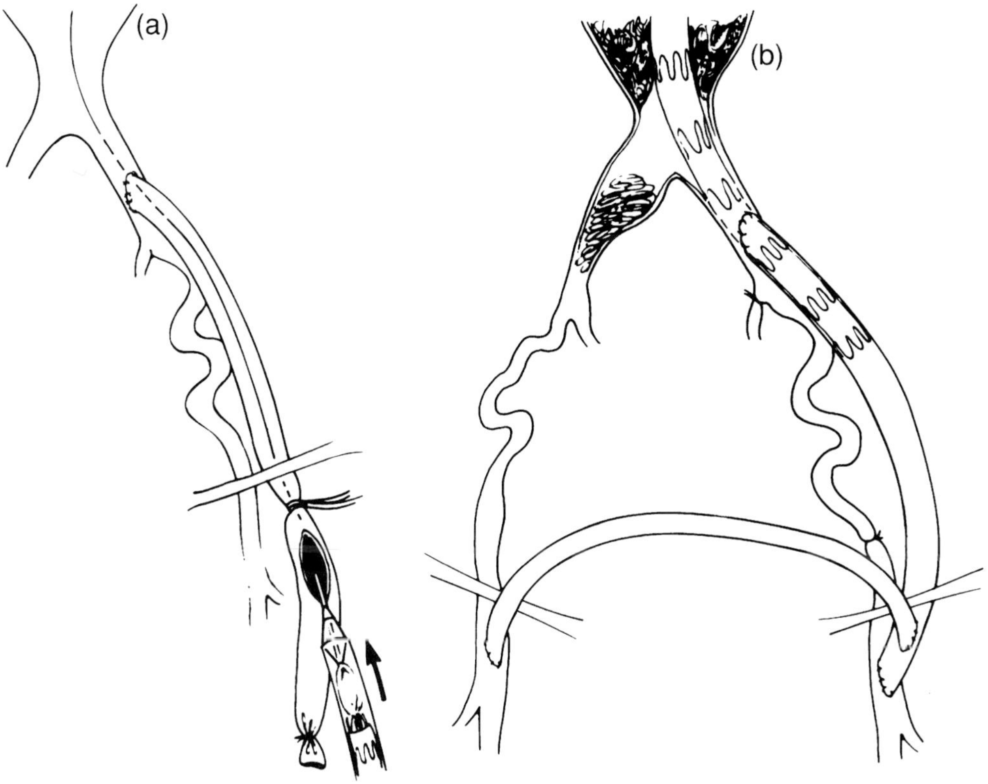

Fig. 12. Artist's rendition of technique that utilizes a 10-mm PTFE iliac conduit anastomosed to the distal common iliac artery or its bifurcation to 'extend' this vessel for easy device delivery (a). The complete procedure includes anastomosis of the iliac conduit to the ipsilateral common femoral artery, ligation of ipsilateral internal and external iliac arteries, cross-over bypass and exclusion of contralateral common iliac artery (b).

Unlike the above-described scenario, *length undersizing* is the recommended policy when doubt exists concerning appropriate length of the device for optimal landing at the level of the common iliac artery; modular grafts can always be extended distally.

In case of a frankly aneurysmal or very large common iliac artery, it is advisable to plan distal landing of the iliac limb at the level of the external iliac artery. This requires preliminary occlusion of the ipsilateral internal iliac artery by transluminal coil embolization, generally done as a percutaneous outpatient procedure a few days before the abdominal aortic aneurysm implant operation. Bilateral internal iliac artery occlusion becomes necessary on occasion; we feel strongly that it should be done as two separate staged interventions prior to endoluminal repair of the aneurysm. To date, we have been fortunate not to have seen any catastrophic ischaemic complication from internal iliac artery occlusion, unilateral or bilateral.

On occasion, aorto-uni-iliac endografting is the best technical approach. This implies the need for exclusion of the contralateral common iliac artery by transluminal coiling or 'wind-sock' endograft, and cross-over femorofemoral bypass to revascularize the contralateral lower extremity. Such situations are likely to require use of an iliac conduit for access and device deployment. The synthetic conduit thus becomes a) the site of distal landing of the endograft iliac limb, and b) the source of inflow for the cross-over bypass (Fig. 12).

TECHNICAL RESULTS AND DURABILITY

More than 2600 Talent aortic endografts have been implanted worldwide since December 1995. Technical results and acute outcome data are available for 745 abdominal aortic aneurysms exclusion procedures. In 596 instances (80%), a bifurcated stent-graft system was employed. Overall, successful technical exclusion of the aneurysm could be achieved with 92% of the implants. Acute (or primary) conversion to standard surgical repair was necessary in 5%. Thirty-day mortality was 4%, which is of special significance given the fact that 60% of the patients were American Society of Anesthesiology (ASA) risk category 3–5.

The Talent endograft is currently undergoing IDE (investigational device exemption) clinical investigation in the USA. Phase I Feasibility Study was conducted between April and December of 1997, and involved 26 patients treated in five different centres. Two-thirds of the patients were 'medical high risk' due to serious cardiac and/or respiratory co-morbidities, and one-third had anatomical high risk situations making them surgically unfit (i.e. 'hostile abdomen'). Thirty-day mortality was 4% (one of 26). Technical success was 88%, with an 8% (two of 26) incidence of endoleaks persisting beyond 3 months.

Phase II of the study has been divided into two arms: high-risk and low-risk patient subgroups. Patient entry is anticipated to be complete by the end of December 1998. By then, a total of nearly 250 patients will have been entered into the study that involves predominantly treatment of aortic aneurysms with a bifurcated system, but also a smaller number of cases with aorto-uni-iliac grafts. Outcome will be compared with that of 100 concurrent surgical controls.

Our own single-centre experience now amounts to over 60 implants (as of 1

Table 4. The Union Memorial Hospital/Helix Health, Baltimore, MD, USA experience of 60 Talent stant grafts for abdominal aortic aneurysms

Technical success	56/60 (93%)
Acute (primary) surgical conversion	1/60 (1.7%)
Unable to complete implant as planned	4/60 (7%)
Unable to deliver main section	2
Surgical conversion	1
Unable to deliver contralateral limb	1
Device migration	1
Subsequent surgical conversion 10 days later (postoperative death at 3 weeks)	
30-Day mortality	1/60 (1.7%)
Average length of hospital stay	3.5 days
Intensive care unit utilization	15%
Endoleaks	
On pre-discharge CT	10
At 30 days	4 (7%)

November 1998). Technical results and acute clinical outcome have been summarized in Table 4. A few patients suffered severe complications from the implant procedure, including renal artery occlusion by the Dacron fabric graft in two instances. One was unilateral, and the other bilateral causing total renal failure and the need for haemodialysis. The latter occurrence took place on a patient with a very short proximal neck who had a huge symptomatic aneurysm; it was felt that the patient was at high risk for fatal rupture and unfit for conventional surgery. Extensive iliac artery dissection occurred in two instances but could be easily treated by stent placement. Nine patients had elevation of serum creatinine post-implant; prolonged (more than 3 weeks) in two. The 'post-implant syndrome' consisting of a flu-like clinical picture including low-grade fever, upper gastrointestinal upset, back pain, and malaise, developed in nine of 56 implanted patients (16%). It is a self-limited condition that usually resolves within 2–3 weeks. Subsequent iliac limb stenosis (from graft infolding) occurred in one patient; percutaneous treatment by balloon dilatation and Wallstent placement easily corrected the problem. One of eight uni-iliac endograft procedures resulted in early postoperative thrombosis of the femorofemoral bypass graft, necessitating axillofemoral graft placement.

The bulk of this experience has occurred within the past 12 months; 'durability' cannot be gauged accurately at this time. Nevertheless, results thus far obtained are very satisfactory and particularly encouraging when taking into account that approximately 70% of the abdominal aortic aneurysm patients we see at present can be treated endoluminally with the Talent stent-graft system. Long-term results and overall clinical efficacy cannot be gleaned from currently available evidence.

Commentary

The authors are extremely fair in saying that as the majority of their experience with the Talent stent graft system for aortic aneurysm is within the last 12 months, that durability cannot be determined. The authors have commented upon some serious complications including covering the renal ostea by Dacron but this has occurred in patients who were unfit for open repair; nevertheless it has been a problem. It is not clear whether this is part of the learning curve of the operators or whether there is a particular difficulty with the Talent system. An impressive feature of this graft system is that it can fit extremely wide diameters and even be used for thoracic aneurysms. It is plain that careful auditing of this graft continues to be vital in order that we shall learn something about it in terms of durability. Clearly it is being used both for patients who could otherwise have an open repair, as well as patients who are unfit for surgery and therefore it would be ideal for this to be used as part of a random controlled trial so that we can learn about how it performs compared with the alternatives. *RMG*

Durability of the Nottingham aorto-uni-iliac custom-built system

SR Walker and BR Hopkinson

INTRODUCTION

Since the 1950s, the standard treatment for abdominal aortic aneurysms thought to be at risk of rupture, and where there were no medical contraindications, has been surgical open repair. Currently the procedure has a low morbidity and mortality rate in selected centres.[1] However, patients at higher risk during open repair of developing complications have been declined surgery. The advent of endovascular repair of abdominal aortic aneurysms in the early 1990s provided a potential therapeutic option in those patients previously declined surgery.[2] In addition, for those patients fit for conventional open repair, there was the possibility of using a technique that may be associated with a faster recovery to normal activities and a reduced complication rate.[3] However, this new technique was associated with its own unique complications and soon questions were being asked as to the durability of the procedure.[4] Certainly there is now ample evidence that the technique is feasible in those patients whose vascular anatomy is suitable for placement of an endovascular graft.[5] The question of long-term durability will require longer follow-up of those patients who have undergone the procedure. However, currently available data may give some clues as to the long-term durability.

Various parameters can be used to indicate an unsuccessful endovascular aneurysm repair (Table 1). These are also the main parameters that can be used to assess long-term durability, the most important parameter being prevention of aneurysm rupture. Aneurysm rupture will most likely arise from the development of an endoleak. An endoleak can arise from three mains sites:

1. The top of the stent graft, the bottom of the stent graft, or in the case of the aorto-uni-iliac device, from the occluder. These endoleaks are usually the result of an incorrect stent/graft size being used, inappropriate landing zones or migration of the graft from its deployment (or intended deployment) site.
2. Mid-graft leak. These may arise from components of modular grafts becoming dislodged from one another or from manufacturing defects in graft materials.
3. Lumbar or inferior mesenteric artery endoleaks. There is no satisfactory way at present to predict preoperatively which patients will develop such endoleaks and they are not related to the graft design.[6]

The first endovascular repair of an abdominal aortic aneurysm in Nottingham, UK, was performed in March 1994. Since then over 250 repairs have been performed. Most of these used an aorto-uni-iliac custom-built system. The original stent graft system used in Nottingham was the Chuter system, designed and developed by Tim

Table 1. Features indicating unsuccessful endovascular aneurysm repair

Perioperative death	
Failure to preserve organ function e.g.	Renal failure
Failure of aneurysm exclusion	Endoleak
	Aneurysm rupture
Failure to successfully deploy graft endovascularly	Early or late conversion to open repair

Chuter. From this original concept, Nottingham has developed its own aorto-uni-iliac graft based on the Ivancev (Malmo) system, the design of which has undergone a number of modifications. The aim of this chapter is to describe the design, the changes that have occurred in the design and to present the results of each design prototype. Thus, although follow-up is short, the durability of each design will be analysed separately so that any changes in features can be discussed.

THE NOTTINGHAM AORTO-UNI-ILIAC CUSTOM-BUILT SYSTEM

Each stent graft is individually designed and constructed for the individual patient. All patients undergo preoperative aneurysm assessment with contrast enhanced spiral CT scan to assess the anatomic suitability for endovascular repair. On the reconstructed images accurate measurements of the aortic and iliac artery dimensions can be made. In our early experience patients also had conventional calibrating angiography which was felt to be particularly useful in length measurements but as experience has grown this has now been abandoned. More recently we have used magnetic resonance imaging to obtain the aortic and iliac dimensions. On the basis of these measurements, the stent graft is designed and constructed in-house.

The first Chuter-designed stent grafts were of Verisoft (Meadox Medicals, Oakland, New Jersey USA) for the graft material and modified Gianturco-z-stents, self-expanding stainless steel stents (William Cook Europe, Denmark). A single 2.5-cm long stent with additional hooks and barbs soldered to four of the stent struts was placed inside the top of the graft and anchored in place with Gore-Tex sutures (Fig. 1). It was felt that the radial force of the self-expanding stent would produce a seal between graft and arterial wall and the hooks and barbs would prevent migration of the stent. An additional stent was placed inside the graft at the bottom end of the graft to produce a seal at the bottom end of the graft. The top and bottom graft diameter was matched very closely to the luminal dimensions as measured preoperatively. The configurations of the stent graft were of either aorto–aortic, bifurcated or aorto-uni-iliac in design. In patients undergoing aorto-uni-iliac repair, contralateral common iliac occlusion was initially achieved by coil embolization and subsequently by inserting a single graft-covered stent which had been sutured along one orifice to produce a small sac.

The first true Nottingham stent graft was the same design as the Chuter stent grafts but the graft delivery system was different. There was also a change to the

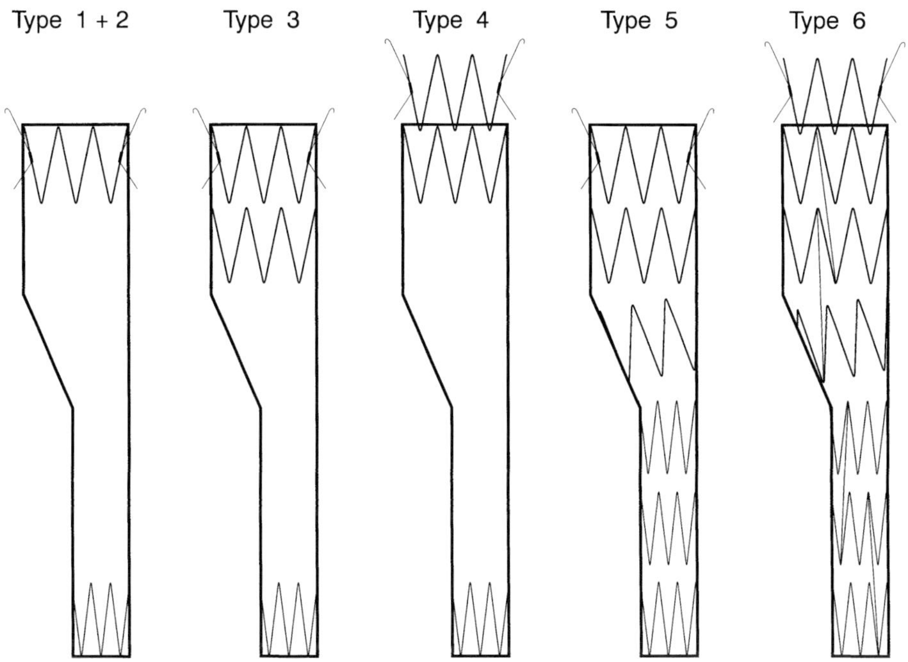

Fig. 1. The various stent graft designs used for the Nottingham aorto-uni-iliac device.

uncrimped Dacron graft (Vascutek, UK). The stent graft consisted of a single stent at the top and bottom of the graft. Subsequent modifications have resulted in an increase in the number of stents within the graft and in the use of a suprarenal uncovered Gianturco stent which has the hocks and barbs attached (Fig. 1).

RESULTS

Between March 1994 and September 1998, 220 Nottingham-style grafts were used. Table 2 shows a summary of the various types of graft used and initial results with duration of follow-up in perioperative survivors. The graphs in Fig. 3 illustrate the greater duration of follow-up for the early type of grafts. To our knowledge, there has been no graft breakage and no separation of graft from stent. There have been cases in which Chuter-deployed grafts have migrated inferiorly and resulted in separation of the hooks from the Gianturco stent. Half of the Chuter-deployed grafts have migrated distally, resulting in an endoleak in six, with four patients requiring open revision of the top end (Table 3). The interval before detection of graft migration is shown in Fig. 3.

Of the two graft migrations in the type 2 stent graft, one was the proximal migration of the distal end of an aorto–aortic stent graft back into the aneurysm. This resulted in an endoleak and the patient underwent endovascular conversion to a commercially available bifurcated endovascular graft.

Table 2. Results of the Nottingham aorto-uni-iliac custom-built system

	Type 1	*Type 2*	*Type 3*	*Type 4*	*Type 5*	*Type 6*
First case	March 1994	February 1995	May 1995	November 1996	December 1996	May 1997
No. of cases	23 Aorto-aortic 1 Aorto-uni-iliac 8 Bifurcated 14	55 Aorto-aortic 1 Aorto-uni-iliac 54	33 All aorto-uni-iliac	19 Aorto-aortic 1 Aorto-uni-iliac 18	49 Aorto-aortic 2 Aorto-uni-iliac 47	41 All aorto-uni-iliac
No. of high risk cases (%)	8 (35)	29 (53)	24 (73)	8 (42)	30 (61)	32 (78)
Perioperative surgical interventions	3	6	6	1	3	3
Perioperative deaths (%)	3 (13)	6 (11)	6 (18)	2 (11)	3 (6)	7 (17)
Duration of follow-up (months) in perioperative survivors (range)	38 (48–24)	23 (36–3)	13 (36–2)	12 (16–10)	4 (14–1)	2 (12–1)

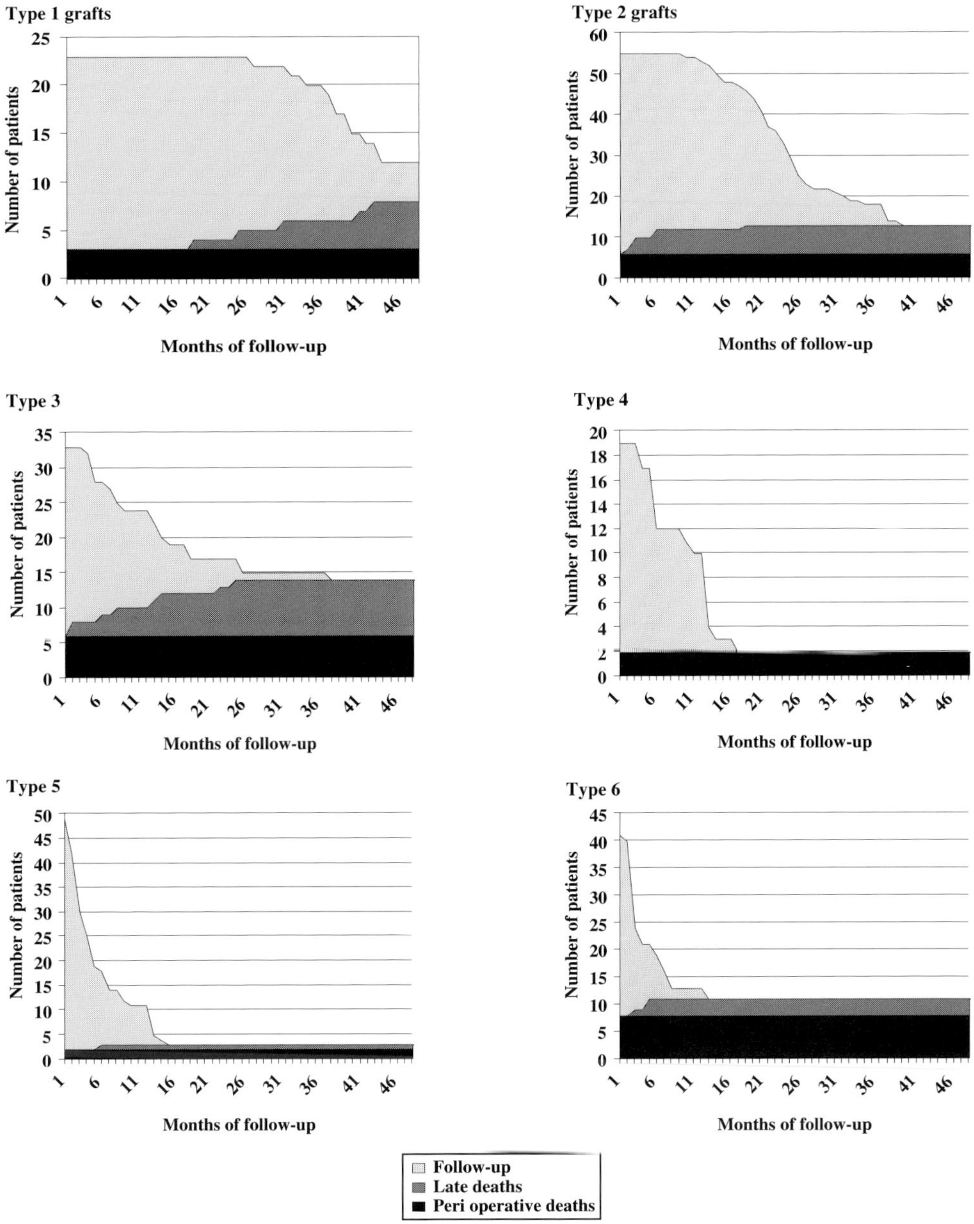

Fig. 2. Graphs to illustrate the follow-up for the various graft types as illustrated in Fig. 1.

There has only been one graft migration in types 3–6. A type 6 graft was noted to have a top endoleak on the completion angiogram and this was confirmed at the 1-week contrast enhanced computed tomography (CT) scan. The patient was not fit for an open conversion and was therefore observed. At the 6-month contrast enhanced CT scan no evidence of an endoleak or graft migration was noted. However, the 1-year CT scan demonstrated both a recurrence of the top endoleak and a 15-mm graft migration.

Table 3. Late complications and interventions

	Type 1	*Type 2*	*Type 3*	*Type 4*	*Type 5*	*Type 6*
Endoleaks	6	3	3	1	5	7
Stent graft migration	10	2	2			
Late surgical interventions	Open revision of top end – 4 Conversion of aorto-aortic graft to bifurcated endovascular graft – 1 Femoro femoral cross-over graft for limb occlusion of bifurcated graft – 1	Open revision of top end – 1 Common iliac artery ligation – 1 Conversion of aorto-aortic to bifurcated graft – 1		Open revision of top end – 2		Packing of aneurysm sac for top endoleak and occluded aortic graft – 1
Causes of late deaths	Carcinoma – 2 Gastrointestinal bleed – 1 Renal failure – 1 Liver failure – 1	Cardiac – 2 Sepsis – 2 Stroke – 1 Respiratory failure – 1 Renal failure – 1 Unknown cause – 1	Carcinoma – 3 Renal failure – 1 Cardiac – 1 Ruptured AAA – 1 Ruptured thoracic aneurysm – 1 Renal failure – 1 Unknown cause – 1		Carcinoma – 1	Ruptured AAA – 1

(a)

(b)

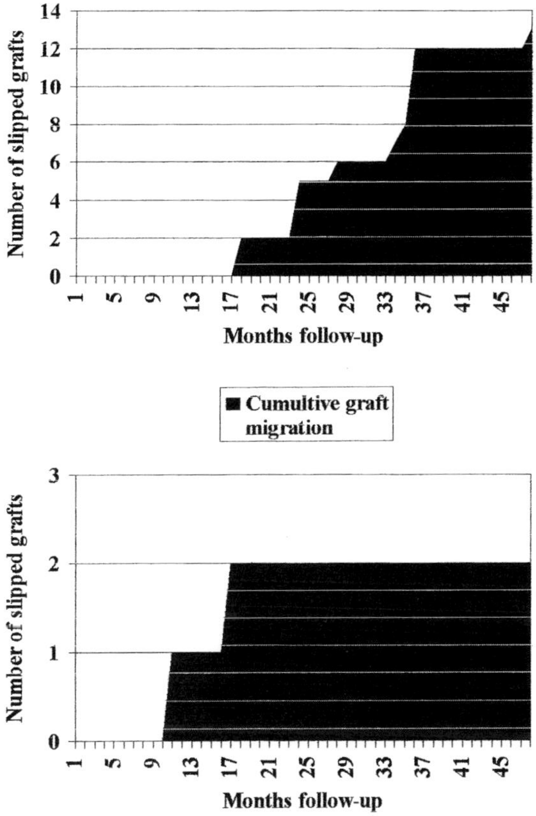

Fig.3. Graphs to show the time interval before detection of graft migration in type 1 (a) and type 2 (b) stent grafts. No migrations have been detected in any of the remaining graft types.

Two patients in this series have died outside the perioperative period from ruptured abdominal aortic aneurysms. The first case was performed in July 1996 using a type 3 stent graft. A CT scan at 6 months showed the top stent to be at the level of the lowest renal artery and there was no endoleak. The 14-month CT scan showed that the top stent had slipped distally by 10mm. Although there was no endoleak, the aneurysm had increased in size by 10mm when compared with the preoperative maximum diameter and therefore a conservative approach was taken. However, the patient presented to his local hospital at 22 months in cardiovascular shock from which he could not be resuscitated. A post-mortem examination reported extensive haemorrhage in relation to the bed of the aorta but no obvious source could be found. We have to assume this was a ruptured AAA. The second patient who ruptured had undergone endovascular repair performed in March 1998. The 1-week CT scan demonstrated a large top endoleak and an attempt was made to treat this endovascularly with an extension piece. However, this did not seal the endoleak and in retrospect this proximal neck was probably not suitable for endovascular repair.

The patient was not fit for a laparotomy. Following discharge, he too presented to his local hospital with cardiovascular shock from which he died. Although no post-mortem examination was performed, his death should be attributed to a ruptured abdominal aortic aneurysm.

DISCUSSION

It would seem reasonable to look at patients with the longest follow-up for evidence of durability. The difficulty with extrapolating such figures to currently used devices is that the stent graft design has changed significantly in order to reduce the incidence of leakage, slippage and rupture. In addition we are still on the steep part of the learning curve, particularly with regards to the patient selection for endovascular repair. As we have modified the stent graft we have performed endovascular repair on patients who would previously have been considered unsuitable for it. Finally, the sizing of the stent grafts has undergone a major revision. Initially it was felt that the graft should be matched very precisely to the proximal and distal vascular dimensions. This meant that there was no room for measurement errors and there was no allowance for any potential future vessel dilatation. This may explain the high number of graft migration and endoleaks in the Chuter-type grafts. We now routinely oversize the graft by 10–20% in order to overcome these problems.

A further difficulty in assessing the long-term durability of the Nottingham aorto-uni-iliac device is the nature of the patient population on which these procedures are being performed. Over half the patients undergoing endovascular repair of abdominal aortic aneurysm in Nottingham have been referred from other hospitals where they have been deemed to be unfit for conventional open surgery due most often to medical co-morbidities. In addition, some patients have been referred because of their anatomic unsuitability for commercially available endovascular repair devices. We are therefore dealing with a rather select patient group. Indeed, some patients who have undergone endovascular repair have not survived the procedure due to their medical co-morbidity and in the future we would have to consider it unwise to offer patients with similarly poor prognosis an endovascular repair. For this reason we are currently working on the development of a scoring system which takes into account both the medical condition of the patient and the anatomic suitability of the patient for endovascular repair. There will be some patients who have abdominal aortic aneurysms but who also have other medical conditions. The difficulty is in predicting which patients would have their survival prolonged by having the aneurysm repaired.

Unlike stent graft systems employed in many other centres, the Nottingham stent graft uses a long established, unaltered vascular graft. There is now increasing evidence of the frailty of expanded polytetrafluoroethylene and other newer textiles that have been used in endovascular grafts.[4] The Dacron used in the Nottingham graft has been shown to have the potential to dilate over a period of time[7] but reports of graft material failure causing leakage are rare.[8,9]

The change from stents simply at the top and bottom of the graft to the fully stented graft was instituted for two reasons. The column of stents was employed to add columnar strength to the stent graft and this may be a factor in the reduction in the incidence of graft migration. In addition, many patients who had type 1-4 grafts required additional Wallstents in order to treat or prevent graft kinking and occlusion. The use of a fully stented graft has almost abolished the use of Wallstents in these patients.

In order to treat patients with short (<1.5cm) or conical necks a good landing zone is required for the top stent. Therefore in these patients an uncovered stent has been added to the top of the graft. The uncovered stent is used to cross the renal arteries. This topic will be discussed further in the chapter by Michael Lawrence-Brown (pp. 375–386). Briefly, our experience of using such uncovered stents has been favourable and allows patients with difficult proximal necks to be treated. We have not experienced any renal complications from this approach but we are currently looking very closely at any changes in renal function with the use of such stents.

CONCLUSION

We believe that the use of a traditional tried and tested vascular graft material supported in its entire length and anchored to the aorta by both hooks and barbs will provide a durable stent graft for the exclusion of abdominal aortic aneurysms. Although the follow-up for this design is limited, the combination has evolved from our initial early experience. There will doubtlessly be further modifications in the future as experience in both the implantation technique and patient selection grows.

REFERENCES

1. Johnson KW, Scobie TK: Multicentre prospective study of nonruptured abdominal aortic aneurysms. 1. Population and operative management. *J Vasc Surg* **7**: 69–81, 1988
2. Parodi JC, Palmaz JC, Barone HD: Transfemoral intraluminal graft implantation for abdominal aortic aneurysm. *Ann Vasc Surg* **5**: 491–499, 1991
3. Boyle JR, Thompson JP, Thompson MM *et al.*: Improved respiratory function and analgesia control after endovascular AAA repair. *J Endovasc Surg* **4**: 62–65, 1997
4. Chakfe N, Riepe G, Beaufigeau M *et al.*: Endovascular treatment of abdominal aortic aneurysms: A promising technique that requires stable devices. *Endocardiovasc Multimedia Magazine* **2**: 23–27, 1998
5. Woodburn KR, May J, White G: Endoluminal abdominal aortic aneurysm surgery. *Br J Surg* **85**: 435–443, 1998
6. Walker SR, Halliday K, Yusuf SW *et al.*: A study on the patency of the inferior mesenteric and lumbar arteries in the incidence of endoleaks following endovascular repair of infrarenal aortic aneurysms. *Clin Radiol* **53**: 593–595, 1998
7. Nunn DB, Freeman MH, Hudgkins PC: Postoperative alterations in size of Dacron aortic arterial grafts. An ultrasonic evaluation. *Ann Surg* **189**: 741–745, 1979
8. Chakfe N, Urban E, Dieval F *et al.*: Les ruptures longitudinales des prostheses vasculaires en polyester. *Ann Vasc Surg* 1999 (in press)
9. Riepe G, Loos J, Iming H *et al.*: Long-term *in vivo* alterations of polyester vascular grafts in humans. *Eur J Vasc Endovasc Surg* **13**: 540–548, 1997

Commentary

In the United Kingdom, the Nottingham group have more long-standing data than many other centres and can truly give us some feeling for durability of the stent graft technique for abdominal aortic aneurysm. Originally they used the Cook stent for an aorto-uni-iliac device which they constructed themselves to great effect. This group has worked closely with those in Malmo and Perth to develop the new Cook Zenith Perth system. Tim Chuter was a Nottingham graduate and the Nottingham Centre has indeed played an important pioneering role in these early years. Simon Whitaker is an extremely capable radiologist working in Nottingham and has played a most important role in bringing together the two disciplines to produce optimal results. *RMG*

Durability of the Leicester-built system

Matthew M Thompson, Guy Fishwick and Peter RF Bell

INTRODUCTION

The immediate results of endovascular aneurysm repair are now available for a substantial number of patients and the feasibility of the technique has been well established by numerous centres.[1–3] Early data suggest that endovascular aneurysm repair may be performed with similar mortality and morbidity to conventional repair, although comparisons between the two procedures are difficult due to differing patient cohorts.[4]

Theoretically, the principle advantages of endoluminal aortic surgery are largely confined to the perioperative period due to the avoidance of a large abdominal incision and a reduction in the duration of cross-clamping. Comparative studies have demonstrated significant physiological advantages to endovascular repair in both respiratory and cardiovascular systems,[5,6] and these changes might be expected to result in improved perioperative mortality rates. However, no randomized studies have been performed to date,[7] although a National Health Service Research and Development sponsored trial is due to commence in early 1999.

Although recent evidence has begun to support the potential advantages of endovascular aneurysm repair in the perioperative period, few data are available concerning the durability of aortic endografts. The long-term results of surgical aneurysm resection have been extensively documented,[8,9] and the combination of modern prosthetic materials with conventional inlay grafting, may be expected to result in an aneurysm repair which will endure for at least 10 years. Conversely, the maximum individual follow-up for patients with endovascular aneurysm repair is unlikely to exceed 5 years and therefore all results are likely to be intermediate at best.

However, in spite of limited follow-up, the durability of endovascular aneurysm repair is a legitimate cause for concern. Doubts have been raised concerning the structural integrity of the endograft itself and over the fate of the excluded aneurysm sac. In recent presentations to the European Vascular Society for Vascular and Endovascular Surgery, Brennan and Dimitri, on behalf of the Eurostar collaboration,[10] demonstrated that 50% of selected nitinol-based endografts demonstrated structural failure and that 55% showed signs of severe distortion. Additionally, Riepe revealed that many explanted nitinol endografts had fractures in the structure of the stent, which is obviously worrying for long-term durability. Several authors have also reported paradoxical aneurysm expansion following endoluminal grafting, and rupture of the aneurysm sac after apparently successful endovascular exclusion has been widely reported.[11,12]

Additionally, as with any new procedure, endoluminal aortic surgery is associated with a distinct profile of complications and the occurrence and management of endoleaks present a challenging problem. Endoleaks affecting the proximal and distal implantation sites, together with collateral perfusion of the aneurysm sac, may be encountered after one-fifth of endovascular procedures ,[13,14] and the natural history and subsequent optimum treatment of this complication is still debatable.

The issue of long-term durability in aortic endografts is clearly crucial to the future of this technique. However, at present the number of differing techniques in use, makes meta-analysis of various individual series difficult to interpret, especially with the various configurations of aortic endograft (straight vs bifurcated vs tapered). There clearly may be a difference in failure rates between grafts which use conventional prosthetic materials, compared with those using specially designed ultra-thin porous prostheses. Similarly the incidence of endoleak between self-expanding and balloon-expandable stents must be addressed, as must the rate of structural failure between fully supported and non-supported grafts. This chapter outlines the intermediate results obtained in Leicester, with an aorto-uni-iliac graft consisting of a tapered thin walled expanded polytetrafluoroethylene (ePTFE) graft sutured to a balloon-expandable stent.

TECHNIQUE OF ENDOVASCULAR ANEURYSM REPAIR AND FOLLOW-UP

Endovascular aneurysm repair

The Leicester system of endovascular aneurysm repair, together with morphological requirements has been extensively described in previous publications, and will not be described in detail here.[3,15] Briefly, the system was designed as an aorto-uni-iliac system, which relies on a femorofemoral cross-over graft and iliac occlusion for perfusion of the contralateral limb and pelvis (Fig. 1).

The endograft consists of a tapered ePTFE graft (Impra, Worcs, UK) attached to an extra-large Palmaz stent (Cordis, Brentford, UK), which is in turn mounted on a balloon angioplasty catheter and packaged inside a 21F teflon sheath (Cook, Letchworth, UK). The graft is introduced into the circulation via a temporary iliac or femoral conduit through a 25F sheath. Following contrast examination and withdrawal of the introducer sheath, the endograft is deployed just below the renal arteries by inflation of the angioplasty balloon. The distal limb of the endograft is then anastomosed to the cross-over graft and the procedure is completed by occlusion of the contralateral common iliac artery with a covered Gianturco stent (Cook, Letchworth, UK), detachable balloon or a ligature.

Follow-up

Patients undergo duplex scanning prior to discharge and subsequently at 6 weeks, 3 months, 6 months, 9 months, 12 months and 6-monthly thereafter. During ultrasound examination the maximum diameter of the aneurysm sac is measured and the presence of flow within the aneurysm sac investigated. Flow within the sac is treated as an endoleak and an estimation of the site and magnitude of the leak is made.

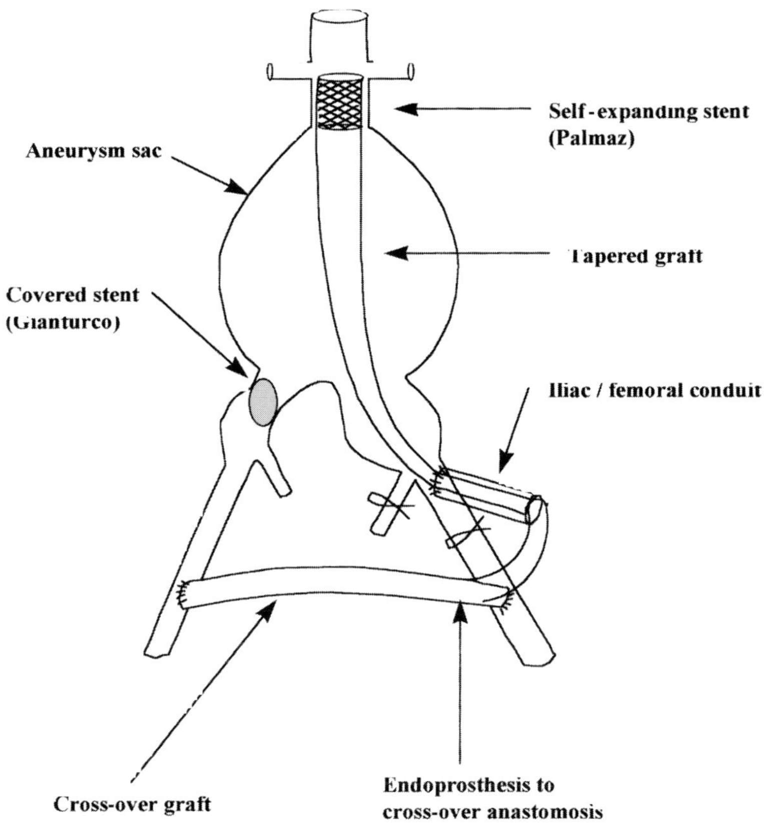

Fig. 1. Diagrammatic illustration of the 'Leicester' custom-built aorto-uni-iliac device. The graft is introduced via a femoral or iliac artery temporary conduit and is deployed in the infrarenal aorta before tapering into the ipsilateral groin and joining the cross-over graft. The revascularization is completed by a femorofemoral cross-over graft accompanied by occlusion of the contralateral common iliac artery.

Patients with evidence of endoleak, or absence of progressive reduction in aneurysm diameter undergo contrast enhanced computed tomography (CT) as previously described.[16] Patients with a CT proven endoleak are subsequently investigated with a diagnostic femoral arteriogram performed with a 6F marker catheter.

RESULTS OF AORTO-UNI-ILIAC ENDOVASCULAR ANEURYSM REPAIR

Immediate results and patient cohort

Sixty patients underwent aorto-uni-iliac grafting at Leicester Royal Infirmary between September 1994 and June 1998. Patients treated at other centres have not been included in this analysis. The overall immediate failure rate, leading to surgical conversion, was 13% (eight of 60) and the 30-day mortality rate was 10% (six of 60). In all, 47 patients were available for long-term review, and the median follow-up for this cohort was 21 months. Additionally there were seven late deaths.

Aortic morphology following endovascular aneurysm repair

Previous studies from our centre have described the fate of the aneurysm sac following endovascular aneurysm repair.[16] Serial duplex scanning revealed that aneurysms successfully excluded from the arterial circulation regressed at a rate of 0.4 cm per year, whereas aneurysms which had a demonstrable endoleak showed an increase in size. The findings from this study are in close agreement with those of others who have described similar changes in aortic morphology.[17,18] Interestingly, we also confirmed the excellent limits of agreement between colour duplex ultrasonography and CT scanning when assessing aneurysm size and the presence of endoleak.[19] We now routinely utilize duplex scanning alone in the follow-up protocol for endovascular aneurysm repair, with CT reserved as a secondary investigative method, in patients with suspected endoleak.

The final results from this imaging study also suggested that the proximal aorta continued to dilate following endovascular aortic surgery at a rate of 1.6 mm per year, a finding which has been reported by several groups.[20,21] This expansion might be expected from the gradual arterial enlargement that occurs during life, but may have important implications in the long-term durability of endovascular grafts. Obviously, if the juxtarenal aorta dilates to a greater diameter than the proximal aortic stent, failure of the endograft will occur.

Immediate endoleaks

In the current series, 52 aorto-uni-iliac grafts were deployed without the need for surgical conversion. In this group, there were five immediate endoleaks, one proximal and the remaining four related to the contralateral common iliac occlusion site or patent lumbar branches. The leaks associated with patent lumbar vessels were diagnosed by contrast examination of the aneurysm sac at the termination of the procedure. The proximal endoleak was treated at time of surgery with deployment of an additional ePTFE-covered Palmaz stent at the proximal attachment site. This manoeuvre abolished the leak.

All immediate distal endoleaks were initially observed for a period of 3 months. At this point, two (due to patent lumbar vessels) had sealed spontaneously and the aneurysm sacs were regressing. Two distal leaks persisted on duplex examination (Fig. 2) and were subsequently investigated by both CT scanning and arteriography. In both cases, the arteriograms demonstrated a leak at the distal common iliac occlusion site (Fig. 3). Both patients were treated with coil embolization (8–10mm platinum coil, Cook, UK, or spirale coil, Balt medical, France) with acceptable immediate results (Fig. 4). On subsequent follow-up, one leak remained sealed, but the other recurred and was treated with surgical ligation.

No patients in this cohort developed a ruptured aneurysm following graft insertion.

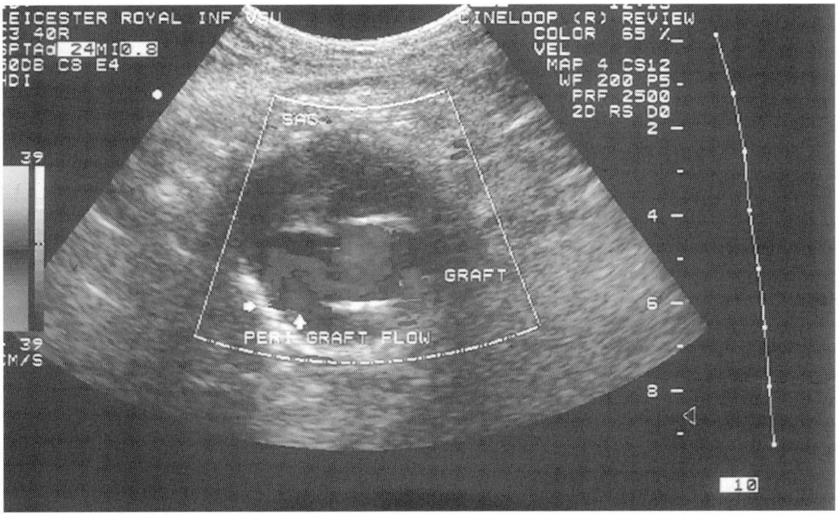

Fig. 2. Colour duplex ultrasound scan demonstrating aorto-uni-iliac endograft within an aneurysm sac. Blood flow can be visualized within the graft and also within the aneurysm sac, which is indicative of an endoleak.

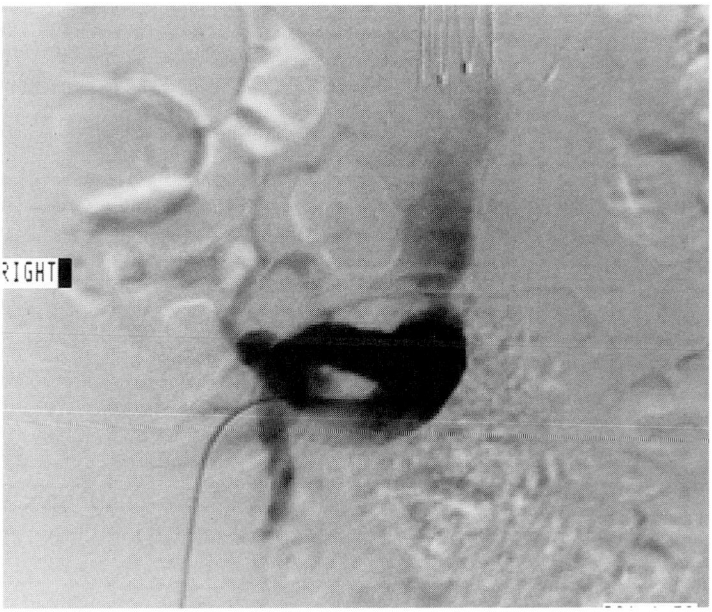

Fig. 3. Retrograde femoral arteriogram to investigate a patient with a distal endoleak. Contrast is seen passing through the common iliac ligation site into the distal aneurysm sac. A covered Gianturco stent which was used to occlude the common iliac artery has been displaced into the proximal common iliac artery and has not effectively occluded the artery.

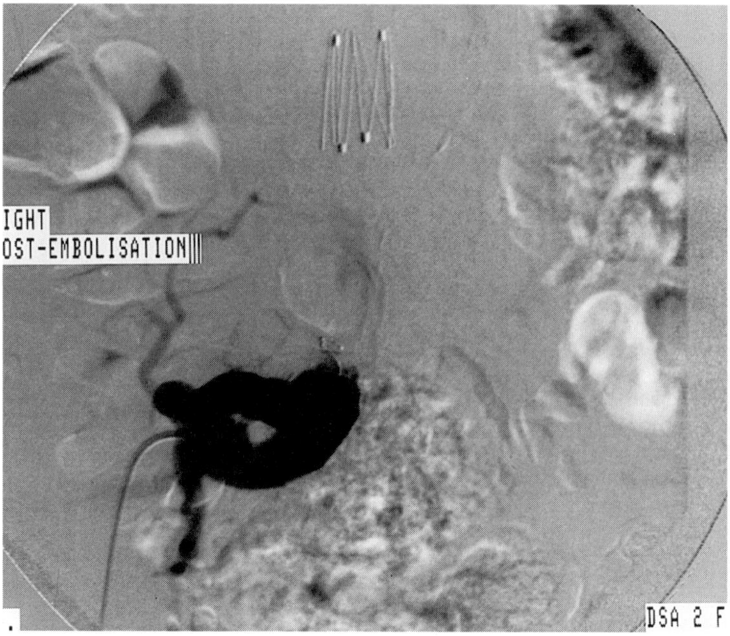

Fig. 4. Distal endoleak (Fig. 3) has been effectively treated by placement of several occluding coils.

Delayed endoleak

Delayed endoleaks were identified in five patients, one related to the proximal stent and four to the distal iliac occlusion site. Three of the four distal leaks have been treated with coil embolization as described previously and all remain sealed at latest review. The remaining distal leak has been investigated but the site of retrograde aneurysm perfusion has not been identified. This patient is currently being observed with 3-monthly duplex scans.

The single patient with a large proximal endoleak demonstrated expansion of the aneurysm sac from 6.5 to 7.0 cm between 12- and 18-month follow-up. The proximal leak was diagnosed on duplex scanning and was confirmed by both CT and arteriography (Figs 5–7). Treatment was attempted by placement of a covered proximal stent. However, the aneurysm neck at the point of the endoleak had expanded to 3.2 cm, from an original diameter of 27 mm. Placement of a 30-mm stent therefore failed to abolish the leak. A custom-built proximal collar is currently under construction (World Medical, USA) and will be implanted in the near future.

The incidence of endoleaks persisting after the initial operation was 17% in this series. This represents a relatively low figure compared with many other series,[22,23] although the overall incidence of endoleaks in all published reports probably averages 25%. Interestingly, the incidence of proximal endoleakage was reassuringly

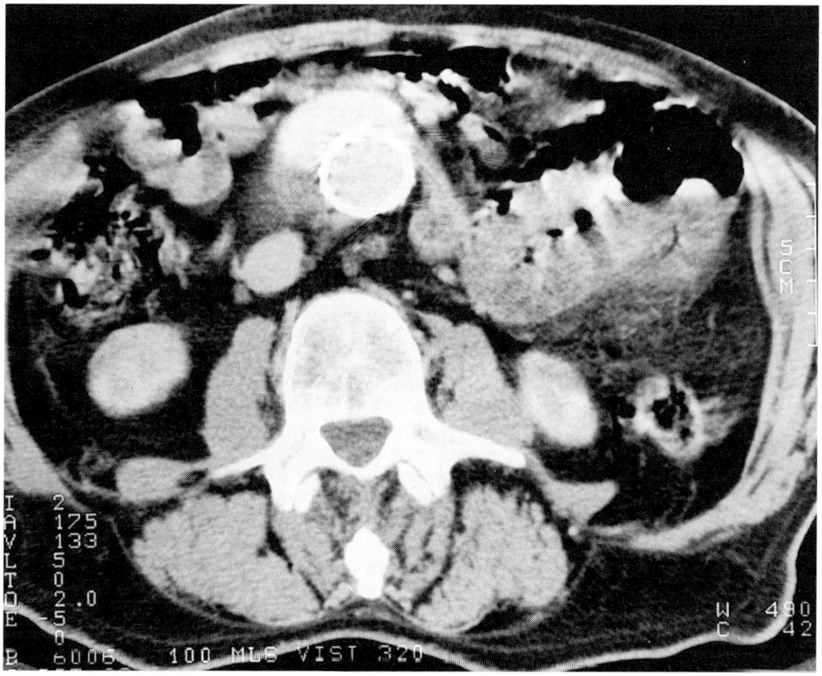

Fig. 5. Computed tomogram demonstrating a large volume of contrast in the aneurysm sac. The leak appears to be related to the anterior aspect of the proximal Palmaz stent.

low in this series (2%), which may reflect the use of a balloon-expandable stent to anchor the proximal extent of the graft. Comparative series have begun to suggest that the incidence of high pressure, high flow, proximal endoleaks may be related to the type of stent used and that balloon-expandable stents may be superior to self-expanding stents. The mechanism responsible for this effect is unknown, but it may be related to the development of intimal hyperplasia as a response to aortic dilation during balloon inflation.

The majority of endoleaks in the current series were related to the contralateral common iliac occlusion site. Throughout the development of the 'Leicester' grafting system, various techniques have been utilized to occlude the iliac system, including detachable balloons, covered Gianturco stents and surgical ligation. Unfortunately, the data are limited at present and it remains impossible to speculate as to the optimum method for occluding the iliac system.

Graft-related complications

The 'Leicester' system uses a commercially available ePTFE graft which is dilated prior to implantation. This process could theoretically lead to disruption of the graft material and predisposition to graft thrombosis or dilatation. However, to date there

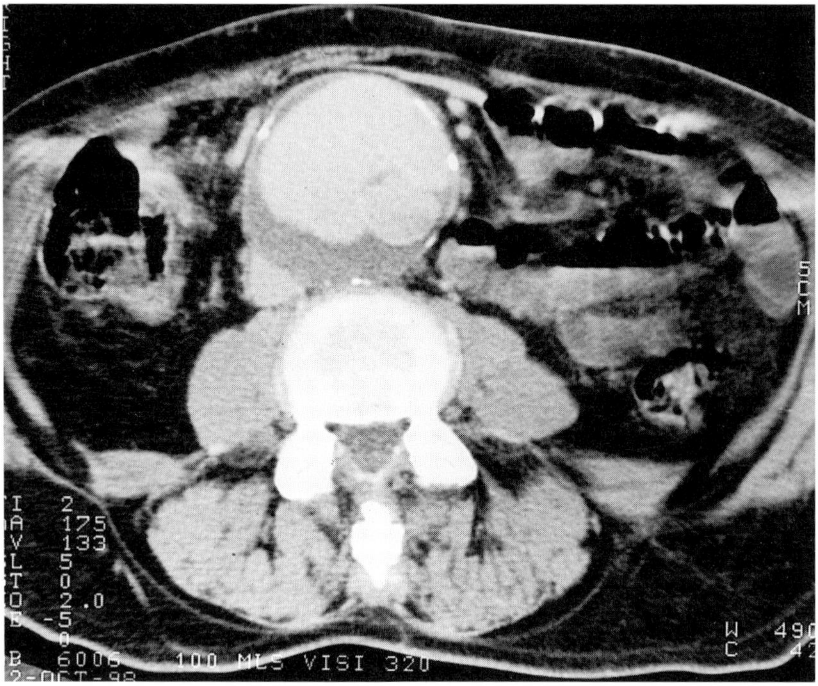

Fig. 6. Computed tomogram demonstrating a large proximal endoleak surrounding the ePTFE graft within a large aneurysm sac.

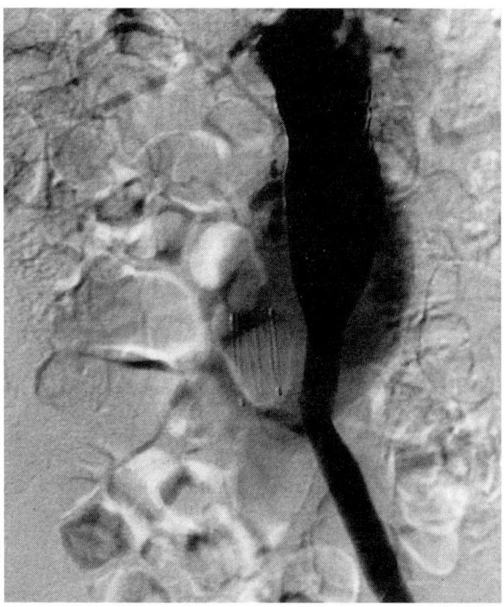

Fig. 7. Arteriogram demonstrating significant perfusion of the aneurysm sac, related to a proximal endoleak. The aorto-uni-iliac tapered graft is demonstrated passing into the left femoral artery.

have been only six graft-related complications. Three patients have presented with acute graft occlusion. Two patients had graft thrombosis, one immediately postoperatively and one 22 months following the procedure. The patient who presented immediately after endografting had a successful thrombectomy whilst the other patient had an axillofemoral graft performed. The remaining patient with graft occlusion had an embolic source and was successfully treated with an open embolectomy. The incidence of graft occlusion in the aorto-uni-iliac grafts performed at our centre was 6%, which is not appreciably different to the graft thrombosis rate reported for bifurcated endovascular systems.[24,25] One graft stenosis has been identified and treated with an intraluminal stent.[26]

One of the potential disadvantages of any aorto-uni-iliac system is the use of a femorofemoral cross-over graft to revascularize the contralateral limb and pelvis. Although this operation has a relatively tarnished reputation in occlusive disease, this graft configuration appears to function well as part of an endovascular aortic procedure. In our series, there has been one graft thrombosis and one graft infection in the 52 successful cases. This experience is similar to that reported by Walker *et al.*[27] who reported two graft infections and one graft thrombosis in 136 patients.

Pelvic revascularization

In the majority of cases, the graft system reported in this article preferentially anastomoses the tapered aortic endograft to the cross-over graft in the groin. This necessitates occlusion of the ipsilateral internal iliac artery to prevent blood flow outside the graft system. The configuration of the graft system determines that the pelvis is perfused by the cross-over graft and retrograde perfusion of the contralateral internal iliac artery. Obviously, with this arrangement, pelvic blood flow may be compromised, if graft flow is inadequate or the perfused internal iliac artery is diseased.

In the patient cohort, there has been one episode of transient ischaemic colitis in the postoperative period which resolved with conservative treatment. Of more concern, is the incidence of buttock claudication in patients having successfully placed endografts. Approximately 40% of patients experience evidence of buttock claudication at 6 weeks. In the majority of cases, claudication resolves over 6 to 12 months, but approximately 10% of patients continue to report lifestyle disabling claudication, which is refractory to treatment. Most patients have normal exercise ankle brachial pressure indices, and it is presumed that their claudication is a result of inadequate pelvic collateralization following internal iliac ligation.

SUMMARY

The 'Leicester' method of aorto-uni-iliac grafting appears to be of comparable durability to other 'in-house' and commercially available grafts. The incidence of graft failure and proximal endoleak are low, but require further evaluation over a prolonged period. The occurrence of buttock claudication remains a significant disadvantage. However, one of the strengths of this system is its flexibility and its applicability to treating ruptured aneurysms. With the durability of the endograft, the evolution of this system will be treat patients with ruptured aneurysms, where the occurrence of subsequent buttock claudication may be more acceptable.

REFERENCES

1. Parodi JC: Endovascular repair of abdominal aortic aneurysms and other arterial lesions. *J Vasc Surg* **21**: 549–555, 1995
2. May J, White GH, Yu W *et al.*: Results of endoluminal grafting of abdominal aortic aneurysms are dependent on aneurysm morphology. *Ann Vasc Surg* **10**: 254–261, 1996
3. Thompson MM, Sayers RD, Nasim A *et al.*: Aortomonoiliac endovascular grafting: difficult solutions to difficult problems. *J Endovasc Surg* **4**: 174–181, 1997
4. May J, White GH, Yu W *et al.*: Concurrent comparison of endoluminal repair vs no treatment for small abdominal aortic aneurysms. *Eur J Vasc Endovasc Surg* **13**: 472–476, 1997
5. Boyle JR, Thompson JP, Thompson MM *et al.*: Improved respiratory function and analgesia control after endovascular AAA repair. *J Endovasc Surg* 4: 62–65, 1997
6. Thompson JP, Boyle JR, Thompson MM: Cardiovascular and catecholamine responses during endovascular and conventional abdominal aortic aneurysm repair. *Eur J Vasc Endovasc Surg* 1999 (in press)
7. Thompson MM, Sayers RD, Bell PR: Endovascular aneurysm repair. [Editorial] *Br Med J* 314: 1139–1140, 1997
8. Matsushita M, Nishikimi N, Sakurai T *et al.*: Late results of surgery for abdominal aortic aneurysm. *Int Angiol* **16**: 158–161, 1997
9. Mohan CR, Hoballah JJ, Martinasevic M *et al.*: The aortic polytetrafluoroethylene graft: further experience. *Eur J Vasc Endovasc Surg* **11**: 158–163, 1996
10. Harris PL, Buth J, Mialhe C *et al.*: The need for clinical trials of endovascular abdominal aortic aneurysm stent-graft repair: The EUROSTAR project. *J Endovasc Surg* **4**: 72–79, 1997
11. Lumsden AB, Allen RC, Chaikof EL *et al.*: Delayed rupture of aortic aneurysms following endovascular stent grafting. *Am J Surg* **170**: 174–178, 1995
12. Torsello G, Kutkuhn B, Kniemeyer H, Sandmann W: [Prevention of acute renal failure in suprarenal aortic surgery. Results of a pilot study]. [German]. *Zentralbl Chir* **118**: 390–394, 1993
13. Holzenbein TJ, Kretschmer G, Dorffner R *et al.*: Endovascular management of 'endoleaks' after transluminal infrarenal abdominal aneurysm repair. *Eur J Vasc Endovasc Surg* **16**: 208–217, 1998
14. White GH, May J, McGahan T *et al.*: Historic control comparison of outcome for matched groups of patients undergoing endoluminal versus open repair of abdominal aortic aneurysms. *J Vasc Surg* **23**: 201–212, 1996
15. Thompson MM, Nasim A, Bell PRF *et al.* (Eds): *Endovascular Surgery for Aortic Aneurysms* pp. 240–253. London: WB Saunders Co., 1997
16. Thompson MM, Boyle JR, Hartshorne T *et al.*: A comparison of computerised tomography and duplex imaging in assessing aortic morphology following endovascular aneurysm repair. *Br J Surg* **85**: 346–350, 1998
17. Resch T, Ivancev K, Lindh M *et al.*: Persistent collateral perfusion of abdominal aortic aneurysm after endovascular repair does not lead to progressive change in aneurysm diameter. *J Vasc Surg* **28**: 242–249, 1998
18. May J, White G, Yu W *et al.*: A prospective study of anatomico-pathological changes in abdominal aortic aneurysms following endoluminal repair: is the aneurysmal process reversed ? *Eur J Vasc Endovasc Surg* **12**: 11–17, 1996
19. Sato DT, Goff CD, Gregory RT *et al.*: Endoleak after aortic stent graft repair: diagnosis by color duplex ultrasound scan versus computed tomography scan. *J Vasc Surg* **28**: 657–663, 1998

20. Sonesson B, Malina M, Ivancev K *et al.*: Dilatation of the infrarenal aneurysm neck after endovascular exclusion of abdominal aortic aneurysm. *J Endovasc Surg* **5**: 195–200, 1998
21. Matsumura JS, Chaikof EL: Continued expansion of aortic necks after endovascular repair of abdominal aortic aneurysms. EVT Investigators. EndoVascular Technologies, Inc. *J Vasc Surg* **28**: 422–430, 1998
22. Matsumura JS, Pearce WH, McCarthy WJ, Yao JS: Reduction in aortic aneurysm size: early results after endovascular graft placement. EVT Investigators. *J Vasc Surg* **25**: 113–123, 1998
23. Malina M, Ivancev K, Chuter TM *et al.*: Changing aneurysmal morphology after endovascular grafting: Relation to leakage or persistent perfusion. *J Endovasc Surg* **4**: 23–32, 1997
24. Dorffner R, Thurnher S, Polterauer P *et al.*: Treatment of abdominal aortic aneurysms with transfemoral placement of stent-grafts: Complications and secondary radiologic intervention. *Radiology* **204**: 79–86, 1997
25. Blum U, Voshage G, Beyersdorf F *et al.*: Two-center German experience with aortic endografting. *J Endovasc Surg* **4**: 137–146, 1997
26. Boyle JR, Thompson MM, Clode-Baker EG *et al.*: Torsion and kinking of unsupported aortic endografts: treatment by endovascular intervention. *J Endovasc Surg* **5**: 216–221, 1998
27. Walker SR, Braithwaite B, Tennant WG *et al.*: Early complications of femorofemoral crossover bypass grafts after aorta uni-iliac endovascular repair of abdominal aortic aneurysms. *J Vasc Surg* **28**: 647–650, 1998

Commentary

The Leicester Centre has knowledge of the building and deployment of aorto-uni-iliac systems and use their own method to great effect. The Leicester system was established in the early days and this centre can also be used for comments in terms of durability. The essential difference between the Leicester system and the Nottingham custom-built system is that with the Leicester system, those who learn the method are taught how to assemble the device. The group have mentioned that the system can be used for treating ruptured aneurysms. The approach to the blood vessels is rather different from the others, but they argue that it is relatively simple to get to the proximal external iliac artery through the extraperitoneal approach and that the whole procedure is simple once this access is achieved. *RMG*

WILL FUTURE DURABILITY OF XENOGRAFTS BE DIFFERENT?

Endothelial manipulation in xenografts

Punit S Ramrakha, Anthony Dorling and Robert I Lechler

INTRODUCTION

Despite the encouraging results from the use of primate organs for clinical xenotransplantation, most of the current attention is focused on the pig as the ideal donor for vascularized organs, for a variety of medical, practical, ethical and financial reasons.[1-3] However, when perfused with human blood, pig organs are rejected almost immediately, a process termed hyperacute rejection (HAR). Much effort has been devoted to elucidating the immunopathological basis of this florid reaction and several innovative therapies have emerged. Unfortunately, even if HAR is averted, other mechanisms of rejection ensue (Fig. 1).

There is a growing appreciation that the endothelium is the gatekeeper regulating the normal interactions of circulating leukocytes, platelets and blood components with tissue, controlling local immune and inflammatory reactions and the processes of vascular injury. When a vascularized xenograft is perfused, the recipient's circulating antibodies, complement and coagulation systems, platelets and leukocytes first encounter foreign antigens on the endothelium and it is here that the rejection response is initiated.[4] In this paper we propose to review what is known

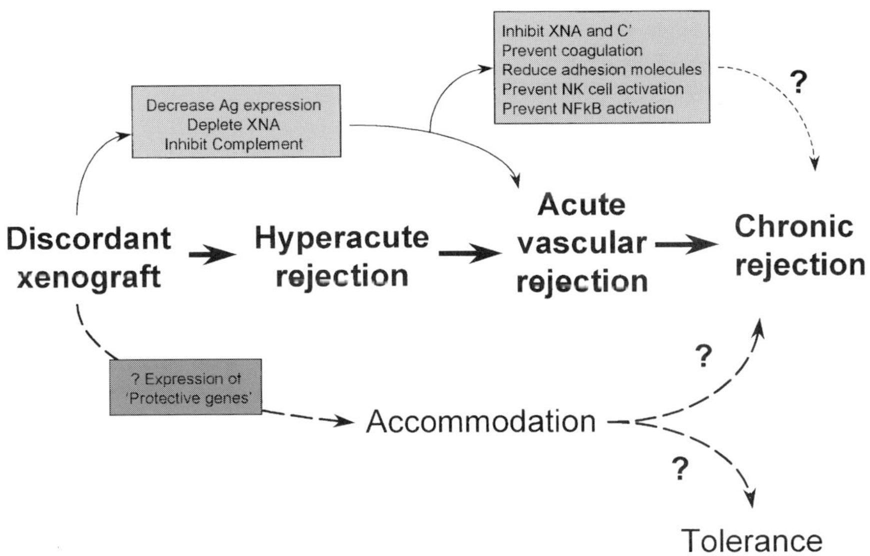

Fig. 1. Fate of discordant xenografts.

about the immunopathology of xenograft rejection. With this understanding comes the possibility of therapies to target the specific molecular mechanisms that precipitate graft destruction. Advances in molecular biology now provide us with the technology to genetically modify the donor animals to ameliorate the rejection response and we will discuss how manipulation of the endothelium may eventually help clinical xenotransplantation become a reality .

HYPERACUTE REJECTION

Perfusion of a pig organ with human blood initiates a cascade of events that results in rejection of the graft within a few minutes to a few hours. This process is associated with 'type I endothelial cell (EC) activation', a rapid change in phenotype, independent of protein synthesis, converting the normally quiescent lining of the vasculature to a pro-coagulant, pro-inflammatory interface. The cells alter in shape and retract, leading to loss of the integrity of the endothelium. Intercellular 'gaps' are created that expose tissue factor, the procoagulant receptor for coagulation factor VII/VIIa,[5] on the subendothelial matrix and provide a nidus for adhesion and aggregation of platelets. There is loss of heparan sulphate[6] and thrombomodulin from the endothelial cell surface, increased expression of P-selectin, and secretion of platelet activating factor and von Willebrand factor. Diffuse intravascular coagulation and thrombosis of the vasculature, haemorrhage, oedema and infarction of interstitial tissues results.[7,8] Over the past decade, the molecular mechanisms underlying this process have been dissected (Fig. 2). There appear to be two prerequisites for initiation of HAR:

1. binding of naturally occurring antibodies (xenoreactive natural antibodies, XNA) to carbohydrate antigens on the glycolipids and glycoproteins of the endothelial cells of the xenograft;
2. incompatibility of complement regulatory proteins of the donor species (pig) with the complement proteins of the recipient, allowing uncontrolled activation of the complement cascade.

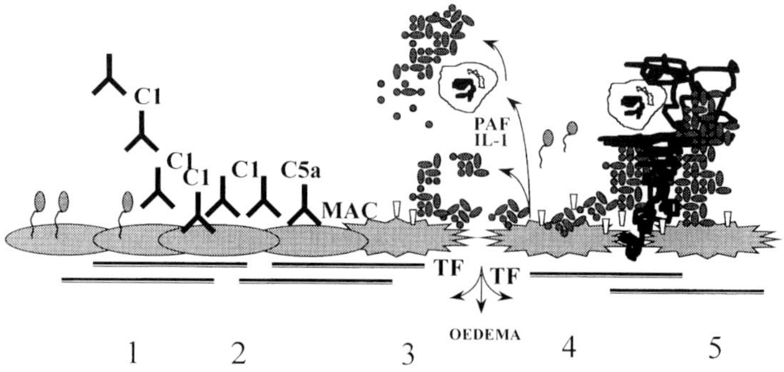

Fig. 2. Pathogenesis of hyperacute rejection.

Inhibition of either of these two events, either by manipulation of the recipient or donor, prior to transplantation, prevents hyperacute xenograft rejection.

Xenoreactive natural antibodies in hyperacute rejection

Old World primates and humans have high levels of pre-existing, 'natural' antibodies (XNA) that react with porcine cells, even in the absence of a known sensitizing event. It is now widely accepted that these XNA are pivotal in initiating HAR of discordant xenografts.[8] Organs undergoing HAR invariably contain immunoglobulin (IgM and IgG) of the recipient deposited along the endothelium, together with components of the classical pathway of complement.[9] Depletion of these antibodies by a variety of means prolongs xenograft survival, even when the complement system of the recipient remains intact,[9–11] and transplantation of a porcine organ into a neonate lacking XNA does not result in HAR.[12]

In attempts to avert HAR, a number of different methods to deplete the XNA have been used and have been shown to be effective, albeit temporarily, in preventing HAR. 'Disposable organ' immunoadsorption,[9] plasmapheresis,[13] infusion of anti-idiotype antibodies,[14] and anti-IgM antibodies,[15] have all been shown to avert HAR, but XNA reduction is temporary: as XNA levels return to normal, rejection of the xenograft is observed.

Identification of the antigenic target of the XNA has opened further avenues for potential therapies. Over 80% of the complement fixing XNA in human serum recognize a single structure – the unfucosylated, terminal non-reducing disaccharide of the aGal-linear B epitope, Galα1-3Galβ1-4GlcNAc-R,* commonly known as the Gal α(1,3)Gal epitope.[16,17] Humans and Old World primates are the only mammals that lack the enzyme α1-3 galactosyl transferase that produces this terminal linkage. It has been suggested that exposure to αGal antigen (e.g. on bacteria in the gastrointestinal tract) triggers the production of these 'natural' xenoantibodies, probably as a defence against these organisms. However, xenogeneic tissues from animals possessing α1,3 galactosyl transferase and expressing the Gal α(1,3)Gal epitope, such as pigs, will also be recognized by these antibodies.

Immunoadsorption through columns containing specific carbohydrates,[18] or systemic administration of synthetic carbohydrate[19] have been shown to prevent HAR. Peptide analogues that mimic Galα(1,3) Gal, identified by screening a bacteriophage display library with XNA,[20] may be used in a similar way. All these methods will certainly achieve short-term reduction in XNA titres but repeated treatments may be required, and it is likely that some form of immunosuppressive drug therapy, to suppress antibody production, will also be necessary.

Modification of the donor to remove the Galα(1,3) Gal epitope is an attractive alternative to these 'systemic' therapies. *In vitro* data suggests that perfusion of the grafts, prior to transplantation, with α-galactosidase is able to enzymatically cleave the carbohydrate epitopes from the endothelial cells, although the effect may only be temporary.[21,22] Genetic modification of the donor would allow more lasting inhibition.

*Abbreviations: Gal = galactose, GlcNAc = N-acetyl glucosmine, R = core structure.

The most logical solution, 'knock-out' of the α1-3 galactosyl transferase gene in the pig, is not as yet technically possible, as porcine embryonic stem cells have proven difficult to isolate. One approach is to overexpress, within the xenogeneic cells, a fucosyl transferase that will compete with α1-3 galactosyl transferase for N-acetyl lactosamine acceptor substrates. This diverts the precursors for Galα(1,3) gal synthesis towards other sugars. This approach decreases the expression of Galα(1,3) gal significantly and prolongs organ survival.[23,24] However, the multiple changes to the pattern of carbohydrate moieties displayed by the porcine cells transfected with fucosyl transferase may limit the utility of this approach. An alternative would be the use of anti-sense techniques to reduce the expression of α1,3 galactosyl transferase.[25] However, in addition to Galα(1,3) gal, XNA recognize other carbohydrate moieties and novel antigenic carbohydrate structures exposed may elicit a different range of antibodies.

Our group has concentrated on the application of a novel technique, 'intracellular knockout' by the expression, within the porcine endothelial cells, of an 'intrabody', an artificial, single-chain antibody,[26] which would target the ligand (the endothelial cell adhesion molecule) for degradation rather than expression on the cell surface. We have generated a number of constructs that target the expression of an α1,3 galactosyl transferase-specific, single-chain antibody, isolated from a synthetic, phage-display antibody library,[27] to the endoplasmic reticulum, fused to a C-terminal signal sequence that retain the antibodies within the endoplasmic reticulum.[28] When transfected into immortalized porcine endothelial cell this was effective in reducing the Galα(1,3) gal epitope expression (A Sepp, RI Lechler, unpublished).

Current estimates suggest that if used in isolation (with current immunosuppressive regimens), prevention of HAR requires over 80% sustained inhibition of the interaction of XNA and xenoantigens, and over 95% reduction may be required for the prevention of the subsequent stages of xenograft rejection.[29,30] Thus, either knock-out of the porcine α1-3 galactosyl transferase gene, or several complementary strategies to prevent expression of the Galα(1,3) gal epitope will be required.

However, depletion of XNA or inhibition of Galα(1,3) gal expression may not need to be permanent. In some circumstances, once HAR has been averted by XNA depletion (or other method), the graft continues to function despite the return of anti-donor antibody and complement back to pre-transplant levels, a phenomenon termed 'accommodation'.[7,8] The mechanisms underlying accommodation are far from clear but as will be discussed later, it may be possible, by genetic manipulation of the graft endothelium, to facilitate the induction of accommodation. This would permit graft survival even in the face of normal circulating levels of XNA.

Complement activation in hyperacute rejection

The development of HAR depends, absolutely, on the activation of complement in all the experimental models of discordant xenotransplantation. Pre-treatment of the recipient with cobra venom factor[31–34] or other anti-complement agents[35,36] prevents HAR, and recipients of xenografts deficient in certain complement components do not exhibit HAR.[37,38] Within minutes of exposure to human serum, XNA (primarily IgM) are deposited and initiate the activation of complement on porcine cells by the classical pathway (IgG XNA are deposited somewhat later than IgM and while they appear not to activate complement, they have been implicated in later phases of xenograft rejection[17,39]). Normally, complement activation and deposition on cells is controlled by membrane-associated regulators of complement activation (RCAs) such as CD55 (decay-accelerating factor), CD46 (membrane cofactor protein) and CD59. However, these appear to function in a species-specific manner; the RCAs of the pig appear to be less efficient than their human homologues in controlling activation of human complement.[40,41]

Once activated, the mechanism by which complement acts to promote HAR is still poorly understood. *Ex vivo* organ perfusion experiments have suggested that inhibiting C5 cleavage can effectively prevent HAR[42,43] suggesting that activation of complement components proximal to C5 in the cascade plays a minor role (if any) in the pathogenesis of HAR. Deposition of the membrane-attack-complex (C5b678) is detectable on porcine endothelium by immunofluorescence. However, lysis of endothelium, though seen in advanced lesions, is not a characteristic feature of HAR suggesting that the terminal complement components trigger HAR through non-cytolytic mechanisms.[44] Complement components appear to alter endothelial cell morphology and function with loss of the anticoagulant phenotype and expression of pro-inflammatory proteins, ultimately resulting in graft destruction.

Suppression of complement activation by manipulation of the recipient (treatment with cobra venom factor,[33,34] soluble complement receptor 1 or other synthetic anti-complement drugs[35,36]) prevents HAR, and prolongs survival of discordant xenografts. However, perhaps the most significant advance in preventing HAR has been the transgenic expression of human RCAs on xenogeneic cells. Transgenic mice expressing human decay accelerating factor and CD59,[45–48] and pigs expressing human decay accelerating factor, CD59 or both,[49–53] have been generated by a number of different groups. Although tissues and organs from these animals bind XNA normally, they are protected from HAR. Organs from decay accelerating factor-transgenic pigs survive up to 60 days in heavily immunosuppressed cynomologus monkeys, without histological evidence of rejection.[54]

It is unlikely that RCAs alone are the solution to the problems of discordant xenotransplantation. Analysis of the survival of xenografts from pigs transgenic for human RCAs has shown that with complement regulation, whereas even minor modulation of the antigens recognized by XNA (or XNA depletion) is effective in preventing HAR, effective prevention of later phases of xenograft rejection requires over 80% inhibition of the interaction of XNA and xenoantigens.[29] Thus, measures to genetically modify the expression of the Galα(1,3) Gal epitope discussed earlier, or strategies to induce accommodation of the endothelial cells to XNA and complement damage (see below), will undoubtedly also be required.

Platelet-endothelial interactions in hyperacute rejection

Under physiological conditions, platelets play an important role in the modulation of the interactions of the endothelium with other blood cells.[55] They release growth factors essential for the integrity of the endothelial monolayer and rapid, efficient clotting depends on platelet activation and aggregation. Endothelial cells regulate platelet aggregation by several mechanisms including release of prostacyclins, generation of nitric oxide, and the action of ecto-adenosine triphosphate (ATP) diphosphohydrolases (ATPDases / CD39) which degrade ATP and platelet-derived adenosine diphosphate (ADP), thus preventing amplification of platelet aggregation. The adenosine monophosphate (AMP) generated by these ecto-ATPDases serves as a substrate for 5′-nucleotidases and generates adenosine, an important platelet 'anti-activator' and vasodilator. In HAR, this carefully regulated system is disrupted and widespread platelet activation and aggregation occur.[56]

The early activation of endothelial cells is associated with expression of P-selectin and the production of platelet activating factor, a lipid mediator that promotes platelet aggregation.[57,58] Endothelial retraction exposes several ligands for platelet surface receptors in the subendothelial matrix including collagen and von Willebrand factor. Interaction of adhesive receptors on the platelet surface with collagen and fibronectin in the subendothelial matrix,[59,60] in concert with thrombin, enhances expression and affinity of platelet GP IIb/IIIa for von Willebrand factor and fibrin(ogen), promoting platelet aggregation.[61–63] Furthermore, there is an increase in P-selectin expression on the platelets promoting adhesion of leukocytes and platelets to the areas of injury, creating additional foci for coagulation.[64–66]

Cross-species polymorphisms in von Willebrand factor may also play a role. Interaction of platelet receptor GPIb with von Willebrand factor is normally highly dependent on shear stresses generated by blood flow.[60,62,67,68] However porcine von Willebrand factor appears to bind to human platelet GP Ib in the apparent absence of shear stress or vascular injury.[69] This and similar as yet uncharacterized interactions may be responsible for the widespread deposition of platelet microthrombi seen within the vasculature of the xenograft undergoing HAR.

Platelet activating factor antagonists prolong xenograft survival and prevent HAR,[58,70] and the combination of platelet activating factor antagonists and anti-P-selectin antibodies reduce platelet aggregation and infiltration of leukocytes into the xenograft in the first few hours after engraftment.[58] In addition, blocking of platelet aggregation with GPIIb/IIIa antagonists or by apyrase results in significant prolongation of xenograft survival.[71] However, each of these treatments results in only modest prolongation of graft survival suggesting that the role of platelets in HAR is secondary to that of XNA and complement.

Graft-specific regulation of platelet activation and aggregation may be achieved by genetically modifying the graft endothelial cell ecto-ATPDase expression. This enzyme not only inhibits platelet aggregation in response to ADP as discussed above, but also prevents platelet aggregation in response to collagen and thrombin.[72] Endothelial cell activation results in loss of ATPDase activity from the surface of porcine endothelial cells.[73] Furthermore, ATPDase activity on the surface of COS-7 cells transfected with the cDNA of human ATPDase was lost following exposure to oxidative stress.[72] By appropriate genetic engineering it may be possible to obtain stable expression of this enzyme on the endothelial cells of the donor organ in a form such that the enzymatic function is retained even in the post-transplant milieu.

DELAYED XENOGRAFT REJECTION

Once considered a daunting barrier for the clinical application of discordant xenotransplantation, HAR can now be averted using a combination of inhibitors of complement activation and inhibition of the XNA/Galα(1,3) Gal interaction. However, over the course of the following days, the xenograft is rejected by a process termed delayed xenograft rejection, sometimes called acute vascular rejection,[34] and occurs even in the absence of TCR$\alpha\beta^+$ cells.[74] This is characterized pathologically by diffuse intravascular coagulation, platelet aggregation, endothelial cell activation and interstitial inflammation with infiltration of host monocytes and natural killer cells into the rejecting organ.[34]

Activation of the vascular endothelium is a prominent feature, and this is now accepted as playing a pivotal role in the pathogenesis of delayed xenograft rejection.[5,75] Unlike type I activation seen in HAR, this type II endothelial cell activation involves transcriptional induction of certain genes and subsequent protein synthesis.[4,76,77] Phenotypically this is characterized by expression of tissue factor, the procoagulant receptor for coagulation factor VII/VIIa[5] and endothelial cell-specific adhesion receptors such as E-selectin.[78,79] In addition chemokines such as IL-8, a neutrophil and lymphocyte chemoattractant, and monocyte-chemoattractant protein membrane cofactor protein-1, are expressed by the activated endothelial cells.[80] Production of chemotactic cytokines by activated endothelium may explain the selective extravasation and activation of leukocytes, and may account for the nature of the cellular infiltrate observed. Upon encountering the foreign endothelium of the xenograft, circulating host monocytes adhere[81–84] and further activate the endothelium[80] thus amplifying the process. In addition, monocytes may exacerbate the already procoagulant environment of the activated vascular endothelium by expressing tissue factor[85] and by inducing the anti-fibrinolytic molecule plasminogen activator inhibitor type 1 in endothelial cells.[80]

As the pathogenesis of delayed xenograft rejection has been investigated, a variety of strategies have been proposed and tested, with varying success, to prevent this.

Xenoreactive natural antibodies and complement in delayed xenograft rejection

There is increasing evidence of the importance of both XNA and complement in the initiation of delayed xenograft rejection. Incomplete inhibition of XNA interactions results in deposition of antibodies with activation of complement (albeit in amounts insufficient to trigger HAR). IgM XNA have been shown to be capable of directly activating porcine endothelial cells, while IgG XNA act as a ligand for Fc-receptors on natural killer or other effector cells;[86] they may also possibly deliver signals for endothelial cell-activation via cell-membrane antigens that bear Galα(1,3) gal epitopes (such as integrins).[87,88] Furthermore, complement has been shown to trigger the synthesis and release of interleukin 1α (IL-1α) which acts in an autocrine and paracrine manner to promote endothelial cell activation.[89] IL-1α stimulates the production of endothelin-1[90] and thromboxane-A2,[91] potent vasoconstrictors that may reduce local blood flow and potentiate the effects of paracrine mediators and promote tissue ischaemia.

The encouraging reports of prolonged survival of decay accelerating factor-transgenic pig hearts transplanted into baboons suggest that controlling complement activation can delay the onset of delayed xenograft rejection significantly.[92] However, there is still evidence of endothelial cell activation in these organs, and this may be related to XNA deposition on the xenogeneic endothelium: depletion of XNA prevented acute vascular rejection of decay accelerating factor/CD59 transgenic porcine cardiac transplants by baboons.[29] Analysis of the survival of xenografts from pigs transgenic for human RCAs has shown that with complement regulation, effective prevention of delayed xenograft rejection requires over 80% inhibition of the interaction of XNA and xenoantigens. Thus measures to genetically modify the expression of Galα(1,3) Gal epitope discussed earlier are also relevant for delayed xenograft rejection.

Coagulation in delayed xenograft rejection

Vascular thrombosis is a prominent feature of xenograft rejection. Whereas platelet microthrombi are prominent in HAR, in delayed xenograft rejection, fibrin-rich microthrombi are a characteristic feature. The generation of thrombin is central to both the amplification of the coagulation process and to platelet aggregation. Modulation of the coagulation cascade, by selective inhibition of thrombin generation or activity may be expected to prolong xenograft survival.[64,65] Use of fibrinolytic agents, thrombin antagonists (D-Phe-Pro-Arg-CH_2Cl or PPACK), blockade of the thrombin receptor with peptide analogues,[93] or systemic administration of recombinant Kunitz-type serine protease inhibitors[94] may control the thrombotic manifestations of xenograft rejection. However, bleeding following systemic administration of these agents will clearly limit their use in the clinical setting. Genetic manipulation of the donor, to express inhibitors of coagulation, is a particularly attractive strategy to allow localized modulation of coagulation within the graft.

Thrombomodulin has been identified as one potential target for genetic intervention. Thrombomodulin is required for the generation of activated protein C, a potent anticoagulant and anti-inflammatory agent.[95] Porcine thrombomodulin on the endothelial cell surface is inefficient at generating activated, human protein C.[96] In addition, xenograft rejection is associated with the loss of thrombomodulin from the endothelial cell surface, by a combination of increased degradation and reduced transcription of the thrombomodulin gene. This functional anticoagulant deficiency in the activated protein C pathway can be reversed *in vitro* by the expression of human thrombomodulin in cultured porcine endothelial cells.[96] Furthermore, it is also possible to obtain supra-physiological expression of human thrombomodulin on the endothelial cell surface, which may well be required for successful xenotransplantation.

An alternative strategy that shows promise is the generation of artificial constructs of normally soluble anticoagulant proteins to anchor them to the endothelial cell membrane, providing a local anticoagulant effect. As discussed earlier, expression of tissue factor by both endothelial cells and infiltrating monocytes is a characteristic feature of delayed xenograft reaction. Tissue factor pathway inhibitor, a protease inhibitor, inhibits the enzyme activity of both factor Xa and the factor VIIa-tissue factor complex by the formation of a quaternary complex in a factor Xa-dependent manner,[97] thereby regulating the initial steps of the intrinsic pathway of coagulation. This is normally tethered to the endothelial cell surface by binding to heparan sulphate. The interaction of XNA and complement with porcine endothelial cells results in a rapid and substantial loss of heparan sulphate from the endothelial cells with loss of tissue factor pathway inhibitor.[6] Along with the observation that porcine tissue factor pathway inhibitor may not be fully interactive with components of the human coagulation cascade,[75] this may contribute significantly to the pro-coagulant environment of HAR and delayed xenograft rejection.

We have generated artificial constructs of human tissue factor pathway inhibitor fused with domains three and four and the carboxy-terminal sequence of human CD4. Transfection of these constructs into porcine endothelial cells results in high expression of tissue factor pathway inhibitor on the endothelial cell surface that is not lost after endothelial cell activation. Furthermore, the coagulation time of human plasma is significantly prolonged when tissue factor pathway inhibitor-CD4 transfectants are compared with control porcine endothelial cells.[98] We have extended these results to hirudin, the leech anticoagulant that is a potent inhibitor of thrombin, and generated constructs similarly fused to the membrane-proximal domains of CD4. The hirudin-CD4 construct, when transfected into porcine endothelial cells, resulted in significant prolongation of the clotting time of human plasma.[98] Combined expression of tissue factor pathway inhibitor and hirudin constructs produced an additive anticoagulant effect.[159] This strategy may be extended to other similar proteins including antithrombin III and fibrinolytics. The expression of these anticoagulant molecules will need to be carefully regulated to ensure that the donor animal retains an intact blood coagulation system, but expression can be 'turned on' immediately prior to transplantation and sustained in the recipient.

Leukocyte–endothelial interactions in delayed xenograft rejection

The first structure that circulating leukocytes come in contact with when blood reperfuses a vascularized graft is the endothelium. The leukocytes must adhere to and cross this endothelial barrier to infiltrate the graft. Recent advances in the understanding of the mechanisms of leukocyte-endothelial cell interactions have revealed a series of adhesion and activation events (the adhesion cascade) that take place during the emigration of leukocytes into tissues[99–101]

Initial rolling on vascular endothelium is mediated by transient interactions between selectins (e.g. L-selectin on leukocytes, E-selectin on activated endothelial cells and P-selectin on both activated endothelial cells and activated platelets) and carbohydrate-bearing counter-structures on the opposite cell (endothelial cells, leukocyte or platelet).[102] However, due to the high on/off rate of these selectin–carbohydrate interactions, this class of receptors cannot support firm adhesion of leukocytes. While rolling, leukocytes become exposed to activating signals which result in an increase in avidity of leukocyte surface integrins. Chemokines are thought to be the likely candidates for this triggering event.[103] This integrin-mediated secondary adhesion results in stable arrest of the leukocyte and is followed by transmigration into the tissues.[101,104] The interaction of vascular cell adhesion molecule (VCAM-1) on endothelial cells with its ligand, the $\alpha4\beta1$ integrin (very late antigen-4 [VLA-4]), on the leukocyte has recently been shown to be the predominant mechanism triggering arrest of rolling monocytes and lymphocytes, and subsequent spreading.[105,106] Transmigration through endothelial tight junctions involves platelet–endothelial cell adhesion molecule (PECAM, CD31), integrin associated protein (IAP, CD47) and integrin αvβ3.[107,108]

Quiescent vascular endothelium expresses an array of molecules that, according to current opinion, should not be sufficient to promote significant binding of leukocytes and subsequent transmigration. However, it is well established that peri-transplant organ ischaemia results in endothelial activation with increased expression of adhesion molecules. In the xenotransplant setting, as has been discussed already, there is widespread endothelial cells activation and adhesion molecule expression. There is a growing body of evidence showing that interfering with the recognition processes mediated by these adhesion molecules (in particular intercellular adhesion molecules (ICAM-1, ICAM-2), lymphocyte function associated antigen-1' (LFA-1), VCAM-1 and CD2) can significantly prolong allogeneic graft survival.[109–117] Furthermore, interfering with the recognition of adhesion molecules in the inductive phase of an immune response may even help to induce tolerance.[110]

Porcine endothelial cells have the capacity to mediate both the initial adhesion as well as the migration and activation of infiltrating human leukocytes[80,118–121] and antibodies against porcine adhesion molecules can inhibit this process.[122,123] Functional interactions between human LFA-1 and pig ICAM, and human VLA-4 and pig VCAM have been documented. Furthermore interaction of human monocytes with porcine endothelium also results in activation of the endothelial cells.[80] This is likely to promote trafficking of human lymphocytes and monocytes into a porcine xenograft and trigger rejection.

Xenotransplantation provides the opportunity to genetically modify the donor and allows the potential for graft-specific inhibition of this cellular rejection process. As mentioned above, targeted disruption or 'knockout' technology is not as yet available for pigs and may not even be desirable for certain endothelial cells adhesion molecules.[124] We have isolated several single chain antibodies against porcine VCAM from a phage display antibody library. These have been genetically engineered to target the expression of the single-chain antibody the endoplasmic reticulum with appropriate signals for retention in the endoplasmic reticulum.[28] These constructs are effective in reducing VCAM expression on immortalized porcine endothelial cells (PS Ramrakha, RI Lechler, unpublished). Our work has so far concentrated on the interaction of porcine VCAM with human VLA-4. However, analysis of the adhesion cascade predicts that inhibition of other molecular interactions should also result in inhibition of leukocyte migration into tissues. Single-chain antibody technology described here may be extended to other endothelial cell adhesion molecules such as ICAM, MAdCAM, PECAM, selectins (P-, L- and E-selectin), LFA-3, CD80/CD86 and thrombospondin. Which individual (or combination of) reagent(s) will be most effective in preventing leukocyte transmigration into the tissues remains to be determined.

Natural killer cells in delayed xenograft rejection

Natural killer cells, along with monocytes, are found in abundance in the cellular infiltrate characteristic of acute vascular rejection of discordant xenografts.[75] Human natural killer cells have been shown to lyse porcine endothelial cells by direct cell-cell contact with the target cell, and the addition of human XNA enhances cytotoxicity, by permitting binding of the natural killer cell Fc-receptor (FcγIII) and subsequent antibody-dependent cellular cytotoxicity.[86,125,126] Cell killing is predominantly by the release of perforin and granzymes, though the expression of Fas ligand by activated natural killer cells provides the potential for a perforin independent mechanism for cytotoxicity.[127,128] Cytotoxicity can be inhibited by major histocompatibility complex expression on the target cell[129,130] but the fact that human natural killer cells readily lyse porcine endothelial cells expressing porcine SLA Class I suggests that porcine class I is unable to interact with human natural killer inhibitory receptors.

Direct contact with human natural killer cells, even in the absence of XNA, induces endothelial cell activation with expression of E-selectin and chemokines (IL-8).[125] Human natural killer cells are activated when exposed to XNA bound to porcine endothelial cells, and secrete a variety of cytokines including interleukins (IL-1, IL-2, IL-3), granulocyte-monocyte colony stimulating factor (GM-CSF), interferons (IFN-α/β/γ), tumour necrosis factor alpha (TNF-α), and lymphotoxin.[131] Whereas IFN-γ and IL-1b are species specific, human TNF-α and lymphotoxin are able to activate porcine endothelial cells to express E-selectin and substantially increase the adherence of natural killer cells to porcine endothelial cells in culture.[118,125]

Treatment of the recipient with immunosuppressive drugs, monoclonal antibodies, lymphoid irradiation and plasmapheresis may all inhibit natural killer cell function and prolong graft survival, but at the cost of significant morbidity and mortality.[132] Attention has focused on genetic manipulation of the donor to inhibit the activation of recipient natural killer cells and subsequent graft destruction.

Strategies aimed at reducing the expression of Galα(1,3) gal expression will reduce the binding of XNA and may reduce natural killer cell mediated rejection. As our understanding of the complex relationship between activating and inhibitory signals through natural killer cell surface receptors grows, it may be possible to identify specific ligands for the inhibitory receptors (such as human major histocompatibility complex class I proteins[133] or single-chain antibodies) which when expressed on the surface of porcine cells will prevent natural killer cell mediated graft destruction.

Endothelial cell activation in delayed xenograft rejection

Endothelial cell activation appears to play a central role in xenotransplant rejection. Interaction of circulating blood components with the xenogeneic endothelial cell results in activation of both the endothelial cells, as well as adherent leukocytes, amplifying the interaction and promoting graft destruction. HAR is associated with an acute change in phenotype over minutes, whereas delayed xenograft rejection is associated with a slower, more sustained change, involving transcriptional induction of pro-inflammatory and pro-coagulant genes. NF-κB, a heterodimeric transcription factor, plays a pivotal role in the activation of essentially all of the genes involved in type II endothelial cell activation. This includes the genes for tissue factor, adhesion molecules (E-selectin, ICAM and VCAM), cytokines (IL-1 and IL-8) and others.[134] One approach to prevent xenograft rejection is to prevent the action of NF-κB and thus prevent type II endothelial cell activation.[135]

In quiescent cells, NF-κB is present in an inactive form in the cytoplasm due to its association with its regulatory counterpart IκB. Following stimuli for endothelial cell activation, IκB is degraded, allowing the NF-κB heterodimer to translocate to the nucleus to interact with the promoter regions of the genes mentioned above.[134,136] Overexpression of IκB in porcine endothelial cells results in sequestration of the NF-κB in the cytoplasm. The IκB-transfected endothelial cells are resistant to activation by lipopolysaccharide,[137] and to natural killer cell-mediated activation.[125] However, the endothelial cells appear to be sensitized to TNF-mediated apoptosis.[138] An alternative strategy that has been employed is the overexpression of a dominant negative mutant of the NF-κB subunit p65 (p65RHD) that lacks the transactivating domain.[139] This does not appear to sensitize the cells to TNF mediated apoptosis.[140] *In vivo* experiments to determine the effect of this manipulation in discordant xenotransplantation are underway.

A complementary strategy to prevent activation of NF-κB is overexpression of so called anti-apoptotic genes (e.g. A20, bcl-2, IL-1-converting enzyme inhibitors, CrmA, p35 or bcl-x_L). Expression of these genes not only prevented apoptosis in endothelial cells but also blocked activation of NF-κB and prevented up-regulation of the pro-inflammatory genes associated with type II endothelial cell activation.[141,142] There is also evidence that expression of these genes plays a role in accommodation.[143] If this is borne out by further investigation, it would allow for the return of XNA of the recipient and obviate the need for severe immunosuppression to prevent antibody synthesis.

T-CELL MEDIATED XENOGRAFT REJECTION

Even if HAR and delayed xenograft rejection are controlled, the next hurdle for survival of a xenograft is T cell mediated rejection. T cells may be sensitized to xenoantigens by either the direct or indirect pathway.[144] *In vitro* studies have demonstrated that porcine tissue promotes vigorous primary proliferative and cytotoxic responses from human T cells, signifying direct recognition of porcine histocompatibility antigens.[118,119,145–149] Recognition of processed porcine antigens via the indirect pathway is particularly strong; human T cells capable of recognizing porcine xenoantigens in association with 'self' major histocompatibility complex are over 100-fold more abundant than T cells that recognize human alloantigens via the indirect pathway.[145] Furthermore there is increasing evidence that these T cells are especially difficult to suppress using standard immunosuppressive regimes,[150,151] and alternative strategies to prevent T cell mediated xenograft rejection are necessary.

Several strategies to overcome or tolerize the direct xeno-response have been reviewed.[152] These include pre-treatment of the recipient with a combination of antibodies and cells to induce graft-specific tolerance, combined with treatment with antibodies to crucial co-stimulatory and accessory molecules. Expression of Fas ligand (FasL) on the endothelium may be another potential strategy. Interactions of Fas with its ligand (FasL) are thought to play a major role in the maintenance of tolerance and immunological homeostasis.[153–156] FasL expression is also the basis of the special status of immune-privileged sites.[157] In one report, co-transplantation of cells genetically engineered to express FasL with allogeneic islets prevented rejection of the islets.[158] Organs from animals transgenic for human FasL expression may be resistant to rejection, and endothelial cells may be one site for expression.

CONCLUSION

Over the past decade there have been several advances in our understanding of the mechanisms involved in rejection of discordant xenografts, and with this understanding comes the possibility of more precisely targeted therapies (Fig. 3). Furthermore, advances in molecular biology now provide us with the technology to genetically modify donor animals to ameliorate the rejection response. The endothelium is the first site where the recipient's circulating leukocytes, platelets and blood components first encounter xenoantigens. Evidence from both *in vitro* and *in vivo* experiments has demonstrated that modulation of this initial interaction is capable of averting xenograft rejection. However, as the pathogenesis of the xenograft rejection process is dissected and solutions found, further layers of complexity are uncovered. The optimal final regimen to allow successful pig-to-human xenotransplantation is likely to require a combination of genes expressed in the donor organ to provide a local therapeutic effect along with systemic administration of immune-modulating agents to the recipient.

HAR →	DXR →	Cellular rejection
Prevent binding of XNA - deplete XNA - decrease Galα(1,3) gal expression	Prevent XNA and complement deposition on endothelium	Prevent EC adhesion and co-stimulating molecule expression
Prevent complement activation - deplete complement in recipient - transgenic expression of RCAs	Prevent intravascular coagulation - expression of thrombomodulin - TFPI / hirudin constructs	Prevent T-cell activation
Prevent platelet aggregation - anti-platelet agents - expression of ecto-ATPDase	Prevent expression of EC adhesion molecules	
	Prevent activation of NK cells	
	Prevent EC activation - Inhibit NF-κB action - Overexpress 'anti-apoptotic' genes	

Fig. 3. Endothelial manipulation in xenotransplantation.

REFERENCES

1. Ramrakha PS, Lechler RI: Cardiac xenotransplantation: a pipe dream ? *Curr Med Lit (Cardiol)* **17**: 31–36, 1998
2. Ye Y, Niekrasz M, Kosanke S *et al.*: The pig as a potential organ donor for man. A study of potentially transferable disease from donor pig to recipient man. *Transplantation* **57**: 694–703, 1994
3. Michaels MG, Simmons RL: Xenotransplant-associated zoonoses. Strategies for prevention. *Transplantation* **57**: 1–7, 1994

4. Pober JS, Cotran RS: The role of endothelial cells in inflammation. *Transplantation* **50**: 537–544, 1990
5. Blakely ML, Van der Werf WJ, Berndt MC *et al.*: Activation of intragraft endothelial and mononuclear cells during discordant xenograft rejection. *Transplantation* **58**: 1059–1066, 1994
6. Platt JL, Vercellotti GM, Lindman BJ *et al.*: Release of heparan sulfate from endothelial cells. Implications for pathogenesis of hyperacute rejection. *J Exp Med* **171**(4): 1363–1368, 1990
7. Platt JL, Vercellotti GM, Dalmasso AP *et al.*: Transplantation of discordant xenografts: a review of progress. *Immunol Today* **11**: 450–456, 1990
8. Parker W, Saadi S, Lin SS *et al.*: Transplantation of discordant xenografts: a challenge revisited. *Immunol Today* **17**: 373–378, 1996
9. Platt JL, Fischel RJ, Matas AJ *et al.*: Immunopathology of hyperacute xenograft rejection in a swine-to-primate model. *Transplantation* **52**: 214–220, 1991
10. Cooper DK, Human PA, Lexer G *et al.*: Effects of cyclosporine and antibody adsorption on pig cardiac xenograft survival in the baboon. *J Heart Transpl* **7**: 238–246, 1988
11. Dalmasso AP, Vercellotti GM, Fischel RJ *et al.*: Mechanism of complement activation in the hyperacute rejection of porcine organs transplanted into primate recipients. *Am J Pathol* **140**: 1157–1166, 1992
12. Kaplon RJ, Michler RE, Xu H *et al.*: Absence of hyperacute rejection in newborn pig-to-baboon cardiac xenografts. *Transplantation* **59**: 1–6, 1995
13. Figueroa J, Fuad SA, Kunjummen BD *et al.*: Suppression of synthesis of natural antibodies by mycophenolate mofetil (RS-61443). Its potential use in discordant xenografting. *Transplantation* **55**: 1371–1374, 1993
14. Geller RL, Bach FH, Turman MA *et al.*: Evidence that polyreactive antibodies are deposited in rejected discordant xenografts. *Transplantation* **55**: 168–172, 1993
15. Soares MP, Latinne D, Elsen M *et al.*: *In vivo* depletion of xenoreactive natural antibodies with an anti-mu monoclonal antibody. *Transplantation* **56**: 1427–1433, 1993
16. Galili U, Macher BA, Buehler J, Shohet SB: Human natural anti-alpha-galactosyl IgG. II. The specific recognition of alpha (1–3)-linked galactose residues. *J Exp Med* **162**: 573–582, 1985
17. Parker W, Bruno D, Holzknecht ZE, Platt JL: Characterization and affinity isolation of xenoreactive human natural antibodies. *J Immunol* **153**: 3791–3803, 1994
18. Good AH, Cooper DK, Malcolm AJ *et al.*: Identification of carbohydrate structures that bind human antiporcine antibodies: implications for discordant xenografting in humans. *Transplant Proc* **24**: 559–562, 1992
19. Ye Y, Neethling FA, Niekrasz M *et al.*: Evidence that intravenously administered alpha-galactosyl carbohydrates reduce baboon serum cytotoxicity to pig kidney cells (PK15) and transplanted pig hearts. *Transplantation* **58**: 330–337, 1994
20. Kooyman DL, McClellan SB, Parker W *et al.*: Identification and characterization of a galactosyl peptide mimetic. Implications for use in removing xenoreactive anti-A Gal antibodies. *Transplantation* **61**: 851–855, 1996
21. Cotterell AH, Collins BH, Parker W *et al.*: The humoral immune response in humans following cross-perfusion of porcine organs. *Transplantation* **60**: 861–868, 1995
22. LaVecchio JA, Dunne AD, Edge AS: Enzymatic removal of alpha-galactosyl epitopes from porcine endothelial cells diminishes the cytotoxic effect of natural antibodies. *Transplantation* **60**: 841–847, 1995
23. Sepp A, Skacel P, Lindstedt R, Lechler RI: Expression of alpha-1,3-galactose and other type 2 oligosaccharide structures in a porcine endothelial cell line transfected with human alpha-1,2-fucosyltransferase cDNA. *J Biol Chem* **272**: 23104–23110, 1997
24. Sandrin MS, Fodor WL, Mouhtouris E *et al.*: Enzymatic remodelling of the carbohydrate surface of a xenogenic cell substantially reduces human antibody binding and complement-mediated cytolysis. *Nat Med* **1**: 1261–1267, 1995
25. Galili U: Interaction of the natural anti-Gal antibody with alpha-galactosyl epitopes: a major obstacle for xenotransplantation in humans. *Immunol Today* **14**: 480–482, 1993
26. Rondon IJ, Marasco WA: Intracellular antibodies (intrabodies) for gene therapy of infectious diseases. *Ann Rev Microbiol* **51**: 257–283, 1997

27. Richardson JH, Waldmann TA, Sodroski JG, Marasco WA: Inducible knockout of the interleukin-2 receptor alpha chain: expression of the high-affinity IL-2 receptor is not required for the *in vitro* growth of HTLV-I-transformed cell lines. *Virology* **237**: 209–216, 1997
28. Munro S, Pelham HR: A C-terminal signal prevents secretion of luminal ER proteins. *Cell* **48**: 899–907, 1987
29. Lin SS, Weidner BC, Byrne GW *et al.*: The role of antibodies in acute vascular rejection of pig-to-baboon cardiac transplants. *J Clin Invest* **101**: 1745–1756, 1998
30. Platt JL: Approaching clinical application of xenotransplantation. *J Card Surg* **12**: 285–293, 1997
31. Gewurz H, Clark DS, Cooper MD *et al.*: Effect of cobra venom-induced inhibition of complement activity on allograft and xenograft rejection reactions. *Transplantation* **5**: 1296–1303, 1967
32. Kemp E, Steinbruchel D, Starklint H *et al.*: Renal xenograft rejection: prolonging effect of captopril, ACE-inhibitors, prostacyclin, and cobra venom factor. *Transplant Proc* **19**: 4471–4474, 1987
33. Hayashi S, Ito M, Yokoyama I, Takagi H: Evidence that combination therapy using cobra venom factor, splenectomy, and deoxyspergualin is effective in guinea pig to rat cardiac xenotransplantation. *Transplantation* **57**: 777–779, 1994
34. Leventhal JR, Matas AJ, Sun LH *et al.*: The immunopathology of cardiac xenograft rejection in the guinea pig-to-rat model. *Transplantation* **56**: 1–8, 1993
35. Miyagawa S, Shirakura R, Matsumiya G *et al.*: Prolonging discordant xenograft survival with anticomplement reagents K76COOH and FUT175. *Transplantation* **55**: 709–713, 1993
36. Pruitt SK, Kirk AD, Bollinger RR *et al.*: The effect of soluble complement receptor type 1 on hyperacute rejection of porcine xenografts. *Transplantation* **57**: 363–370, 1994
37. O'Regan CC, Robitaille P, Pinto Blonde M, Chartrand C: Delayed rejection of cardiac xenografts in C6–deficient rabbits. *Immunology* **38**: 245–248, 1979
38. Zhow XJ, Niesen N, Pawlowski I *et al.*: Prolongation of survival of discordant kidney xenografts by C6 deficiency. *Transplantation* **50**: 896–898, 1990
39. Sandrin MS, Vaughan HA, Dabkowski PL, McKenzie IF: Anti-pig IgM antibodies in human serum react predominantly with Gal(alpha 1–3)Gal epitopes. *Proc Natl Acad Sci USA* **90**: 11391–11395, 1993
40. Miyagawa S, Hirose H, Shirakura R *et al.*: The mechanism of discordant xenograft rejection. *Transplantation* **46**: 825–830, 1988
41. Dalmasso AP, Vercellotti GM, Platt JL, Bach FH: Inhibition of complement-mediated endothelial cell cytotoxicity by decay-accelerating factor. Potential for prevention of xenograft hyperacute rejection. *Transplantation* **52**: 530–533, 1991
42. Kroshus TJ, Rollins SA, Dalmasso AP *et al.*: Complement inhibition with an anti-C5 monoclonal antibody prevents acute cardiac tissue injury in an *ex vivo* model of pig-to-human xenotransplantation. *Transplantation* **60**: 1194–1202, 1995
43. Rollins SA, Matis LA, Springhorn JP *et al.*: Monoclonal antibodies directed against human C5 and C8 block complement-mediated damage of xenogeneic cells and organs. *Transplantation* **60**: 1284–1292, 1995
44. Saadi S, Platt JL: Transient perturbation of endothelial integrity induced by natural antibodies and complement. *J Exp Med* **181**: 21–31, 1995
45. Byrne GW, McCurry KR, Kagan D *et al.*: Protection of xenogeneic cardiac endothelium from human complement by expression of CD59 or DAF in transgenic mice. *Transplantation* **60**: 1149–1156, 1995
46. McCurry KR, Kooyman DL, Diamond LE *et al.*: Transgenic expression of human complement regulatory proteins in mice results in diminished complement deposition during organ xenoperfusion. *Transplantation* **59**: 1177–1182, 1995
47. Somerville C, van Denderen B, Adam B *et al.*: Expression and function of human CD59 and human CD55 in transgenic mice. *Transplant Proc* **27**: 3565–3566, 1995
48. van Denderen BJ, Pearse MJ, Katerelos M *et al.*: Expression of functional decay-accelerating factor (CD55) in transgenic mice protects against human complement-mediated attack. *Transplantation* **61**: 582–588, 1996

49. Cozzi E, White DJ: The generation of transgenic pigs as potential organ donors for humans. *Nat Med* **1**: 964–966, 1995
50. Diamond LE, McCurry KR, Martin MJ *et al.*: Characterization of transgenic pigs expressing functionally active human CD59 on cardiac endothelium. *Transplantation* **61**: 1241–1249, 1996
51. Fodor WL, Williams BL, Matis LA *et al.*: Expression of a functional human complement inhibitor in a transgenic pig as a model for the prevention of xenogeneic hyperacute organ rejection. *Proc Natl Acad Sci USA* **91**: 11153–11157, 1994
52. McCurry KR, Kooyman DL, Alvarado CG *et al.*: Human complement regulatory proteins protect swine-to-primate cardiac xenografts from humoral injury. *Nat Med* **1**: 423–427, 1995
53. Rosengard AM, Cary NR, Langford GA *et al.*: Tissue expression of human complement inhibitor, decay-accelerating factor, in transgenic pigs. A potential approach for preventing xenograft rejection. *Transplantation* **59**: 1325–1333, 1995
54. White DJG: hDAF transgenic pig organs: are they concordant for human transplantation. *Xeno* **4**: 50–54, 1996
55. Marcus AJ, Safier LB: Thromboregulation: multicellular modulation of platelet reactivity in hemostasis and thrombosis. *FASEB J* **7**: 516–522, 1993
56. Robson SC, Kopp C, Lesnikoski B: Platelets and xenograft rejection. *Xeno* **2**: 38–46, 1994
57. Prescott SM, Zimmerman GA, McIntyre TM: Human endothelial cells in culture produce platelet-activating factor (1-alkyl-2-acetyl-sn-glycero-3-phosphocholine) when stimulated with thrombin. *Proc Natl Acad Sci USA* **81**: 3534–3538, 1984
58. Coughlan AF, Berndt MC, Dunlop LC, Hancock WW: *In vivo* studies of P-selectin and platelet activating factor during endotoxemia, accelerated allograft rejection, and discordant xenograft rejection. *Transplant Proc* **25**: 2930–2931, 1993
59. Hynes RO: Integrins: versatility, modulation, and signaling in cell adhesion. *Cell* **69**: 11–25, 1992
60. Roth GJ: Platelets and blood vessels: the adhesion event. *Immunol Today* **13**: 100–105, 1992
61. Smyth SS, Joneckis CC, Parise LV: Regulation of vascular integrins. [published erratum appears in *Blood* **83**: 2013, 1994]. *Blood* **81**: 2827–2843, 1993
62. Ruggeri ZM, Ware J: von Willebrand factor. *FASEB J* **7**: 308–316, 1993
63. Kroll MH, Harris TS, Moake JL *et al.*: von Willebrand factor binding to platelet GpIb initiates signals for platelet activation. *J Clin Invest* **88**: 1568–1573, 1991
64. Furie B, Furie BC: Molecular and cellular biology of blood coagulation. *New Engl J Med* **326**: 800–806, 1992
65. Esmon CT: Cell mediated events that control blood coagulation and vascular injury. *Ann Rev Cell Biol* **9**: 1–26, 1993
66. Edwards RL, Rickles FR: The role of leukocytes in the activation of blood coagulation. *Semin Hematol* **29**: 202–212, 1992
67. Chow TW, Hellums JD, Moake JL, Kroll MH: Shear stress-induced von Willebrand factor binding to platelet glycoprotein Ib initiates calcium influx associated with aggregation. *Blood* **80**: 113–120, 1992
68. Savage B, Shattil SJ, Ruggeri ZM: Modulation of platelet function through adhesion receptors. A dual role for glycoprotein IIb-IIIa (integrin alpha IIb beta 3) mediated by fibrinogen and glycoprotein Ib-von Willebrand factor. *J Biol Chem* **267**: 11300–11306, 1992
69. Legrand C, Thibert V, Dubernard V *et al.*: Molecular requirements for the interaction of thrombospondin with thrombin-activated human platelets: modulation of platelet aggregation. *Blood* **79**: 1995–2003, 1992
70. Makowka L, Chapman FA, Cramer DV *et al.*: Platelet-activating factor and hyperacute rejection. The effect of a platelet-activating factor antagonist, SRI 63–441, on rejection of xenografts and allografts in sensitized hosts. *Transplantation* **50**: 359–365, 1990
71. Candinas D, Lesnikoski BA, Hancock WW *et al.*: Inhibition of platelet integrin GPIIbIIIa prolongs survival of discordant cardiac xenografts. *Transplantation* **62**: 1–5, 1996
72. Kaczmarek E, Koziak K, Sevigny J *et al.*: Identification and characterization of CD39/vascular ATP diphosphohydrolase. *J Biol Chem* **271**: 33116–33122, 1996
73. Robson SC, Kaczmarek E, Siegel JB *et al.*: Loss of ATP diphosphohydrolase activity with endothelial cell activation. *J Exp Med* **185**: 153–163, 1997

74. Candinas D, Belliveau S, Koyamada N *et al.*: T cell independence of macrophage and natural killer cell infiltration, cytokine production, and endothelial activation during delayed xenograft rejection. *Transplantation* **62**: 1920–1927, 1996
75. Bach FH, Winkler H, Ferran C *et al.*: Delayed xenograft rejection. *Immunol Today* **17**: 379–384, 1996
76. Pober JS, Cotran RS: Cytokines and endothelial cell biology. *Physiol Rev* **70**: 427–451, 1990
77. Cotran RS, Pober JS: Effects of cytokines on vascular endothelium: their role in vascular and immune injury. *Kidney Int* **35**: 969–975, 1989
78. Bevilacqua MP, Stengelin S, Gimbrone MA Jr, Seed B: Endothelial leukocyte adhesion molecule 1: an inducible receptor for neutrophils related to complement regulatory proteins and lectins. *Science* **243**: 1160–1165, 1989
79. Ferran C, Peuchmaur M, Desruennes M *et al.*: Implications of *de novo* ELAM-1 and VCAM-1 expression in human cardiac allograft rejection. *Transplantation* **55**: 605–609, 1993
80. Millan MT, Geczy C, Stuhlmeier KM *et al.*: Human monocytes activate porcine endothelial cells, resulting in increased E-selectin, interleukin-8, monocyte chemotactic protein-1, and plasminogen activator inhibitor-type-1 expression. *Transplantation* **63**: 421–429, 1997
81. DiCorleto PE, de la Motte CA: Characterization of the adhesion of the human monocytic cell line U937 to cultured endothelial cells. *J Clin Invest* **75**: 1153–1161, 1985
82. Beekhuizen H, Corsel van Tilburg AJ, van Furth R: Characterization of monocyte adherence to human macrovascular and microvascular endothelial cells. *J Immunol* **145**: 510–518, 1990
83. Beekhuizen H, van Furth R: Monocyte adherence to human vascular endothelium. *J Leukoc Biol* **54**: 363–378, 1993
84. Wang J, Beekhuizen H, van Furth R: Surface molecules involved in the adherence of recombinant interferon-gamma (rIFN-gamma)-stimulated human monocytes to vascular endothelial cells. *Clin Exp Immunol* **95**: 263–269, 1994
85. Edgington TS, Mackman N, Brand K, Ruf W: The structural biology of expression and function of tissue factor. *Thromb Haemost* **66**: 67–79, 1991
86. Inverardi L, Samaja M, Motterlini R *et al.*: Early recognition of a discordant xenogeneic organ by human circulating lymphocytes. *J Immunol* **149**: 1416–1423, 1992
87. Holzknecht ZE, Platt JL: Identification of porcine endothelial cell membrane antigens recognized by human xenoreactive natural antibodies. *J Immunol* **154**: 4565–4575, 1995
88. Lampugnani MG, Resnati M, Dejana E, Marchisio PC: The role of integrins in the maintenance of endothelial monolayer integrity. *J Cell Biol* **112**: 479–490, 1991
89. Saadi S, Holzknecht RA, Patte CP *et al.*: Complement-mediated regulation of tissue factor activity in endothelium. *J Exp Med* **182**: 1807–1814, 1995
90. Yoshizumi M, Kurihara H, Morita T *et al.*: Interleukin 1 increases the production of endothelin-1 by cultured endothelial cells. *Biochem Biophys Res Commun* **166**: 324–329, 1990
91. Conti P, Cifone MG, Alesse E *et al.*: *In vitro* enhanced thromboxane B2 release by polymorphonuclear leukocytes and macrophages after treatment with human recombinant interleukin 1. *Prostaglandins* **32**: 111–115, 1986
92. Zaidi A, Schmoeckel M, Bhatti F *et al.*: Life-supporting pig-to-primate renal xenotransplantation using genetically modified donors. *Transplantation* **65**: 1584–1590, 1998
93. Maraganore JM: Thrombin, thrombin inhibitors, and the arterial thrombotic process. *Thromb Haemost* **70**: 208–211, 1993
94. Jakobs FM, Davis EA, White T *et al.*: Prolonged discordant xenograft survival by inhibition of the intrinsic coagulation pathway in complement C6–deficient recipients. *J Heart Lung Transplant* **17**: 306–311, 1998
95. Grey ST, Tsuchida A, Hau H *et al.*: Selective inhibitory effects of the anticoagulant activated protein C on the responses of human mononuclear phagocytes to LPS, IFN-gamma, or phorbol ester. *J Immunol* **153**: 3664–3672, 1994
96. Kopp CW, Grey ST, Siegel JB *et al.*: Expression of human thrombomodulin cofactor activity in porcine endothelial cells. *Transplantation* **66**: 244–251, 1998
97. Girard TJ, Broze GJ Jr: Tissue factor pathway inhibitor. *Methods Enzymol* **222**: 195–209, 1993

98. Riesbeck K, Dorling A, Kemball Cook G *et al.*: Human tissue factor pathway inhibitor fused to CD4 binds both FXa and TF/FVIIa at the cell surface. *Thromb Haemost* **78**: 1488–1494, 1997
99. Bevilacqua MP: Endothelial-leukocyte adhesion molecules. *Ann Rev Immunol* **11**: 767–804, 1993
100. Butcher EC: Leukocyte-endothelial cell recognition: three (or more) steps to specificity and diversity. *Cell* **67**: 1033–1036, 1991
101. Springer TA: Traffic signals for lymphocyte recirculation and leukocyte emigration: the multistep paradigm. *Cell* **76**: 301–314, 1994
102. Tedder TF, Steeber DA, Chen A, Engel P: The selectins: vascular adhesion molecules. *FASEB J* **9**: 866–873, 1995
103. Tanaka Y, Adams DH, Shaw S: Proteoglycans on endothelial cells present adhesion-inducing cytokines to leukocytes. *Immunol Today* **14**: 111–115, 1993
104. Carlos TM, Harlan JM: Leukocyte-endothelial adhesion molecules. *Blood* **84**: 2068–2101, 1994
105. Jones DA, McIntire LV, Smith CW, Picker LJ: A two-step adhesion cascade for T cell/endothelial cell interactions under flow conditions. *J Clin Invest* **94**: 2443–2450, 1994
106. Alon R, Kassner PD, Carr MW *et al.*: The integrin VLA-4 supports tethering and rolling in flow on VCAM-1. *J Cell Biol* **128**: 1243–1253, 1995
107. Muller WA: The role of PECAM-1 (CD31) in leukocyte emigration: studies *in vitro* and *in vivo*. *J Leukoc Biol* **57**: 523–528, 1995
108. Brown EJ, Lindberg FP: Leucocyte adhesion molecules in host defence against infection. *Ann Med* **28**: 201–208, 1996
109. van Dijken PJ, Ghayur T, Mauch P *et al.*: Evidence that anti-LFA-1 *in vivo* improves engraftment and survival after allogeneic bone marrow transplantation. *Transplantation* **49**: 882–886, 1990
110. Isobe M, Yagita H, Okumura K, Ihara A: Specific acceptance of cardiac allograft after treatment with antibodies to ICAM-1 and LFA-1. *Science* **255**: 1125–1127, 1992
111. Berlin PJ, Bacher JD, Sharrow SO *et al.*: Monoclonal antibodies against human T cell adhesion molecules–modulation of immune function in nonhuman primates. *Transplantation* **53**: 840–849, 1992
112. Fischer A, Griscelli C, Blanche S *et al.*: Prevention of graft failure by an anti-HLFA-1 monoclonal antibody in HLA-mismatched bone-marrow transplantation. *Lancet* **ii**: 1058–1061, 1986
113. Le Mauff B, Hourmant M, Rougier JP *et al.*: Effect of anti-LFA1 (CD11a) monoclonal antibodies in acute rejection in human kidney transplantation. *Transplantation* **52**: 291–296, 1991
114. Kameoka H, Ishibashi M, Tamatani T *et al.*: The immunosuppressive action of anti-CD18 monoclonal antibody in rat heterotopic heart allotransplantation. *Transplantation* **55**: 665–667, 1993
115. Byrne JG, Smith WJ, Murphy MP *et al.*: Complete prevention of myocardial stunning, contracture, low-reflow, and edema after heart transplantation by blocking neutrophil adhesion molecules during reperfusion. *J Thorac Cardiovasc Surg* **104**: 1589–1596, 1992
116. Cosimi AB, Conti D, Delmonico FL *et al.*: *In vivo* effects of monoclonal antibody to ICAM-1 (CD54) in nonhuman primates with renal allografts. *J Immunol* **144**: 4604–4612, 1990
117. Orosz CG, Ohye RG, Pelletier RP *et al.*: Treatment with anti-vascular cell adhesion molecule 1 monoclonal antibody induces long-term murine cardiac allograft acceptance. *Transplantation* **56**: 453–460, 1993
118. Murray AG, Khodadoust MM, Pober JS, Bothwell AL: Porcine aortic endothelial cells activate human T cells: direct presentation of MHC antigens and costimulation by ligands for human CD2 and CD28. *Immunity* **1**: 57–63, 1994
119. Rollins SA, Kennedy SP, Chodera AJ *et al.*: Evidence that activation of human T cells by porcine endothelium involves direct recognition of porcine SLA and costimulation by porcine ligands for LFA-1 and CD2. *Transplantation* **57**: 1709–1716, 1994
120. Pleass HC, Forsythe JL, Proud G *et al.*: Xenotransplantation: an examination of the

adhesive interactions between human lymphocytes and porcine renal epithelial cells. *Transpl Immunol* **2**: 225–230, 1994
121. Dorling A, Lechler RI: Prospects for xenografting. *Curr Opin Immunol* **6**: 765–769, 1994
122. Dorling A, Stocker C, Tsao T *et al.*: *In vitro* accommodation of immortalized porcine endothelial cells: resistance to complement mediated lysis and down-regulation of VCAM expression induced by low concentrations of polyclonal human IgG antipig antibodies. *Transplantation* **62**: 1127–1136, 1996
123. Mueller JP, Evans MJ, Cofiell R *et al.*: Porcine vascular cell adhesion molecule (VCAM) mediates endothelial cell adhesion to human T cells. Development of blocking antibodies specific for porcine VCAM. *Transplantation* **60**: 1299–1306, 1995
124. Gurtner GC, Davis V, Li H *et al.*: Targeted disruption of the murine VCAM1 gene: essential role of VCAM-1 in chorioallantoic fusion and placentation. *Genes Dev* **9**: 1–14, 1995
125. Goodman DJ, Von Albertini M, Willson A *et al.*: Direct activation of porcine endothelial cells by human natural killer cells. *Transplantation* **61**: 763–771, 1996
126. Schaapherder AF, Daha MR, te Bulte MT *et al.*: Antibody-dependent cell-mediated cytotoxicity against porcine endothelium induced by a majority of human sera. *Transplantation* **57**: 1376–1382, 1994
127. Kagi D, Ledermann B, Burki K *et al.*: Cytotoxicity mediated by T cells and natural killer cells is greatly impaired in perforin-deficient mice. *Nature* **369**: 31–37, 1994
128. Kagi D, Vignaux F, Ledermann B *et al.*: Fas and perforin pathways as major mechanisms of T cell-mediated cytotoxicity. *Science* **265**: 528–530, 1994
129. Lanier LL, Phillips JH: Inhibitory MHC class I receptors on NK cells and T cells. *Immunol Today* **17**: 86–91, 1996
130. Lanier LL: NK cell receptors. *Ann Rev Immunol* **16**: 359–393, 1998
131. Robertson MJ, Ritz J: Biology and clinical relevance of human natural killer cells. *Blood* **76**: 2421–2438, 1990
132. Loughran TP Jr, Deeg HJ, Storb R: Inhibition of canine NK activity by anti-CD18 monoclonal antibody, UV irradiation and cyclosporine. *Exp Hematol* **21**: 411–413, 1993
133. Seebach JD, Comrack C, Germana S *et al.*: HLA-Cw3 expression on porcine endothelial cells protects against xenogeneic cytotoxicity mediated by a subset of human NK cells. *J Immunol* **159**: 3655–3661, 1997
134. Baeuerle PA, Henkel T: Function and activation of NF-kappa B in the immune system. *Ann Rev Immunol* **12**: 141–179, 1994
135. Bach FH, Robson SC, Ferran C *et al.*: Endothelial cell activation and thromboregulation during xenograft rejection. *Immunol Rev* **141**: 5–30, 1994
136. Siebenlist U, Franzoso G, Brown K: Structure, regulation and function of NF-kappa B. *Ann Rev Cell Biol* **10**: 405–455, 1994
137. Wrighton CJ, Hofer Warbinek R, Moll T *et al.*: Inhibition of endothelial cell activation by adenovirus-mediated expression of I kappa B alpha, an inhibitor of the transcription factor NF-kappa B. *J Exp Med* **183**: 1013–1022, 1996
138. Wrighton CJ, McShea A, deMartin R *et al.*: Prevention of NF-κB activtion in porcine aortic endothelial cells renders them sensitive to TNFα-induced programmed cell death. (Abstract) *Third Int Congr Xenotransplantation Boston, MA*, 1995.
139. Anrather J, Csizmadia V, Brostjan C *et al.*: Inhibition of bovine endothelial cell activation in vitro by regulated expression of a transdominant inhibitor of NF-kappa B. *J Clin Invest* **99**: 763–772, 1997
140. Soares M, Anrather J, Kaczmarek E *et al.*: Inhibition of endothelial cell activation by adenovirus mediated overexpression of a transdominant mutant of relA does not sensitize to TNF-α mediated apoptosis. (Abstract) *Fourth Intl Congr Xenotransplantation Nantes, France*, 1997: O17.
141. Cooper JT, Stroka DM, Brostjan C *et al.*: A20 blocks endothelial cell activation through a NF-kappaB-dependent mechanism. *J Biol Chem* **271**: 18068–18073, 1996
142. Ferran C, Stroka DM, Badrichani AZ *et al.*: A20 inhibits NF-kappaB activation in endothelial cells without sensitizing to tumor necrosis factor-mediated apoptosis. *Blood* **91**: 2249–2258, 1998

143. Bach FH, Ferran C, Hechenleitner P *et al.*: Accommodation of vascularized xenografts: expression of 'protective genes' by donor endothelial cells in a host Th2 cytokine environment. *Nat Med* **3**: 196–204, 1997
144. Dorling A, Lechler RI: The passenger leukocyte, dendritic cell and antigen-presenting cells (APC). In: Tilney NL, Strom TB, Paul LC (Eds), *Transplantation Biology; Cellular and Molecular Aspects*. Philadelphia: Lippincott-Raven, 1996
145. Dorling A, Lombardi G, Binns R, Lechler RI: Detection of primary direct and indirect human anti-porcine T cell responses using a porcine dendritic cell population. *Eur-J-Immunol* **26**: 1378–1387, 1996
146. Kirk AD, Li RA, Kinch MS *et al.*: The human antiporcine cellular repertoire. *In vitro* studies of acquired and innate cellular responsiveness. *Transplantation* **55**: 924–931, 1993
147. Bravery CA, Batten P, Yacoub MH, Rose ML: Direct recognition of SLA- and HLA-like class II antigens on porcine endothelium by human T cells results in T cell activation and release of interleukin-2. *Transplantation* **60**: 1024–1033, 1995
148. Yamada K, Sachs DH, DerSimonian H: Human anti-porcine xenogeneic T cell response. Evidence for allelic specificity of mixed leukocyte reaction and for both direct and indirect pathways of recognition. *J Immunol* **155**: 5249–5256, 1995
149. Lucas PJ, Shearer GM, Neudorf S, Gress RE: The human antimurine xenogeneic cytotoxic response. I. Dependence on responder antigen-presenting cells. *J Immunol* **144**: 4548–4554, 1990
150. Auchincloss H Jr, Sachs DH: Xenogeneic transplantation. *Ann Rev Immunol* **16**: 433–470, 1998
151. Auchincloss H Jr: Why is cell-mediated xenograft rejection so strong? *Xeno* **3**: 19–22, 1995
152. Dorling A, Riesbeck K, Lechler RI: The T-cell response to xenografts: molecular interactions and graft specific immunosuppression. *Xeno* **4**: 68–76, 1996
153. Yagita H, Hanabuchi S, Asano Y *et al.*: Fas-mediated cytotoxicity–a new immunoregulatory and pathogenic function of Th1 CD4+ T cells. *Immunol Rev* **146**: 223–239, 1995
154. Golstein P, Marguet D, Depraetere V: Fas bridging cell death and cytotoxicity: the reaper connection. *Immunol Rev* **146**: 45–56, 1995
155. Lynch DH, Ramsdell F, Alderson MR: Fas and FasL in the homeostatic regulation of immune responses. *Immunol Today* **16**: 569–574, 1995
156. Nagata S: Fas and Fas ligand: a death factor and its receptor. *Adv Immunol* **57**: 129–144, 1994
157. Bellgrau D, Gold D, Selawry H *et al.*: A role for CD95 ligand in preventing graft rejection. *Nature* **377**: 630–632, 1995
158. Lau HT, Yu M, Fontana A, Stoeckert CJ Jr: Prevention of isl*et al*lograft rejection with engineered myoblasts expressing FasL in mice. *Science* **273**: 109–112, 1996
159. Riesbeck K, Chen D, Kemball-Cook G *et al.* Expression of hirudin fusion proteins in mammalian cells: a strategy for prevention of intravascular thrombosis. *Circulation* **98**: 2744–2752, 1998

Commentary

Surgeons are skilled in the use of a variety of materials for vascular reconstruction procedures. In large diameter vessels, e.g. the aorta, Dacron and its derivatives are used. For reconstruction of small diameter arteries, autologous conduits, particularly saphenous vein are used. Where no autologous vein is available small bore conduits of polytetrafluorethylene and other man-made materials may be used. In the very difficult situations of infected aortic grafts or aortoenteric fistula, cyopreserved homografts have been used with some success.[1] Homografts have also been used for femorodistal reconstruction, these grafts including glutaraldehyde-tanned umbilical vein (Dardik Biograft) and crypopreserved saphenous vein.[2,3] Historically, glutaraldehyde-fixed heterografts have been tested and bovine aortic grafts remain on the marketplace. Do vascular surgeons need the development of new grafts, including xenografts? If the early process of hyperacute rejection can be resolved by manipulation of the endothelium, will longer-term immunological problems arise, to diminish the mechanical strength of the graft?

There are at least two situations where vascular surgeons might welcome the availability of xenografts. I have already referred to the first situation, where a major vascular infection leads to a communication between the aorta, or an aortic prosthesis, and the bowel, oesophagus or lung. Current surgical treatments of aorta-enteric fistulae are associated with a very high mortality rate.[4] Fresh arterial allografts for the correction of aortoenteric fistulae have been attempted, but abandoned because of the late complications of graft dilatation and rupture.[5] Graft dilatation and rupture also has proved a serious problem associated with placement of Dardik grafts for infrainguinal reconstruction.[6] In both these situations, it appears as though an immune response against the connective tissue framework of the grafts developed.

The second situation where xenografts could be advantageous is for femorodistal reconstructions where no autologous vein is available and the distal anastomosis has to be below the knee. Prothetic grafts which cross the knee have miserable 1-year patency rates: ~ 50%.[7] Some surgeons will seek and use brachiocephalic vein for distal reconstructions, if saphenous vein is unavailable. The use of cephalic vein for coronary artery bypass surgery has gained a poor reputation, but for revascularization of the leg, arm vein bypass grafts have been reported to have a 1-year patency of 74%.[8] However, in many patients the arm veins may have been damaged by repeated venepuncture. Where the distal anastomosis lies below the knee, cryopreserved vein homografts used to alleviate critical ischaemia had a 1-year patency rate of 68%.[3] Biodegradation of these grafts is common, with aneurysms being found in 58% of grafts after 5 years. Late aneurysmal dilatation complicates the long-term function of all non-autologous grafts of biological origin. Why?

The extracellular matrix is a critical component of blood vessels, contributing to mechanical strength, determining elasticity, guiding cell migration, controlling the phenotype of the cellular elements and influencing cell–cell communications. There is important evidence to indicate that in arterial xenografts the extracellular matrix is immunogenic. Allaire and colleagues have investigated the function of decellularized arterial allografts and xenografts.[9,10] Using rats these workers have shown that allograft immunologic injury and subsequent remodelling was dependent on the presence of arterial wall cells.[9] In arterial xenografts (guinea pig to rat), which had been decellularized, after 8 weeks the grafts were aneurysmal.[10] These aneurysmal grafts had been invaded by macrophages and T cells, with deposition of immunoglobulins and histological evidence of elastin resorption. In contrast for decellularized rat allografts, the media was devoid of inflammatory cells, with intact elastic lamallae after 8 weeks. This is important evidence to indicate that immunological injury to the connective tissue of arterial xenografts is likely to cause aneurysmal dilatation.

Vascular surgeons have built up considerable experience of the use of biological grafts in man. Their rich combined experience should sound a warning note to those pushing forward the barriers to xenotransplantation. Beware of late aneurysmal dilatation resulting from direct immunological injury to the connective tissue. *JTP*

References

1. Vogt RR, Pfammetter T, Schlumpf R *et al.*: *In situ* repair or aortobronchial, aortoesophageal and aortoenteric fistulae with cryopreserved homografts. *J Vasc Surg* **26**: 11–17, 1997
2. Dardik H, Ibrahim IM, Darkik I: Evaluation of glutaraldehyde-tanned human umbilical cord vein as a vascular prosthesis for bypass to the popliteal tibial and peroneal arteries. *Surgery* **83**: 577–588, 1978
3. Van Reet Dortlund RWH, van Leeuwen MS, Steijling JJF *et al.*: Long-term results with vein homograft in femoro-distal reconstructions. *Eur J Vasc Surg* **5**: 557–564, 1991
4. Bahnini A, Plissonier D, Koskas F, Kieffer E: Traitement des fistules protheto-digestives par allogreffe arterielle. *J Med Vasc* **21**: 167–170, 1996
5. Szilagyi DE, Rodgriguez FJ, Smith FR, Elliott JP: Late fate of arterial allografts: observation 6–15 years after implantation. *Arch Surg* **101**: 721–733, 1970
6. Boontje AH: Aneurysm formation in human umbilical vein grafts used as arterial substitutes. *J Vasc Surg* **2**: 524–529, 1985
7. McCollum C, Kenchington G, Alexander C *et al.*: PTFE or HUV for femoropopliteal bypass: a multi-centre trial. *Eur J Vasc Surg* **5**: 435–443, 1991
8. Andros G, Harris RW, Salles-Cunha SK *et al.*: Arm veins for arterial revascularization of the leg: Arteriographic and clinical observations. *J Vasc Surg* **4**: 416–427, 1986
9. Allaire E, Guettier C, Bruneval P *et al.*: Cell-free arterial grafts: morphologic characteristics of aortic isografts, allografts and xenografts in rats. *J Vasc Surg* **19**: 446–456, 1994
10. Allaire E, Bruneval P, Mandet C *et al.*: The immunogenicity of the extracellular matrix in arterial xenografts. *Surgery* **122**: 73–81, 1997

SOME HISTORICAL OBSERVATIONS ON DURABILITY

A historical look at grafts introduced into the human circulation: what we have learned about durability

Nigel J Standfield

'In this work, when it shall be found that much is omitted, let it not be forgotten that much likewise is performed'

Samuel Johnson (1755)[1]

INTRODUCTION

Vascular surgery is still very much in its infancy, despite all the progress of the past 50 years. One of the main challenges has been the development of vascular grafts and, in particular, suitable synthetic materials that are durable *in vivo*. This chapter charts the progress of vascular surgery from simple ligation through to the use of bypass grafts. As patients live longer following reconstructive surgery, the durability of these grafts takes on more and more importance.

ARTERIAL LACERATION – FROM LIGATION TO ANASTOMOSIS

Vascular surgery originated with the first attempt to control a bleeding vessel and it was probably Sushruta, the famous surgeon of ancient India, who first ligated blood vessels with hemp fibres. There is debate as to exactly when Sushruta lived, but it was between 800 and 600 BC. His was not a universally accepted technique for controlling haemorrhage as many surgeons through history used cautery or styptics and bandage. Ambroise Paré's major undertaking was the reintroduction of the ligature as the preferred treatment for blood vessel injury. Born in 1510 in France, Paré gained his experience in military surgery and greatly improved results by discouraging the use of hot irons and boiling oil.

Very little progress was made in vascular surgery until 15 June 1759 when Richard Lambert, a surgeon in Newcastle upon Tyne, persuaded his colleague, Hallowell, to attempt repairing a brachial artery aneurysm rather than proximal and distal ligation. This was performed successfully and the patient maintained a viable extremity with a palpable pulse at the wrist. Lambert was encouraged to describe the operation by William Hunter and thus the first lateral arteriorrhaphy was performed.

Arteriorrhaphy, however, remained unfashionable as a result of the unsuccessful experiments performed by Assmann of Gronigen. His attempts at repairing lacerations in canine femoral arteries resulted in thrombosis of the vessel and he concluded that the suturing of the laceration was effective in stopping haemorrhage alone and the irritation to the blood vessel resulted in thrombosis. Assmann only performed four experiments but his conclusion that operative repair of arteries with preservation of the lumen was not possible was widely accepted and progress in vascular repair and anastomoses would be delayed for almost another century.

In 1877 Nicolai Eck[2] was studying liver blood flow in Pavlov's laboratory in Leningrad. He performed experiments on more than 60 dogs and anastomosed the portal vein and inferior vena cava using a continuous silk suture. This is the first documented anastomosis of two blood vessels and as the first portacaval shunt became known as the Eck fistula.

In 1889, Alexander Jassinowsky of Dorpat published his results of direct suture of lacerations in the carotids of dogs, calves and horses. Of 26 experiments, 22 were successful with a patent lumen and no thrombosis and there were no cases of secondary haemorrhage or aneurysm formation in the successful cases.

Following this, several surgeons repeated these experiments and interest evolved in the use of rigid prostheses to approximate completely divided arteries. In 1894, Robert Abbe[3] a New York surgeon, reported his results using a glass tube. He divided the femoral arteries of dogs and the aorta of a cat and then placed a fine glass tube, half an inch in diameter and shaped like an hour-glass, into the proximal and distal lumens and secured the vessel over the glass with a fine silk suture. Thrombosis occurred in the femoral vessels of the dogs but the aorta of the cat remained patent. This was the first experimental use of a prosthesis in vascular surgery. Other surgeons performed similar experiments and different materials were used to construct the tubes. Emoin Payr[4,5] used a magnesium tube in 1901 following the resection of a tumour in the groin. A segment of the femoral vein had to be removed and continuity was restored with the magnesium tube. Payr assumed that since magnesium is soluble *in vivo* a patent lumen would result and at autopsy 3 days later the prosthesis was indeed patent. Further experiments went on to show, however, that Payr's magnesium tubes ultimately resulted in thrombosis and could not therefore be used.

While interest continued in finding the best material from which to construct these rigid tube prostheses, John Murphy[6] of Chicago experimented on direct end-to-end anastomoses of cat and calf aortas, carotids and femorals. On 7 October 1896, he operated on a false aneurysm in the groin following a gunshot injury. Murphy resected the aneurysm with a portion of the common femoral artery and sutured the ends with an invagination technique. The patient survived with an intact distal circulation. This was the first successful case of end-to-end arterial anastomosis.

ANEURYSMS – FROM LIGATION TO REPAIR

Ligation of aneurysms of the brachial and popliteal arteries had been performed by Anel, Desault and others during the eighteenth century and John Hunter[7,8] became known for his treatment of popliteal aneurysms. Many surgeons, however, did not agree and felt that amputation should be performed as a primary operation to prevent the gangrene or exsanguinating haemorrhage that sometimes followed ligation. In December 1785, John Hunter successful ligated a popliteal aneurysm in a coachman who subsequently returned to work. Hunter performed this operation on four other patients with complete success in three. One patient survived for 50 years after Hunter's operation and at autopsy the superficial femoral and popliteal arteries were solid cords and the aneurysm had reduced to a small fibrous nodule.

In 1805, Astley Cooper performed one of the earliest carotid artery ligations for an aneurysm of the right common carotid artery in a 44-year-old woman, Mary Edwards. She died 16 days postoperatively and at autopsy there was suppuration within and surrounding the large aneurysm sac. There was compression of the larynx and trachea. Cooper felt that the operation would be successful if it were performed on smaller aneurysms. On 22 June 1808, Cooper double ligated and divided the common carotid artery of Humphrey Humphreys, a 51-year-old porter. He had a left carotid aneurysm 'the size of a walnut'. Humphreys recovered well from the operation and returned to work, eventually dying in 1821 from a left-sided cerebral haemorrhage. Cooper described the post-mortem findings in the first issue of the Guy's Hospital Reports, 1836: 'The disease of which he died sufficiently attested the freedom of the circulation as well as its force in the cerebral vessels on the side of which the carotid has been tied.'

The day after Humphrey's operation, Cooper ligated the external iliac artery in a 39-year-old man with a large femoral aneurysm. He survived and lived until 1826. Cooper also performed his post-mortem and reported the findings in the first issue of the Guy's Hospital Reports. Cooper performed this operation on nine further occasions.

In 1817, Cooper performed a remarkable operation when he ligated the aorta of a 38-year-old porter, Charles Hutson, in his bed when his external iliac artery aneurysm ruptured through the skin and began bleeding externally. Hutson appeared well the following day but died 40 hours postoperatively.

It was not until 1923 that the first successful abdominal aortic ligation was performed by Rudolph Matas.[9]

Rudolph Matas was also famed for performing an endoaneurysmorrhaphy[10] on a traumatic brachial artery aneurysm in May 1888.

Matas' ingenuity resulted in him developing and describing three types of aneurysmorrhaphy: obliterative, restorative and reconstructive. In the obliterative operation, sutures were used inside the sac to occlude all the branches arising from the sac including the proximal and distal artery. The other two types were modifications resulting in a patent lumen. He would place a catheter into the main arteries and the sac was obliterated by suturing it over the catheter.

In 1900, Matas attempted to treat an abdominal aortic aneurysm with wire and an electric current. This was unsuccessful. In 1923 he successfully ligated the infrarenal aorta for a large aneurysm and this was the first time proximal ligation for aneurysm was successful.

In 1940 Matas[11] reported his personal experience of operations on 620 aneurysms. Of these, 101 were variations of his endoaneurysmorrhaphy technique and it had a very low mortality rate of less than 5% with no cases of gangrene.

In the 1940s surgery to correct coarctation of the aorta played an important role in the development of aortic surgery in general. In 1944, Blalock and Park hypothesized that a coarctation could be bypassed from the left subclavian artery, but it was Clarence Crafoord[12] of Sweden who first successfully corrected a coarctation. In October 1944 he resected coarctations in two patients and anastomosed by an end-to-end technique described by Carrel. Both patients made excellent recoveries. During the next few years, surgical correction of coarctation of the aorta was performed in many centres around the world and in 1947 Shumacker[13] excised a 4-cm aneurysm adjacent to a coarctation and successfully maintained continuity with end-to-end anastomosis.

Since the work of Abbe in 1894, surgical research had tried to find ways of replacing missing segments of arteries although it was accepted that the use of rigid arterial prostheses was not feasible. Between 1904 and 1906 Carrel and Guthrie in Chicago implanted preserved blood vessels into cats' aortas that had been harvested several weeks earlier and preserved near the freezing point of a saline solution. One graft remained patent for 77 days. It was not until 1948 that Gross[14] reported the use of preserved arterial grafts in humans with cyanotic heart disease and coarctation. Several other reports followed and this led quickly to the use of homografts in treating aortoiliac occlusive disease. In 1950 Jacques Oudot[15] replaced a thrombosed aortic bifurcation and in 1951 Charles Dubost,[16,17] also of France, resected an abdominal aortic aneurysm and inserted a thoracic artery homograft to maintain continuity. There was great enthusiasm for the use of homografts[18–23] initially but it was only short-lived because of the degenerative changes resulting in poor long-term patency and the difficulties harvesting and preserving them. It led directly to attempts to use synthetic fabrics to restore continuity or to bypass obstructions.

The very first fabric prosthesis was a silk handkerchief fashioned into a tube on a sewing machine by Voorhees and sutured into the abdominal aorta of a dog with silk sutures for the anastomosis. The graft remained patent for 1 hour but the dog eventually died from haemorrhage through the prosthesis and anastomosis.

The Union Carbide Company donated a bolt of vinyon-N cloth, the material from which parachutes were manufactured and Voorhees continued experimenting, soon realising that pore size in the fabric was critical to the ingrowth of fibroblasts and that without the ingrowth there would be no support for a neoendothelium. Haematoma formation around the graft also prevented proper healing. By the end of 1950, vinyon-N grafts had been implanted in approximately 40 dogs and 75% survived the operation to allow autopsy study.[24–26]

The first human implant of man-made fibre was in 1952 when a patient presented with a ruptured abdominal aortic aneurysm at Columbia and the artery bank at New York Hospital had no grafts available. Voorhees constructed a vinyon-N tube and it was successfully implanted, functioning well for 30 minutes, before the patient died from a myocardial infarction, secondary to haemorrhagic shock and coagulopathy. In 1954[27] Voorhees reported the outcome of vinyon-N cloth tubes in 17 abdominal aortic and one popliteal aneurysms. Different centres started exploring different materials and when Union Carbide eventually stopped production of vinyon-N, the use of Orlon, Teflon, Nylon and Dacron was investigated. Mass production of fabric prostheses soon followed and we now entered the modern era of vascular surgery.

THE VENOUS AUTOGRAFT

The first experiments using venous autografts in the arterial circulation were performed by Alfred Exner, in Austria, and Alexis Carrel, in France, at the beginning of the twentieth century. Carrel[28,29] first conceived the idea in 1901 at the University of Lyon and then collaborated closely with Charles Guthrie in Chicago. Their results were successful because they used a direct suture technique of vein to artery under meticulous aseptic conditions.[30] Exner's[31] experiments resulted in graft thrombosis because he used Payr's magnesium tubes to place canine external jugular veins into the carotid artery.

The first clinical anastomosis of a venous graft into the arterial circulation was performed by Jose Goyanes in Madrid in 1906.[32] Goyanes' patient had a syphilitic popliteal aneurysm and on 12 June Goyanes excised the aneurysm and because he was unable to primarily repair the defect he used an adjacent segment of popliteal vein to bridge the gap. This operation also represents the first *in situ* vein graft.

In 1907[33] Stitch reported his experimental results with venous autografts. Eric Lexer of Königsberg read these results with interest and used a reversed 10-cm segment of long saphenous vein to restore arterial continuity having excised a pseudoaneurysm of the axillary artery in a 69-year-old man. Although the patient died on the 5th postoperative day, the venous graft was found to be patent at post-mortem. Unaware of Goyanes' case the previous year, Lexer[34] reported this case, claiming to be the first to use a venous autograft to replace an artery.

In 1913, Bertram Bernheim[35] encouraged by his associate William Halstead, published a textbook on vascular surgical techniques based upon his own experience of venous autografts in animals. In 1915, Bernheim[36] successful repaired a 15-cm defect in the popoliteal artery after excision of a syphilitic aneurysm in a 43-year-old man using a segment of long saphenous vein. This was the beginning of clinical arterial reconstruction in the USA.

In 1913, Hogarth Pringle[37] reported two cases of reversed saphenous vein grafts at the Royal Infirmary of Glasgow.

A major problem confronting many of the early attempts at venous bypass was graft thrombosis. Heparin was first discovered in 1916 by Jay McLean,[38] a medical student. Heparin, however, was too toxic at this stage for clinical use. Best and Scott[39] described the purification of heparin in 1933 and in 1938, Murray[40] demonstrated that it could prevent suture line thrombosis in arteries and vein.

On 3 June 1948, Jean Kunlin in Paris[41] performed an end-to-side reversed vein bypass from the femoral to the popliteal arteries in a patient with painful arterial ulcers. The concept of an end-to-side anastomosis was new but it was very important as the side branches on the remaining native vessel could be preserved. The results were dramatic with healing of the ulcers in 2 weeks. In 1951, Kunlin[42] reported 17 cases of autogenous venous bypasses.

William Holden[43] performed the first successful femoropopliteal bypass in the USA 6 months after Kunlin.

There were few advances in bypass surgery for vascular injuries caused in wars until Hughes[44] reported 34 cases of autogenous vein grafts for vascular injury during the Korean War. The limb salvage rate was approximately 90%. Rich[45] found similar results during the Vietnam War.

The principles of arterial reconstruction using autogenous venous bypasses was gaining wide acceptance and Fontaine[46] reported 28 cases with 10 patent at 1-year follow-up. Julian[47] also reported 19 cases with 12 patent. Further series followed from Lord and Stone[48] 1957, Dale and DeWeese[49] 1959 and Linton and Darling[50] 1962.

Whilst reverse vein grafting was becoming accepted, some centres were exploring the concept of *in situ* grafting. In 1959, Paul Cartier of Montreal and Karl Hall,[51] working with Charles Rob in St Mary's Hospital, London, began the first clinical trials of *in situ* vein bypass. Cartier used a retrograde valve stripper and Hall resorted to direct excision of the valve cusps initially but eventually developed his own retrograde valve stripper in 1968. Hall[52] reported excellent results with 75% patency rates. However other centres did not feel that the *in situ* technique offered any advantages over reversed vein bypass.

In 1979, Leather[53] revived the technique by utilizing a simplified atraumatic method of destroying the valves and since then *in situ* grafting has been the method of choice in many centres.

Although there remains debate as to which is the superior technique for venous bypass grafting, there is no doubt that autogenous vein is presently the conduit of choice for lower extremity revascularization.

THE SYNTHETIC ARTERIAL PROSTHESIS

Once Union Carbide stopped production of vinyon-N, other prosthetic materials were investigated and Dacron has become the preferred material for aortic reconstruction. When arterial bypass is considered for disease in arteries distal to the inguinal ligament, the treatment of choice in most cases is arterial bypass with autologous vein. When the patient's own vein is unavailable or unsuitable, a vascular prosthesis is selected. These prostheses have been manufactured from a variety of materials, both synthetic and biological, but none are as durable as autologous vein. Dacron and expanded polytetrafluoroethylene (PTFE) have been used as synthetic materials and a whole range of collagen tubes derived from human umbilical vein, bovine carotid artery, and composite vascular prostheses such as the Omniflow vascular graft, which comprises a polyester mesh and tanned biological tissue (ovine collagen). However, none of the prostheses for infrainguinal reconstruction have proven entirely satisfactory with poor long-term patency as a serious consequence.

There are several factors which lead to failure of these small bore prostheses. The lack of an antithrombotic lining will lead to graft thrombosis if flow is inadequate, possibly as a result of poor distal runoff. Incompliant walls, poor handling characteristics and the development of myointimal hyperplasia at the distal anastomosis all contribute to the relative poor performance of these infrainguinal bypass grafts as well as an increased risk of graft infection. A number of techniques have been used and are still being evaluated to overcome these variable problems. Heparin bonding and endothelial seeding may reduce surface thrombogenicity but are still experimental. The use of vein 'cuff' or 'patch' at the distal anastomosis and interposition of vein between synthetic graft and arterial wall have all been tried and whilst offering an advantage still result in relatively poor graft survival. Attempts at finding a truly compliant prosthesis which overcomes the tissue's response to an implanted synthetic graft which results in an indistensable fibrous capsule neutralizing any initial radial compliance have to date still proven unsatisfactory.

In considering the durability of infrainguinal bypass grafts there are many variables influencing the short-term and long-term outcome which have little to do with the bypass graft itself. Poor distal runoff, myointimal hyperplasia, intentional or inadvertent endarterectomy of the distal anastomosis, the passage of the graft across a joint, distal sepsis, disease progression and inactivity of the patient will all influence the graft survival or failure. These do not have a significant part to play in aortoiliac reconstruction and discussion relating to the durability of these grafts very much focuses on narrower issues such as the graft material and the graft–vessel interface. For the rest of this discussion, I have therefore concentrated on aortoiliac reconstruction.

AORTOILIAC GRAFTS

Since 1952, many centres around the world have explored different materials for replacing or bypassing the aorta and Dacron is now universally preferred as the material of choice. Replacement or bypass of the abdominal aorta with a Dacron prosthesis is now a common procedure giving excellent short- and long-term results.[54,55] However, complications inherent to such Dacron prostheses are being reported with increasing frequency[56–75] and arise from defects in the prosthetic fabric. Reported defects include focal and multifocal deterioration of prosthetic fibres with discrete aneurysmal defects as well as generalized prosthetic dilatation. These defects have resulted in a variety of complications including disruption of the prosthesis with exsanguination,[69] massive transinterstices bleeding,[70,71] false aneurysms arising from holes or tears in the prosthesis,[57,59,69,70,72,73] anastomotic false aneurysms,[71,74,75] prosthesis-enteric fistulae,[57,59,70] and thrombosis or embolization of the prosthesis.[59,60,69,73,75]

Dilatation of Dacron vascular grafts continues to be a problem and directly or indirectly results in fabric failure and complications such as those previously described. Graft dilatation for knitted Dacron ranges from 14.8 to 85.7%[66,76,76–80] although the three parts of an aortobifemoral graft (aortic segment, right and left limbs) may not necessarily dilate uniformly to the same degree.[79] There are three different reasons for this dilatation phenomenon in textile structures.

First, there is an increase in the length and diameter of the prosthesis due to flattening of the crimps as the graft is pressurized. Second, there is a rearrangement of the yarns within the textile structure. Woven fabrics with interlacing yarns have a comparatively high initial modulus and exhibit little in the way of dilatation under arterial pressure. Knitted structures, however, have a looped construction and hence can easily straighten and thus are prone to dilatation. Grafts with greater loop length, lightweight fabrics, weft knits and l-bar warp knits are prone to greater dilatation. Third, the fibres and yarns experience elongation and permanent deformation due to fatigue and biodegradation, manufacturing flaws, damage to the material during graft processing (compaction, crimping, clearing) inappropriate surgical handling of the graft, and improper resterilization and/or storage.[76,77]

Because of the characteristics of their manufacture, woven grafts not only have better dimensional stability and are much less prone to dilatation,[76] but also are less porous and have a greater ability to control blood loss. In order to limit the blood loss from knitted Dacron grafts, the grafts either have to be preclotted with the patient's own blood or they come prepared and the structure sealed to zero porosity with either gelatine, collagen or albumin. It would seem that the woven graft would be preferable to the knitted. However, the woven grafts are less easy to handle, less easy to suture and are prone to fray at the cut end. The continued challenge is to create a knitted prosthesis that is easy to handle and suture, is zero porous and has good dimensional stability so that it is less likely to dilate.

Dilatation rates in the first 6 months after implantation are up to 25% and most of the observed dilatation appears to occur in the first 1–2 months.[81] In a study from an implant retrieval programme in animals,[82] the tendency for grafts to dilate early confirmed the findings in human implants although the tendency to dilatation does continue with time but at a slower rate. Despite earlier claims of biological stability there is increasing evidence that Dacron implanted in humans does undergo some degradation with consequent loss of strength as a result of a combination of physical and chemical factors,[83] and in hypertensive patients dilatation could conceivably become a greater problem.

Uncomplicated graft dilatation does not necessarily equate with graft failure. The reduction in velocity of blood flow and the consequent potential for thrombus formation associated with dilatation, does not seem to be a significant problem with large vessel prostheses.[84]

Manufacturers perform lot-to-lot testing of grafts to ensure uniformity based on the following characteristics:[85]

1. Permeability
2. Strength
3. Nominal internal diameter (in a resting stage)
4. Nominal internal diameter under physiological pressure (defined as 120 mmHg)
5. Usable length
6. Nominal wall thickness
7. Suture retention strength.

However, there is no uniform strength test to try to predict grafts that may fail. The radial tensile strength test and a modified burst test are currently used to evaluate graft strength but do not predict graft dilatation.

Commercial prostheses have a bursting strength 10–50 times greater than a normal artery.[86,87] However there is a progressive loss of bursting strength (2% per year) for Dacron arterial prostheses in humans[83,87] and hence lightweight prostheses with a low initial burst strength, susceptibility to yarn damage, fatigue and degradation after implantation may not offer acceptable safety margins to justify their use in all patients.

ANASTOMOTIC ANEURYSMS

The reported incidences of anastomotic aneurysms vary widely from 1 to 24%.[88–92] These differences may be explained by:

1. Major differences in the types of cases and types of arterial reconstructions performed. In some studies the location of the anastomosis is not considered although it is well established that anastomoses onto the femoral artery are most prone to developing anastomotic aneurysms.[89,92]
2. The different techniques and their varying accuracy for detecting aneurysmal dilatation, such as palpation alone, CT-scanning or ultrasonography.
3. Major differences in the length of follow-up.
4. End-to-end or end-to-side anastomoses. End-to-end anastomoses provide a more haemodynamically stable flow for the prevention of anastomotic aneurysms.[92,93]

The mechanism of anastomotic false aneurysm formation is open to speculation. Sutures may be intact on the prosthesis[94] and have thus torn from the artery, possibly as a result of graft dilatation[95] and the consequent increases in tension and force at the anastomosis. Infection does not appear to play a role.[92,93]

CONCLUSION

Crimped knitted Dacron prostheses have been commonly used for over 30 years as arterial substitutes in the aortoiliofemoral vessels. Although graft failures and anastomotic aneurysms have occurred and may be associated with very serious complications, such as rupture and haemorrhage, these prostheses have proven highly effective and relatively durable. The future lies in continuing to identify ways to improve the durability of vascular grafts.

REFERENCES

1. Johnson S: *Dictionary of the English Language* 1755
2. Child CG: Eck's fistula. *Surg Gyn Obstet* **96:** 375–376, 1953
3. Abbe R: The surgery of the hand. *NY Med J* **59:** 33–40, 1894
4. Payr E: Zw frage der circulaeren vereinigung von blutgefaessen mit resorbirbaren prothesen. *Arch Klin Chir* **62:** 67–93, 1900
5. Payr E: Weitere mittheilungen veber verwendung des magnesiums bei der naht der blutgefaessen. *Arch Klin Chir* **64:** 726, 1901
6. Murphy JB: Resection of arteries and veins injured in continuity – end-to-end suture – experimental and clinical research. *Med Rec* **51:** 73–88, 1897
7. Chitwood WR Jr: John and William Hunter on aneurysms. *Arch Surg* **112:** 829–836, 1977
8. Schechter DC, Bergan JJ: Popliteal aneurysm: A celebration of the bicentennial of John Hunter's operation. *Ann Vasc Surg* **1:** 118, 1986
9. Matas R: Ligation of the abdominal aorta. *Ann Surg* **81:** 457, 1925
10. Matas R: Traumatic aneurysm of the left brachial artery. *Med News Phil* **53:** 462, 1888.
11. Matas R: Personal experiences in vascular surgery. A statistical synopsis. *Ann Surg* **112:** 802–839, 1940
12. Crafoord C, Nylin G: Congenital coarctation of the aorta and its surgical treatment. *J Thorac Surg* **14:** 347–361, 1945
13. Shumacker MB Jr: Coarctation and aneurysm of the aorta. Report of a case treated by excision and end-to-end suture of aorta. *Ann Surg* **127:** 655–665, 1948
14. Gross RE, Humoitt ES, Bill AH Jr *et al.*: Preliminary observations on the use of human

arterial grafts in the treatment of certain cardiovascular defects. *New Engl J Med* **239:** 578–579, 1948
15. Oudot J: La greffe vasculaire dans les thromboses du carrefour aortique. *Presse Med* **59:** 234–236, 1951
16. Dubost C: First successful resection of an aneurysm of an abdominal aorta with restoration of the continuity by a human arterial graft. *World J Surg* **6:** 256–257, 1982
17. Dubost C, Allary M, Oeconomos N: Resection of an aneurysm of the abdominal aorta: Re-establishment of the continuity by a preserved human arterial graft, with results after five months. *Arch Surg* **64:** 405–408, 1952
18. DeBakey ME, Cooley DA: Successful resection of aneurysm of thoracic aorta and replacement by graft. *J Am Med Assoc* **152:** 673–676, 1953
19. Deterling RA JR, Coleman C Jr, Parshley MS: Experimental studies of the frozen homologous aortic graft. *Surgery* **29:** 419–440, 1951
20. Gross RE: Treatment of certain aortic coarctations by homologous grafts. A report of nineteen cases. *Ann Surg* **134:** 753–768, 1951
21. Julian OC, Dye WS, Olwin JH *et al.*: Direct surgery of arteriosclerosis. *Ann Surg* **136:** 459–474, 1952
22. Lan CR, Aran HH: Resection of the descending thoracic aorta for aneurysm. A report of the use of a homograft in a case and an experimental study. *Ann Surg* **134:** 743, 1951
23. Szilagyi DE: Ten years' experience with aorto-iliac and femoro-popliteal arterial reconstruction. *J Cardiovasc Surg* **5:** 502–508, 1964
24. Voorhees AB Jr: The development of arterial prostheses. A personal view. *Arch Surg* **120:** 289–295, 1985
25. Voorhees AB Jr: The origins of the permeable arterial prosthesis. A personal reminiscence. *Surg Rounds* **11:** 79, 1988
26. Voorhees AB JR, Jaretzki A, Blakemore AH: The use of tubes constructed from vinyon 'N' cloth in bridging arterial defects. A preliminary report. *Ann Surg* **135:** 332–336, 1952.
27. Blakemore AH, Voorhees AB Jr: The use of tubes constructed from vinyon 'N' cloth in bridging arterial defects – experimental and clinical. *Ann Surg* **140:** 324–334, 1954
28. Carrel A: La technique opératoire des anastonoses vasculaires et la transplantation des viscères. *Lyon Med* **98:** 859–864, 1902
29. Carrel A, Morel A: Anastanose bout à bout de la jugulaire et de la carotide primitive. *Lyon Med* **99:** 114, 1902
30. Carrel A, Guthrie CC: Uniterminal and biterminal venous transplantation. *Surg Gyn Obstet* **2:** 266, 1906
31. Exner A: Einige tierversuche ueber vereinigung und transplantation von blutgefaessen. *Wien Klin Wschr* **16:** 273, 1903
32. Goyanes J: Nuevous trabajos de cirugia vascular. Sustritucion plastica de las arterias por las venas, o arterioplastia venosa, applicada, como nuevo metodo, al tratamiento de los aneurismas. *El Sigo Med* **53:** 561–564, 1906
33. Stitch R, Makkas M, Dowman CE: Beitrage zur gefaesschirurgie; cirkulaere arteriennaht und gefaesstransplantationen. *Beitr Klin Chir* **53:** 113, 1907
34. Lexer E: Die ideale operation des arteriellen und des arteriellvenoesen aneurysma. *Arch Klin Chir* **83:** 459, 1907
35. Bernheim BM: *Surgery of the Vascular System.* Philadelphia: JB Lippincott Co, 1913
36. Bernheim BM: The ideal operation for aneurysm of the extremity. Report of a case. *Bull Johns Hopkins Hosp* **27:** 93, 1916
37. Pringle H: Two cases of vein grafting for the maintenance of direct arterial circulation. *Lancet* **i:** 1795, 1913
38. MacLean J: The thromboplastic action of cephalin. *Am J Physiol* **41:** 250, 1916
39. Best CH, Scott C: The purification of heparin. *J Biol Chem* **102:** 425, 1933
40. Murray G: Heparin in surgical treatment of blood vessels. *Arch Surg* **40:** 307–325, 1940
41. Kunlin J: Le traitement de l'artérite obliterarte par la greffe veineuse. *Arch Mal Coeur* **42:** 371–372, 1949
42. Kunlin J: Le traitment de l'ischemie artéritique par la greffe veineuse longue. *Rev Chir* **70:** 206, 1951

43. Holden WD: Reconstruction of the femoral artery for arteriosclerotic thrombosis. *Surgery* **27:** 417, 1950
44. Hughes CW: Arterial repair during the Korean war. *Ann Surg* **147:** 555–561, 1958
45. Rich NM: Vascular trauma in Vietnam. *J Cardiovasc Surg* **11:** 368–377, 1970
46. Fontaine R, Buck P, Riveaux R *et al.*: Treatment of arterial occlusion, comparative value of thrombectomy, thromboendarterectomy, arteriovenous shunt and vascular grafts (fresh venous autografts). *Lyon Chir* **46:** 73–94, 1951
47. Julian OC, Dye WS, Olwin JH: Direct surgery of arteriosclerosis. *Ann Surg* **136:** 459, 1952
48. Lord JW, Stone DW: The use of autologous venous grafts in the peripheral arterial system. *Arch Surg* **74:** 71–79, 1957
49. Dale WA, DeWeese JA, Merle Scott WJ: Autogenous venous shunt grafts. Rationale and report of 31 for atherosclerosis. *Surgery* **46:** 145–153, 1959
50. Linton RR, Darling RC: Autogenous saphenous vein bypass grafts in femoropopliteal obliterative arterial disease. *Surgery* **51:** 62–73, 1962
51. Hall KV: The great saphenous vein used *in situ* as an arterial shunt after extirpation of the vein valves. *Surgery* **51:** 492–495, 1962
52. Hall KV: The saphenous vein used *in situ* as an arterial bypass. *Am J Surg* **136:** 123, 1978
53. Leather RP, Powers SR JR, Karmody AM: A reappraisal of the *in situ* saphenous vein arterial bypass: its use in limb salvage. *Surgery* **86:** 453–461, 1979
54. Crawford ES, Bomberger RA, Glaeser DH *et al.*: Aortoiliac occlusive disease: factors influencing survival and function following reconstructive operation over a twenty-five year period. *Surgery* **90:** 1055–1067, 1981
55. Malan E, Ruberti U, Tiberio G *et al.*: Abdominal aortic aneurysms. Results from surgical treatment in 198 cases. *J Cardiovasc Surg* **13:** 576–583, 1972
56. Wesolowski SA, Fries CC, Hennigar G *et al.*: Factors contributing to long-term failures in human vascular prosthetic grafts. *J Cardiovasc Surg* **38:** 544–567, 1964
57. Perry MO: Early failure of Dacron prosthetic grafts. *J Cardiovasc Surg* **16:** 318–321, 1975
58. Hayward RH, Korompai FL: Degeneration of knitted Dacron grafts. *Surgery* **79:** 581–583, 1976
59. Yashar JJ, Richman MH, Dyckman J *et al.*: Failure of Dacron prostheses caused by structural defect. *Surgery* **84:** 659–663, 1978
60. Greenhalgh RM: Dilatation and stretching of knitted Dacron grafts associated with failure. In Bergan JJ, Yao JSJ (Eds) *Surgery of the Aorta and its Body Branches* pp. 621–626. New York: Grune and Stratton, 1979
61. Koopmann MDE, Brands LC: Degenerative changes in Dacron external velour vascular prostheses. *J Cardiovasc Surg* **21:** 159–162, 1980
62. Greenhalgh RM: Mechanical and biochemical factors influencing arterial reconstruction. *Ann Roy Coll Surg Engl* **63:** 399–404, 1981
63. Berger K, Sauvage LR: Late fiber deterioration in Dacron arterial grafts. *Ann Surg* **139:** 477–491, 1981
64. Watanabe T, Kusaba A, Kuma H *et al.*: Failure of Dacron arterial prostheses caused by structural defects. *J Cardiovasc Surg* **24:** 95–100, 1983
65. Ratto GB, Trunini M, Sacco A *et al.*: Multiple aneurysmal dilatations in a knitted Dacron velour graft. *J Cardiovasc Surg* **26:** 589–591, 1985
66. Lundquist B, Almgren B, Bowald S *et al.*: Deterioration and dilatation of Dacron prosthetic grafts. *Acta Chir Scand* **529:** 81–85, 1985
67. Sladen JG, Gerein AN, Miyagishima RT: Late rupture of prosthetic aortic grafts. *Am J Surg* **153:** 453–458, 1987
68. Mager HR, Teague CA: Late rupture of knitted velour Dacron arterial prostheses. *Aust NZ J Surg* **58:** 549–553, 1988
69. Cooke PA, Nobis PA, Stoney RJ: Dacron aortic graft failure. *Arch Surg* **108:** 101–103, 1974
70. Blumenberg RM, Gelfand ML: Failure of knitted Dacron as an arterial prosthesis. *Surgery* **81:** 493–496, 1977
71. Ottinger LW, Darling C, Wirthlin LS, Linton RR: Failure of ultraweight knitted Dacron grafts in arterial reconstruction. *Arch Surg* **111:** 146–149, 1976
72. May J, Stephen M: Multiple aneurysms in Dacron velour grafts. *Arch Surg* **113**: 320–321, 1978

73. Rais O, Lundstrom B, Anqquist KA, Hallmans G: Bilateral aneurysms of Dacron graft following aorto-femoral graft operation. *Acta Chir Scand* **142:** 479–482, 1976
74. Gaylis H: Pathogenesis of anastomotic aneurysms. *Surgery* **90:** 509–515, 1981
75. Kim GE, Imparto, AM, Nathan I, Riles TS: Dilatation of synthetic grafts and junctional aneurysms. *Arch Surg* **114:** 1296–1303, 1979
76. Alimi Y, Juhan C, Morati N *et al.*: Dilatation of woven and knitted aortic prosthetic grafts: CT scan evaluation. *Ann Vasc Surg* **8:** 238–242, 1994
77. Blumenberg RM, Gelfand ML, Barton EA *et al.*: Clinical significance of aortic graft dilation. *J Vasc Surg* **14:** 175–180, 1991
78. Clagett GP, Salander JM, Eddleman WL *et al.*: Dilatation of knitted Dacron aortic prostheses and anastomotic false aneurysms; etiologic considerations. *Surgery* **93:** 9–16, 1983
79. Nunn DB, Carter MM, Donohue MT, Hudgins PC: Postoperative dilation of knitted Dacron aortic bifurcation graft. *J Vasc Surg* **12:** 291–297, 1990
80. Nunn DB, Freeman MH, Hudgins PC: Postoperative alterations in size of Dacron aortic grafts. An ultrasonic evaluation. *Ann Surg* **189:** 741–744, 1979
81. Nunn DB, Carter MM, Donohue MT, Powdeyhimi B: Dilative characteristics of Microvel and Vasculow-II aortic bifurcation grafts. *J Biomed Mater Res* **30:** 41–46, 1996
82. Mary C, Marois Y, King MW *et al.*: *In vitro* and *in vivo* studies of a polyester arterial prosthesis with a warp-knitted sharkskin structure. *J Biomed Mater Res* **35:** 459–472, 1997
83. King MW, Guidoin R, Blais P *et al.*: Degradation of polyester arterial prostheses: a physical or chemical mechanism? In: Fraker AC, Griffin CD (Eds) *Corrosion and Degradation of Implant Materials: Second Symposium* ASTM STP 859 pp. 295–307. Philadelphia: American Society for Testing and Materials, 1985
84. Powdeyhimi B, Wagner D: On the correlation between the failure of vascular grafts and their structural and material properties: a critical analysis. *J Biomed Mater Res* **20:** 375–409, 1987
85. American National Standard for vascular graft prostheses: Developed by the Association for the Advancement of Medical Instrumentation. Approved 7 July 1986 by the American National Standards Institute, Inc.
86. Snyder RW, Tenney B, Guidoin R: Strength and endurance of vascular grafts. In: Kanbic ME, Kartrowitz A, Sung P (Eds) *Vascular Graft Update: Safety and Performance*, ASTM STP 898 pp. 108–121. Philadelphia: 1986
87. King MW, Guidoin RG, Gunasekera KR, Gosselin C: Designing polyester vascular prostheses for the future. *Med Progr Technol* **9:** 217–226, 1983
88. Sieswerda C, Skotnicki SH, Barentsz JO *et al.*: Anastomotic aneurysms – an underdiagnosed complication after aorto-iliac reconstructions. *Eur J Vasc Surg* **3:** 233–238, 1989
89. Van Den Akker PJ, Brand R: False aneurysms after prosthetic reconstructions for aorto-iliac obstructive disease. *Ann Surg* **210:** 658–666, 1989
90. Briggs RM, Bruce SJ, Collins GJ: Anastomotic aneurysms. *Am J Surg* **146:** 770–773, 1983
91. Kalsbeek HL: False aneurysms in patients with an aortic bifurcation prosthesis. *Ned Tijolscht Geneeskd* **133:** 681–683, 1989
92. den Hoed PT, Veen HF: The late complications of aorto-ilio-femoral Dacron prostheses: Dilatation and anastomic aneurysm formation. *Eur J Vasc Surg* **6:** 282–287, 1992
93. Szilaqyi DE, Whitcomb JG, Schenker W *et al.*: The laws of fluid flow and arterial grafting. *Surgery* **47:** 55, 1960
94. Clagett GP, Salander JM *et al.*: Dilation of knitted Dacron aortic prostheses and anastomotic false aneurysms: Etiologic considerations. *Surgery* **93:** 9–16, 1983
95. Nichols WK, Stanton M, Silver D, Keitzer WF: Anastomotic aneurysms following lower extremity revascularisation. *Surgery* **88:** 366–374, 1980

Commentary

Dr Michael DeBakey was very much involved with the introduction of prosthetic materials for arterial grafts and once told me how he happened upon Dacron for the purpose. He went to a ladies wear shop and describes that he felt embarrassed about this particularly as he asked for some material, for example Prolon or Nylon and he attracted some strange looks! The shop assistant suggested that he should try Dacron because no other material was available. DeBakey had not heard of this material, but decided that he had better take it or his visit would have been in vain. He returned home and this Dacron material was easily sewn into a tube, as DeBakey's mother was a seamstress. The Dacron was sewn into dogs, 'it worked in dogs and so we tried it in humans', DeBakey told me. He attributes the introduction of Dacron to pure serendipity. It seems that by pure chance, Dacron was available in the shop and was used and has been so extremely durable and inert.

The introduction of the Dacron man-made fibre, in particular, has been the most extraordinary stroke of luck and its durability has far exceeded the durability of homografts and heterografts. The early surgeons loved the use of arterial homograft and said how perfect a material it was to sew into place. They were horrified when the homograft soon dilated as a result of loss of the strength of the material through rejection. In time, virtually all homografts and worse than that, heterografts, have lost their connective tissue strength and dilated and caused problems. The exception might be bovine pericardium which is used by cardiac surgeons for coarctation of the aorta in place of a Dacron patch, although follow-up is short compared with our knowledge of the Dacron material. Cardiothoracic surgeons also use animal heart valves and think nothing of it and seem to have durable results.

It is comforting to be able to look back for approximately 50 years on the durability of arterial grafts with the knowledge of the success of autologous saphenous vein and the man-made fibre, Dacron. Against that we have learned how relatively unsuccessful are homografts and heterografts. Unfortunately we have to take a view on the introduction of endovascular procedures without such knowledge of durability and it will be decades before we can be absolutely sure of some of these novel techniques. *RMG*

Index

Abbreviations used in subheadings are: AAA = abdominal aortic aneurysm; CLI = critical limb ischaemia; PTFE = polytetrafluoroethylene; PVD = peripheral vascular disease; RETA = Registry of Endovascular Treatment of Aneurysms.